For EU product safety concerns:
IN TECH d.o.o., Prolaz Marije Krucifikse Kozulić 3, 51000 Rijeka, Croatia,
info@intechopen.com or visit our website at intechopen.com.

Meet the editor

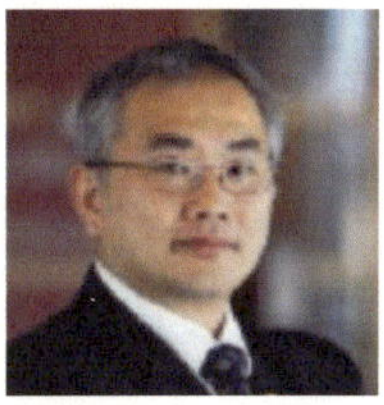

Clark C. Chen received his B.S. from Stanford University in 1992, M.S. from Columbia University in 1993, and his M.D.-Ph.D. from Harvard Medical School in 2001. He completed his neurosurgery training at the Massachusetts General Hospital and subsequently completed independent fellowships in stereotactic neurosurgery and radiosurgery. Dr. Chen previously served as the director of Clinical Neuro-Oncology at the Beth Israel Deaconess Medical Center before his current role as the Director of Stereotactic and Radiosurgery and Co-Director of Surgical Neuro-Oncology at the University of California, San Diego. Dr. Chen's research is directed at identifying alterations in DNA repair pathways as they relate to brain cancer therapy. Dr. Chen is the recipient of the Damon Runyon Fellowship Award, the James Kerr Award, American Brain Tumor Association Investigator Award, Paul Calabresi Scholar Award, Burroughs Wellcome Career Award, William Guy Forbeck Scholar Award, the Doris Duke Clinical Scientist Award, and the Kimmel Scholar Award.

Contents

Preface

DNA repair processes are of fundamental importance to all aspects of cell biology. It is through these processes and their critical interfaces to DNA replication, transcription, cell cycle, telomere maintenance, and other essential cellular processes that genomic stability is maintained. The aims of this edition are three-fold. The first section of the book aims to illustrate novel mechanistic insights into the various forms of DNA repair. The second section of the book describes works that elucidate the interfaces between DNA repair and the various essential processes. The final section of the book outlines strategies for clinical translation of the vast reservoir of knowledge on this topic into therapeutic, prognostic, and predictive platforms.

Clark C. Chen, M.D., Ph.D.
University of California, San Diego

Section 1

Novel Insights into DNA Repair

Chapter 1

Recombination Hot-Spots and Defense Players – Maintenance of Genomic Integrity

Radhika Pankaj Kamdar and Basuthkar J. Rao

Additional information is available at the end of the chapter

http://dx.doi.org/10.5772/54016

1. Introduction

Internal factors and external agents are a source of constant genomic stress in living organisms leading to instability in the form of chromosomal deletions, duplications and translocations. These erroneous rearrangements of the chromosome alter the normal functioning of the genes harbored on them leading to genetic birth defects, intellectual disabilities, premature ageing and even cancer predisposition in humans [1]. Such chromosomal aberrations occur at gaps within the genome or at breakpoint junctions on double stranded DNA motifs known as fragile sites. Preventing or repairing these DNA damages is pivotal for the normal physiological function of a human body. However, prevention or total abolition of DNA damage from an organism is impossible as it is a constant and spontaneous phenomenon occurring in a physiological environment, stalling DNA replication. Therefore, focus on mechanisms that could stabilize such breakage-prone motifs and repair the damage on DNA could grant an insight into understanding and enhancing them for maintenance of genomic integrity.

2. Mechanisms of DNA repair

Estimation studies suggest that each mammalian cell genome is subject to several hundreds of DNA strand breaks within the normal physiological setting [2]. Hence, prokaryotes and especially eukaryotes are equipped with defense mechanisms against genotoxic stress in order to constantly repair and restore the genome, bringing the replication process back in order from its attenuated state. Efficient timely repair can restore a near-zero status of damages at a steady-state level in a eukaryotic cell.

DNA repair pathways in higher eukaryotes such as yeast are constantly operational throughout the various phases of the cell cycle. Homologous Recombination (HR) is the most commonly known pathway to be predominant in the late S and G2 phases of the cell cycle [3]. It requires a pair of sister chromatids as template for adequate homology to recombine the broken DNA ends and hence is seen mostly in these two phases of the cell cycle where such templates are available. HR creates new combination of DNA sequences during sister chromatid exchange in meiosis, a cell division process carried out in germ cells in eukaryotes.

Intriguingly, mammalian DNA also undergoes constant damage and the first mechanism to sense these damages and respond to them is the Non-Homologous End-Joining pathway (NHEJ) [4]. As the name suggests, it has almost no regard for homology while rejoining the broken DNA ends and hence can occur throughout the cell-cycle regardless of the cycle phase. It is therefore depicted as an error-prone mechanism as opposed to HR which operates based on homology and hence is considered to be error-proof. A modified version of NHEJ is MMEJ (Microhomology-Mediated End-Joining) which requires a 5 – 25 bp homology for end-joining which is likely to be available in the S phase in contrast to G0/G1 and early S phase of the cell cycle where NHEJ is more predominant [5].

3. NHEJ

Mammalian system undergoes spontaneous DNA damage which is responded immediately by NHEJ, making it the first choice for DNA repair mechanism. The three core steps include detection, processing and ligation. According to the classical NHEJ pathway, Ku70/80 heterodimer detects these damages and is believed to act as early sensors binding the broken ends followed by recruitment of DNA dependent protein kinase (DNA-PK) which brings these ends in synapsis and activates the downstream substrates by phosphorylation. Several nucleases and polymerases then trim the overhangs or fill-in the gaps to create adequate homology for ligation by XRCC4-DNA Ligase IV-XLF complex [6].

NHEJ causes insertions or deletions of DNA sequences at the broken regions leading to chromosomal translocations which are frequently found in leukemia and lymphoid malignancies. Immunoglobulin (Ig)/T-cell receptor (TCR) recombinase is known to be involved in such aberrant chromosomal rearrangements because of its recognition of target heptamer-nonamer V(D)J signal sequences. Other non-resembling sequences also direct recombination. One such example was found in a patient with acute T-cell lymphoblastic leukemia (ALL) carrying t(8;14) (q24;q11) and t(1;14) (p32;q11) translocations [7]. The novel conserved sequences, GCAGC[A/T]C and CCCA[C/G]GAC, identified at recombination hot-spots led to the speculation that site-specific recombination events might occur mediated by proteins.

Recombination associated factor (ReHF-1) was identified to bind specifically to the 8q24 and 1p32 breakpoint junctions [8]. BCLF-1, another analogous protein was identified to bind to breakpoint clusters in Bcl-2 oncogene in patients with follicular lymphoma carrying t(14;18) (q32;q21) translocations [9]. Recombinant BCLF-1 protein demonstrated strong binding affinity towards single-stranded oligonucleotides representing the breakpoint junctions [10]. Thus the activity of the two proteins, ReHF-1/BCLF-1 was inseparable inferring them to be identical or nearly identical at consensus target sequences in chromosomal translocations in human lymphoid neoplasms. The protein was therefore renamed as Translin, derived from translocation [10].

4. Orthologues of Translin

4.1. Human Translin

Translin was identified to bind several breakpoint junctions, found in patients carrying chromosomal translocations t(8;14)(q24;q11), t(1;14)(p32;q11) and t(14;18)(q32;21), revealing similarity to consensus target sequences, ATGCAG and GCCC[A/T][G/C][G/C][A/T] [10]. The gene, assigned 2q21.1 as the chromosomal locus by fluorescence *in situ* hybridization (FISH) studies, was cloned and the cDNA predicted to code for a polypeptide chain consisting of 228 amino acids, whose sequence did not possess any significant similarity to then known proteins. Nucleotide and amino acid sequence analysis revealed a heptad repeat of hydrophobic amino acids, five leucines and one valine, which is consistent with the hypothetical structure of a "leucine zipper" [11]. Also, amino acids spanning from 54 – 64 and 86 – 97 were predicted as two basic regions upstream to the leucine zipper [12] (Figure1).

The purified recombinant protein migrated as a 27 kDa monomer under reducing conditions and as a 54 kDa dimer under non-reducing conditions on SDS-PAGE [10]. These results indicated that two polypeptide chains were bound together by disulphide bonds which could be easily separated under the presence of reducing agents such as β-mercaptoethanol or dithiotritol. Gel filtration analysis and native gel electrophoresis revealed the native state of translin as a 220 kDa octamer with the formation of higher order multimeric structure, probably connected via the leucine zipper motifs from each dimer [13].

4.2. Testis/Brain – RNA Binding Protein (TB – RBP)

Mouse testicular extracts revealed a RNA-protein complex that bound to the Y and H elements of 3′ UTR of protamine-2 [14]. A similar protein was also found in brain extracts and termed as Testis/Brain – RNA binding protein [15]. The open reading frame consisted of 228 amino acids coding for a molecular weight of 26 kDa. The heptad repeat of leucine zipper motif spanned from amino acids 177 – 212. Yeast 2-hybrid assays later confirmed that like translin, TB/RBP also dimerized via the C-terminal, housing the leucine zipper and a cystine at 225th position forming disulphide bridges [16].

It also shared a 90% and a 99% identity with Translin nucleotide and amino acid sequence respectively and was thus deemed as the mouse orthologue of the human protein [17]. Only three amino acids that differ in TB-RBP are alanine – threonine at 49th, glycine – serine at 66th and valine – glycine at 226th positions respectively. Analysis of the human and mouse translin revealed that each of them consisted of six exons, five introns and a GC-rich region

[12]. TB - RBP also harbors potential phosphorylation sites for protein kinase C and tyrosine kinase.

4.3. Drosophila Translin

The fly orthologue of translin was identified, cloned, purified and characterized by our group [18]. The gene from *Drosophila melanogaster* was recognized to have five exons as annotated by the Berkeley *Drosophila* Genome Project (BDGP). The 28 kDa monomer, established by MALDI-TOF, shared only 52% sequence identity with the corresponding human protein. As opposed to the 54 kDa dimer of human translin, the fly protein existed as a 56 kDa in its dimeric state. The dimer of translin existed in relative abundance as compared to that of the *Drosophila* protein laying differences in the stability of the two dimers. Although the fly protein shares a high sequential identity with that of the vertebrates, the extreme C-terminal varies in sequence and length (Figure 2). The putative leucine zipper domain may be responsible for multimerization, but the two basic regions are less conserved in *Drosophila* translin [18].

4.4. *S.pombe* Translin

Schizosaccharomyces pombe and human translin, both forming octameric ring, share an overall 36% identity and 54% similarity, with higher degrees in the C-terminal region [19].

4.5. Orthologues in other vertebrates

Another orthologue of translin was also identified in *Xenopus laevis*, annotated as X-translin [20]. Based on gel filtration studies, chicken translin was believed to exist as a decamer [13]. Translin was also identified as one of the structural proteins in 2D and MALDI-TOF profiling of the skeletal muscle of Takifugu rubripes, a kind of pufferfish [21]. It was thus established that translin was largely conserved across evolution, consisting of the leucine zipper and at least one of the short basic regions which was speculated as the DNA-binding domain.

5. Structure of Translin and orthologues

Electron microscopic studies and single-particle analysis reconstructed a three-dimensional structure of translin. The eight subunits appeared to assemble in an octameric ring with two distinct basic domains and a funnel shaped central channel [22] (Figure 1). This creates a binding interface for nucleotides. Ultracentrifugation and sedimentation equilibrium studies further established that the predominant species of translin was a hydrodynamic oblate ellipsoid structure of octamer which is also the basic binding unit for DNA at chromosomal breakpoints [23]. This was later confirmed by X-ray diffraction and crystallization at 2.2 Å that presented two tetramers to form an octamer by two-fold symmetry mainly brought about by hydrophobic interactions (Figure 1) [24]. These results suggest that the higher order structure of translin is not based on strong intermolecular hydrogen interactions rendering the whole molecule to be rather flexible in order to change the relative positions of monomer for nucleic acid binding with better accessibility of the central core. In the presence or absence of DNA or RNA, translin forms chiral or pin-wheel shaped rings which are similar to that of human Dmc1 protein, a meiosis specific recombinase [22]. Crystallization of TB-RBP resulted in the formation of orthorhombic crystals [25]. Dynamic light scattering (DLS) recognized equilibrium between tetramers and octamers of TB-RBP in solution. Wild-type *Drosophila* translin existed as an octamer/decamer whereas at high resolution crystallization parameters, the mutant P168S exhibited two identical tetrameric forms (Figure 2) [26].

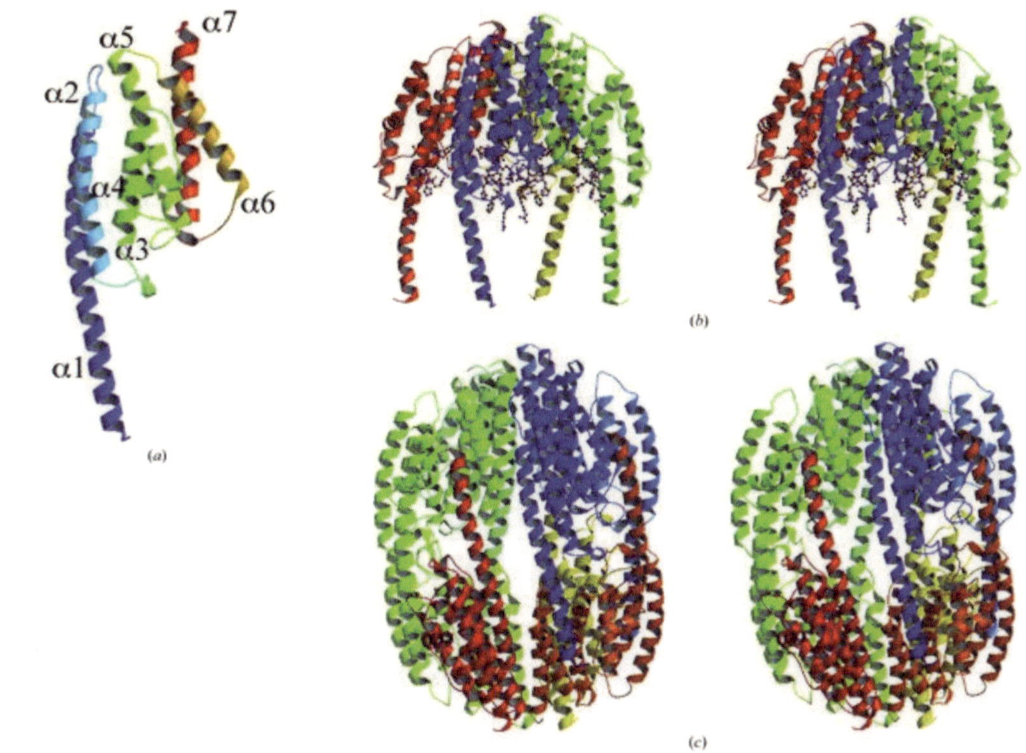

Figure 1. Overall architecture of human Translin. (a) Ribbon representation of residues Met1±Phe217 of a translin monomer. (b) Translin tetramer or `two dimers' in the asymmetric unit. The regions with side chains are `basic regions' that are supposed to bind to the target *©2004 International Union of Crystallography* DNA/RNA. They are located in the inner surface of the tetramer. (c) Translin octamer, which is the two tetramers related by a crystallographic two fold symmetry. *Reproduced with permission from Acta Crystallographica Section D60, Sugiura et. al., 2004, 674-679 [24].*

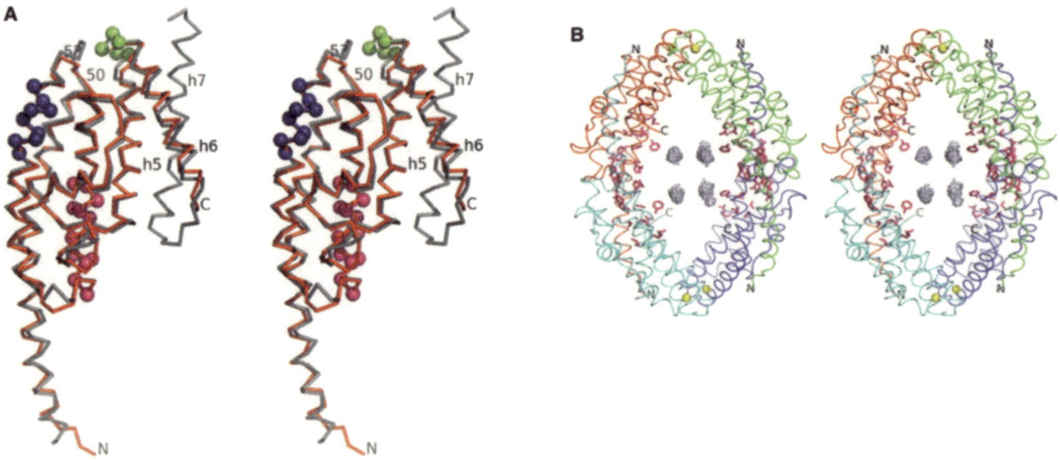

Figure 2. A) Stereo-view of the C^{α} trace of the *Drosophila* P168S mutant translin monomer structure (red) (residues 3 and 187 are identified with N and C labels, respectively) super-posed onto the structure of human translin protein (grey). The basic-1, basic-2 and putative GTP-binding motifs of human translin sequence are shown as blue, magenta and green spheres, respectively. The shortened loop 1 of *Drosophila* translin is identified by residues numbered 50 and 53. The α 7 helix of human translin (labeled h7) is not modeled in *Drosophila* mutant translin structures as it is disordered in the crystals. Also marked are the α5 and α 6 helices (labeled h5 and h6). (B) Cartoon of the *Drosophila* P168S mutant translin tetramer. The translin molecules of the tetramer are shown in cyan, red, green and blue, respectively, with the N- and C-termini of each marked as N and C. The amino acids of the basic-2 motifs are shown in magenta. The positions of the four columns of unaccounted electron density observed at the center of the tetramer cavity are shown as gray contours. The amino acid residue at position 168 is marked with yellow sphere for each monomer. *Reproduced with permission from Dr.Vinay Kumar, BARC, FEBS Journal, Gupta et. al., 2008, 4235-4249 [26]. Journal compilation©2008 FEBS*

6. Localization of Translin and orthologues

Translin was mainly found to be localized in the cytoplasm as it comprises of a hydrophobic nuclear export signal in its C-terminal [10]. Both, the nuclear export signal and the putative GTP binding domain also seemed to be conserved among human, mouse and fly translin [27-29], although the GTP binding ability of the fly protein was lower than that of its mammalian counterpart [29].

TB-RBP was encoded by a single copy gene in mouse, but three different RNA transcripts of 1.2, 1.7 and 3 kb each were found during spermatogenesis in pre-pubertal and sexually active testes. Additionally, expression of the different sizes of TB-RBP mRNAs was also found in other tissues such as heart, liver, kidney and spleen [30]. Translin staining was found to be intense in the cytoplasm of cerebral cortex/purkinje cells establishing its somatodendritic localization which is also consistent with the studies performed in spermatocytes [31]. Non-hematopoietic mammalian cells, eg., HeLa treated with DNA damaging agents such as mitomycin C and etoposide increased the nuclear localization of TB-RBP, thereby indicating a signaling cascade that initiated the nuclear transport of the molecule following exposure to DNA damaging agents [32].

Drosophila translin was ubiquitously localized in the cytoplasm, in the early embryonal syncytial stage, but later enriched in ventral neuroblasts as demonstrated from our florescence studies; probably depicting the metaphase of the cell cycle. Cells around the tracheal pits in the embryo and oenocytes in the third instar larva also exhibited elevated levels of protein. RNA in situ hybridization displayed an increased expression in the ventral midline cells of the larval brain, suggesting a neuronal expression, which was corroborated by protein immunostaining. In adult flies, translin was localized in the brain neuronal cell bodies and in early spermatocytes. Interestingly, *Drosophila* translin mutants exhibited a sex specific impaired motor response i.e. only in females [18].Taken together, the multiple cellular localizations, the high neuronal expression and the attendant locomotor defect of the translin mutant indicated that the fly protein may have multiple roles in neuronal development.

7. Interactors of Translin and their physiological significance

Choromosomal translocations are widespread among a diverse group of neoplasms and other genetic disorders. Hence, the mechanism to repair and stabilize such anomalous rearrangements at recombination hot-spots presumably involved several other factors which could act as functional interactors of translin.

7.1. Translin associated factor – X (TRAX)

In order to isolate other recombination hot-spot proteins, yeast 2-hybrid system was employed by Aoki and co-workers using human translin as bait. It led to the identification of a 33 kDa protein which shared 28% overall and 38% C-terminal sequence identity with translin It was therefore nomenclatured as the Translin-associated factor – X (TRAX) [33]. The N-terminal encased the bipartite nuclear targeting signal comprising of two basic regions separated by a spacer sequence and supposed to be responsible for the nuclear transport of translin. Human TRAX gene composed of six exons with a putative CpG island at the 5′ end, mapped at least 35 kb proximal to DISC1 and within approximately 150–250 kb of the translocation breakpoint at 1q42.1 [34]. Mouse trax gene was later isolated by Devon et. al. and mapped by FISH on chromosome locus 1q41. It was identified as a gene encoding for a 290 amino acid protein and because of its shared sequential identity with that of the human protein, was presumed to be the mouse orthologue [35]. It was expressed in various tissues, such as spleen, testis, ovary, thymus, etc. and primarily cytoplasmic in localization [36]. The isoforms were transcribed at equal ratios in kidney, testis and heart. The open reading frame was largely conserved across evolution sharing 90%, 35%, 34% and 30% identity with human, *D. melanogaster*, *A. thaliana* and *S. pombe* respectively. In addition to coding sequence, conservation was also observed in the 3′UTR region. Mouse trax being an interactor, could also be considered as a paralog of translin due to its 29% identity and 41% similarity to the mouse protein. The bipartite nuclear localization signal in human trax was absent in the fly protein.

7.2. GADD34

DNA damage, in mammalian cells, is capable of activating a cascade of cell-cycle checkpoints and also triggering an apoptotic response in the cells. GADD34 or growth-arrest and DNA-damage inducible gene is one such example which was inducted in response to rapid UV radiation in Chinese hamster ovary (CHO) cell lines. *In vitro* as well as *in vivo* studies established a strong interaction with translin in the cytoplasm, although the exact role of GADD34 in translin regulation is unclear [37]. However, one possibility could be the transport of translin from cytoplasm to nucleus as observed in lymphoid lineages with rearranged Ig/TCR loci. Evidence supports that GADD34 and translin play a role in stress response since DNA damaging drugs elevate the GADD34 levels in mammalian cultured cells.

7.3. TER-ATPase

Transcriptional endoplasmic reticulum ATPase (TER-ATPase), γ-actin and Trax co-immunoprecipitated with TB-RBP from mouse testicular extracts [38]. TB-RBP was further found to interact with mRNAs encoding for myelin basic protein and calmodulin kinase II as well as protamines 1 and 2 in brain and testicular extracts respectively. Based on confocal microscopic investigation, TB-BRP co-localized with microtubules throughout the cytoplasm in mouse germ cells [39].TER-ATPase is known to transport membrane vesicles to Golgi apparatus [40] whereas actin is a cytoskeletal structural protein of microfilaments [41]. Immunocytochemical analyses in the nervous system indicate that the interactions between TB-RBP and TER-ATPase facilitate them as two components of a larger complex facilitating mRNA transport and localization. Another possibility is that TB-RBP functions as an anchoring protein for RNA to dock onto microtubules, and, in association with other proteins such as the TER-ATPase and Trax, it translocates specific mRNAs [38].Thus, it is likely that TB-RBP functions in both intracellular and intercellular mRNA transport in testis [30] as well as facilitating its storage until the time of translation.

7.4. HCV

Another interactor of translin found by yeast assays and confirmed *in vitro* by co-immunoprecipitation was Hepatitis C virus core protein from liver hepatocellular carcinoma Hep G2 cell lines [42].Translin function can be triggered by chromosomal translocations in normal lymphocytes [43].Therefore, the interaction between HCV core protein and translin protein may trigger the B-cell progressing into lymphoma in patients infected with HCV. This molecular mechanism could at least partially explain for tumorigenesis of HCV.

7.5. GRBP

Glycolytic pathway is co-ordinated by a key enzyme L-type pyruvate kinase that is regulated by carbohydrates at transcriptional and post-transcriptional levels [44, 45]. A novel pro-

http://dx.doi.org/10.5772/54016

tein binding factor bound to glucose response element (GRE) was isolated from rat liver cytosol and nuclei [46]. This glucose response binding protein (GRBP) complex revealed translin/trax 240 and 420 kDa heteromeric complex in the nuclear and cytosolic extracts respectively. The amount of GRBP complex was increased in liver nuclear extract by a high carbohydrate diet and decreased by starvation, high fat, and high protein diet. The levels in cytosol were dependent on carbohydrate availability [47]. The constituents of the GRBP complex could be designated to bind to the glucose response element of the pyruvate kinase gene as a function of high fat diet.

7.6. KIF17b and KIF2Aβ

A testis-enriched kinesin KIF17b coimmunoprecipitated with TB-RBP in a RNA–protein complex containing specific cAMP-responsive element modulator (CREM)-regulated mRNAs. This complex was temporally and sequentially expressed indicating a separation of the processes of transport and translation in mammalian male germ cells [48]. Another kinesin KIF2Aβ, also enriched in testes, colocalized with trax in the perinuclear region such as Golgi complex, thereby indicating some role in spermatogenesis [49].Testis mRNAs encoding protamine 1 and 2 (Prm1 and 2), transition protein 1 and 2 (Tnp1 and 2), A-kinase anchoring protein 4 (Akap4), and glyceraldehyde 3-phosphate dehydrogenase-S (Gapds), and brain mRNAs encoding tau, Ca2+-calmodulin-dependent protein kinase II, and myelin basic protein have been reported to be target mRNAs of translin [39, 50-52]. These are transcribed in post meiotic germ cells by (CREM)-tau and are subcellularly transported in association with the kinesin KIF17b [53]. Other examples of translin target mRNAs encoding diazepam-binding inhibitor–like 5, arylsulfatase A, a tetratricopeptide repeat structure-containing protein and ring finger protein 139 were initially expressed in pachytene spermatocytes [54]. In addition, two non-coding RNAs, Nct1 and 2, abundant in nuclei of the spermatocytes were also identified adjacent to recombination hot-spot motif GGA [55].

8. Interactors of TRAX and their physiological significance

Trax has been co-purified with translin on numerous occasions. In one of our own studies, we attempted the purification of recombinant human TRAX and were presented with a highly unstable and insoluble protein. It was stabilized by co-expression with translin and it co-purified as a soluble translin-trax heteromeric complex. This purified complex was assessed for its functional activity by DNA-binding gel shift assays. Translin gave rise to a distinct DNA gel-shift complex with duplex DNA unlike that of the translin-trax heteromeric complex. However, the complex like that to translin formed a stable protein-DNA complex demonstrating specific ssDNA binding activity. The gel shift complex was excised and analyzed for its composition on SDS-PAGE. Stoichiometrically, it was found that the minimum binding unit for ssDNA was a dimer of translin and monomer of trax which existed nearly in a ratio of 1:1, similar to that of a purified recombinant complex [56]. All these results, put together, suggested that heteromeric complex exhibits relatively more stable binding to ssDNA. trax contains three functional properties: a nuclear localization signal, RNA binding activity, and the ability to interact with translin. The ability of trax to form a heteromeric complex with translin and the bipartite nuclear localization signal on trax may be the most vital properties to transport translin from cytoplasm to nucleus. Therefore, it will not be inconsequential to assume that there could be other molecules interacting with trax for translin transport and function in the nucleus.

8.1. C1D

A large number of proteins control gene expression by binding to repetitive sequences of genomic DNA and targeting a subset to nuclear matrix [57]. C1D is one such non-histone protein which is also an activator of DNA-PK [58], that plays an important role in DNA double-strand break (DSB) repair mechanism through NHEJ and V(D)J recombination, a process specific to lymphocytes for the development of immune system [59]. Yeast 2-hybrid screens established that trax interacts specifically with C1D via its putative leucine zipper. Immunoflorescence staining showed that C1D is predominantly localized in the nucleus with some diffused pattern observed in the cytoplasm. Moreover, whilst translin also interacts with trax via its leucine zipper, to stabilize the protein, C1D-TRAX interaction is enhanced or induced in response to γ-irradiation, thus deeming the interaction of both translin and C1D with trax as mutually independent events [60]. In this regard, it should be noted that Trax has been shown to enhance the DNA binding capacity of TB-RBP (translin), while decreasing its RNA-binding ability [36]. One biological consequence of trax-C1D interaction could be the regulation of translin – trax interaction rather than regulating any pre-formed heteromeric complex. Trax's ability to change protein partners between translin and C1D could act as a switch *in vivo* regulating the preference of translin binding to nucleic acids. This theory appeared to be consistent with the model proposed by Hecht and co-workers that trax is a vital regulator for Translin's sub-cellular locale [61].

Disruption of CID in yeast strains resulted in increased temperature sensitivity, but insensitivity towards DNA damaging agents such as methylmethanosulphate (MMS) or UV and only mild sensitivity to γ-irradiation. This phenomenon is highly reminiscent to that of YKu70p [62]. Further rejoining and recombination assays exhibited defects in NHEJ and HR pathways in yc1d mutants, thus implicating the role of C1D in both the DSB repair pathways [60]. This hypothesis is supported by the established interaction between C1D and DNA-PK [58].

8.2. A_2A adenosine receptor (A_2A-R)

p53 is a nuclear phosphoprotein and tumor suppressor that regulates the cell cycle [63]. $p53^{+/-}$ mice exhibit brain malformations whereas $p53^{-/-}$mice exhibit neuronal developmental abnormalities, including that of neural tube closure [64]. Adenosine with its four receptors is known to modulate neuronal function [65]. One of its receptorsA_2A-R can be stimulated in the presence of inhibitors against protein kinase A and C, in order to rescue the impairment of nerve growth factor (NGF) followed by inhibition of cell proliferation. Trax was found to be interacting with the cytoplasmic region of A_2A-R and its over-expression also demonstrated a similar rescue effect [66]. It can thus be inferred that A_2A-R might exert its rescue effect mediated as a function of negative proliferation signal by trax. It was later discovered that the p53 blockage rescue effect was critically dependent on the functional interaction of trax and KIF2A [67].

8.3. GAP – 43

Trax was shown to co-express and function as an operational switch to regulate the transcription of the growth-associated protein (GAP-43) during post-natal development. Following trax switch-off, axonal growth was upregulated as a result of increased levels of GAP-43 [68]. Thus, it can be speculated that trax may have potent therapeutic potential against neuronal injuries associated with the inability of axons to regrow, as usually occurs within long neuronal pathways such as the optic nerve and spinal tracts.

8.4. PLCβ1

Mammalian phospholipase Cβ1 (PLCβ1) is mainly localized on the cytosolic plasma membrane surface where it is associated with its membrane-bound activator $G\alpha_q$ [69]. PLCβ1 interacts with trax specifically through its C-terminal and allows trax to directly compete with its functional interactor $G\alpha_{q.}$ PLCβ1-trax complex is observed mostly in the cytosol and a small amount is seen in the nucleus thereby revealing yet another role of trax as a regulator for the cellular compartmentalization of its interactors [70]. The mode of stabilization of PLCβ1 could be attributed to two main factors; (i) activation of PKC through phosphorylation, which is directly downstream of PLCβ1 and (ii) interaction with trax [71] that regulates its cellular localization. A latest study also linked the interaction between PLCβ1 and trax in the regulation of genes by RNA interference [72].

9. Functional characterization of Translin/TB-RBP and Trax

9.1. DNA/RNA binding mode of Translin

Electron microscopic and X-ray diffraction studies have characterized translin as an assembly of eight polypeptide chains that form ring-shaped octameric structure (Figure 1) [22, 24]. Crystal structure showed that each monomer of translin/TB-RBP is composed of about 70% R-helices, 25% random coils, and 5% beta-sheets [24, 25, 73].The hydrophobic heptad repeats consisting of the leucine zippers form the core of the octamer. The DNA-binding activity is attributed to the two relatively short basic amino acid regions, 56 – 64 and 86 – 97, found upstream to the leucine zipper. The latter one was deemed responsible for creating the DNA binding domain on the ring structure and even a point mutation in this region could completely inhibit the DNA binding activity of the protein [13].

Amino acid sequence analysis of TB-RBP also demonstrated a leucine zipper and stretch of basic amino acid residues on two different peptides that were identical to the human protein and indexed for chromosomal translocation in lymphoid cells. GST–tagged TB-RBP recombinant protein also interacted *in vitro* with DNA oligo sequences representing the target recognition motifs from clustered breakpoint region of Bcl2 oncogene found in follicular lymphoma patients [17]. These studies further confirmed single-stranded DNA binding ability of translin.

The DNA-RNA binding function of the protein is attributed to its C-terminal, encasing the motif of basic amino acids, with a minimum requirement of a dimer [16]. Additionally, the RNA-binding ability of the protein was observed only in brain and meiotic germ cells of mouse testis [30].

The mouse orthologues of human translin, and trax, respectively, also interact to form a heterodimer. This heterodimeric unit enhances the TB-RBP binding to ssDNA, but inhibits its interaction with RNA. In addition, analogous to translin-DNA binding, only one of the two basic regions is essential to bind to ssDNA interaction, but both the domains are required for RNA binding [36]. However, the absence of common RNA recognition motifs in TB-RBP sets it apart from other RNA-binding proteins [74]. Other RNA-binding proteins, such as the human teratocarcinoma protein p40, which binds to LINE-1 RNA [75], an AU-rich sequence-binding protein [76], thymidylate synthase [77], and one of the iron responsive element-binding proteins (IRE-BP1) [78], all lack common RNA-binding domains but are known to regulate stored mRNAs during spermatogenesis and facilitate transport of specific mRNAs in the nervous system [14, 50].

Electrophoretic mobility gel-shift assays (EMSA) based on interaction studies between translin and target DNA sequences from broken hot-spot regions on chromosome 18q21, clearly indicated that translin binds to DNA from ends and hence requires single-stranded ends to load onto staggered DNA break-points [43]. Studies from our lab further complied with these observations. According to our results, we were able to put forth a model stating that free translin octamer undergoes a conformational change, leading to either compaction or dissociation of the molecule and loads onto DNA duplexes via its free ends resulting into a tighter clamping of the duplex ends [79].

9.2. GTP acts as a "switch" to regulate Translin-DNA/RNA binding

Sequence analysis of mouse TB-RBP revealed several domains, one of it being the putative GTP-binding domain, VTAGD, in the C-terminal, that shares substantial homology with sequence, DTAGQ on G-proteins [27]. This domain is also fairly conserved differing in only one amino acid among *Drosophila*, human & *Xenopus* translin. Radiolabeled EMSA revealed that only GTP, but neither GDP, GDP-γS nor ATP, decreased the RNA binding ability of TB-RBP. A mutation in the GTP binding site altered only the RNA binding ability of the protein but did not influence its DNA binding ability. This mutation also did not interfere with the dimerization of the protein, its interaction with wild-type TB-RBP or also with trax, since these interactions are mostly dependent on the leucine zipper. Moreover, mammalian cell lines transfected with the GTP mutated TB-RBP resulted in cell death indicating a dominant negative role in cultured cells [28].

In order to further understand the mechanism of GTP modulation on translin, we performed several biochemical and biophysical experiments on human translin and its *Droso-*

phila orthologue which was cloned and characterized in our laboratory [18]. Our studies using circular dichroism (CD) spectroscopy showed that addition of GTP reduced the ellipticity from the secondary structure of human translin whereas the response was not similar for that of the *Drosphila* orthologue. MALDI-TOF analyses of the total tryptic profile for both the proteins showed that the liberated proteolyzed fragments predominantly belonged to 24 – 27 and 6 – 8 kDa size categories. GTP addition further enhanced the C-terminal cleavages in the former category, specifically in translin. Isothermal calorimetric studies probed the heat changes associated with GTP-mediated effects, distributed in two distinct phases for human and fly translin protein. In the first phase, the GTP : protein monomer ratio increased from 0:1 to 1:1 showing an initial exothermic curve followed by an endothermic change. However, in the final phase of titration, as the ratio increased beyond 1:1, the heat changes observed with translin were markedly different from that of the *Drosophila* protein. Human translin showed an exponential decrease in enthalpy, whereas the *Drosophila* protein showed a monotonic rise in enthalpy. These two sets of sites seemed independent models as per curve-fitting analysis and hence their binding patterns could not be correlated as either parallel or sequential. Our findings led us to hypothesize a model. As the GTP : protein ratio increases beyond 1:1, the occupancy of the putative final site on translin with GTP induces dissociative change within the translin octamer, as evidenced by the exponential decrease in the enthalpy curve in the second stage of titration. Interestingly, under similar conditions, the heat changes recovered from GTP titration with *Drosophila* translin were similar to that of human translin in the first part but different in the second stage affirming that the fly translin oligomer may be smaller than the octamer, perhaps a tetramer or hexamer, which can dissociate into stable dimers as evidenced from gel filtration studies. Human translin exhibits a stable octameric state and binds ssDNA/RNA/dsDNA targets, in sequential order of binding ability, all of which get attenuated when GTP is added. Conversely, *Drosophila* translin exhibits a stable dimeric state that assembles into a sub-octameric (tetramer/hexamer) form and fails to bind ssDNA and RNA targets [29]. We predicted that this phenomenon could likely be a manifestation of a structural dissociation, i.e., "loosening or slackening" in the ellipsoidal ring that lowers the nucleic acid tethering by the protein. These observations were compliant with our earlier hypothesis for translin loading onto free DNA ends due to conformational changes [79]. Furthermore, enhanced C-terminal cleavages by the protease action in the presence of GTP are a reflection of structural reorganization in the human translin ring, and the lack of the same in *Drosophila* protein is consistent with the model that oligomeric status may be critical for the "switchability" by GTP. A parallel inference has been drawn from the well-characterized RAG1and RAG2 proteins that perform critical DNA recognition and cleavage functions in V(D)J recombination, where physiological concentrations of GTP strongly and selectively inhibit the RAG-mediated transposition reaction [80]. This further encouraged us to believe that GTP binding might similarly impinge on the proposed chromosomal breakage-rejoining function of translin, *in vivo*.

Not only translin, but also tanslin-trax complex has been investigated substantially for its nucleic acid binding properties, but trax, a rather unstable protein was not known to bind DNA or RNA independently. Very recently, Gupta and Kumar successfully identified two novel nucleic acid binding motifs in trax, nomenclatured as B2 and B3 (B2,115QFHRA119;

B3,237YEVSKKL243) [81]. Intriguingly, the binding activity displayed by the translin-traxB2 complex was comparable to that of the wild type translin-trax complex,, but that of the translin-traxB3 complex was markedly reduced. The motifs seemingly contributed towards the DNA-binding ability of the tanslin-trax heteromeric complex.

10. Physiological role of Translin and its implications in genetic disorders

Translin was identified as a novel DNA binding protein at chromosomal breakpoint junctions in several lymphoid malignancies [10]. Since then several biochemical and molecular studies have been carried out in order to characterize the protein for its physiological relevance across evolution.

Cellular processes such as cell signaling, trafficking, and targeting are governed by protein interactions occurring through short peptide segments that share a common "motif". Two such protein binding modules are; DxxDxxxD protein phosphatase 1 binding motif and a VxxxRxYS motif that binds to translin [82].

10.1. Cell cycle proliferation

Translin was contemplated as a part of cell division machinery when mammalian cells were treated with DNA damage inducing agents, such as, doxycycline, which led the protein synthesis to become maximal during the G2/M phase. The protein was also found to be associated with γ-tubulin and less markedly with α-tubulin, in agreement with the presence of γ-tubulin in the centrosome, the spindle poles and the microtubule bundles of the mid-bodies during mitosis. Translin localizes to mitotic spindle microtubules during metaphase and shifts to mid-bodies in late telophase [83].

Mutation in Atm gene leads to a recessive human genetic disorder, Ataxia telangiectasia (AT), characterized by progressive neurodegeneration, immunologic defects, cancer predisposition, and hypersensitivity to ionizing radiation [84]. AT cells show irradiation-induced cell cycle checkpoint defects, since wild type ATM activates p53, which in turn is known to induce the downstream apoptosis cascade $p21^{WAF1/CIP1}$ [85]. Intriguingly, mice spleen cells, defective in ATM gene exhibited intermediate translin levels in response to γ-irradiation, associating altered protein expression with cell cycle proliferation.

TB-RBP heterozygous mice were phenotypically indistinguishable from their wild-type littermates. Normal T-cell development and V(D)J recombination supported that absence of TB-RBP was not essential for its function but had an influence on the behavioral pattern. However, the birth weight was 10-30% lower for TB-RBP deficient homozygotes with a coordinated reduced sperm count and high level of apoptosis indicating abnormal spermatogenesis. Also, the females produced smaller and fewer litters [53]. The TB-RBP-deficient mouse embryonic fibroblasts (MEFs) exhibited a reduced growth rate compared with MEFs from littermates which was remedied with the reintroduction of TB-RBP. Trax was also found to be absent in these cells in spite of normal mRNA levels, probably a consequence of ubiquitination [86]. Complementing the deficiency with a wild-type TB-RBP molecule regulated the trax protein expression levels, indicating that they both existed proportionally for normal cell proliferation. This phenomenon was also corroborated by shRNA against trax in HeLa cells that exhibited sluggish proliferation due to loss of trax mRNA [86]. On the other hand, deletion of translin in the yeast gene, did not alter the growth rate or phenotypic changes in cell morphology or size, but rather a double mutant of translin-trax slightly stimulated the cell growth [19]. Thus, both these genes can be deemed non-essential in *S.pombe*. Translin also exhibited a higher affinity for homologous RNA sequences, such as (GU)n and (GUU)n, suggesting its primary role in functions related to RNA metabolism [19]. In addition, X-translin exhibited a weak and diffused nuclear staining, but a prominent granular cytoplasmic staining during interphase. Interestingly, it refers that a part of the protein underwent a remarkable redistribution throughout mitosis and associated with centrosomes, thus mystifying its role in cell cycle [20].

10.2. mRNA regulation

Immunocytochemical studies showed that translin/TB-RBP was distributed in the nucleus and the cytoplasm of the developing rat hippocampal cells whereas it localized only in the nuclei of the glial cells [87]. Mouse cerebellar extracts demonstrated that both translin and trax were predominantly localized in the cytosolic fraction as components of the GS1 complex, which also consists of RNA oligonucleotides [88]. The translin-trax heteromeric complex was found to be enriched in brain following UV radiation. This led to a speculation that the complex may somehow be responsible for increase in the basal levels of GS1, thus implying a role in DNA repair.

Paradoxically, immunoblot analysis demonstrated levels of translin and trax in kidney, lung and cerebellum equal to that of brain and testis. Interestingly, gel-shift analysis of kidney extracts revealed that the expression of these proteins was masked by endogenous RNA; asserting that the TB/RBP-trax complex bound to RNA *in vivo*, implicating its role in RNA processing [89]. Translin knock-out mice exposed multiple behavioral abnormalities and alterations in levels of transcripts encoding synaptic proteins [90].

Neural BC1 RNA complex is expressed in the brain and distributed in the dendrites in the form of ribonucleoproteins [91]. Pur α and β are single stranded DNA/RNA binding proteins that have been known to play a role in transcription and replication [92, 93]. These proteins linked the BC1 RNA, distributed in the neuronal dendrites as ribonucleoproteins (RNPs) and consisted of translin, to microtubules. Mouse translin and a like partner protein, assumingly trax co-purified, from brain, with BC1 RNA as a 138 kDa complex suggesting that it is a molecular scaffolding assembly required for translin transport along dendritic microtubules, probably with a transient interaction with RNPs [94] and with the ability to repress mRNA translation [14]. Thus translin could possibly play a role in regulation of mRNA translation within dendrites during transport. Another example of translin/trax complex binding to RNA is its interaction with 3′UTR of protamine-2 comprising of Y and H elements. Mutation studies found that a minimum cluster of 8 G residues with an oligo length of 24 nucleotides was vital for high binding affinity [95]. This further supported the translin – BC1 RNA interactions at its 5′ end, rich in G-clusters. A confluence of localization, biochemical and RNA trafficking studies supports the view that this complex mediates dendritic trafficking of RNAs, a process thought to play a critical role in synaptic plasticity. Another study showed translin binding to ssDNA of Tetrahymena telomerase, (TTGGGG)n and human telomeric repeats, (TTAGGG)n also rich in G residues, probably by unwinding the hairpins formed by hydrogen bonding between non-canonical structures [96].

Another brain derived neurotropic factor (BDNF) mRNA is targeted to dendrites where it plays a key role in mediating synaptic plasticity [97]. Translin has been shown to bind to this mRNA and regulate its dendritic trafficking which is impaired due a mutation G196A (Val66Met) in BDNF [98]. Thus, the abnormal targeting can lead to pathologic neuropsychiatric disorders.

Similarly, TB-RBP was also observed in the nuclei of neurons and dendrons in the mouse hypothalamus [99]. Other RNA-binding proteins such as FMR1 and FXR1 and 2, responsible for mental retardation and Fragile X syndrome, are also expressed differentially in the cytoplasm of neurons during brain development [100]. This puts forth a theory based on co-existence of translin with factors accountable for mental disorders wherein TB-RBP/translin functions in the neurons binding mRNA for its cytoplasmic export followed by storage, localization and regulation of translation.

Translin also co-operates in the activation of steroidogenic factor – 1 (SF–1) for transcriptional regulation in rat leydig cells [101].

RNA interference (RNAi) is a biological mechanism in order to degrade the dsRNA and also the concomitant degradation of the homologous mRNA [102]. Mechanistic studies revealed that when dsRNA enters a cell, it is first digested into ~22 bp short dsRNA (small interference RNA or siRNA) by Dicer, a RNase III family member that is also responsible for miRNA formation. siRNA fragments, usually 5′-phosphorylated, then bind to the RNA-induced silencing complex (RISC) where they are unwound and directed to mRNA. One of the components of RISC is Argonaute2 (Ago2), which is believed to bind to the 3′ overhang of siRNA through a PAZ domain capable of binding single-stranded RNA with relatively low affinity [103, 104]. Another protein tightly bound to siRNA was identified to be TB-RBP and discovered to possess both ssRNase and dsRNase activities from two open ends of the corresponding RNA molecules [105]. A complex of translin-trax purified from the Dicer-R2D2-Ago2 reconstituted system from *Drosophila* was termed as C3PO. It enhanced the RISC activity of the recombinant complex [106], thus acting as a key activator in regulation of RNAi machinery. Only C3PO complex, neither translin nor trax alone, could function together with hAgo2 to reconstitute duplex siRNA-initiated RISC activity. Crystallization studies of hC3PO revealed two translin-trax heterodimers and two translin-translin homodimers tetramerizing side-by-side, in a stoichiometry of 6:2 to form an asymmetric octameric barrel. This asymmetric assembly proved pivotal for the function of C3PO as a novel endonuclease that cleaves RNA at the interior surface [107]. Truncated C3PO in *Drosophila* adopts a hexameric topology composed of four translin and two trax molecules according to the crystal structure, which is consistent with gel filtration and light scattering studies. The truncated complex, like full-length, exhibits endoribonuclease activity on the siRNA passenger strand, leaving 3′ hydroxyl-cleaved ends in order to activate RISC [108].

R2D2, dsRNA-binding protein and an essential component in the siRNA pathway in *Drosophila,* was expressed at minimal levels in silk moth tissues. The silk moth-derived Bm5 cell line was also deficient in expression of mRNA encoding full-length Bm translin, an RNA-binding factor that has been shown to stimulate the efficiency of RNAi [109], thereby explaining variable success of RNAi technology in lepidopteram insects.

A most recent study in the filamentous fungus, *Neurospora crassa,* showed that C3PO does not play a significant role in RNAi, but rather functions as an RNase that removes the 5′ pre-tRNA fragments which were identified as the major substrates for translin-trax complex in the fungus [110]. In the translin knock-out and trax knock-out mutants, tRNA levels, protein translation efficiency and cell growth were elevated which was consistent with the increase of cell proliferation rates of translin knock-out and trax knock-out mutant cells observed in fission yeast [19]. In addition, both translin and trax are known to be required for normal cell proliferation of mouse embryonic stem cells [86]. Because the changes in tRNA levels can differentially affect expression of various proteins, the roles of translin and trax in tRNA processing and other RNA processing may provide a potential explanation for its many biological roles in several organisms.

10.3. Regulation in meiotic germ cells

Similar to the human and mouse protein, *Xenopus* translin also binds to single stranded DNA encompassing the chromosomal breakpoint consensus sequences. It has been described as capable to inhibit paternal mRNA translation, indicating that it could play an important role in maternal mRNA translation and control during *Xenopus* oogenesis and embryogenesis [20].

Interestingly, western blot analysis of germ cell protein extracts demonstrated an increased ratio of trax to TB-RBP in meiotic pachytene spermatocytes compared to the post-meiotic round and elongated spermatids, resulting in nuclear localization due to a functional nuclear localization signal on trax; whereas elevated levels of TB-RBP prompted trax to remain in the cytoplasm due to functional nuclear export signal on TB-RBP. This indicates that the localization of the two proteins in male germ cells is modulated by their relative ratios [111].

Based upon the specificity of translin binding to consensus sequences of breakpoints in chromosome translocations, it can be proposed that TB-RBP functions in the nuclei of germ cells in meiotic recombination or DNA repair in addition to serving as an RNA- and microtubule binding protein in the cytoplasm of testicular cells. Gapds mRNA was also found to be present in the adult testis extract and its translation was inhibited by the TB-RBP according to *in vitro* translation assays [52].

Drosophila translin was also found to be essential for normal trax expression substantiating a report in a parallel study that trax expression was lost in translin knock-out mice [53]. Loss of translin and trax in *Drosophila* did not seem to have an effect either on oogenesis or meiotic recombination rates and chromosome segregation. In addition, no evidence was found for an increased sensitivity for DNA double-strand damage in embryos and developing larvae [32].

10.4. Hemotopoietic regeneration

Pluripotent human leukemia cell line K562 exhibited decrease in translin levels as a response to DNA damaging drugs such as etoposide and mitomycin C [43]. p53 is known to increase in response to ionizing radiation, but also nuclear levels of translin were elevated. This referred to the activation of signal transduction pathways to arrest cells at specific checkpoints in the cell cycle, allowing translin to localize in the nucleus and carry out the repair of damaged DNA [112]. In order to address the functional significance of translin in the hematopoietic generation system with reference to acute radiation-responses, translin homozygous and heterozygous mice were assessed for hematopoietic colony formation. In response to 4 Gy IR, 1 week later, extramedullary hematopoietic colonies were observed in translin$^{+/-}$ mice, whereas those in translin$^{-/-}$ mice were delayed for more than two weeks as compared to their wild type comtemporaries [113]. Thus, it can be assumed that translin somehow contributes to hematopoietic regeneration by acting as a sensor protein for radiation-induced damage. Neonatal translin $^{-/-}$ mice also exhibit delayed chondrocyte development linked to differentiation of mesenchymal stem cells. This can be further linked to the maintenance of constant number of hematopoietic progenitors by self renewal [114]. Their differentiation from hematopoietic stem cells, which is a critical phenomena in bone marrow hemtapoeisis, is shown to be perturbed in the absence of translin and trax [115].

10.5. Inherited genetic disorders and neoplasms

Inverted repeats, minisatellites, and the chi (χ) recombination hotspots are some of the DNA motifs that have been associated with gene conversion in human genes causing inherited diseases. DNA breakage could be more prominent in such gene conversion events that tend to occur within the G-rich or CpG-islands that can potentially form non-B-DNA structures [116]. Maximal converted tracts were enriched in a truncated version of the χ-element (TGGTGG motif), immunoglobulin heavy chain class switch repeats, translin target sites and several novel motifs including (or overlapping) the classical meiotic recombination hotspot, CCTCCCCT. It was thus postulated that the high density of recombination-related motifs served as target binding sites for protein complexes, such as translin and RAG-associated proteins, or arrest sites for DNA polymerases, which may assist, induce or indeed be required for the recombination-repair process [117].

10.5.1. Muscular dystrophy

Muscular dystrophies are allelic disorders caused by a mutation in the dystrophin gene [118]. Two deletion hot-spots in this gene locus were comprehensively analyzed for target recognition consensus sequences. Among other elements, such as chi, Pur α, minisatellite sequences, translin-binding sites were also identified in the muscular dystrophy gene at chromosomal breakpoint junctions [119]. This further validates the involvement of gene rearrangement in genetic disorders.

http://dx.doi.org/10.5772/54016

10.5.2. Sotos syndrome

Sotos syndrome (SoS), a rare congenital dysmorphic disorder, is characterized by overgrowth in childhood, distinctive craniofacial features, and mental retardation [120]. It is caused by mutations in NSD1 gene flanked by low copy repeats (LCRs). Translin target motifs were significantly higher in and around these breakpoint regions [121].

10.5.3. Fragile X syndrome

Mutations in the Fragile X mental retardation protein (FMRP) is responsible for Fragile X syndrome resulting in behavioral and neurochemical alterations in mice [122]. Like FMRP, translin is present in neuronal dendrites and associates with microtubules and motor proteins. Translin knock-out mice also exhibit behavioral, locomotor and sex-related variations [123]. These evidences suggest that both the proteins may act in the same neuronal pathway thus leading to a speculation that mutations in one or both the proteins are likely to contribute to neuronal illnesses such as fragile X-like syndrome, mental retardation, attention deficit hyperactivity disorder, epilepsy, and autism spectrum disorders in humans.

10.5.4. Schizophrenia

Disrupted in Schizophrenia 1 locus (DISC1) was first identified from a large Scottish family with a balanced translocation t(1;11) (q42.2;q14.3) responsible for schizophrenia and bipolar disorder (BP). Translin-associated factor X (TRAX), has been shown to undergo intergenic splicing with DISC1 and thus may also be affected by the translocation [124]. Locus 1q42 encompasses, DISC1 and 2 and trax that occur as an enriched complex with Translin in brain thus making it highly relevant for etiology of psychotic disorders [125]. These haplotypes were also associated with several quantitative endophenotypic traits including impairments in short- and long-term memory functioning and reduced gray matter density in the prefrontal cortex. The effects were consistent with their production of proteins that play roles in neurotic outgrowth, neuronal migration, synaptogenesis, and glutamatergic neurotransmission [126].

10.5.5. Sarcoma

Rhabdomyosarcoma occurs in connective tissue, presumably arising from progenitors of skeletal muscle. It is a common malignant tumor among young children and adolescents. Another variant of rhabdomyosarcoma is alveolar rhabdomyosarcoma and is characterized by a specific chromosomal translocation t(2;13)(q35;q14) [127] generating the PAX3-FKHR fusion gene. The t(2;13) breakpoint lies within the PAX3 and FKHR genes on chromosomes 2 and 13 respectively. The sequences flanking the breakpoint sites in these genes were found to be 62% homologous to the consensus sequence alleged to be the target recognition sequence of translin at the translocations [128].

Another example of reciprocal translocation, t(12;16)(q32;q16), is a common genetic event occurring in myxoid and round-cell liposarcomas, a malignant adipose tissue neoplasm. It is the result of a novel chimera formed by TLS/FUS and CHOP genes [129]. *In silico* sequence analysis revealed more than 70% homologous sequences possessing translin-binding motifs adjacent to TLS/CHOP breakpoint junctions. Also, topoisomerase II consensus cleavage sites were found at these regions suggesting a role of the enzyme in creating staggered ends and recruiting one of the several factors such as translin in the process of chromosomal translocation. [130]. Furthermore, sequences highly homologous to consensus translin-binding motifs were also found at the breakpoints generated by translocation t(X;18) in synovial sarcoma [131].

10.5.6. Leukemia

Chronic myelogenic leukemia, associated with unregulated growth of myeloid cells in bone marrow is the result of a somatic gene rearrangement forming a fusion by two-way exchange between 2 genes; BCR on chromosome 22 and ABL on chromosome 9 to form BCR-ABL. Consequently, t(9;22)(q34;q11) is the chromosomal translocation and the small derivative chromosome 22 product is well known as the Philadelphia or Ph chromosome [132]. Clinical studies also demonstrated these breakpoints in most patients with topoisomerase II inhibitor therapy-related acute myeloid leukemia (tAML) [133]. Breakpoint sequence patterns on this region of the BCR gene shared 80% identity with the translin consensus recognition sites. These were also positively identified in acute lymphoblastic leukemia cases with BCR-ABL hybrid. Alu sequences, the most repetitive regions of the human genome possess a high frequency of involvement in BCR recombination. Surprisingly, they also shared a close homology to translin consensus sequences, thereby indicating that the protein might be able to bind to one of the most ubiquitous regions of the genome [134].

10.5.7. Lymphoma

Burkitt's lymphoma cells that are deficient in component(s) of NHEJ pathway exhibit a large number of translocations resembling the classic translocations [135]. Further investigation may lead to a novel pathway employing translin and interactors for rejoining the breakpoints at these junctions that resemble translin recognition motifs.

10.5.8. Carcinoma

Translin-like protein was also detected in the proteomic analysis of human colorectal carcinoma cell lines along with other proteins, such as endothelial cell growth factor 1 (platelet-derived), rhotekin protein (RTKN), septin 1, cyclin dependent kinase 1, and sialic acid binding Ig-like lectin 11, tyrosinase-related protein. All of these are known to be involved in cell growth, motility, invasion, adhesion, apoptosis and tumor immunity, which is associated with distinct aspects of tumour metastasis [136].

10.5.9. Dysgerminoma

Dysgerminoma, arising from gonad cells, is a rare form of ovarian tumor in adolescent women [137]. RNF139/TRC8 is a potential tumor suppressor gene and its post-transcriptional regulation is disrupted by a balanced translocation t(8;22)(q24.13;q11.21). Translin was found to be involved in posttranscriptional regulation of TRC8, which could be related to the interaction between translin and TRC8 to dysgerminoma. Thereby, a model was proposed wherein one copy of TRC8 was disrupted by palindrome-mediated translocation followed by further loss of TCR8 expression through suppression by translin, thus setting the stage for deregulated proliferation [138].

Monosomy 1p36 is the most common terminal deletion in newborns [139]. Two interstitial deletions were further discovered within the same chromosome generating balanced reciprocal translocation t(1;9)(p36.3;q34). Alignments of these junctions did not exhibit any sequence similarities suggesting the involvement of NHEJ in the ligation of broken ends. Further analysis of the breakpoint regions, even from solid tumors, revealed sequences similar to that of translin consensus binding motifs, GCCCWSSW [140]. Although the translin recognition sequences are frequent in the human genome, due to their repetitive nature, DNA breakage can still not be considered a random event. These results could support the hypothesis that either the translin-binding sites are more prone to breakage or are involved in rejoining the broken chromosomes furthering the mechanism of NHEJ.

11. Translin and NHEJ

It will be worth investigating as to how translocations are generated in compromised cases of NHEJ. One theory proposed by our group states that molecules such as translin, trax and their partners/interactors who do not appear to directly function in either of the predominant repair pathways, NHEJ or HR, might somehow deceptively lead the cells into misrepair functions and leading to chromosomal translocations. A possible mechanism that could function like the NHEJ would involve recruitment of translin and parallel factors onto damaged DNA ends, rejoining the staggered DNA DSBs followed by ligation of broken ends. The result would be a DNA sequence comprising of deletions and insertions at the repaired breakpoint junctions [141]. The mechanism is analogous to the study which demonstrated XRCC4-DNA Ligase IV complex as the most critical factor in rejoining the broken DNA ends though NHEJ. However, the recruitment and assembly of the NHEJ core factors was strikingly diverse from the known classical hierarchy of the molecules [142].

Various biochemical and genetics studies have demonstrated that even in the absence of one or more core components of NHEJ, broken ends of DNA are joined. These mechanisms are referred to as alternative end-joining (EJ) or back-up pathways [143]. In this case, the rejoining of DNA DSBs occurs at slower kinetics and can be erroneous which is incompatible with the concept of HR mechanism. Hence, it can be inferred that there are two possible signaling cascades in an event of DNA DSB, once which is the classical NHEJ (C-NHEJ), also known as DNA-PK – dependent NHEJ (D-NHEJ) involving Ku-DNA-PK complex as well as XRCC4-DNA Ligase IV complex which is effective in class switch recombination (CSR) in normal B lymphocytes. The other is the back-up NHEJ (B-NHEJ) which takes over the repair task on the occasion of deficiency of the core factors such as Ku heterodimer, DNA-PK and XRCC4-DNA Ligase IV [144]. Boboila et. al. have demonstrated that CSR is mediated by alternative end-joining (A-EJ) in the event of combined deficiency of Ku 70 and DNA Ligase IV. IgH-c-myc chromosomal translocations were also augmented in this case [145]. Another study demonstrated that the characteristics of translocation breakpoint junctions in wild-type mammalian cells and those deficient in XRCC4-DNA Ligase IV were similar, further implying that A-EJ pathway could be the primary mediator of chromosomal translocation in mammalian cells [146].

All of these recent evidences suggest that chromosomal translocations are rather suppressed when canonical NHEJ in involved in repair of DNA DSBs. But they become more common when A-EJ takes over. One of the speculation is that there is a rare probability for concurrent DSBs as one is usually repaired and restored to original chromosomal configuration by immediate sensing of Ku-DNA-PK-XRCC4-DNA Ligase IV complex before the next one occurs. Thus the temporal opportunity for translocations to occur is reduced [147]. On the occasion of inefficient C-NHEJ, the rejoining is slower by A-EJ, widening the time frame before each DSB closure, thus increasing the chance of two or multiple DSBs at the same time, leading to chromosomal translocations. However, which enzymes participate in this pathway is not quite certain. There are mounting evidences depicting Mre11-Rad50-NBS1, pol β, PARP, PALF and DNA Ligase I or III as some of the players carrying out A-EJ. However, no set rules governing the hierarchy of this mechanism are brought to light. Several of these translocations possess translin recognition motifs. Therefore, one theory could be postulated, wherein, translin might be the early sensory molecule binding to recognition sequences and recruiting the downstream nucleases and ligases.

Several other pathways which are ATM-dependent or MRN-dependent are also highlighted by other groups. Since any physiological mechanism is less likely to be exclusively independent, there is a high probability of cross-talk even among the DSB repair pathways: HR, C-NHEJ, A-EJ, or other pathways involving the core and alternative components. However, this discussion is beyond the scope of this review.

12. Conclusions

Detailed analysis of breakpoint junction consensus sequences suggested that they were not simple and could possess a diverse amount of variations. Translin has been found to bind at translocation break points and proposed to be involved in DNA recombination and repair and in the regulation of telomere length [148]. Surprisingly, AT and GC repeat sequences which had almost no homology with known breakpoint sequences such as ATGCAG and GCCC(A/T)(G/C)(G/C)(A/T) showed a high binding affinity to translin. Translin also binds d(GT)n and (TTAGGG)n overhangs linked to Ds DNA which forms unusual structures such as DNA quadruplexes or that inhibits their binding to the protein unless unwound and the binding domains are accessible per octamer [96]. This leads to a proposition that translin might be involved in the control of recombination at microsatellites and in the maintenance of telomeres which are highly repetitive structures. The binding of translin to oligonucleotides *in vitro* has been demonstrated to increase the extension of telomeres [96]. Amplification of telomerase and increased telomere length is associated with the invasive and metastatic potential of murine and human tumors [149]. Translin transcripts are also at an elevated level in mouse lung adenocarocinoma indicating an early event in carcinogenesis [150].

Other than DNA/RNA regulation, translin might also be considered a responsible factor in one of the benchmark obese phenotypes in mice [151].

13. Future directives

Long-term administration of imipramine, an anti-depressant drug, downregulated translin presumably playing a vital role in the segregation of chromosomes and cytokinesis as well as accelerating cell proliferation [152]. tsnΔ and traxΔ cells were not responsive to several DNA damaging agents indicating that neither protein was required for recovery from DNA damage, dispelling the suggestion that these proteins are evolutionarily conserved due to a fundamental role in the DNA damage response [153]. The finding that trax and translin seem to regulate cell proliferation in higher eukaryotes, but not in *S. pombe*, where the biochemical function is conserved, indicates that there is not a clear correlation between the conserved biochemical function and regulation of cell proliferation, suggesting that the two are not linked. Further analysis in this simple eukaryote will provide insight into the nature of this process.

Trax harbors a nuclear localization signal and interacts with translin to transport it to the nucleus when required. Once in the nucleus, translin–trax can interact with DNA to carry out the repair function along with several other co-factors. Thereafter, trax dissociates from the complex, exchanging translin for C1D, and freeing translin to interact with mRNAs marked for export from the nucleus via translin's nuclear export signal [60, 86]. Once translin has re-entered the cytoplasm, it can remain bound to the mRNA until a cellular signal for release and subsequent translation of the message has been received (Figure 3). The ability to act as a shuttling protein is a hallmark of the RNA-binding proteins that traffic mRNAs in neuronal cells [154]. Based on studies of translin-trax involved in dendritic targeting of BDNF mRNA, it is conceivable that heteromeric translin/trax complexes mediate dendritic trafficking of mRNAs, but that its nuclease activity is suppressed during mRNA transport [155] and activated when functioning as components of RISC complex. Accordingly, it will be of interest in future studies to test these models of translin's dual role in mRNA transport and silencing.

The influence of translin on proliferation, DNA repair, chromosome segregation and cytokinesis, RNA stability and transport, and translation of proteins as well as telomere elongation may be critical in tumor formation and progression.

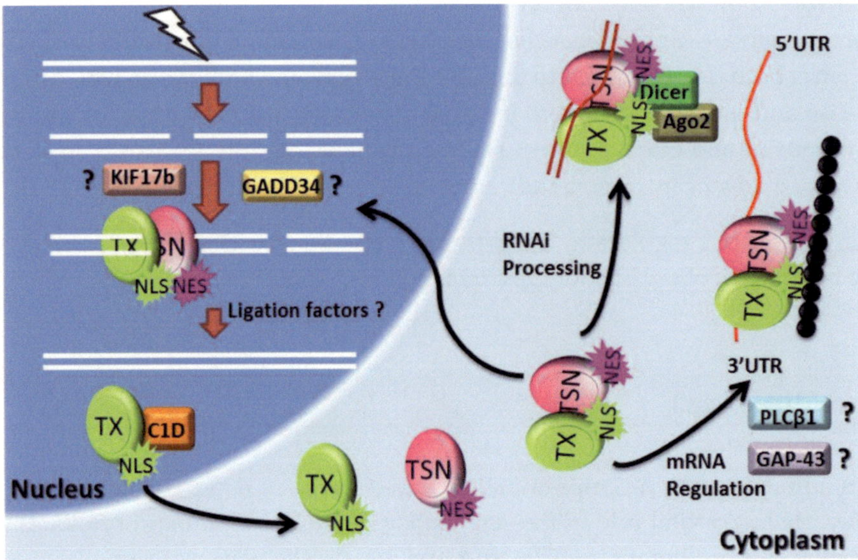

Figure 3. Proposed model for shuttling mechanism of Translin-Trax complex

Acknowledgements

I would like to thank the Journal of Acta Crystallographica Section D, Biological Crystallography and Dr. Masataka Kasai, for granting me permission to reproduce the crystal structure of Translin, in order to better emphasize the significance of the oligomeric state. RPK is also greatly appreciative of Dr. Vinay Kumar and his group, BARC, India, for consenting to the re-use of the crystal structure of the *Drosophila* mutant translin and its oligomeric status from his publication, Gupta et. al., (2008) FEBS Journal. I would also like to thank Dr. Sunil Saroj, Emory University, USA, for his kind help in graphic designing of the model.

Author details

Radhika Pankaj Kamdar[1] and Basuthkar J. Rao[2]

1 Department of Human Genetics, Emory University School of Medicine, Atlanta, Georgia, USA

2 Department of Biological Sciences, Tata Institute of Fundamental Research, Mumbai, Maharashtra, India

References

[1] Biesecker LG. The end of the beginning of chromosome ends. American journal of medical genetics. 2002;107(4):263-6.

[2] Vilenchik MM, Knudson AG, Jr. Inverse radiation dose-rate effects on somatic and germ-line mutations and DNA damage rates. Proceedings of the National Academy of Sciences of the United States of America. 2000;97(10):5381-6.

[3] Bressan DA, Baxter BK, Petrini JH. The Mre11-Rad50-Xrs2 protein complex facilitates homologous recombination-based double-strand break repair in Saccharomyces cerevisiae. Molecular and cellular biology. 1999;19(11):7681-7.

[4] Hefferin ML, Tomkinson AE. Mechanism of DNA double-strand break repair by non-homologous end joining. DNA repair. 2005;4(6):639-48.

[5] McVey M, Lee SE. MMEJ repair of double-strand breaks (director's cut): deleted sequences and alternative endings. Trends in genetics : TIG. 2008;24(11):529-38.

[6] Kamdar RP. DNA double strand break repair through non-homologus end-joining : Recruitment and assembly of the players. In: Inna kruman (ed.) DNA Repair. Intech; 2011. P477-502.

[7] Kasai M, Maziarz RT, Aoki K, Macintyre E, Strominger JL. Molecular involvement of the pvt-1 locus in a gamma/delta T-cell leukemia bearing a variant t(8;14)(q24;q11) translocation. Molecular and cellular biology. 1992;12(10):4751-7.

[8] Kasai M, Aoki K, Matsuo Y, Minowada J, Maziarz RT, Strominger JL. Recombination hotspot associated factors specifically recognize novel target sequences at the site of interchromosomal rearrangements in T-ALL patients with t(8;14)(q24;q11) and t(1;14)(p32;q11). International immunology. 1994;6(7):1017-25.

[9] Aoki K, Nakahara K, Ikegawa C, Seto M, Takahashi T, Minowada J, et al. Nuclear proteins binding to a novel target sequence within the recombination hotspot regions of Bcl-2 and the immunoglobulin DH gene family. Oncogene. 1994;9(4):1109-15.

[10] Aoki K, Suzuki K, Sugano T, Tasaka T, Nakahara K, Kuge O, et al. A novel gene, Translin, encodes a recombination hotspot binding protein associated with chromosomal translocations. Nature genetics. 1995;10(2):167-74.

[11] Landschulz WH, Johnson PF, McKnight SL. The leucine zipper: a hypothetical structure common to a new class of DNA binding proteins. Science. 1988;240(4860):1759-64.

[12] Aoki K, Inazawa J, Takahashi T, Nakahara K, Kasai M. Genomic structure and chromosomal localization of the gene encoding translin, a recombination hotspot binding protein. Genomics. 1997;43(2):237-41.

[13] Aoki K, Suzuki K, Ishida R, Kasai M. The DNA binding activity of Translin is mediated by a basic region in the ring-shaped structure conserved in evolution. FEBS letters. 1999;443(3):363-6.

[14] Kwon YK, Hecht NB. Binding of a phosphoprotein to the 3' untranslated region of the mouse protamine 2 mRNA temporally represses its translation. Molecular and cellular biology. 1993;13(10):6547-57.

[15] Han MK, Lin P, Paek D, Harvey JJ, Fuior E, Knutson JR. Fluorescence studies of pyrene maleimide-labeled translin: excimer fluorescence indicates subunits associate in a tail-to-tail configuration to form octamer. Biochemistry. 2002;41(10):3468-76.

[16] Wu XQ, Xu L, Hecht NB. Dimerization of the testis brain RNA-binding protein (translin) is mediated through its C-terminus and is required for DNA- and RNA-binding. Nucleic acids research. 1998;26(7):1675-80.

[17] Wu XQ, Gu W, Meng X, Hecht NB. The RNA-binding protein, TB-RBP, is the mouse homologue of translin, a recombination protein associated with chromosomal translocations. Proceedings of the National Academy of Sciences of the United States of America. 1997;94(11):5640-5.

[18] Suseendranathan K, Sengupta K, Rikhy R, D'Souza JS, Kokkanti M, Kulkarni MG, et al. Expression pattern of Drosophila translin and behavioral analyses of the mutant. European journal of cell biology. 2007;86(3):173-86.

[19] Laufman O, Ben Yosef R, Adir N, Manor H. Cloning and characterization of the Schizosaccharomyces pombe homologs of the human protein Translin and the Translin-associated protein TRAX. Nucleic acids research. 2005;33(13):4128-39.

[20] Castro A, Peter M, Magnaghi-Jaulin L, Vigneron S, Loyaux D, Lorca T, et al. Part of Xenopus translin is localized in the centrosomes during mitosis. Biochemical and biophysical research communications. 2000;276(2):515-23.

[21] Lu J, Zheng J, Liu H, Li J, Chen H, Chen K. Protein profiling analysis of skeletal muscle of a pufferfish, Takifugu rubripes. Molecular biology reports. 2010;37(5):2141-7.

[22] VanLoock MS, Yu X, Kasai M, Egelman EH. Electron microscopic studies of the translin octameric ring. Journal of structural biology. 2001;135(1):58-66.

[23] Lee SP, Fuior E, Lewis MS, Han MK. Analytical ultracentrifugation studies of translin: analysis of protein-DNA interactions using a single-stranded fluorogenic oligonucleotide. Biochemistry. 2001;40(46):14081-8.

[24] Sugiura I, Sasaki C, Hasegawa T, Kohno T, Sugio S, Moriyama H, et al. Structure of human translin at 2.2 A resolution. Acta crystallographica Section D, Biological crystallography. 2004;60(Pt 4):674-9.

[25] Pascal JM, Chennathukuzhi VM, Hecht NB, Robertus JD. Mouse testis-brain RNA-binding protein (TB-RBP): expression, purification and crystal X-ray diffraction. Acta crystallographica Section D, Biological crystallography. 2001;57(Pt 11):1692-4.

[26] Gupta GD, Makde RD, Rao BJ, Kumar V. Crystal structures of Drosophila mutant translin and characterization of translin variants reveal the structural plasticity of translin proteins. The FEBS journal. 2008;275(16):4235-49.

[27] Takai Y, Sasaki T, Matozaki T. Small GTP-binding proteins. Physiological reviews. 2001;81(1):153-208.

[28] Chennathukuzhi VM, Kurihara Y, Bray JD, Yang J, Hecht NB. Altering the GTP binding site of the DNA/RNA-binding protein, Translin/TB-RBP, decreases RNA binding and may create a dominant negative phenotype. Nucleic acids research. 2001;29(21): 4433-40.

[29] Sengupta K, Kamdar RP, D'Souza JS, Mustafi SM, Rao BJ. GTP-induced conformational changes in translin: a comparison between human and Drosophila proteins. Biochemistry. 2006;45(3):861-70.

[30] Gu W, Wu XQ, Meng XH, Morales C, el-Alfy M, Hecht NB. The RNA- and DNA-binding protein TB-RBP is spatially and developmentally regulated during spermatogenesis. Molecular reproduction and development. 1998;49(3):219-28.

[31] Finkenstadt PM, Kang WS, Jeon M, Taira E, Tang W, Baraban JM. Somatodendritic localization of Translin, a component of the Translin/Trax RNA binding complex. Journal of neurochemistry. 2000;75(4):1754-62.

[32] Claussen M, Koch R, Jin ZY, Suter B. Functional characterization of Drosophila Translin and Trax. Genetics. 2006;174(3):1337-47.

[33] Aoki K, Ishida R, Kasai M. Isolation and characterization of a cDNA encoding a Translin-like protein, TRAX. FEBS letters. 1997;401(2-3):109-12.

[34] Meng G, Aoki K, Tokura K, Nakahara K, Inazawa J, Kasai M. Genomic structure and chromosomal localization of the gene encoding TRAX, a Translin-associated factor X. Journal of human genetics. 2000;45(5):305-8.

[35] Devon RS, Taylor MS, Millar JK, Porteous DJ. Isolation and characterization of the mouse translin-associated protein X (Trax) gene. Mammalian genome : official journal of the International Mammalian Genome Society. 2000;11(5):395-8.

[36] Chennathukuzhi VM, Kurihara Y, Bray JD, Hecht NB. Trax (translin-associated factor X), a primarily cytoplasmic protein, inhibits the binding of TB-RBP (translin) to RNA. The Journal of biological chemistry. 2001;276(16):13256-63.

[37] Hasegawa T, Isobe K. Evidence for the interaction between Translin and GADD34 in mammalian cells. Biochimica et biophysica acta. 1999;1428(2-3):161-8.

[38] Wu XQ, Lefrancois S, Morales CR, Hecht NB. Protein-protein interactions between the testis brain RNA-binding protein and the transitional endoplasmic reticulum ATPase, a cytoskeletal gamma actin and Trax in male germ cells and the brain. Biochemistry. 1999;38(35):11261-70.

[39] Wu XQ, Hecht NB. Mouse testis brain ribonucleic acid-binding protein/translin co-localizes with microtubules and is immunoprecipitated with messenger ribonucleic acids encoding myelin basic protein, alpha calmodulin kinase II, and protamines 1 and 2. Biology of reproduction. 2000;62(3):720-5.

[40] Zhang L, Ashendel CL, Becker GW, Morre DJ. Isolation and characterization of the principal ATPase associated with transitional endoplasmic reticulum of rat liver. The Journal of cell biology. 1994;127(6 Pt 2):1871-83. Epub 1994/12/01.

[41] Frixione E. Recurring views on the structure and function of the cytoskeleton: a 300-year epic. Cell motility and the cytoskeleton. 2000;46(2):73-94.

[42] Li K, Wang L, Cheng J, Lu YY, Zhang LX, Mu JS, et al. Interaction between hepatitis C virus core protein and translin protein--a possible molecular mechanism for hepatocellular carcinoma and lymphoma caused by hepatitis C virus. World journal of gastroenterology : WJG. 2003;9(2):300-3.

[43] Kasai M, Matsuzaki T, Katayanagi K, Omori A, Maziarz RT, Strominger JL, et al. The translin ring specifically recognizes DNA ends at recombination hot spots in the human genome. The Journal of biological chemistry. 1997;272(17):11402-7.

[44] Vaulont S, Munnich A, Decaux JF, Kahn A. Transcriptional and post-transcriptional regulation of L-type pyruvate kinase gene expression in rat liver. The Journal of biological chemistry. 1986;261(17):7621-5.

[45] Decaux JF, Antoine B, Kahn A. Regulation of the expression of the L-type pyruvate kinase gene in adult rat hepatocytes in primary culture. The Journal of biological chemistry. 1989;264(20):11584-90.

[46] Hasegawa J, Osatomi K, Wu RF, Uyeda K. A novel factor binding to the glucose response elements of liver pyruvate kinase and fatty acid synthase genes. The Journal of biological chemistry. 1999;274(2):1100-7.

[47] Wu RF, Osatomi K, Terada LS, Uyeda K. Identification of Translin/Trax complex as a glucose response element binding protein in liver. Biochimica et biophysica acta. 2003;1624(1-3):29-35.

[48] Chennathukuzhi V, Morales CR, El-Alfy M, Hecht NB. The kinesin KIF17b and RNA-binding protein TB-RBP transport specific cAMP-responsive element modulator-regulated mRNAs in male germ cells. Proceedings of the National Academy of Sciences of the United States of America. 2003;100(26):15566-71.

[49] Bray JD, Chennathukuzhi VM, Hecht NB. KIF2Abeta: A kinesin family member enriched in mouse male germ cells, interacts with translin associated factor-X (TRAX). Molecular reproduction and development. 2004;69(4):387-96.

[50] Han JR, Gu W, Hecht NB. Testis-brain RNA-binding protein, a testicular translational regulatory RNA-binding protein, is present in the brain and binds to the 3' untranslated regions of transported brain mRNAs. Biology of reproduction. 1995;53(3):707-17.

[51] Han JR, Yiu GK, Hecht NB. Testis/brain RNA-binding protein attaches translationally repressed and transported mRNAs to microtubules. Proceedings of the National Academy of Sciences of the United States of America. 1995;92(21):9550-4.

[52] Yang J, Chennathukuzhi V, Miki K, O'Brien DA, Hecht NB. Mouse testis brain RNA-binding protein/translin selectively binds to the messenger RNA of the fibrous sheath protein glyceraldehyde 3-phosphate dehydrogenase-S and suppresses its translation in vitro. Biology of reproduction. 2003;68(3):853-9.

[53] Chennathukuzhi V, Stein JM, Abel T, Donlon S, Yang S, Miller JP, et al. Mice deficient for testis-brain RNA-binding protein exhibit a coordinate loss of TRAX, reduced fertility, altered gene expression in the brain, and behavioral changes. Molecular and cellular biology. 2003;23(18):6419-34.

[54] Cho YS, Iguchi N, Yang J, Handel MA, Hecht NB. Meiotic messenger RNA and noncoding RNA targets of the RNA-binding protein Translin (TSN) in mouse testis. Biology of reproduction. 2005;73(4):840-7.

[55] Iguchi N, Xu M, Hori T, Hecht NB. Noncoding RNAs of the mammalian testis: the meiotic transcripts Nct1 and Nct2 encode piRNAs. Annals of the New York Academy of Sciences. 2007;1120:84-94.

[56] Gupta GD, Makde RD, Kamdar RP, D'Souza JS, Kulkarni MG, Kumar V, et al. Coexpressed recombinant human Translin-Trax complex binds DNA. FEBS letters. 2005;579(14):3141-6.

[57] Pfutz M, Gileadi O, Werner D. Identification of human satellite DNA sequences associated with chemically resistant nonhistone polypeptide adducts. Chromosoma. 1992;101(10):609-17.

[58] Yavuzer U, Smith GC, Bliss T, Werner D, Jackson SP. DNA end-independent activation of DNA-PK mediated via association with the DNA-binding protein C1D. Genes & development. 1998;12(14):2188-99.

[59] Smith GC, Jackson SP. The DNA-dependent protein kinase. Genes & development. 1999;13(8):916-34.

[60] Erdemir T, Bilican B, Oncel D, Goding CR, Yavuzer U. DNA damage-dependent interaction of the nuclear matrix protein C1D with Translin-associated factor X (TRAX). Journal of cell science. 2002;115(Pt 1):207-16.

[61] Yang S, Cho YS, Chennathukuzhi VM, Underkoffler LA, Loomes K, Hecht NB. Translin-associated factor X is post-transcriptionally regulated by its partner protein TB-RBP, and both are essential for normal cell proliferation. The Journal of biological chemistry. 2004;279(13):12605-14.

[62] Erdemir T, Bilican B, Cagatay T, Goding CR, Yavuzer U. Saccharomyces cerevisiae C1D is implicated in both non-homologous DNA end joining and homologous recombination. Molecular microbiology. 2002;46(4):947-57.

[63] Sabbatini P, Chiou SK, Rao L, White E. Modulation of p53-mediated transcriptional repression and apoptosis by the adenovirus E1B 19K protein. Molecular and cellular biology. 1995;15(2):1060-70.

[64] Armstrong JF, Kaufman MH, Harrison DJ, Clarke AR. High-frequency developmental abnormalities in p53-deficient mice. Current biology : CB. 1995;5(8):931-6.

[65] Daval JL, Nehlig A, Nicolas F. Physiological and pharmacological properties of adenosine: therapeutic implications. Life sciences. 1991;49(20):1435-53.

[66] Sun CN, Cheng HC, Chou JL, Lee SY, Lin YW, Lai HL, et al. Rescue of p53 blockage by the A(2A) adenosine receptor via a novel interacting protein, translin-associated protein X. Molecular pharmacology. 2006;70(2):454-66.

[67] Sun CN, Chuang HC, Wang JY, Chen SY, Cheng YY, Lee CF, et al. The A2A adenosine receptor rescues neuritogenesis impaired by p53 blockage via KIF2A, a kinesin family member. Developmental neurobiology. 2010;70(8):604-21.

[68] Schroer U, Volk GF, Liedtke T, Thanos S. Translin-associated factor-X (Trax) is a molecular switch of growth-associated protein (GAP)-43 that controls axonal regeneration. The European journal of neuroscience. 2007;26(8):2169-78.

[69] Suh PG, Park JI, Manzoli L, Cocco L, Peak JC, Katan M, et al. Multiple roles of phosphoinositide-specific phospholipase C isozymes. BMB reports. 2008;41(6):415-34.

[70] Aisiku OR, Runnels LW, Scarlata S. Identification of a novel binding partner of phospholipase cbeta1: translin-associated factor X. PloS one. 2010;5(11):e15001.

[71] Aisiku O, Dowal L, Scarlata S. Protein kinase C phosphorylation of PLCbeta1 regulates its cellular localization. Archives of biochemistry and biophysics. 2011;509(2): 186-90.

[72] Philip F, Guo Y, Aisiku O, Scarlata S. Phospholipase Cbeta1 is linked to RNA interference of specific genes through translin-associated factor X. FASEB journal : official publication of the Federation of American Societies for Experimental Biology. 2012.

[73] Pascal JM, Hart PJ, Hecht NB, Robertus JD. Crystal structure of TB-RBP, a novel RNA-binding and regulating protein. Journal of molecular biology. 2002;319(5): 1049-57.

[74] Burd CG, Dreyfuss G. Conserved structures and diversity of functions of RNA-binding proteins. Science. 1994;265(5172):615-21.

[75] Hohjoh H, Singer MF. Cytoplasmic ribonucleoprotein complexes containing human LINE-1 protein and RNA. The EMBO journal. 1996;15(3):630-9.

[76] Nakagawa J, Waldner H, Meyer-Monard S, Hofsteenge J, Jeno P, Moroni C. AUH, a gene encoding an AU-specific RNA binding protein with intrinsic enoyl-CoA hydratase activity. Proceedings of the National Academy of Sciences of the United States of America. 1995;92(6):2051-5.

[77] Chu E, Koeller DM, Casey JL, Drake JC, Chabner BA, Elwood PC, et al. Autoregulation of human thymidylate synthase messenger RNA translation by thymidylate synthase. Proceedings of the National Academy of Sciences of the United States of America. 1991;88(20):8977-81.

[78] Klausner RD, Rouault TA, Harford JB. Regulating the fate of mRNA: the control of cellular iron metabolism. Cell. 1993;72(1):19-28.

[79] Sengupta K, Rao BJ. Translin binding to DNA: recruitment through DNA ends and consequent conformational transitions. Biochemistry. 2002;41(51):15315-26.

[80] Tsai CL, Schatz DG. Regulation of RAG1/RAG2-mediated transposition by GTP and the C-terminal region of RAG2. The EMBO journal. 2003;22(8):1922-30.

[81] Gupta GD, Kumar V. Identification of nucleic acid binding sites on translin-associated factor X (TRAX) protein. PloS one. 2012;7(3):e33035.

[82] Neduva V, Linding R, Su-Angrand I, Stark A, de Masi F, Gibson TJ, et al. Systematic discovery of new recognition peptides mediating protein interaction networks. PLoS biology. 2005;3(12):e405.

[83] Ishida R, Okado H, Sato H, Shionoiri C, Aoki K, Kasai M. A role for the octameric ring protein, Translin, in mitotic cell division. FEBS letters. 2002;525(1-3):105-10.

[84] Savitsky K, Bar-Shira A, Gilad S, Rotman G, Ziv Y, Vanagaite L, et al. A single ataxia telangiectasia gene with a product similar to PI-3 kinase. Science. 1995;268(5218): 1749-53.

[85] Taylor AM, Byrd PJ, McConville CM, Thacker S. Genetic and cellular features of ataxia telangiectasia. International journal of radiation biology. 1994;65(1):65-70.

[86] Yang S, Hecht NB. Translin associated protein X is essential for cellular proliferation. FEBS letters. 2004;576(1-2):221-5.

[87] Kobayashi S, Takashima A, Anzai K. The dendritic translocation of translin protein in the form of BC1 RNA protein particles in developing rat hippocampal neurons in primary culture. Biochemical and biophysical research communications. 1998;253(2): 448-53.

[88] Taira E, Finkenstadt PM, Baraban JM. Identification of translin and trax as components of the GS1 strand-specific DNA binding complex enriched in brain. Journal of neurochemistry. 1998;71(2):471-7.

[89] Finkenstadt PM, Jeon M, Baraban JM. Masking of the Translin/Trax complex by endogenous RNA. FEBS letters. 2001;498(1):6-10.

[90] Li Z, Wu Y, Baraban JM. The Translin/Trax RNA binding complex: clues to function in the nervous system. Biochimica et biophysica acta. 2008;1779(8):479-85.

[91] Muramatsu T, Ohmae A, Anzai K. BC1 RNA protein particles in mouse brain contain two y-,h-element-binding proteins, translin and a 37 kDa protein. Biochemical and biophysical research communications. 1998;247(1):7-11.

[92] Chang CF, Gallia GL, Muralidharan V, Chen NN, Zoltick P, Johnson E, et al. Evidence that replication of human neurotropic JC virus DNA in glial cells is regulated by the sequence-specific single-stranded DNA-binding protein Pur alpha. Journal of virology. 1996;70(6):4150-6.

[93] Du Q, Tomkinson AE, Gardner PD. Transcriptional regulation of neuronal nicotinic acetylcholine receptor genes. A possible role for the DNA-binding protein Puralpha. The Journal of biological chemistry. 1997;272(23):14990-5.

[94] Ohashi S, Kobayashi S, Omori A, Ohara S, Omae A, Muramatsu T, et al. The single-stranded DNA- and RNA-binding proteins pur alpha and pur beta link BC1 RNA to microtubules through binding to the dendrite-targeting RNA motifs. Journal of neurochemistry. 2000;75(5):1781-90.

[95] Li Z, Baraban JM. High affinity binding of the Translin/Trax complex to RNA does not require the presence of Y or H elements. Brain research Molecular brain research. 2004;120(2):123-9.

[96] Cohen S, Jacob E, Manor H. Effects of single-stranded DNA binding proteins on primer extension by telomerase. Biochimica et biophysica acta. 2004;1679(2):129-40.

[97] Soule J, Messaoudi E, Bramham CR. Brain-derived neurotrophic factor and control of synaptic consolidation in the adult brain. Biochemical Society transactions. 2006;34(Pt 4):600-4.

[98] Chiaruttini C, Vicario A, Li Z, Baj G, Braiuca P, Wu Y, et al. Dendritic trafficking of BDNF mRNA is mediated by translin and blocked by the G196A (Val66Met) mutation. Proceedings of the National Academy of Sciences of the United States of America. 2009;106(38):16481-6.

[99] Wu XQ, Petrusz P, Hecht NB. Testis-brain RNA-binding protein (Translin) is primarily expressed in neurons of the mouse brain. Brain research. 1999;819(1-2):174-8.

[100] Tamanini F, Willemsen R, van Unen L, Bontekoe C, Galjaard H, Oostra BA, et al. Differential expression of FMR1, FXR1 and FXR2 proteins in human brain and testis. Human molecular genetics. 1997;6(8):1315-22.

[101] Mellon SH, Bair SR, Depoix C, Vigne JL, Hecht NB, Brake PB. Translin coactivates steroidogenic factor-1-stimulated transcription. Molecular endocrinology. 2007;21(1): 89-105.

[102] Hannon GJ. RNA interference. Nature. 2002;418(6894):244-51.

[103] Song JJ, Liu J, Tolia NH, Schneiderman J, Smith SK, Martienssen RA, et al. The crystal structure of the Argonaute2 PAZ domain reveals an RNA binding motif in RNAi effector complexes. Nature structural biology. 2003;10(12):1026-32.

[104] Hammond SM, Boettcher S, Caudy AA, Kobayashi R, Hannon GJ. Argonaute2, a link between genetic and biochemical analyses of RNAi. Science. 2001;293(5532):1146-50.

[105] Wang J, Boja ES, Oubrahim H, Chock PB. Testis brain ribonucleic acid-binding protein/translin possesses both single-stranded and double-stranded ribonuclease activities. Biochemistry. 2004;43(42):13424-31.

[106] Liu Y, Ye X, Jiang F, Liang C, Chen D, Peng J, et al. C3PO, an endoribonuclease that promotes RNAi by facilitating RISC activation. Science. 2009;325(5941):750-3.

[107] Ye X, Huang N, Liu Y, Paroo Z, Huerta C, Li P, et al. Structure of C3PO and mechanism of human RISC activation. Nature structural & molecular biology. 2011;18(6): 650-7.

[108] Tian Y, Simanshu DK, Ascano M, Diaz-Avalos R, Park AY, Juranek SA, et al. Multimeric assembly and biochemical characterization of the Trax-translin endonuclease complex. Nature structural & molecular biology. 2011;18(6):658-64.

[109] Swevers L, Liu J, Huvenne H, Smagghe G. Search for limiting factors in the RNAi pathway in silkmoth tissues and the Bm5 cell line: the RNA-binding proteins R2D2 and Translin. PloS one. 2011;6(5):e20250.

[110] Li L, Gu W, Liang C, Liu Q, Mello CC, Liu Y. The translin-TRAX complex (C3PO) is a ribonuclease in tRNA processing. Nature structural & molecular biology. 2012;19(8): 824-30.

[111] Cho YS, Chennathukuzhi VM, Handel MA, Eppig J, Hecht NB. The relative levels of translin-associated factor X (TRAX) and testis brain RNA-binding protein determine their nucleocytoplasmic distribution in male germ cells. The Journal of biological chemistry. 2004;279(30):31514-23.

[112] Weinert T. DNA damage and checkpoint pathways: molecular anatomy and interactions with repair. Cell. 1998;94(5):555-8.

[113] Fukuda Y, Ishida R, Aoki K, Nakahara K, Takashi T, Mochida K, et al. Contribution of Translin to hematopoietic regeneration after sublethal ionizing irradiation. Biological & pharmaceutical bulletin. 2008;31(2):207-11.

[114] Spangrude GJ, Heimfeld S, Weissman IL. Purification and characterization of mouse hematopoietic stem cells. Science. 1988;241(4861):58-62.

[115] Ishida R, Aoki K, Nakahara K, Fukuda Y, Ohori M, Saito Y, Kano K, Matsuda J, Asano S, Maziarz RT, Kasai M. Translin/TRAX Deficiency Affects Mesenchymal Differentiation Programs and Induces Bone Marrow Failure. In: R.K. Srivastava and S. Shankar (eds.), Stem Cells and Human Diseases. Springer Link; 2012. 467. DOI 10.1007/978-94-007-2801-1_21

[116] Xu C, Bian C, Lam R, Dong A, Min J. The structural basis for selective binding of non-methylated CpG islands by the CFP1 CXXC domain. Nature communications. 2011;2:227.

[117] Chuzhanova N, Chen JM, Bacolla A, Patrinos GP, Ferec C, Wells RD, et al. Gene conversion causing human inherited disease: evidence for involvement of non-B-DNA-forming sequences and recombination-promoting motifs in DNA breakage and repair. Human mutation. 2009;30(8):1189-98.

[118] Nishio H, Takeshima Y, Narita N, Yanagawa H, Suzuki Y, Ishikawa Y, et al. Identification of a novel first exon in the human dystrophin gene and of a new promoter located more than 500 kb upstream of the nearest known promoter. The Journal of clinical investigation. 1994;94(3):1037-42.

[119] Sironi M, Pozzoli U, Cagliani R, Giorda R, Comi GP, Bardoni A, et al. Relevance of sequence and structure elements for deletion events in the dystrophin gene major hot-spot. Human genetics. 2003;112(3):272-88.

[120] Cole TR, Hughes HE. Sotos syndrome: a study of the diagnostic criteria and natural history. Journal of medical genetics. 1994;31(1):20-32.

[121] Visser R, Shimokawa O, Harada N, Kinoshita A, Ohta T, Niikawa N, et al. Identification of a 3.0-kb major recombination hotspot in patients with Sotos syndrome who carry a common 1.9-Mb microdeletion. American journal of human genetics. 2005;76(1):52-67.

[122] Dobkin C, Rabe A, Dumas R, El Idrissi A, Haubenstock H, Brown WT. Fmr1 knockout mouse has a distinctive strain-specific learning impairment. Neuroscience. 2000;100(2):423-9.

[123] Stein JM, Bergman W, Fang Y, Davison L, Brensinger C, Robinson MB, et al. Behavioral and neurochemical alterations in mice lacking the RNA-binding protein translin. The Journal of neuroscience : the official journal of the Society for Neuroscience. 2006;26(8):2184-96.

[124] Blackwood DH, Muir WJ. Clinical phenotypes associated with DISC1, a candidate gene for schizophrenia. Neurotoxicity research. 2004;6(1):35-41.

[125] Hennah W, Tuulio-Henriksson A, Paunio T, Ekelund J, Varilo T, Partonen T, et al. A haplotype within the DISC1 gene is associated with visual memory functions in families with a high density of schizophrenia. Molecular psychiatry. 2005;10(12): 1097-103.

[126] Cannon TD, Hennah W, van Erp TG, Thompson PM, Lonnqvist J, Huttunen M, et al. Association of DISC1/TRAX haplotypes with schizophrenia, reduced prefrontal gray matter, and impaired short- and long-term memory. Archives of general psychiatry. 2005;62(11):1205-13.

[127] Douglass EC, Valentine M, Etcubanas E, Parham D, Webber BL, Houghton PJ, et al. A specific chromosomal abnormality in rhabdomyosarcoma. Cytogenetics and cell genetics. 1987;45(3-4):148-55.

[128] Chalk JG, Barr FG, Mitchell CD. Translin recognition site sequences flank chromosome translocation breakpoints in alveolar rhabdomyosarcoma cell lines. Oncogene. 1997;15(10):1199-205.

[129] Kanoe H, Nakayama T, Hosaka T, Murakami H, Yamamoto H, Nakashima Y, et al. Characteristics of genomic breakpoints in TLS-CHOP translocations in liposarcomas suggest the involvement of Translin and topoisomerase II in the process of translocation. Oncogene. 1999;18(3):721-9.

[130] Gubin AN, Njoroge JM, Bouffard GG, Miller JL. Gene expression in proliferating human erythroid cells. Genomics. 1999;59(2):168-77.

[131] Wei Y, Sun M, Wang J, Hou Y, Zhu X. (Sequence analysis of translocation t (X; 18) genomic breakpoints characterized in synovial sarcoma). Zhonghua bing li xue za zhi Chinese journal of pathology. 2002;31(5):411-5.

[132] Fitzgerald PH, Morris CM. Complex chromosomal translocations in the Philadelphia chromosome leukemias. Serial translocations or a concerted genomic rearrangement? Cancer genetics and cytogenetics. 1991;57(2):143-51.

[133] Atlas M, Head D, Behm F, Schmidt E, Zeleznik-Le NH, Roe BA, et al. Cloning and sequence analysis of four t(9;11) therapy-related leukemia breakpoints. Leukemia : official journal of the Leukemia Society of America, Leukemia Research Fund, UK. 1998;12(12):1895-902.

[134] Jeffs AR, Benjes SM, Smith TL, Sowerby SJ, Morris CM. The BCR gene recombines preferentially with Alu elements in complex BCR-ABL translocations of chronic myeloid leukaemia. Human molecular genetics. 1998;7(5):767-76.

[135] Korsmeyer SJ. Chromosomal translocations in lymphoid malignancies reveal novel proto-oncogenes. Annual review of immunology. 1992;10:785-807.

[136] Ying-Tao Z, Yi-Ping G, Lu-Sheng S, Yi-Li W. Proteomic analysis of differentially expressed proteins between metastatic and non-metastatic human colorectal carcinoma cell lines. European journal of gastroenterology & hepatology. 2005;17(7):725-32.

[137] Ulbright TM. Germ cell tumors of the gonads: a selective review emphasizing problems in differential diagnosis, newly appreciated, and controversial issues. Modern pathology : an official journal of the United States and Canadian Academy of Pathology, Inc. 2005;18 Suppl 2:S61-79.

[138] Gimelli S, Beri S, Drabkin HA, Gambini C, Gregorio A, Fiorio P, et al. The tumor suppressor gene TRC8/RNF139 is disrupted by a constitutional balanced translocation t(8;22)(q24.13;q11.21) in a young girl with dysgerminoma. Molecular cancer. 2009;8:52.

[139] Shaw CJ, Lupski JR. Implications of human genome architecture for rearrangement-based disorders: the genomic basis of disease. Human molecular genetics. 2004;13 Spec No 1:R57-64.

[140] Gajecka M, Pavlicek A, Glotzbach CD, Ballif BC, Jarmuz M, Jurka J, et al. Identification of sequence motifs at the breakpoint junctions in three t(1;9)(p36.3;q34) and delineation of mechanisms involved in generating balanced translocations. Human genetics. 2006;120(4):519-26.

[141] Gajecka M, Glotzbach CD, Shaffer LG. Characterization of a complex rearrangement with interstitial deletions and inversion on human chromosome 1. Chromosome research : an international journal on the molecular, supramolecular and evolutionary aspects of chromosome biology. 2006;14(3):277-82.

[142] Kamdar RP, Matsumoto Y. Radiation-induced XRCC4 association with chromatin DNA analyzed by biochemical fractionation. Journal of radiation research. 2010;51(3):303-13.

[143] Nevaldine B, Longo JA, Hahn PJ. The scid defect results in much slower repair of DNA double-strand breaks but not high levels of residual breaks. Radiation research. 1997;147(5):535-40.

[144] Wang H, Perrault AR, Takeda Y, Qin W, Iliakis G. Biochemical evidence for Ku-independent backup pathways of NHEJ. Nucleic acids research. 2003;31(18):5377-88.

[145] Boboila C, Jankovic M, Yan CT, Wang JH, Wesemann DR, Zhang T, et al. Alternative end-joining catalyzes robust IgH locus deletions and translocations in the combined absence of ligase 4 and Ku70. Proceedings of the National Academy of Sciences of the United States of America. 2010;107(7):3034-9.

[146] Simsek D, Jasin M. Alternative end-joining is suppressed by the canonical NHEJ component Xrcc4-ligase IV during chromosomal translocation formation. Nature structural & molecular biology. 2010;17(4):410-6.

[147] Lieber MR. NHEJ and its backup pathways in chromosomal translocations. Nature structural & molecular biology. 2010;17(4):393-5.

[148] Jacob E, Pucshansky L, Zeruya E, Baran N, Manor H. The human protein translin specifically binds single-stranded microsatellite repeats, d(GT)n, and G-strand telomeric repeats, d(TTAGGG)n: a study of the binding parameters. Journal of molecular biology. 2004;344(4):939-50.

[149] Multani AS, Ozen M, Sen S, Mandal AK, Price JE, Fan D, et al. Amplification of telomeric DNA directly correlates with metastatic potential of human and murine cancers of various histological origin. International journal of oncology. 1999;15(3):423-9.

[150] Sargent LM, Ensell MX, Ostvold AC, Baldwin KT, Kashon ML, Lowry DT, et al. Chromosomal changes in high- and low-invasive mouse lung adenocarcinoma cell strains derived from early passage mouse lung adenocarcinoma cell strains. Toxicology and applied pharmacology. 2008;233(1):81-91.

[151] Brommage R, Desai U, Revelli JP, Donoviel DB, Fontenot GK, Dacosta CM, et al. High-throughput screening of mouse knockout lines identifies true lean and obese phenotypes. Obesity. 2008;16(10):2362-7.

[152] Palotas M, Palotas A, Puskas LG, Kitajka K, Pakaski M, Janka Z, et al. Gene expression profile analysis of the rat cortex following treatment with imipramine and citalopram. The international journal of neuropsychopharmacology / official scientific journal of the Collegium Internationale Neuropsychopharmacologicum. 2004;7(4): 401-13.

[153] Jaendling A, Ramayah S, Pryce DW, McFarlane RJ. Functional characterisation of the Schizosaccharomyces pombe homologue of the leukaemia-associated translocation breakpoint binding protein translin and its binding partner, TRAX. Biochimica et biophysica acta. 2008;1783(2):203-13.

[154] Besse F, Ephrussi A. Translational control of localized mRNAs: restricting protein synthesis in space and time. Nature reviews Molecular cell biology. 2008;9(12): 971-80.

[155] Wu YC, Williamson R, Li Z, Vicario A, Xu J, Kasai M, et al. Dendritic trafficking of brain-derived neurotrophic factor mRNA: regulation by translin-dependent and -independent mechanisms. Journal of neurochemistry. 2011;116(6):1112-21.

Chapter 2

The Role of Multimerization During Non-Homologous End Joining

Michelle Rubin, Jonathan Newsome and
Albert Ribes-Zamora

Additional information is available at the end of the chapter

http://dx.doi.org/10.5772/53982

1. Introduction

In order to sustain life, cells must protect their genetic information from the constant threat posed by mutagenic agents such as ultraviolet light, irradiation or reactive oxygen species, as well as from mistakes introduced during the replication of their genomes [1]. To deal with this problem, natural selection has favored a system that repairs the damage caused by these DNA lesions while allowing the highly infrequent but steady production of mutations that constitute the source for adaptive changes during evolution. To repair damaged DNA, cells have developed a myriad of highly specialized pathways that recognize and repair specific types of injuries produced by specific types of mutagenic events [2, 3]. For instance, while base excision repair detects and repairs chemically damaged nucleotide bases typically produced by oxygen radicals or alkylating agents, nucleotide excision repair is responsible for the removal of thymine dimers caused by ultraviolet light exposure. Additionally, the mismatch repair pathway specializes in fixing errors introduced during DNA replication. More globally, these pathways are part of the DNA damage response (DDR), a signal transduction cascade coordinated by the ATM/ATR kinases in mammalian cells that halts cell cycle progression while DNA is being repaired, and it can trigger apoptosis when the damage is deemed non-repairable [4]. The importance of these pathways is underlined by their high conservation, both in prokaryotes and eukaryotes, and it is emphasized by the role that they play in disease when impaired. Malfunctioning DNA repair pathways are associated with several disorders such as Xeroderma pigmentosum or Nijmegen syndrome as well as with increased cancer risk, as they boost the formation of spontaneous mutations that can lead to tumorigenesis [5].

For any type of cell, one of the more toxic DNA injuries is the double-strand break (DSB). This form of lesion can arise as a consequence of mechanical stress, exposure to irradiation or as a result of a replication fork encountering a single-strand nick [6]. DSBs can induce translocations, aneuploidy and global genome instability that can ultimately render cells either unviable or tumorigenic [5]. To repair a DSB, mammalian cells can take advantage of the presence of homologous chromosomal copies and use homologous recombination (HR) to faithfully amend the break [7]. In the cell cycle phases where identical chromosomal copies are not available, the preferred repair pathway is non-homologous end joining (NHEJ) which seams the two ends of the break with mostly minimal alteration of the DNA sequence [1, 8-10]. NHEJ requires the completion of three major steps: (1) protection and synapsis of both DNA ends, (2) processing of the DNA termini and (3) the final ligation of the ends [9, 10]. The DNA-PK complex, formed by the Ku heterodimer and DNA-PKcs, is responsible for the initial protection and synapses of the ends and recruits other NHEJ factors to the DSB. These factors include the nuclease Artemis and polymerases Polμ and Polλ that will remove and add nucleotides to replace possible damaged bases generated during the breaking process. The final ligation step is performed by DNA ligase IV (LigIV), whose recruitment to DSBs depends on its close association with XRCC4, a process aided by XLF. The regulation of these steps is still not clear but it is known that DNA-PKcs phosphorylates several NHEJ factors and can induce its own removal from DSBs, and that ubiquitination also plays a role in disassembling complexes once the damage has been repaired [11-14]. Furthermore, ATM can phosphorylate NHEJ factors, although their role during NHEJ remains to be elucidated [15].

During evolution, the end protection properties of some NHEJ factors were recycled into protecting the natural ends of chromosomes. How telomeres manage to harbor NHEJ factors to protect their ends while preventing them from triggering end-to-end fusions is still an open question [16]. Later on, NHEJ was again recycled into joining physiologically programmed DSBs that occur during V(D)J recombination and class switch recombination (CSR) in B- and T- lymphocytes. These pathways ensure antigen-binding diversity in antibodies as well as the presence of different antibody isotypes capable of binding different downstream effectors. Consistent with a role of NHEJ in these pathways, mutations in several NHEJ factors are associated with diseases in which the immune system is compromised. For instance, mutations in XLF, DNA-PKcs and Artemis are present in patients suffering from severe combined immunodeficiency or SCID [17].

2. Multimerization of NHEJ factors

For the last two decades, research in NHEJ has mostly focused on the identification of genes involved in this pathway and the dissection of their enzymatic activities [9]. The structures of most NHEJ factors have been solved and this is starting to unravel how NHEJ is regulated throughout the cell cycle [18]. Despite these advances, we are still lacking a clear model of how all these factors assemble at DSBs and whether different complexes form depending on the type of damage, the location of the break or the cell cycle phase when the injury occurs [10]. One of the emerging themes in the field is the assembly of NHEJ factors as multimers at DSB. This multimerization has been reported for several NHEJ proteins and occurs with varying degrees of complexity. The simplest form of multimerization is seen with DNA-PKcs, where monomers bound to opposing ends of a DSB can dimerize and effectively synapse the DNA break [19]. Similarly, two Ku heterodimers are capable of forming a heterotetramer that can tether the ends of a DSB. More intricate multimerization can be observed in the MRN heterotrimer, a complex composed of Mre11, Rad50 and Nbs1 that can form either heterohexamers, where two molecules of each subunit combine into a larger structure, or multimers of four MRN complexes at DSBs [20]. Most recently, a complex multimerization of NHEJ proteins has been observed in the form of long filaments created by the polymerization of multiple alternating copies of XLF and XRCC4 homodimers [21-23]. Combined, this data suggests that formation of multimers is a constant theme in the assembly of NHEJ proteins at DSBs. Below we review current literature on this topic, identifying questions that remain to be answered while laying out possible new research directions. While NHEJ can be divided into classical NHEJ (c-NHEJ) or alternative NHEJ (a-NHEJ) depending on the factors required for completion, here we focus on c-NHEJ and will refer to it as NHEJ.

2.1. The Ku heterodimer

Once a break forms, one of the first responders is the Ku heterodimer, an abundant protein (~400,000 molecules per cell) formed by the Ku70 and Ku80 subunits [24]. Ku is an obligate dimer as in the absence of one subunit the other subunit disappears from cell extracts, presumably due to lack of proper folding [25, 26]. Despite showing low sequence similarities, both Ku70 and Ku80 contain nearly identical domains and have very similar secondary and tertiary structures. Both subunits share a vonWillebrand domain (vWA, also referred to as the a/b domain) in their N-termini followed by a central dimerization domain that can also bind DNA [27]. The only divergence between both subunits is the presence of a C-terminus SAP domain (SAF-A/B, Acinus and PIAS) exclusively in Ku70, which is replaced in KU80 by a domain that is involved in recruiting DNA-PKcs to DSBs [24, 27, 28].

The structure of Ku shows a quasi-symmetrical configuration with both central domains dimerizing and forming a DNA binding ring flanked by the two vWA domains on opposite sides of the ring [27]. This creates a toroidal structure with a basket-like shape that can thread onto DNA (Figure 1A). Ku binds duplex DNA ends with great affinity (Kd~10^{-9} M) and in a sequence independent manner, hence its role as the first DSB recognition factor [29-31]. Ku needs at least 14bp to bind DNA and since the DNA binding ring is preformed, Ku requires a free end to associate with DNA [27]. Consistent with this, the affinity of Ku to circular DNA is orders of magnitude lower compared with linear DNA [32]. Similarly, Ku's affinity to single-stranded DNA (ssDNA) is lower than to double-stranded DNA (dsDNA), which presumably favors HR over NHEJ once resection of ends becomes too extensive to hold Ku [7].

Resolution of the X-ray structure of DNA bound Ku indicated that binding occurs with a preferred orientation that places the Ku70 vWA domain closest to the end and the Ku80 vWA furthest from the end [27]. In the budding yeast *S. cerevisae*, mutations in α-helix5 ($\alpha5$), the most outer structure in the vWA domain had opposite effects in each subunit [33]. Whereas Yku80-a5 mutations disrupt Ku's telomeric silencing function without perturbing DNA repair abilities, mutations in Yku70-$\alpha5$ impair NHEJ while preserving Ku's telomeric functions [33]. This suggests that Ku is spatially organized in two faces with distinct roles in NHEJ and telomeric functions, a hypothesis termed the two-face model. In essence, this model states that the inward face, composed mostly of the Ku80 vWA and Ku70 C-terminal domain (CTD), is oriented towards internal tracks of DNA and has telomeric roles. In contrast, the outward face of Ku is the closest to the DNA end and its main role is to engage the nearby DNA end in NHEJ. Consistent with this, mutations in both the Ku70 vWA domain and the Ku80 CTD, the two major components of the outer face, impair NHEJ [33, 34]. The most recent discovery that mutations in human Ku70-$\alpha5$ also diminish NHEJ suggests that the two-face model may also be conserved in mammalian cells [35].

A

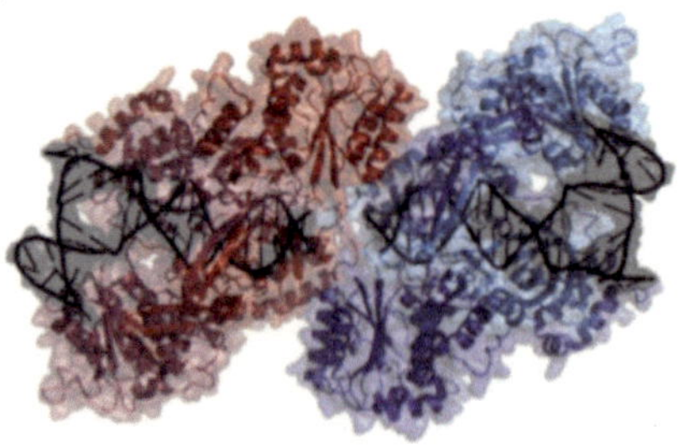

B

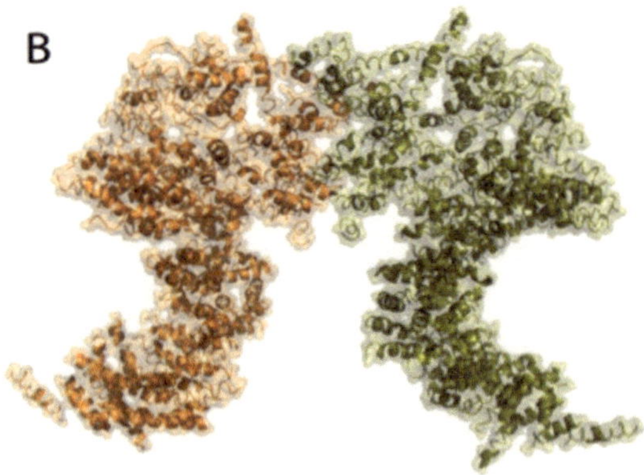

Figure 1. Molecular modeling of Ku and DNA-PKcs dimerization. A Possible Ku tetramer formation through outward face interactions. Each Ku dimer is represented in red and blue, whereas DNA is depicted as black line (Adapted from 1JEY). B Possible Head-to-Head mediated dimerization of two DNA-PKcs molecules (Adapted from 3KGV).

Ku plays multiple roles during NHEJ. Initially, Ku not only binds and detects DSB but also protects the ends from nucleolytic degradation and tilts the choice of DSB repair towards NHEJ and away from HR [7, 36]. Perhaps the most extensive role for Ku is to recruit NHEJ factors to DSB sites. The Ku80 CTD recruits DNA-PKcs to DSBs and binds a long list of NHEJ factors including XRCC4, LigIV, XLF, Polμ, and Polλ [9, 10]. Moreover, Ku's requirement for the recruitment of DNA-PKcs, XLF and XRCC4 has been demonstrated *in vivo* [37, 38]. In addition, Ku possesses some catalytic activities and can function as a deubiquitylating enzyme or as a 5′-dRP/AP lyase which suggests that Ku may aid in processing DNA ends before the final ligation [39].

The ability of the Ku heterodimer to self-associate and create higher order multimers was already apparent in early studies. Seminal work from Cary *et al* using gel filtration chromatography showed that while recombinant Ku exists as a single heterodimer in solution, the addition of 24bp DNA fragments promotes the appearance of Ku multimers whose sizes correspond to that of a heterotetramer [40]. More importantly, using a combination of electron microscopy (EM) and atomic force microscopy (AFM), they visualized Ku-dependent end-to-end bridging events involving either ends of two DNA fragments or loops within a single DNA fragment. Ku was found forming higher order multimers in the junction of those events, which suggests that Ku multimerization is responsible for its end bridging properties. To note, this was not the result of non-specific aggregation of Ku as multimers could only be detected with DNA-bound Ku and not with free Ku molecules. The ability of Ku to synapse two ends was later confirmed by Ramsden *et al* using a mix of biotinylated DNA fragments with ^{32}P-radiolabeled dsDNA [41]. When streptavidin beads were used to pull down biotinylated DNA, researchers could recover radiolabeled DNA only when recombinant Ku was also present in the mix. This co-precipitation could not be explained by a single Ku molecule binding and stabilizing the junction of two DNA fragments with complementary ends as similar results were obtained when DNA fragments with non-compatible ends were used. This result suggests that synapses were achieved through the interaction of at least two Ku molecules each bound to a differently labeled DNA. More recently, DNA-bound Ku heterotetramers have been demonstrated as supershifts in electromobility shift assays (EMSA) and EM studies have visualized formation of end bridges using recombinant yeast Ku protein, indicating that multimerization-dependent synapses may be evolutionarily conserved [42].

Recent work with the Ku80 CTD suggests that Ku heterotetramerization may occur through the interaction of two outward faces [42]. This long and flexible domain interacts with the Ku core domain and upon binding to DNA it undergoes a conformational change that relocates it to the outward face [43]. Researchers have now shown that the Ku80 CTD can dimerize and thus, can putatively mediate Ku-Ku interactions across a DSB enabling the tethering of two DNA ends [42]. In fact, Ku proteins bearing Ku80 CTD truncations have reduced ability to form heterotetramers as shown by reduced supershift EMSA signals compared with wild type [42]. Ku80 CTD truncations impair NHEJ, but this result cannot be fully attributed to reduced heterotetramer formation as the Ku80 CTD is also involved in recruiting DNA-PKcs to DSBs. Intriguingly, a mutation in the outward face located Ku70-α5 also impairs NHEJ, although the effect of this mutation on Ku heterotetramerization remains to be investigated [35].

While the presence of Ku multimers of higher order than heterotetramers has been detected in EM and AFM using recombinant Ku proteins, its functional significance remains to be elucidated and evidence for its existence in living cells is lacking [40, 44-46]. A single heterotetramer is sufficient to create a synaptic complex across DSB and it is difficult to envision how higher order Ku complexes may aid in this process. Since Ku can slide towards internal tracks of DNA, one possibility is that multiple Ku molecules threaded into a single DNA end could form filaments held by interactions between inward and outward faces. However, fluorescence anisotropy studies do not support this model [47].

2.2. The DNA-PKcs

With over 400 kDa, the DNA-PKcs is one of the largest kinases in mammalian cells. Along with ATM and ATR, it belongs to the phosphatidylinositol-3-OH kinase (PI3K)-related kinase (PIKK) family that preferentially phosphorylates serines and threonines followed by a glutamine [48]. Although DNA-PKcs can bind directly to DNA, during NHEJ it is recruited to DSBs by the Ku80 CTD flexible domain, which increases the affinity of DNA-PKcs to DNA by 100 fold [49-51]. Therefore, assembly of the DNA-PK complex only occurs at DSBs where it induces Ku displacement one helix turn away from the end and positions DNA-PKcs at the very tip of the break [44]. The DNA-PK complex performs two major roles during NHEJ: it forms a synaptic complex across DSBs and serves as a scaffold for the recruitment of all other NHEJ factors [52]. DNA-PKcs is responsible for the recruitment of Artemis to DSBs, which provides the NHEJ machinery with a variety of end processing activities including 5′ endonuclease, 3′ endonuclease and hairpin opening [53]. In addition, DNA-PKcs directly binds XRCC4 and stimulates the ligase activity of XRCC4/Ligase IV complex [52, 54, 55]. Both dimerization and XRCC4 interaction induces DNA-PKcs kinase activity which is known to phosphorylate several NHEJ factors such as Ku, Artemis, XRCC4, LigIV and XLF, although the role of these phosphorylation events in NHEJ remains to be elucidated [56, 57]. More importantly, DNA-PKcs possesses over 15 autophosphorylation sites that become phosphorylated after formation of the synaptic complex and that are involved in releasing DNA-PKcs from Ku and DSB [11]. Consistent with this, non-autophosphorylatable mutations or kinase-dead DNA-PKcs mutants still localize to DSBs but are retained longer at sites of DNA damage [43].

Given its large size, the complete structure of DNA-PKcs has been elusive at the atomic level. Single particle cryo-EM, small-angle X-ray scattering (SAXS) experiments and more recently, the crystal structure at 6.6 angstroms resolution, have shown that multiple N-terminus HEAT repeats, encompassing ~66 helices, form a ring-like structure with a gap at one end (Figure 1B) [58-60]. This structure is usually referred to as the `palm′ region and it also encloses a globular DNA binding domain, although a clear picture of how DNA-PKcs interacts with DNA is missing. The top of the palm houses the so-called `crown′ or `head′ that includes the globular C-terminus kinase domain, along with FAT and FATC domains. Also missing is the exact location of the Ku80 CTD interaction and the details of how the whole Ku heterodimer is accommodated by the DNA-PKcs structure to create the DNA-PK complex [61]. Several pieces of evidence indicate that DNA-PKcs undergoes conformational changes as a result of autophosphorylation [43, 62, 63]. SAXS analysis has detected a phosphorylation-driven conformational change that repositions the head with respect to the palm [43], whereas the crystal structure suggests that auto-transphosphorylation widens the gap at the end of the palm and facilitates disassembly of DNA-PKcs from Ku and DSBs [58].

During NHEJ, DNA-PKcs multimerization is limited to the dimerization of the two DNA-PKcs located at opposite ends of a DSB to create a synaptic complex. Early studies demonstrated the ability of DNA-PK to mediate co-immunoprecipitation of biotinylated DNA fragments with radiolabeled probes [64]. In agreement, initial EM experiments visualized the ability of DNA-PKcs to circularize DNA fragments and detected synaptic complexes whose size was consistent with that of a DNA-PKcs dimer. While DNA-PKcs was sufficient to create a synaptic complex, these were significantly more abundant when Ku was present [64]. Importantly, end-to-end bridges still occurred in the presence of kinase inhibitors, indicating that autophosphorylation events were not required for synaptic complex formation [64]. Further single particle EM, cryo-EM and SAXS studies have visualized dimers of DNA-PKcs molecules that form in a concentration dependent manner and in a process that is highly enhanced in the presence of Ku [43, 60, 63]. These techniques detected two types of DNA-PKcs dimers with different orientations depending on the DNA molecules used. In the presence of 40bp Y-shaped DNA fragments, DNA-PKcs dimers formed in a palm-to-palm fashion whereas, in the presence of a 40bp hairpin DNA, DNA-PKcs dimers had the opposite orientation and formed through head-to-head interactions [43, 60, 63]. These two kinds of DNA-PKcs dimers were observed in the presence or absence of Ku. The reason for the existence of two DNA-PKcs dimer subspecies is not clear but authors speculate that the Y-shape DNA induced orientation may be caused by the binding of two DNA-PKcs molecules to the same DNA fragment, suggesting that dimers generated by head-to-head interactions may be the only ones capable of bridging two DNA fragments [43]. Corroborating this hypothesis, DNA-PKcs dimers with a head-to-head orientation were the only type of dimers observed in the absence of DNA [43]. Overall, the current model proposes that Ku recruits DNA-PKcs to sites of DNA damage where it dimerizes through head-to-head interactions, creating synaptic complexes across DSBs [10]. DNA-PKcs dimerization at breaks stimulates auto-transphosphorylation, which in turn induces conformational changes that disassemble the DNA-PK complex and promotes its timely release from DNA ends [11].

2.3. The MRN complex

The association of the conserved Mre11 and Rad50 subunits along with Nbs1 (a protein whose functional homolog in *S. cerevisiae* is Xrs2), makes up the mammalian MRN complex, also known as the MRX complex in yeast [65-68]. This complex plays vital roles in multiple DNA repair pathways, including HR and NHEJ, and is responsible for the co-activation of the DDR in the presence of DNA injury [68-70]. Analysis of the domain composition and enzymatic activities of each subunit suggest possible mechanistic roles for the MRN complex during DNA repair. Rad50 is a member of the SMC protein family whose members play roles in chromosome condensation and cohesion [71, 72]. A key feature of these proteins is the presence of long coiled-coil domains that can fold on themselves via an antiparallel manner, bringing the N- and C-terminus in close proximity [73]. In Rad50, folding of the coiled-coil domain permits the reconstitution of a bipartite ATP-binding cassette (ABC)-type ATPase globular domain made of N-terminal Walker A and C-terminal Walker B nucleotide binding motifs [74, 75]. In other complexes, binding and hydrolysis of ATP by similar ABC-ATPase domains, mediate large conformational changes that can be transmitted to other members of the complex [71, 76]. Crystallography and SAXS data support a similar role for the Rad50 ABC-ATPase domain in the MRN complex [74, 77, 78].

As is the case for Rad50, Mre11 can bind DNA and possesses a specific region capable of capping DNA ends [20, 79]. Mre11 contains a phosphoesterase domain in its N-terminus that endows the MRN complex with ssDNA endonuclease and 3′ to 5′ dsDNA exonuclease enzymatic activities. Mre11 is the only subunit that interacts with all components of the complex as it also binds Nbs1 whose main function is to recruit DNA repair factors to DSB. For instance, the Nbs1 N-terminus is responsible for bringing ATM and ATR to DNA damage locations and hence, acts as a DSB sensor during the initiation of the DDR [80, 81]. Similarly, the Nbs1 N-terminus contains BRCT and FHA domains that bind and recruit CtIP (Sae2 in *S. cerevisiae*), an important nuclease during DNA repair, to DSBs [28, 82] as well as MDC1 [83, 84] and ATR[85], and the WRN helicase [86].

The MRN complex is at the center of the decision process that governs whether a DSB is repaired by NHEJ or HR [87, 88]. The current model indicates that, in the presence of DNA injury, recruitment of CtIP to DSB provides the MRN complex with the 5′ to 3′ exonuclease activity necessary to chew away part of the DNA ends and create an initial ~50-100nt ssDNA 3′ overhang [18, 82, 89-92]. This overhang is a poor binding substrate for Ku but an ideal substrate for the HR initiation factor RPA and thus, it favors DSB repair by HR over NHEJ [32, 93]. Since CtIP activity and recruitment to DSBs is dependent upon CDK phosphorylation of both CtIP and Nbs1 during S and G2 phases [93-95], the lack of these post-translational modifications during G1 prevents overhang formation at DSB ends in this phase and tilts the choice of DNA repair pathway towards NHEJ. Therefore, and according to this model, NHEJ remains active throughout the cell cycle but is overpowered by HR during S and G2 due to CDK-dependent 3′ overhang formation by the MRN/CtIP complex. This system ensures that HR is only active when an identical copy of the damaged DNA is available.

Despite favoring HR, the MRN complex also plays essential roles during NHEJ when HR is inhibited. Yeast defective for any MRX subunit are inviable in the presence of a single HO–induced break that can only be repaired by NHEJ [96]. Similarly, mammalian cells depleted of Mre11 display reduced end-joining activities [97], impaired NHEJ [69, 98] and, in the case of B-lymphocytes, markedly reduced CSR [99]. Intriguingly, yeast nuclease-dead Mre11 mutants can carry end-joining activity near wild type levels [100] and B lymphocytes only show mild defects in CSR in the presence of a Mre11 mutation lacking nuclease activity [99]. These results indicate that the MRN complex mostly plays a signaling and structural role during NHEJ, and that its end processing capabilities are dispensable or can be compensated by other nucleases. Scanning force microscopy (SFM) and AFM have demonstrated the ability of the MRN complex to create long range bridges across DNA molecules [101, 102] implicating DNA end tethering as the most likely structural role for MRN during NHEJ.

Formation of higher order multimers is essential to our understanding of the mechanistic roles of MRN during NHEJ. The MRX complex assembles as a heterohexamer where two Mre11 molecules bind simultaneously to two Rad50 and two Nbs1 subunits (Figure2A) [70, 103]. A combination of SAXS with X-ray crystallography has shown that, through interactions of the N-terminus globular domain, Mre11 form very stable dimers capable of forming bridges between two DNA molecules [20, 104]. Rad50 can also form dimers through two different dimerization regions located at opposite poles of the molecule [74]. At the end of the coiled-coil region, Rad50 contains a $C_{XX}C$ motif that can dimerize through the formation of two zinc-hook (Zn-hook) domains that lock in a single Zn(2+) ion [103]. At the opposite pole, two globular

ABC-ATPase domains bound to ATP can dimerize in head-to-tail fashion between N- and C-terminal domains, trapping two ATP molecules in the process [74]. Moreover, Mre11 dimers bind ABC-ATPase dimers forming the so-called M2R2 head region. In this disposition, a heterohexamer has a circular shape formed by two coiled-coil regions as semicircles are united at one end by the Zn-hook domain and by interactions within the M2R2 head at the other end (Figure 2C). Mre11 also contains a helix-loop-helix domain in its C-terminus that extends away from the N-terminal globular region and binds the base of the Rad50 coiled-coil region in the vicinity of the ABC-ATPase domain, further reinforcing the interaction between Mre11 and Rad50 dimers (Figure 2A). In contrast, Nbs1 does not form dimers nor does it contribute to heterohexamer-ization. Recent studies indicate that the MRN heterohexamer presents two distinct configurations [77, 78, 105, 106]. In the absence of ATP binding, the MRN complex adopts an `open' conformation where Mre11 dimers localize in between the two Rad50 ABC-ATPase domains, preventing their dimerization (Figure 2A). In this `open' configuration, Rad50 can only dimerize through the Zn-hook domain. Upon ATP binding, a conformational change allows displacement of the Mre11 dimers and dimerization of two Rad50 ABC-ATPase domains (Figure 2B). This `close' configuration is substantially more rigid and may promote DNA binding by Rad50 [77, 78, 105, 106]. Subsequent ATP hydrolysis disrupts ABC-ATPase mediated Rad50 dimerization and stimulates Mre11 nuclease activity [107].

A

B

C

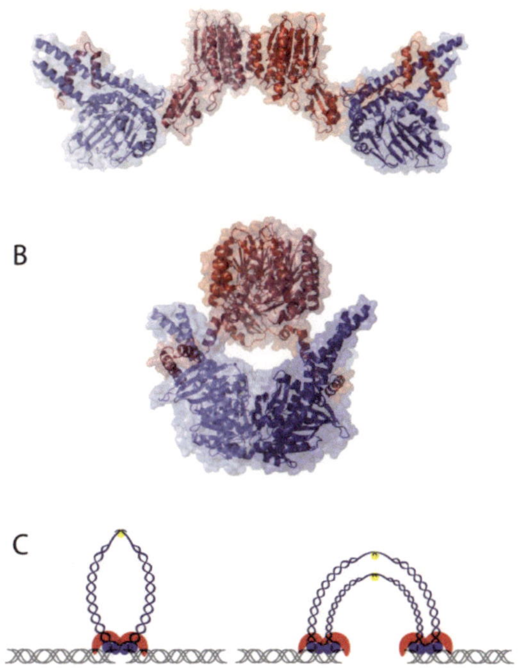

Figure 2. The MRN complex undergoes ATP-Driven conformational changes. A Molecular structure of the open state where Mre11 dimer is depicted in red and Rad50 in blue (Adapted from 3QG5). B Closed conformation of the MRN complex. (Adapted from 3QF7 and 3THO). C Tethering of DSB ends by different multimerization states of the MRN complex.

In the MRN complex, multimerization regulates formation of DNA bridges, with increasing order of multimers providing longer range tethering capabilities. Short range bridges can be achieved by single heterohexamers, where each Mre11 subunit is bound to a different DNA end (Figure 2C) [103]. In contrast with Ku heterotetramers and DNA-PKcs dimers, where multimerization occurs after the assembly of subunits located at each end of a DSB, short range bridges mediated by single heterohexamers must be achieved without disruption of the MRN complex as heterohexamers are predicted to be pre-assembled before binding DNA ends. Therefore, single heterohexamers may only bridge ends that are in close proximity (~100 angstroms) as to allow simultaneous binding of each end to the MRN complex without disrupting the M2R2 head [20, 103]. The role that DNA binding activity of the Rad50 dimers may play in synapse formation by heterohexamers remains to be elucidated but SFM has shown that Rad50 is also able to bind and tether DNA molecules in the absence of Mre11 [108].

Longer range bridges can be achieved through the formation of higher order multimers where two heterohexamers, each bound to a different end, combine to form a structure capable of tethering DNA molecules as far as 1200 angstroms apart [20, 103]. This configuration has been confirmed by AFM and EM and consists of two M2R2 heads separated by two long coiled-coil regions held together by two Zn-hooks (Figure 2C) [102, 103]. Consistent with this, AFM has demonstrated that upon DNA binding, heterohexamers extend their two coiled-coil regions in a parallel fashion that disrupts Zn-hook mediated dimerization within the heterohexamer and favors formation of Zn-hook interactions with other heterohexamers [102]. These assemblies have been proposed to mediate long distance tethering of homologous sequences during HR and to hold DNA ends in close proximity during NHEJ, preventing them from going astray and facilitating DSB repair by the rest of the NHEJ machinery [70, 109]. Consistent with this, in yeast, loss of the Rad50 CxxC Zn-hook motif abolishes DNA repair while replacing it with a *FKBP* homodimerization domain has no major effect [110]. Similarly, truncations of the coiled-coil region in Rad50 impairs DNA repair [109]. Since heterohexamers could potentially form Zn-hook interactions with more than one heterohexamer at a time, further higher order arrangements have been proposed to form multiple interactions to secure bridges across DNA molecules, a possibility whose biological significance remains to be investigated.

2.4. XLF and XRCC4

Although neither of them have any intrinsic enzymatic activity, XLF (also known as Cernnunos) and XRCC4 are involved in the final ligation step catalyzed by LigIV. XRCC4 binds tightly to LigIV and drives its localization to sites of DNA damage, whereas XLF stimulates the ability of the XRCC4-LigIV complex to ligate DSBs 20-200 fold, especially in the presence of non-cohesive ends [111-114]. XRCC4 is also capable of binding several other NHEJ factors including XLF, DNA-PKcs and the Ku heterodimer, while known interactions for XLF include XRCC4 and the Ku heterodimer. In addition, both XLF and XRCC4 can bind DNA, although their localization to sites of DNA damage is dependent on their interaction with members of the DNA-PK complex. While DNA-PKcs can recruit the XRCC4-LigIV complex to DSBs, Ku is capable of bringing both XRCC4-LigIV and XLF to sites of DNA damage in the absence of DNA-PKcs [37, 38, 54, 115, 116].

Both XLF and XRCC4 are obligated homodimers that have very similar structures where the presence of an N-terminal globular domain, or `head', is followed by a coiled-coil region that mediates homodimerization [112, 117, 118]. In this disposition, the two head domains on each homodimer face each other with opposite orientation. Given its heterogeneity and flexible nature, the structure of the C-terminal domain for both XRCC4 and XLF remain to be resolved. Nevertheless, XRCC4 SAXS analysis is consistent with the C-terminal domain folding backwards and interacting with the head domain [119]. Likewise, XLF's structure resolution revealed a fold back in the coiled-coil region that shortens the helix and creates a kink that likely positions the C-terminal domain in close proximity to the head domain [118]. The presence of discrete regions in both XRCC4 and XLF correlates with the spatial organization of their interactions with NHEJ factors. While their N-terminal domains mediate XRCC4-XLF interaction, the XRCC4-LigIV interaction maps to the XRCC4 coiled-coil region and the C-terminal domain of XLF interacts with Ku [22, 38, 116, 119-122]. In addition, both XRCC4 and XLF can bind DNA. EMSA analysis has identified the upper part of the XRCC4 coiled-coil domain and the XLF C-terminus as their respective DNA binding regions [22, 23, 118].

Besides forming homodimers, XRCC4 also exists as tetramers and higher order multimers in solution [119, 123]. Although coiled-coil mediation of tetramerization was initially proposed, SAXS analyses have demonstrated that tetramerization is mostly mediated by the interaction of two N-terminal domains in a way that leaves the stalks of each dimer pointing in opposite directions [119, 124, 125]. These head-to-head interactions can also drive formation of XRCC4 filaments, as detected by SAXS [119]. Interestingly, while full length XRCC4 mostly exists as tetramers and filaments in solution, truncation of the C-terminus makes homodimers the predominant XRCC4 form, suggesting that the C-terminus also contributes to tetramerization and filament formation. The presence of a LigIV BRCT region responsible for binding the XRCC4 coiled-coil region also made XRCC4 filaments unstable, indicating that the XRCC4-LigIV complex does not exist as part of a filament and suggesting that under physiological conditions, XRCC4 remains in multiple configurations [119]. Given the fact that mammalian cells contain six times more XRCC4 molecules than LigIV, XRCC4 filaments may constitute a protein reservoir that can readily be mobilized in the presence of DNA damage. The ability of XLF to form higher order assemblies in solution suggests that XLF filaments may also exist in cells [118].

In addition, XRCC4 can also form filaments through its interaction with XLF. SAXS analysis, EM, SFM and crystallography have all detected long filaments of alternating XRCC4 and XLF molecules bound through head-to-head interactions (Figure 3) [21-23, 119, 126]. In this conformation, XRCC4 and XLF stalks are both oriented towards the same direction, albeit with a 30-degree offset from each other. Furthermore, two filaments can intertwine through XRCC4-XRCC4 interactions to form a left-handed helix with a ~220 angstrom diameter where head domains reside in the interior while coiled-coil regions stick out to the exterior. Higher order multimers where several filaments constitute a thicker fiber have also been proposed [22, 23, 126]. Importantly, mutations in residues directly involved in XRCC4-XLF interaction not only disrupt filament formation but also disrupt NHEJ and render cells radiosensitive, indicating that XRCC4-XLF filaments are functionally relevant structures during DSB repair [23, 126]. Futhermore, during NHEJ, XRCC4-XLF filament formation is likely to be regulated as *in vitro* experiments have shown that DNA-PKcs dependent phosphorylation of XRCC4 and XLF disassembles XRCC4-XLF filaments [126].

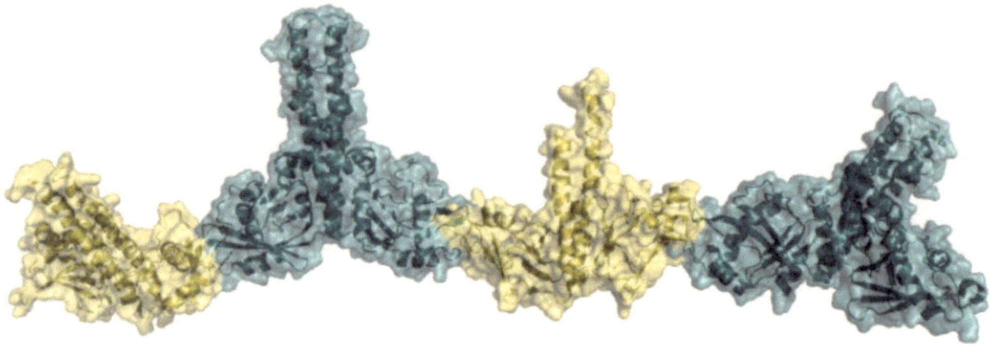

Figure 3. Sequential interactions between the N-terminal domains of XRCC4 and XLF can create multimeric filaments. XRCC4 is colored yellow and XLF is colored teal (Adapated from 3RWR).

Given the ability of XRCC4 and XLF to bind DNA, it is likely that the XRCC4-XLF complex forms nucleoprotein filaments. In agreement, EMSA experiments in the presence of XRCC4 and XLF can detect supershifts consistent with formation of large nucleoprotein complexes [23, 126]. How DNA interacts with XLF-XRCC4 filaments is not clear, but EMSA supershifts are lost in the absence of the XLF C-terminus domain but not when the XRCC4 DNA binding region has been removed, suggesting that the XLF C-terminus plays a greater role than XRCC4 in nucleoprotein filament formation. Recently, HDX studies have revealed that the interface between XRCC4 and XLF in the filament may accommodate DNA, although the details of this interaction remain to be elucidated [22]. These nucleoprotein filaments are highly reminiscent of Rad51 filaments that form during HR and suggest that XRCC4-XLF filaments may also coat dsDNA ends to protect and prepare them for processing and ligation. It is also possible that they facilitate DNA repair by 'peeling' away nucleosomes from DSBs and making DNA ends more accessible to other NHEJ factors. In addition, due to their length and ability to bind DNA, XRCC4-XLF filaments can form bridges across DSBs, as demonstrated by their ability to mediate co-immunoprecipitation of two different DNA fragments [23, 126]. Importantly, conditions that disrupt XRCC4-XLF filament formation, such as mutations in the XRCC4-XLF interface, presence of LigIV BRCT domains, lack of the XLF C-terminal domain or DNA-PKcs phosphorylation, also prevent DNA bridging *in vitro* [23, 126].

While LigIV uses its BRCT domains to bind the XRCC4 coiled-coil region, its catalytic domain interacts with the XRCC4 N-terminus domain and therefore, the presence of LigIV bound to XRCC4 is not compatible with XRCC4-XLF filament formation [127]. These data suggest that XRCC4 may be present in different configurations at DSB: as an XRCC4 filament, as part of an XRCC4-XLF nucleofilament and as a separate XRCC4-LigIV complex. Since LigIV can only interact with one head of the XRCC4 homodimer, it is also possible that the other head may be free to start polymerization of a LigIV-free XRCC4-XLF filament. In this conformation, a single XRCC4-LigIV at the tip of a DSB may cap an XRCC4-XLF filament that extends inward and away from the end [22]. Other possibilities include DNA-PK acting both as the DNA end cap of an XRCC4-XLF filament and as the recruiter of an XRCC4-LigIV complex or a single filament that expands across the DSB, allowing other NHEJ factors to reach the DNA ends [22, 126]. Further experiments are required to discern among these possibilities and to investigate how and when XRCC4-XLF filaments assemble, and to investigate the additional functions that they play during NHEJ.

3. Conclusions and new directions

The evidence presented here strongly indicates that multimerization of Ku, DNA-PKcs, the MRN complex and the XRCC4/XLF complex play crucial functions during NHEJ. In contrast, while more than one molecule of other NHEJ components like Artemis, LigIV, Polμ and Polλ are likely to be present at DSBs, neither the presence of higher order multimers nor a functional role for the accumulation of their subunits at breaks has been demonstrated. In other DNA repair pathways, several examples of multimerization can also be found. For instance, during HR the RPA complex polymerizes along ssDNA ends forming filaments that protect ends from degradation and are readily substituted by Rad51 filaments to catalyze strand exchange. Other notable examples include WRN, a member of the RecQ helicases involved in DNA damage response and telomere maintenance, which contains a coiled-coil region that serves as a multimerization domain to create trimers and hexamers required for full protein function and BLM, a member of the same protein family that functionally exists as homohexameric rings [128, 129]. Recent studies have demonstrated that CtIP dimerization is also required for its recruitment to DSB and subsequent HR [130].

During NHEJ, the most prevalent role for multimerization is to ensure the formation of protein bridges across a DSB. When bound to both ends of a break, either DNA-PKcs, the Ku heterodimer or the MRX complex can form multimerization-driven synapses that hold the two ends together and facilitate DNA damage repair. In addition, XRCC4-XLF filaments can also form bridges across two DNA fragments and may contribute to end synapses. How NHEJ factors assemble at DSB and the stoichiometry of such assemblies remain to be elucidated. The high redundancy of NHEJ factors capable of bridging ends may reflect the presence of different subcomplexes that are formed depending on the type or location of the damage. Alternatively, different NHEJ proteins may be involved in synapsing DNA ends at different steps during NHEJ. For example, initial Ku-mediated DNA bridges may be disrupted and replaced by DNA-PKcs as recruitment of DNA-PKcs to DSBs is known to displace Ku internally away from the ends [131]. Further investigations on how multimerization influences NHEJ are likely to provide insights not only on the stoichiometry of NHEJ complexes at DSBs but also on the different progression steps of the DNA repair process. An important aspect to consider is the diversity that exists among NHEJ bridging proteins with respect to the distance between DNA ends once the bridge is formed. While multimers of MRX complex can establish long-range bridges between DNA ends, DNA-PKcs and the Ku heterodimer bridges are limited to short-range synapses. It is possible that different synaptic complexes may modulate the separation of DNA ends during different NHEJ steps to allow the timely access of DNA processing factors while, at the same time, holding the two ends together. In addition, there may be differences in the strength by which each synaptic complex holds the two DNA ends. For instance, Ku mediated synapses can only be observed at high concentrations of Ku protein, which may partially explain why its detection was missed in several studies. The weakness of Ku mediated synapses may facilitate its replacement by putatively stronger synapses via DNA-PKcs. Future experiments are needed to delineate other possible transitions between synapses of different strength during each NHEJ step and to establish whether different DNA bridges can occur simultaneously at the same DSB.

It could also be insightful to dissect the multimerization state of NHEJ proteins at the end of chromosomes. Telomeres use the shelterin complex to protect the natural chromosome end from being acted upon as a DSB, which could result in deleterious chromosome end-to-end fusions and generalized genomic instability [132]. Surprisingly, telomeres also harbor several members of the NHEJ machinery such as Ku, the MRX complex and DNA-PKcs [16]. How these proteins are prevented from engaging in NHEJ at telomeres is not fully understood but it is possible that interactions with shelterin components not only recruit NHEJ proteins to telomeres but also impair their multimerization. Therefore, delineating how NHEJ proteins interact with sheltering components could provide information on how their DNA repair properties are blocked at telomeres.

Another untapped area of investigation is the role that NHEJ multimerization may play during V(D)J recombination and CSR. These programmed physiological cuts generate different DNA end substrates that support the formation of different subcomplexes depending on their end processing needs. While Ku and LigIV are sufficient to join blunt signal ends, ligation of coding ends necessitates the action of DNA-PKcs, Artemis, XRCC4 and XLF to open the hairpin formed by the RAG1/RAG2 complex. It is possible that multimerization requirements between these two substrates are different and thus, it would be insightful to test the effect that multimerization impairing mutations, like those on Ku80-CTD or in the XRCC4-XLF interaction region, have on V(D)J recombination and CSR. These studies may potentially reveal differences in the requirement for multimerization between programmed DSBs and radiation-induced DNA breaks.

3.1. Therapeutical uses

Due to the accumulation of mutations that they produce, defects in DNA repair mechanisms are associated with the development of several types of cancer. For instance, between 5-15% of hereditable breast, ovarian or pancreatic cancer contain mutations in HR genes whereas 3-4% of familial colon cancers contain mutations in mismatch repair genes [133, 134]. On the other hand, during tumor progression, cancerous cells become ever more dependent on DNA repair mechanisms to prevent their genome instability from inducing cell death. As a result, overexpression of DNA repair genes is frequently found in advanced stage cancers. For example,

DNA-PKcs is overexpressed in nasopharyngeal, colorectal and non-small cell lung carcinomas and its level of expression correlates with advanced tumor stages [135]. The use of chemo- and radio-therapy to treat tumors exacerbates this effect by further selecting cancerous cells with overactivated DNA repair mechanisms that can deal with the newly inflicted DNA damage, especially DSB, the most toxic type of lesion produced by these treatments.

A recent study has shown that Ku and XRCC4 expression can be used to predict the effectiveness of chemo- and radiotherapy in hypopharyngeal cancers. Tumors with lower Ku70 and XRCC4 expression correlated with higher survival rates after treatment [136]. Similar high correlations were obtained when studying DNA-PKcs and Mre11 expression in tumors treated with radiotherapy [137]. These results exemplify how strategies aimed at impairing NHEJ could radiosensitize tumor cells, increase treatment efficacy and improve patients' outcomes. For instance, targeting DNA-PKcs with small molecule inhibitors (SMI) has hypersensitized cells to ionizing irradiation, and it has successfully delayed tumor growth in mice treated with radiotherapy [138].

The emerging role of multimerization during NHEJ raises the possibility of radiosensitizing cancerous cells by means of preventing multimerization of NHEJ factors. Therapeutic reagents designed to block important sites for multimerization are likely to impair NHEJ and thus enhance the sensitivity of cancerous cells to radiation and possibly others to DNA damaging chemicals. In this context, it would be paramount to investigate how multi-merization of NHEJ factors differs at telomeres and at DSB. These differences could be exploited to design reagents that block NHEJ without affecting their telomeric roles. This is particularly relevant for the Ku heterodimer, as human cell lines lacking Ku expression quickly die due to massive telomere loss [139]. A reagent that impairs Ku's NHEJ without affecting its telomeric functions could radiosensitize tumor cells without compromising the viability of healthy cells. Similarly, possible differences between multimerization of NHEJ factors at sites of DNA damage with respect to physiologically programmed cuts during V(D)J and CS recombination could be used to generate molecular targeted therapeutic reagents that radiosensitize cancer cells without adversely affecting the patient's immune system.

Acknowledgements

We would like to express our sincere gratitude to Dr. Alison Bertuch, Dr. Sandra Indiviglio, Dr. Jill Dewey and Katherina Alsina for their insightful revisions to this manuscript.

Author details

Michelle Rubin, Jonathan Newsome and Albert Ribes-Zamora*

*Address all correspondence to: ribesza@stthom.edu

Biology Department, University of St.Thomas, Houston, Texas, USA

References

[1] Jackson SP. Sensing and repairing DNA double-strand breaks. Carcinogenesis. 2002 May;23(5) 687-696.

[2] Mladenov E, Iliakis G. Induction and repair of DNA double strand breaks: the increasing spectrum of non-homologous end joining pathways. Mutat Res. 2011 Jun 3;711(1-2) 61-72.

[3] Hiom K. Coping with DNA double strand breaks. DNA Repair (Amst). 2010 Dec 10;9(12) 1256-1263.

[4] Bensimon A, Aebersold R, Shiloh Y. Beyond ATM: the protein kinase landscape of the DNA damage response. FEBS Lett. 2011 Jun 6;585(11) 1625-1639.

[5] Lieber MR, Gu J, Lu H, Shimazaki N, Tsai AG. Nonhomologous DNA end joining (NHEJ) and chromosomal translocations in humans. Subcell Biochem. 2010;50 279-296.

[6] Rouse J, Jackson SP. Interfaces between the detection, signaling, and repair of DNA damage. Science. 2002 Jul 26;297(5581) 547-551.

[7] Symington LS, Gautier J. Double-strand break end resection and repair pathway choice. Annu Rev Genet. 2011;45 247-271.

[8] Mahaney BL, Meek K, Lees-Miller SP. Repair of ionizing radiation-induced DNA double-strand breaks by non-homologous end-joining. Biochem J. 2009 Feb 1;417(3) 639-650.

[9] Lieber MR. The mechanism of double-strand DNA break repair by the nonhomologous DNA end-joining pathway. Annu Rev Biochem. 2010;79 181-211.

[10] Ochi T, Sibanda BL, Wu Q, Chirgadze DY, Bolanos-Garcia VM, Blundell TL. Structural biology of DNA repair: spatial organisation of the multicomponent complexes of nonhomologous end joining. J Nucleic Acids. 2010;2010.

[11] Dobbs TA, Tainer JA, Lees-Miller SP. A structural model for regulation of NHEJ by DNA-PKcs autophosphorylation. DNA Repair (Amst). 2010 Dec 10;9(12) 1307-1314.

[12] Markkanen E, van Loon B, Ferrari E, Hubscher U. Ubiquitylation of DNA polymerase lambda. FEBS Lett. 2011 Sep 16;585(18) 2826-2830.

[13] Postow L. Destroying the ring: Freeing DNA from Ku with ubiquitin. FEBS Lett. 2011 Sep 16;585(18) 2876-2882.

[14] Rathaus M, Lerrer B, Cohen HY. DeubiKuitylation: a novel DUB enzymatic activity for the DNA repair protein, Ku70. Cell Cycle. 2009 Jun 15;8(12) 1843-1852.

[15] Yu Y, Mahaney BL, Yano K, Ye R, Fang S, Douglas P, Chen DJ, Lees-Miller SP. DNA-PK and ATM phosphorylation sites in XLF/Cernunnos are not required for repair of DNA double strand breaks. DNA Repair (Amst). 2008 Oct 1;7(10) 1680-1692.

[16] Riha K, Heacock ML, Shippen DE. The role of the nonhomologous end-joining DNA double-strand break repair pathway in telomere biology. Annu Rev Genet. 2006;40 237-277.

[17] Gennery AR. Primary immunodeficiency syndromes associated with defective DNA double-strand break repair. Br Med Bull. 2006;77-78 71-85.

[18] You Z, Bailis JM. DNA damage and decisions: CtIP coordinates DNA repair and cell cycle checkpoints. Trends Cell Biol. 2010 Jul;20(7) 402-409.

[19] Rivera-Calzada A, Maman JD, Spagnolo L, Pearl LH, Llorca O. Three-dimensional structure and regulation of the DNA-dependent protein kinase catalytic subunit (DNA-PKcs). Structure. 2005 Feb;13(2) 243-255.

[20] Williams RS, Moncalian G, Williams JS, Yamada Y, Limbo O, Shin DS, Groocock LM, Cahill D, Hitomi C, Guenther G, Moiani D, Carney JP, Russell P, Tainer JA. Mre11 dimers coordinate DNA end bridging and nuclease processing in double-strand-break repair. Cell. 2008 Oct 3;135(1) 97-109.

[21] Ropars V, Drevet P, Legrand P, Baconnais S, Amram J, Faure G, Marquez JA, Pietrement O, Guerois R, Callebaut I, Le Cam E, Revy P, de Villartay JP, Charbonnier JB. Structural characterization of filaments formed by human Xrcc4-Cernunnos/XLF complex involved in nonhomologous DNA end-joining. Proc Natl Acad Sci U S A. 2011 Aug 2;108(31) 12663-12668.

[22] Hammel M, Rey M, Yu Y, Mani RS, Classen S, Liu M, Pique ME, Fang S, Mahaney BL, Weinfeld M, Schriemer DC, Lees-Miller SP, Tainer JA. XRCC4 protein interactions with XRCC4-like factor (XLF) create an extended grooved scaffold for DNA ligation and double strand break repair. J Biol Chem. 2011 Sep 16;286(37) 32638-32650.

[23] Andres SN, Vergnes A, Ristic D, Wyman C, Modesti M, Junop M. A human XRCC4-XLF complex bridges DNA. Nucleic Acids Res. 2012 Feb;40(4) 1868-1878.

[24] Downs JA, Jackson SP. A means to a DNA end: the many roles of Ku. Nat Rev Mol Cell Biol. 2004 May;5(5) 367-378.

[25] Chen F, Peterson SR, Story MD, Chen DJ. Disruption of DNA-PK in Ku80 mutant xrs-6 and the implications in DNA double-strand break repair. Mutat Res. 1996 Jan 2;362(1) 9-19.

[26] Errami A, Smider V, Rathmell WK, He DM, Hendrickson EA, Zdzienicka MZ, Chu G. Ku86 defines the genetic defect and restores X-ray resistance and V(D)J recombination to complementation group 5 hamster cell mutants. Mol Cell Biol. 1996 Apr; 16(4) 1519-1526.

[27] Walker JR, Corpina RA, Goldberg J. Structure of the Ku heterodimer bound to DNA and its implications for double-strand break repair. Nature. 2001 Aug 9;412(6847) 607-614.

[28] Falck J, Coates J, Jackson SP. Conserved modes of recruitment of ATM, ATR and DNA-PKcs to sites of DNA damage. Nature. 2005 Mar 31;434(7033) 605-611.

[29] Mimori T, Hardin JA. Mechanism of interaction between Ku protein and DNA. J Biol Chem. 1986 Aug 5;261(22) 10375-10379.

[30] Blier PR, Griffith AJ, Craft J, Hardin JA. Binding of Ku protein to DNA. Measurement of affinity for ends and demonstration of binding to nicks. J Biol Chem. 1993 Apr 5;268(10) 7594-7601.

[31] Falzon M, Fewell JW, Kuff EL. EBP-80, a transcription factor closely resembling the human autoantigen Ku, recognizes single- to double-strand transitions in DNA. J Biol Chem. 1993 May 15;268(14) 10546-10552.

[32] Dynan WS, Yoo S. Interaction of Ku protein and DNA-dependent protein kinase catalytic subunit with nucleic acids. Nucleic Acids Res. 1998 Apr 1;26(7) 1551-1559.

[33] Ribes-Zamora A, Mihalek I, Lichtarge O, Bertuch AA. Distinct faces of the Ku heterodimer mediate DNA repair and telomeric functions. Nat Struct Mol Biol. 2007 Apr; 14(4) 301-307.

[34] Palmbos PL, Daley JM, Wilson TE. Mutations of the Yku80 C terminus and Xrs2 FHA domain specifically block yeast nonhomologous end joining. Mol Cell Biol. 2005 Dec; 25(24) 10782-10790.

[35] Fell VL, Schild-Poulter C. Ku regulates signaling to DNA damage response pathways through the Ku70 von Willebrand A domain. Mol Cell Biol. 2012 Jan;32(1) 76-87.

[36] Shao Z, Davis AJ, Fattah KR, So S, Sun J, Lee KJ, Harrison L, Yang J, Chen DJ. Persistently bound Ku at DNA ends attenuates DNA end resection and homologous recombination. DNA Repair (Amst). 2012 Mar 1;11(3) 310-316.

[37] Mari PO, Florea BI, Persengiev SP, Verkaik NS, Bruggenwirth HT, Modesti M, Giglia-Mari G, Bezstarosti K, Demmers JA, Luider TM, Houtsmuller AB, van Gent DC. Dynamic assembly of end-joining complexes requires interaction between Ku70/80 and XRCC4. Proc Natl Acad Sci U S A. 2006 Dec 5;103(49) 18597-18602.

[38] Yano K, Morotomi-Yano K, Wang SY, Uematsu N, Lee KJ, Asaithamby A, Weterings E, Chen DJ. Ku recruits XLF to DNA double-strand breaks. EMBO Rep. 2008 Jan;9(1) 91-96.

[39] Roberts SA, Strande N, Burkhalter MD, Strom C, Havener JM, Hasty P, Ramsden DA. Ku is a 5'-dRP/AP lyase that excises nucleotide damage near broken ends. Nature. 2010 Apr 22;464(7292) 1214-1217.

[40] Cary RB, Peterson SR, Wang J, Bear DG, Bradbury EM, Chen DJ. DNA looping by Ku and the DNA-dependent protein kinase. Proc Natl Acad Sci U S A. 1997 Apr 29;94(9) 4267-4272.

[41] Ramsden DA, Gellert M. Ku protein stimulates DNA end joining by mammalian DNA ligases: a direct role for Ku in repair of DNA double-strand breaks. EMBO J. 1998 Jan 15;17(2) 609-614.

[42] Bennett SM, Woods DS, Pawelczak KS, Turchi JJ. Multiple protein-protein interactions within the DNA-PK complex are mediated by the C-terminus of Ku 80. Int J Biochem Mol Biol. 2012;3(1) 36-45.

[43] Hammel M, Yu Y, Mahaney BL, Cai B, Ye R, Phipps BM, Rambo RP, Hura GL, Pelikan M, So S, Abolfath RM, Chen DJ, Lees-Miller SP, Tainer JA. Ku and DNA-dependent protein kinase dynamic conformations and assembly regulate DNA binding and the initial non-homologous end joining complex. J Biol Chem. 2010 Jan 8;285(2) 1414-1423.

[44] Yaneva M, Kowalewski T, Lieber MR. Interaction of DNA-dependent protein kinase with DNA and with Ku: biochemical and atomic-force microscopy studies. EMBO J. 1997 Aug 15;16(16) 5098-5112.

[45] Merkle D, Douglas P, Moorhead GB, Leonenko Z, Yu Y, Cramb D, Bazett-Jones DP, Lees-Miller SP. The DNA-dependent protein kinase interacts with DNA to form a protein-DNA complex that is disrupted by phosphorylation. Biochemistry. 2002 Oct 22;41(42) 12706-12714.

[46] Grob P, Zhang TT, Hannah R, Yang H, Hefferin ML, Tomkinson AE, Nogales E. Electron microscopy visualization of DNA-protein complexes formed by Ku and DNA ligase IV. DNA Repair (Amst). 2012 Jan 2;11(1) 74-81.

[47] Arosio D, Costantini S, Kong Y, Vindigni A. Fluorescence anisotropy studies on the Ku-DNA interaction: anion and cation effects. J Biol Chem. 2004 Oct 8;279(41) 42826-42835.

[48] Llorca O. Electron microscopy reconstructions of DNA repair complexes. Curr Opin Struct Biol. 2007 Apr;17(2) 215-220.

[49] Singleton BK, Torres-Arzayus MI, Rottinghaus ST, Taccioli GE, Jeggo PA. The C terminus of Ku80 activates the DNA-dependent protein kinase catalytic subunit. Mol Cell Biol. 1999 May;19(5) 3267-3277.

[50] Hammarsten O, Chu G. DNA-dependent protein kinase: DNA binding and activation in the absence of Ku. Proc Natl Acad Sci U S A. 1998 Jan 20;95(2) 525-530.

[51] West RB, Yaneva M, Lieber MR. Productive and nonproductive complexes of Ku and DNA-dependent protein kinase at DNA termini. Mol Cell Biol. 1998 Oct;18(10) 5908-5920.

[52] Meek K, Dang V, Lees-Miller SP. DNA-PK: the means to justify the ends? Adv Immunol. 2008;99 33-58.

[53] Ma Y, Schwarz K, Lieber MR. The Artemis:DNA-PKcs endonuclease cleaves DNA loops, flaps, and gaps. DNA Repair (Amst). 2005 Jul 12;4(7) 845-851.

[54] Costantini S, Woodbine L, Andreoli L, Jeggo PA, Vindigni A. Interaction of the Ku heterodimer with the DNA ligase IV/Xrcc4 complex and its regulation by DNA-PK. DNA Repair (Amst). 2007 Jun 1;6(6) 712-722.

[55] van Heemst D, Brugmans L, Verkaik NS, van Gent DC. End-joining of blunt DNA double-strand breaks in mammalian fibroblasts is precise and requires DNA-PK and XRCC4. DNA Repair (Amst). 2004 Jan 5;3(1) 43-50.

[56] Weterings E, Chen DJ. The endless tale of non-homologous end-joining. Cell Res. 2008 Jan;18(1) 114-124.

[57] Douglas P, Gupta S, Morrice N, Meek K, Lees-Miller SP. DNA-PK-dependent phosphorylation of Ku70/80 is not required for non-homologous end joining. DNA Repair (Amst). 2005 Aug 15;4(9) 1006-1018.

[58] Sibanda BL, Chirgadze DY, Blundell TL. Crystal structure of DNA-PKcs reveals a large open-ring cradle comprised of HEAT repeats. Nature. 2010 Jan 7;463(7277) 118-121.

[59] Williams DR, Lee KJ, Shi J, Chen DJ, Stewart PL. Cryo-EM structure of the DNA-dependent protein kinase catalytic subunit at subnanometer resolution reveals alpha helices and insight into DNA binding. Structure. 2008 Mar;16(3) 468-477.

[60] Spagnolo L, Rivera-Calzada A, Pearl LH, Llorca O. Three-dimensional structure of the human DNA-PKcs/Ku70/Ku80 complex assembled on DNA and its implications for DNA DSB repair. Mol Cell. 2006 May 19;22(4) 511-519.

[61] Rivera-Calzada A, Spagnolo L, Pearl LH, Llorca O. Structural model of full-length human Ku70-Ku80 heterodimer and its recognition of DNA and DNA-PKcs. EMBO Rep. 2007 Jan;8(1) 56-62.

[62] Boskovic J, Rivera-Calzada A, Maman JD, Chacon P, Willison KR, Pearl LH, Llorca O. Visualization of DNA-induced conformational changes in the DNA repair kinase DNA-PKcs. EMBO J. 2003 Nov 3;22(21) 5875-5882.

[63] Morris EP, Rivera-Calzada A, da Fonseca PC, Llorca O, Pearl LH, Spagnolo L. Evidence for a remodelling of DNA-PK upon autophosphorylation from electron microscopy studies. Nucleic Acids Res. 2011 Jul;39(13) 5757-5767.

[64] DeFazio LG, Stansel RM, Griffith JD, Chu G. Synapsis of DNA ends by DNA-dependent protein kinase. EMBO J. 2002 Jun 17;21(12) 3192-3200.

[65] Usui T, Ohta T, Oshiumi H, Tomizawa J, Ogawa H, Ogawa T. Complex formation and functional versatility of Mre11 of budding yeast in recombination. Cell. 1998 Nov 25;95(5) 705-716.

[66] Dolganov GM, Maser RS, Novikov A, Tosto L, Chong S, Bressan DA, Petrini JH. Human Rad50 is physically associated with human Mre11: identification of a conserved multiprotein complex implicated in recombinational DNA repair. Mol Cell Biol. 1996 Sep;16(9) 4832-4841.

[67] Stracker TH, Petrini JH. The MRE11 complex: starting from the ends. Nat Rev Mol Cell Biol. 2011 Feb;12(2) 90-103.

[68] Lamarche BJ, Orazio NI, Weitzman MD. The MRN complex in double-strand break repair and telomere maintenance. FEBS Lett. 2010 Sep 10;584(17) 3682-3695.

[69] Xie A, Kwok A, Scully R. Role of mammalian Mre11 in classical and alternative non-homologous end joining. Nat Struct Mol Biol. 2009 Aug;16(8) 814-818.

[70] Williams GJ, Lees-Miller SP, Tainer JA. Mre11-Rad50-Nbs1 conformations and the control of sensing, signaling, and effector responses at DNA double-strand breaks. DNA Repair (Amst). 2010 Dec 10;9(12) 1299-1306.

[71] Hopfner KP, Tainer JA. Rad50/SMC proteins and ABC transporters: unifying concepts from high-resolution structures. Curr Opin Struct Biol. 2003 Apr;13(2) 249-255.

[72] Kinoshita E, van der Linden E, Sanchez H, Wyman C. RAD50, an SMC family member with multiple roles in DNA break repair: how does ATP affect function? Chromosome Res. 2009;17(2) 277-288.

[73] de Jager M, Trujillo KM, Sung P, Hopfner KP, Carney JP, Tainer JA, Connelly JC, Leach DR, Kanaar R, Wyman C. Differential arrangements of conserved building blocks among homologs of the Rad50/Mre11 DNA repair protein complex. J Mol Biol. 2004 Jun 11;339(4) 937-949.

[74] Hopfner KP, Karcher A, Shin DS, Craig L, Arthur LM, Carney JP, Tainer JA. Structural biology of Rad50 ATPase: ATP-driven conformational control in DNA double-strand break repair and the ABC-ATPase superfamily. Cell. 2000 Jun 23;101(7) 789-800.

[75] Hopfner KP, Karcher A, Craig L, Woo TT, Carney JP, Tainer JA. Structural biochemistry and interaction architecture of the DNA double-strand break repair Mre11 nuclease and Rad50-ATPase. Cell. 2001 May 18;105(4) 473-485.

[76] Moncalian G, Lengsfeld B, Bhaskara V, Hopfner KP, Karcher A, Alden E, Tainer JA, Paull TT. The rad50 signature motif: essential to ATP binding and biological function. J Mol Biol. 2004 Jan 23;335(4) 937-951.

[77] Lammens K, Bemeleit DJ, Mockel C, Clausing E, Schele A, Hartung S, Schiller CB, Lucas M, Angermuller C, Soding J, Strasser K, Hopfner KP. The Mre11:Rad50 structure shows an ATP-dependent molecular clamp in DNA double-strand break repair. Cell. 2011 Apr 1;145(1) 54-66.

[78] Williams GJ, Williams RS, Williams JS, Moncalian G, Arvai AS, Limbo O, Guenther G, SilDas S, Hammel M, Russell P, Tainer JA. ABC ATPase signature helices in Rad50 link nucleotide state to Mre11 interface for DNA repair. Nat Struct Mol Biol. 2011 Apr;18(4) 423-431.

[79] de Jager M, Dronkert ML, Modesti M, Beerens CE, Kanaar R, van Gent DC. DNA-binding and strand-annealing activities of human Mre11: implications for its roles in

DNA double-strand break repair pathways. Nucleic Acids Res. 2001 Mar 15;29(6) 1317-1325.

[80] Petrini JH, Stracker TH. The cellular response to DNA double-strand breaks: defining the sensors and mediators. Trends Cell Biol. 2003 Sep;13(9) 458-462.

[81] Lloyd J, Chapman JR, Clapperton JA, Haire LF, Hartsuiker E, Li J, Carr AM, Jackson SP, Smerdon SJ. A supramodular FHA/BRCT-repeat architecture mediates Nbs1 adaptor function in response to DNA damage. Cell. 2009 Oct 2;139(1) 100-111.

[82] Williams RS, Dodson GE, Limbo O, Yamada Y, Williams JS, Guenther G, Classen S, Glover JN, Iwasaki H, Russell P, Tainer JA. Nbs1 flexibly tethers Ctp1 and Mre11-Rad50 to coordinate DNA double-strand break processing and repair. Cell. 2009 Oct 2;139(1) 87-99.

[83] Spycher C, Miller ES, Townsend K, Pavic L, Morrice NA, Janscak P, Stewart GS, Stucki M. Constitutive phosphorylation of MDC1 physically links the MRE11-RAD50-NBS1 complex to damaged chromatin. J Cell Biol. 2008 Apr 21;181(2) 227-240.

[84] Hari FJ, Spycher C, Jungmichel S, Pavic L, Stucki M. A divalent FHA/BRCT-binding mechanism couples the MRE11-RAD50-NBS1 complex to damaged chromatin. EMBO Rep. 2010 May;11(5) 387-392.

[85] Olson E, Nievera CJ, Lee AY, Chen L, Wu X. The Mre11-Rad50-Nbs1 complex acts both upstream and downstream of ataxia telangiectasia mutated and Rad3-related protein (ATR) to regulate the S-phase checkpoint following UV treatment. J Biol Chem. 2007 Aug 3;282(31) 22939-22952.

[86] Kobayashi J, Okui M, Asaithamby A, Burma S, Chen BP, Tanimoto K, Matsuura S, Komatsu K, Chen DJ. WRN participates in translesion synthesis pathway through interaction with NBS1. Mech Ageing Dev. 2010 Jun;131(6) 436-444.

[87] Huertas P. DNA resection in eukaryotes: deciding how to fix the break. Nat Struct Mol Biol. 2010 Jan;17(1) 11-16.

[88] Langerak P, Russell P. Regulatory networks integrating cell cycle control with DNA damage checkpoints and double-strand break repair. Philos Trans R Soc Lond B Biol Sci. 2011 Dec 27;366(1584) 3562-3571.

[89] You Z, Shi LZ, Zhu Q, Wu P, Zhang YW, Basilio A, Tonnu N, Verma IM, Berns MW, Hunter T. CtIP links DNA double-strand break sensing to resection. Mol Cell. 2009 Dec 25;36(6) 954-969.

[90] Gravel S, Chapman JR, Magill C, Jackson SP. DNA helicases Sgs1 and BLM promote DNA double-strand break resection. Genes Dev. 2008 Oct 15;22(20) 2767-2772.

[91] Sartori AA, Lukas C, Coates J, Mistrik M, Fu S, Bartek J, Baer R, Lukas J, Jackson SP. Human CtIP promotes DNA end resection. Nature. 2007 Nov 22;450(7169) 509-514.

[92] Paull TT. Making the best of the loose ends: Mre11/Rad50 complexes and Sae2 promote DNA double-strand break resection. DNA Repair (Amst). 2010 Dec 10;9(12) 1283-1291.

[93] Huertas P, Cortes-Ledesma F, Sartori AA, Aguilera A, Jackson SP. CDK targets Sae2 to control DNA-end resection and homologous recombination. Nature. 2008 Oct 2;455(7213) 689-692.

[94] Huertas P, Jackson SP. Human CtIP mediates cell cycle control of DNA end resection and double strand break repair. J Biol Chem. 2009 Apr 3;284(14) 9558-9565.

[95] Falck J, Forment JV, Coates J, Mistrik M, Lukas J, Bartek J, Jackson SP. CDK targeting of NBS1 promotes DNA-end resection, replication restart and homologous recombination. EMBO Rep. 2012 May 8.

[96] Moore JK, Haber JE. Cell cycle and genetic requirements of two pathways of nonhomologous end-joining repair of double-strand breaks in Saccharomyces cerevisiae. Mol Cell Biol. 1996 May;16(5) 2164-2173.

[97] Huang J, Dynan WS. Reconstitution of the mammalian DNA double-strand break end-joining reaction reveals a requirement for an Mre11/Rad50/NBS1-containing fraction. Nucleic Acids Res. 2002 Feb 1;30(3) 667-674.

[98] Rass E, Grabarz A, Plo I, Gautier J, Bertrand P, Lopez BS. Role of Mre11 in chromosomal nonhomologous end joining in mammalian cells. Nat Struct Mol Biol. 2009 Aug; 16(8) 819-824.

[99] Dinkelmann M, Spehalski E, Stoneham T, Buis J, Wu Y, Sekiguchi JM, Ferguson DO. Multiple functions of MRN in end-joining pathways during isotype class switching. Nat Struct Mol Biol. 2009 Aug;16(8) 808-813.

[100] Zhang X, Paull TT. The Mre11/Rad50/Xrs2 complex and non-homologous end-joining of incompatible ends in S. cerevisiae. DNA Repair (Amst). 2005 Nov 21;4(11) 1281-1294.

[101] de Jager M, van Noort J, van Gent DC, Dekker C, Kanaar R, Wyman C. Human Rad50/Mre11 is a flexible complex that can tether DNA ends. Mol Cell. 2001 Nov;8(5) 1129-1135.

[102] Moreno-Herrero F, de Jager M, Dekker NH, Kanaar R, Wyman C, Dekker C. Mesoscale conformational changes in the DNA-repair complex Rad50/Mre11/Nbs1 upon binding DNA. Nature. 2005 Sep 15;437(7057) 440-443.

[103] Hopfner KP, Craig L, Moncalian G, Zinkel RA, Usui T, Owen BA, Karcher A, Henderson B, Bodmer JL, McMurray CT, Carney JP, Petrini JH, Tainer JA. The Rad50 zinc-hook is a structure joining Mre11 complexes in DNA recombination and repair. Nature. 2002 Aug 1;418(6897) 562-566.

[104] Park YB, Chae J, Kim YC, Cho Y. Crystal structure of human Mre11: understanding tumorigenic mutations. Structure. 2011 Nov 9;19(11) 1591-1602.

[105] Wyman C, Lebbink J, Kanaar R. Mre11-Rad50 complex crystals suggest molecular calisthenics. DNA Repair (Amst). 2011 Oct 10;10(10) 1066-1070.

[106] Mockel C, Lammens K, Schele A, Hopfner KP. ATP driven structural changes of the bacterial Mre11:Rad50 catalytic head complex. Nucleic Acids Res. 2012 Jan;40(2) 914-927.

[107] Lim HS, Kim JS, Park YB, Gwon GH, Cho Y. Crystal structure of the Mre11-Rad50-ATPgammaS complex: understanding the interplay between Mre11 and Rad50. Genes Dev. 2011 May 15;25(10) 1091-1104.

[108] van der Linden E, Sanchez H, Kinoshita E, Kanaar R, Wyman C. RAD50 and NBS1 form a stable complex functional in DNA binding and tethering. Nucleic Acids Res. 2009 Apr;37(5) 1580-1588.

[109] Hohl M, Kwon Y, Galvan SM, Xue X, Tous C, Aguilera A, Sung P, Petrini JH. The Rad50 coiled-coil domain is indispensable for Mre11 complex functions. Nat Struct Mol Biol. 2011 Oct;18(10) 1124-1131.

[110] Wiltzius JJ, Hohl M, Fleming JC, Petrini JH. The Rad50 hook domain is a critical determinant of Mre11 complex functions. Nat Struct Mol Biol. 2005 May;12(5) 403-407.

[111] Hentges P, Ahnesorg P, Pitcher RS, Bruce CK, Kysela B, Green AJ, Bianchi J, Wilson TE, Jackson SP, Doherty AJ. Evolutionary and functional conservation of the DNA non-homologous end-joining protein, XLF/Cernunnos. J Biol Chem. 2006 Dec 8;281(49) 37517-37526.

[112] Ahnesorg P, Smith P, Jackson SP. XLF interacts with the XRCC4-DNA ligase IV complex to promote DNA nonhomologous end-joining. Cell. 2006 Jan 27;124(2) 301-313.

[113] Tsai CJ, Kim SA, Chu G. Cernunnos/XLF promotes the ligation of mismatched and noncohesive DNA ends. Proc Natl Acad Sci U S A. 2007 May 8;104(19) 7851-7856.

[114] Grawunder U, Zimmer D, Leiber MR. DNA ligase IV binds to XRCC4 via a motif located between rather than within its BRCT domains. Curr Biol. 1998 Jul 16;8(15) 873-876.

[115] Drouet J, Delteil C, Lefrancois J, Concannon P, Salles B, Calsou P. DNA-dependent protein kinase and XRCC4-DNA ligase IV mobilization in the cell in response to DNA double strand breaks. J Biol Chem. 2005 Feb 25;280(8) 7060-7069.

[116] Yano K, Morotomi-Yano K, Lee KJ, Chen DJ. Functional significance of the interaction with Ku in DNA double-strand break recognition of XLF. FEBS Lett. 2011 Mar 23;585(6) 841-846.

[117] Junop MS, Modesti M, Guarne A, Ghirlando R, Gellert M, Yang W. Crystal structure of the Xrcc4 DNA repair protein and implications for end joining. EMBO J. 2000 Nov 15;19(22) 5962-5970.

[118] Andres SN, Modesti M, Tsai CJ, Chu G, Junop MS. Crystal structure of human XLF: a twist in nonhomologous DNA end-joining. Mol Cell. 2007 Dec 28;28(6) 1093-1101.

[119] Hammel M, Yu Y, Fang S, Lees-Miller SP, Tainer JA. XLF regulates filament architecture of the XRCC4.ligase IV complex. Structure. 2010 Nov 10;18(11) 1431-1442.

[120] Yano K, Chen DJ. Live cell imaging of XLF and XRCC4 reveals a novel view of protein assembly in the non-homologous end-joining pathway. Cell Cycle. 2008 May 15;7(10) 1321-1325.

[121] Malivert L, Ropars V, Nunez M, Drevet P, Miron S, Faure G, Guerois R, Mornon JP, Revy P, Charbonnier JB, Callebaut I, de Villartay JP. Delineation of the Xrcc4-interacting region in the globular head domain of cernunnos/XLF. J Biol Chem. 2010 Aug 20;285(34) 26475-26483.

[122] Sibanda BL, Critchlow SE, Begun J, Pei XY, Jackson SP, Blundell TL, Pellegrini L. Crystal structure of an Xrcc4-DNA ligase IV complex. Nat Struct Biol. 2001 Dec;8(12) 1015-1019.

[123] Recuero-Checa MA, Dore AS, Arias-Palomo E, Rivera-Calzada A, Scheres SH, Maman JD, Pearl LH, Llorca O. Electron microscopy of Xrcc4 and the DNA ligase IV-Xrcc4 DNA repair complex. DNA Repair (Amst). 2009 Dec 3;8(12) 1380-1389.

[124] Modesti M, Junop MS, Ghirlando R, van de Rakt M, Gellert M, Yang W, Kanaar R. Tetramerization and DNA ligase IV interaction of the DNA double-strand break repair protein XRCC4 are mutually exclusive. J Mol Biol. 2003 Nov 21;334(2) 215-228.

[125] Dahm K. Role and regulation of human XRCC4-like factor/cernunnos. J Cell Biochem. 2008 Aug 1;104(5) 1534-1540.

[126] Roy S, Andres SN, Vergnes A, Neal JA, Xu Y, Yu Y, Lees-Miller SP, Junop M, Modesti M, Meek K. XRCC4's interaction with XLF is required for coding (but not signal) end joining. Nucleic Acids Res. 2012 Feb;40(4) 1684-1694.

[127] Ochi T, Wu Q, Chirgadze DY, Grossmann JG, Bolanos-Garcia VM, Blundell TL. Structural Insights into the Role of Domain Flexibility in Human DNA Ligase IV. Structure. 2012 Jul 3;20(7) 1212-1222.

[128] Perry JJ, Asaithamby A, Barnebey A, Kiamanesch F, Chen DJ, Han S, Tainer JA, Yannone SM. Identification of a coiled coil in werner syndrome protein that facilitates multimerization and promotes exonuclease processivity. J Biol Chem. 2010 Aug 13;285(33) 25699-25707.

[129] Bernstein KA, Gangloff S, Rothstein R. The RecQ DNA helicases in DNA repair. Annu Rev Genet. 2010;44 393-417.

[130] Wang H, Shao Z, Shi LZ, Hwang PY, Truong LN, Berns MW, Chen DJ, Wu X. CtIP Protein Dimerization Is Critical for Its Recruitment to Chromosomal DNA Double-stranded Breaks. J Biol Chem. 2012 Jun 15;287(25) 21471-21480.

[131] Yoo S, Dynan WS. Geometry of a complex formed by double strand break repair proteins at a single DNA end: recruitment of DNA-PKcs induces inward translocation of Ku protein. Nucleic Acids Res. 1999 Dec 15;27(24) 4679-4686.

[132] Palm W, de Lange T. How shelterin protects mammalian telomeres. Annu Rev Genet. 2008;42 301-334.

[133] Goggins M, Schutte M, Lu J, Moskaluk CA, Weinstein CL, Petersen GM, Yeo CJ, Jackson CE, Lynch HT, Hruban RH, Kern SE. Germline BRCA2 gene mutations in patients with apparently sporadic pancreatic carcinomas. Cancer Res. 1996 Dec 1;56(23) 5360-5364.

[134] Lynch HT, de la Chapelle A. Hereditary colorectal cancer. N Engl J Med. 2003 Mar 6;348(10) 919-932.

[135] Hsu FM, Zhang S, Chen BP. Role of DNA-dependent protein kinase catalytic subunit in cancer development and treatment. Transl Cancer Res. 2012 Jun 1;1(1) 22-34.

[136] Hayashi J, Sakata KI, Someya M, Matsumoto Y, Satoh M, Nakata K, Hori M, Takagi M, Kondoh A, Himi T, Hareyama M. Analysis and results of Ku and XRCC4 expression in hypopharyngeal cancer tissues treated with chemoradiotherapy. Oncol Lett. 2012 Jul;4(1) 151-155.

[137] Yuan SS, Hou MF, Hsieh YC, Huang CY, Lee YC, Chen YJ, Lo S. Role of MRE11 in Cell Proliferation, Tumor Invasion, and DNA Repair in Breast Cancer. J Natl Cancer Inst. 2012 Aug 22.

[138] Saenz JB, Doggett TA, Haslam DB. Identification and characterization of small molecules that inhibit intracellular toxin transport. Infect Immun. 2007 Sep;75(9) 4552-4561.

[139] Wang Y, Ghosh G, Hendrickson EA. Ku86 represses lethal telomere deletion events in human somatic cells. Proc Natl Acad Sci U S A. 2009 Jul 28;106(30) 12430-12435.

Chapter 3

Epimutation in DNA Mismatch Repair (MMR) Genes

Kouji Banno, Iori Kisu, Megumi Yanokura,
Yuya Nogami, Kiyoko Umene, Kosuke Tsuji,
Kenta Masuda, Arisa Ueki, Nobuyuki Susumu and
Daisuke Aoki

Additional information is available at the end of the chapter

http://dx.doi.org/10.5772/53812

1. Introduction

Generally, disease susceptibility is determined based on changes not only in DNA sequences but also in the activities of genes and chromosomal regions. Epigenetic regulation has attracted attention as a mechanism underlying changes of activities of genes and chromosomal regions. Epigenetic modification regulates gene activity and is essential for cell division and histogenesis. Genetically, phenotype diversity of identical cells is thought to be caused by differences in epigenetic profiles. Epimutations have also recently been recognized as the first step of tumorigenesis of cancers and are thought to be direct dispositions to cancers [1].

2. What is epimutation?

Epimutation affects one or both alleles and decreases the gene product by inhibiting transcription. Tumor cells are typical examples of the results of epimutation that occurs at a high frequency in mammals. Epimutation in cancer generally occurs in somatic cells with tumor progression. Various epimutations are present in cancers and are frequently observed in tumor suppressor genes [1-4].

Germline epimutation which occurs in germ cells is defined as those changes maintained in fertilization and embryogenesis and present in all somatic cells in the mature body. Transmission of epigenetic characteristics through generations has been reported. The cancer risk is similar in individuals carrying a germline epimutation. However, epimutation is not necessarily inherited, and inheritance patterns that do not follow Mendel's laws have been reported [5-8]. Complete elimination of epimutation in spermatogenesis has also been shown [9]. Only inheritance of maternal epimutation has been confirmed, suggesting that elimination of epimutation in oogenesis is less likely to occur [8-9]. Several genomic imprinting-associated somatic cell abnormalities are thought to be caused by germline epimutation [4]. Constitutional epimutation is defined as those changes observed in all tissues in the body due to occurrence in an early step of embryogenesis before differentiation into the three germ layers. Not all cells possess this type of epimutation, leading to a mosaic pattern at the cell level, and it is unclear if this epimutation is transmitted from the previous generation. All epimutation types are a first step leading to tumorigenesis and may be direct causes of carcinogenesis [1].

3. Germline epimutation and disease

Epimutation is not only involved in cancer, but is also observed in genomic imprinting (Table 1). Since a gene transmitted from one parent is selectively expressed in genomic imprinting, a hereditary disease develops when the gene is defective, even though the allelic gene is normal. The characteristic phenotype of genomic imprinting is maintained by imprinting control centers (ICs). ICs are short sequences present in the gene to be imprinted. Hemiallelic methylation of ICs results in transcription of the other allele, controlling imprinting [1]. Diverse gene aberrations in these ICs, such as micro defects, have been discovered, and these are considered to be the causes of epimutations observed in very rare neurobehavioral congenital familial diseases such as Angelman syndrome (AS), Prader-Willi syndrome (PWS), and Beckwith-Wiedemann syndrome (BWS). PWS is characterized by hypotonia in the neonatal period, increased appetite, overeating and subsequent obesity after infancy, characteristic desires, mild mental retardation, and hypoplasia of the external genitalia. In contrast, AS is characterized by severe mental retardation, epilepsy, and awkward movement. However, the causative genetic locus is located in the q11-q13 region on the long arm of chromosome 15 in both diseases. PWS and AS are caused by chromosomal 15q11q13 deletion in many cases, but there are a few cases of imprinting mutation causing abnormal genomic imprinting. In imprinting mutation, the parental chromosome is normal, but the imprinting of 15q11-q13 is changed to the opposite pattern. Familial cases of imprinting mutations are known, and minute deletions upstream of the *SNURF-SNRPN* gene, which has ICs in PWS and AS, have been described [10]. However, ICs are resistant to minute changes or contain several extra elements, and most imprinting mutations are thought to occur due to epimutation after fertilization [11].

BWS is a congenital disease with a high reported risk of embryonal fetal tumors, such as Wilms tumor, hepatoblastoma, and rhabdomyosarcoma. The p15.5 region on the short arm of chromosome 11 (11p15.5) has been identified as the causative locus. There are two imprinting domains in 11p15.5: the *Cyclin-dependent kinase inhibitor 1C/KCNQ1 opposite antisense transcript 1(CDKN1C/KCNQ1OT1)* domain and the *Insulin-like growth factor 2(IGF2)/H19* domain, and expression of the imprinting gene near the domain is controlled by the respective imprinting regulation region. *CDKN1C* expression is decreased due to DNA hypomethylation of the *CDKN1C/KCNQ1OT1* domain in about 30-50% of BWS cases, and *IGF2* expression is enhanced due to DNA hypermethylation of the *IGF2/H19* domain in about 5-10% [12]. Silver-Russell syndrome (SRS) is characterized by intrauterine growth restriction and severe failure to thrive after birth, and epimutation of the *H19* gene in 11p15.5 is the cause of this disease [13]. *IGF2* and *H19* are regulated by a common enhancer present in the terminal end of the short arm of chromosome 11. Normally, sperm-derived *H19–DMR* is methylated and ovum-derived *H19–DMR* is not methylated. The enhancer acts on *IGF2* because CTCF protein cannot bind to methylated DMR in the former case, whereas it acts on *H19* because CTCF protein binds to non-methylated DMR in the latter. Hypomethylation of sperm-derived H19-DMR due to epimutation causes the gene to behave similarly to the maternal domain and induces underexpression of *IGF2* and overexpression of *H19*, causing SRS due to *IGF2* underexpression [14]. Thus, these diseases are thought to develop due to aberration in ICs.

Gene name	Epimutation type	Disease
hMLH1	germline, constitutional	Lynch syndrome
hMSH2	germline	Lynch syndrome
DAPK1	unknown	B-cell CLL
HBA2	unknown	α-Thalassemia
BRCA2	constitutional	Sporadic breast cancer
KIP2/LIT1	unknown	Beckwith-Wiedemann syndrome
IGF2	unknown	Beckwith-Wiedemann syndrome
H19	unknown	Silver-Russell syndrome

Table 1. Epimutation and disease

Epimutation also occurs due to genomic changes, such as insertion, deletion, and changes in the length of tandem repeat sequences, which are termed copy number variations (CNVs) [15]. In α-thalassemia, another well-known epimutation-associated disease, the deleted region of the *LUC7-like (LUC7L)* gene is close to an α-globin gene, *hemoglobin alpha 2 (HBA2)*, leading to methylation of the *HBA2* gene promoter [16].

4. Epimutation of DNA mismatch repair genes

A study on familial cancer showed that a gene group inactivated by mutation in characteristic regions produces a predisposition to cancer. Mutation of a tumor suppressor gene, *Retinoblastoma (RB)*, provided the first evidence of a causative gene in hereditary cancer [17]. Subsequently, Nishishou et al. reported mutation of *Adenomatous polyposis coli (APC)* in familial adenomatous polyposis [17] and Hussussian et al. found mutation of *Cyclin-dependent kinase inhibitor2A (CDKN2A)* in familial melanoma [19]. As more mutations have been identified in tumor suppressor genes, the various cancer-associated mechanisms of these genes have been elucidated. Relationships of *Breast cancer susceptibility gene 1(BRCA1), MutL protein homolog 1 (MLH1),* and *MutS homologue 2 (MSH2),* all of which are DNA repair genes (DNA mismatch repair: MMR), with predispositions to familial cancers have also been found. Mutation-induced gene inactivation in hereditary cancer is recessively inherited and many carriers have no abnormal phenotype. However, the cancer prevalence shows marked dominant inheritance because mutation, inactivation, and loss of heterozygosity readily occur in the normal allele [1].

Methylation of *RB* was the first reported cancer-inducing epimutation [19-20]. Later, methylation of many other oncogenes, such as *Von Hippel-Lindau (VHL), MLH1, APC,* and *BRCA1,* was shown in sporadic cancers [22-24]. *VHL* mutation is related to primary ciliary function, hemostasis of the extracellular matrix, tumor metabolism, and particularly to clear cell carcinoma [25]. Vaziri et al. examined the *VHL* gene in an analysis of the clonal relationship between the primary tumor and metastatic lesions of clear cell carcinoma in 10 patients. The gene status differed between the primary tumor and the metastatic lesions in 4 patients. In addition, even when the *VHL* genotype differed in another renal primary tumor or among several metastatic lesions within a patient, the *VHL* germline genotype in adjacent normal tissue was always the wild-type germline *VHL* gene in the primary tumor. These findings indicated that the status of *VHL* may differ between the primary tumor and metastatic lesions in clear cell carcinoma [26].

Regarding DNA repair genes, methylation of *MLH1* and *MSH2* has been reported to cause Lynch syndrome (hereditary non-polyposis colorectal cancer (HNPCC)). This methylation is also known as a predisposition to characteristic cancers, such as those in the endometrium, small intestine, and ovary, in addition to colon cancer. Both genes encode mismatch repair proteins and inactivation of these proteins is thought to induce microsatellite instability (MSI) in tumors [27]. MSI frequently occurs in endometrial cancer and accumulation of MSI-induced gene mutations plays a major role in carcinogenesis [28]. It has since been discovered that *MLH1* may also be methylated in sporadic colorectal cancer. In an investigation of methylation of the *MLH1* promoter in 110 patients with sporadic early-onset colorectal cancer, Auclair et al. found methylation in 55 (50%) and also observed decreased *MLH1* expression due to hypermethylation, which was present in 7.4% of all patients, suggesting that constitutional epimutation is the fundamental mechanism inducing early-onset colorectal cancer [29]. The phenotype of sporadic colorectal cancer with *MLH1* methylation is the same as that of mismatch repair defects, and the clinicopathological characteristics are similar to those of a hereditary tumor. *MLH1* methylation occurs in sporadic colorectal cancer at a high frequency [23] and is strongly related to cancers showing the CpG island methylator phenotype (CIMP). Methylation of CpG islands, which are characteristic of promoter regions, has been shown to occur at a high frequency in CIMP-positive cancer [30]. These cancers arise mainly from the ascending colon and have a particularly high incidence in elderly women.

Gazzoli et al. first demonstrated that *MLH1* may be methylated in peripheral blood, as in tumors, in colorectal cancer patients [31]. In an investigation of 14 Lynch syndrome patients with MSI, no mismatch repair gene methylation was noted in any patient, but hypermethylation (about 50%) of *MLH1* was discovered in normal blood DNA in a 25-year-old female patient [31]. This allelic methylation in unrelated tissue derived from the embryologically different germ layer indicated that the methylation may be constitutional or germline. No conclusion could be reached with regard to the heredity of this epimutation because no mutation was detected in parental tissue, but the occurrence of methylation so early in life is of interest. A later study clarified that constitutional methylation occurs in colorectal cancer patients with hemiallelic methylation of *MLH1* [32], in 2 colorectal cancer patients. Tissues from parents were unavailable, but no methylation was observed in tissues in 4 of 5 children of these patients.

It remains unclear whether constitutional epimutation is transmitted from the mother or father or occurs *de novo* in early embryogenesis [1]. Crepin et al. investigated constitutional epimutations of *MLH1* and *MSH2* and defective *EPCAM* in 134 germline mutation-free patients with suspected Lynch syndrome, and found *MLH1* constitutional epimutation in 2 patients. One was a female patient, and her 2 children (one male and one female) developed early-onset colorectal cancer, suggesting that *MLH1* constitutional epimutation is related to inheritance. In addition, somatic cell *BRAF* mutation was found in one child, indicating that cancers in patients *with MLH1* constitutional epimutation are similar to *MSI-high* sporadic cancers [33]. In addition to reports supporting inheritance from the mother, Goel et al. described cases of epimutation of the paternal allele, in which analysis of the genotype showed that the inactivated T allele was inherited from the father [34]. Miyukura et al. showed that complete methylation of the *MLH1* promoter region plays an important role in inactivation of *MLH1* in sporadic colorectal cancer patients with high MSI [35]. This complete methylation was induced in both alleles, and methylation upstream of the *MLH1* promoter region was also observed in normal large intestinal mucosa adjacent to the cancer in one-third of colorectal cancer patients with complete methylation [36]. Subsequently, Miyukura et al. surveyed methylation of the *MLH1* promoter region in peripheral blood lymphocytes in 30 patients with sporadic early-onset colorectal cancer or multiple primary cancers, and found complete methylation of the *MLH1* promoter region in peripheral blood lymphocytes (PBLs) in 4 patients (early-onset sporadic colorectal cancer: 2, multiple cancers including colorectal cancer: 1, multiple cancers including cancer of the uterine body: 1) [37]. This was hemiallelic methylation. In one of the patients with early-onset sporadic colorectal cancer, no methylation was detected in a sister's PBLs. MSI was confirmed in all patients and methylation was also observed in the normal large intestine, gastrointestinal mucosa, endometrium, and bone marrow in 3. Interestingly, loss of heterozygosity (LOH), loss of the G allele of the *MLH1* locus in somatic cells, and biallelic methylation were observed when both alleles of *MLH1* in colorectal cancer were investigated, and these findings are consistent with the germline epimutation-associated cancerization mechanism based on Knudsen's "two hit" hypothesis proposed by Suter et al. (Figure 1) [31]. Furthermore, according to Kantelinen et al., variants of uncertain significance (VUS) of the mature hereditary MMR gene present in some colorectal cancer patients may form pairs with other MMR gene VUS and indirectly induce MMR deficiency. An analysis of 8 pairs of MMR gene mutations carried by cancer patients showed aberrations in 2 pairs. Pairs with *MSH2* may increase the cancer risk by reducing the repair ability of the *wild-type MSH2* by half. Two *MSH6* mutations were MMR defects [38]. *MLH1* VUS has also been reported to influence mRNA transcription and impair MMR activity [39].

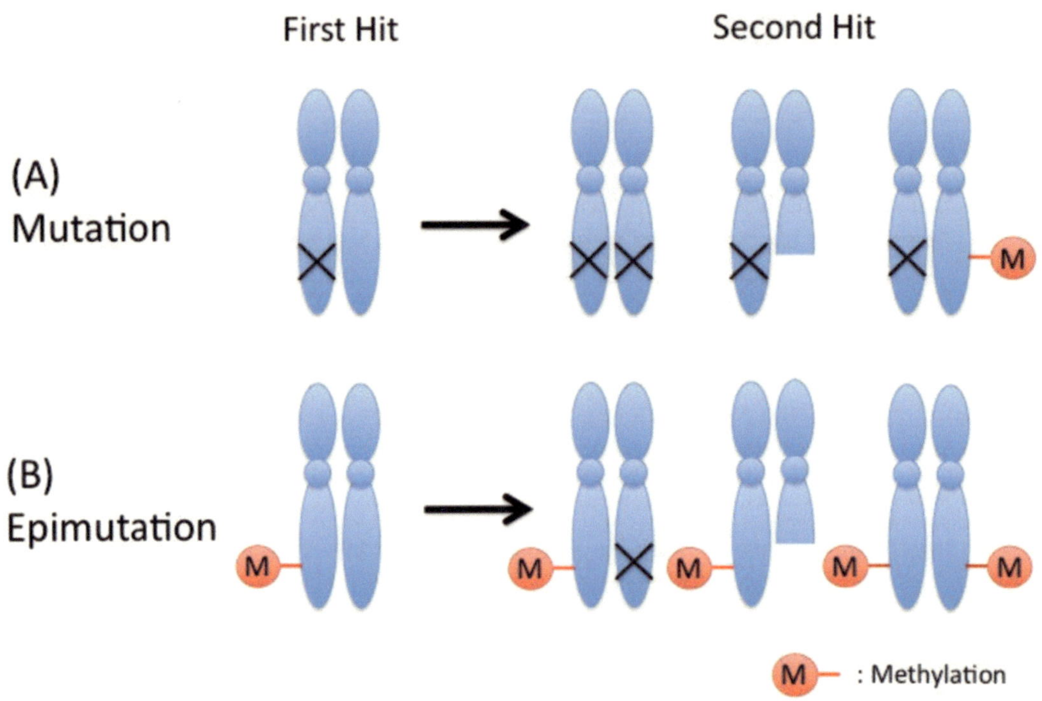

Figure 1. Mechanisms of epimutation in induction of cancer. (A) Germ cell mutation of tumor suppressor genes. (B) Germ cell epimutation of tumor suppressor genes. Somatic cell mutation, heterozygote loss, and other allele epimutations are triggers that induce tumorigenesis.

Allelic methylation is noted in many cases of Lynch syndrome, but there are some exceptions. Wu et al. investigated germline methylation of *MLH1* in 140 gastric cancer patients with a familial medical history. *MLH1* promoter methylation was detected in peripheral blood DNA in only 0.7% of the gastric cancer patients, and the methylation pattern of these patients was mosaic. Mosaic germline epimutation of *MLH1* occurs in familial gastric cancer, although the incidence is low [40]. Hitchins et al. found allelic *MLH1* epimutation in 2 cases in an investigation of constitutional *MLH1* methylation in white blood cell DNA in 122 ethnically diverse South African subjects aged ≤50 years old with early-onset colorectal cancer, with a few alleles showing a mosaic pattern [41].

Epimutation is not always inherited and inheritance patterns that do not follow Mendel's laws have been reported [5-8]. Complete elimination of epimutation in spermatogenesis has also been shown. Only inheritance of maternal epimutation has been found in previous reports, suggesting that elimination of epimutation in oogenesis is less likely to occur [8-9]. In a cohort study of 160 Lynch syndrome patients without germline mutation of mismatch repair genes, constitutive *MLH1* methylation was induced in only one patient, and no *MLH1* methylation was found in the parents or siblings of this patient, indicating that clinicopathological characteristics are better indices than familial medical history for identification of constitutional epimutation of tumor suppressor genes in cancer patients [5]. In addition, Pineda et al. reported that it is useful to screen for *MLH1* methylation in lymphocyte DNA in patients with Lynch syndrome-related tumor with early *MLH1* methylation to judge the presence of epimutation [42].

Epimutation is also related to chronic lymphocytic leukemia (CLL), in which apoptosis of leukemia cells is strongly inhibited. Apoptosis inhibition in CLL is caused by enhanced B-cell lymphoma 2 (BCL2) production and methylation of the *Death-associated protein kinase1* (*DAPK1*) promoter region [44]. *DAPK1* was identified as a familial tumor suppressor gene and the *DAPK1* promoter region is methylated in CLL [44]. This methylation increases Homeobox B7 (HOXB7) protein binding upstream of the promoter region and 75% of *DAPK1* genes in the allele are downregulated. Methylation-induced *DAPK1* inactivation causes both familial and sporadic CLL, whereas hypomethylation of *DAPK1* in peripheral blood mononuclear cells (PBMCs) of healthy subjects has been reported [45]. An association of this hypomethylation with CLL has yet to be shown.

A recent study showed that a specific MMR gene is involved in regulation of cellular dynamics, such as apoptosis. Therefore, the action of specific MMR gene expression of *MSH2* and *MLH1* may also be important in resistance to cytotoxic drugs used in chemotherapy, such as cisplatin [46]. However, it has also been shown that MMR inactivation is not related to inherent cisplatin resistance of cells, suggesting that MMR inactivation may have a role in acquired drug resistance [47]. Involvement of impairment of the MMR pathway in aging of hematopoietic stem and precursor cells has also been reported. Kenyon et al. investigated MSI and MMR gene expression in hematopoietic stem, precursor, and colony-forming cells, and found that there were many *CD34(+)* precursors with MSI lacking *MLH1* expression and protein in hematopoietic colony-forming cells in subjects aged ≥45 years old, compared to younger subjects [48].

There have been many reports on the relationship of breast cancer with *BRCA1* mutation. Armes and Lakhani et al. showed that breast cancer arising in patients with germline *BRCA1* mutation has histological characteristics such as a high mitotic count and lymphocyte infiltration. This morphology is now referred to as the basal-like type, and Foulkes et al. found that this type accounted for 80-90% of cancers arising in germline *BRCA1* mutation carriers [49]. Methylation in the *BRCA1* promoter region in sporadic breast cancer was subsequently discovered [50] and this led to many studies on the association between *BRCA1* mutation and methylation. Under the hypothesis that a sporadic tumor with *BRCA1* methylation should be similar to tumors with *BRCA1* mutation if *BRCA1* methylation induces tumorigenesis, Cattear and Morris et al. reported that sporadic tumors with *BRCA1* methylation have pathological characteristics similar to those of hereditary breast cancer with *BRCA1* mutation [51].

Hedenfalk et al. also showed that the overall phenotypes of the gene were similar between the two breast cancer types [52]. Tumors accompanied by *BRCA1* methylation have a high grade, are negative for estrogen and progesterone receptors, and have a high incidence in young women. These features are referred to as *BRCA1*-like characteristics. Hedenfalk et al. also found *BRCA1* methylation at high frequencies of 67% in medullary carcinoma and 55% in mucinous carcinoma, and these histologic types were noted at high frequency in family lines carrying *BRCA1* mutations [52]. Recently, Snell et al. discovered methylation of the *BRCA1* promoter region in normal tissue of breast cancer patients with the *BRCA1*-like characteristic histologic type [53]. No germline mutation of *BRCA1* or *BRCA2* was detected in these patients. These findings suggest constitutional epimutation of *BRCA1* in breast cancer patients. It is thought that *BRCA1* methylation is the first hit and subsequent deletion of both *BRCA1* genes then leads to the characteristic tumor pathology [1].

MMR gene mutation-induced breast cancer in Lynch syndrome has also recently been described by Buerki et al. [54] in an investigation of 70 unrelated families with Lynch syndrome. The subjects were 632 females, of whom 51 and 40 carried *MLH1* and *MSH2* mutations, respectively. MMR impairment was detected in 85.7% (6/7) of molecular test-applicable breast cancer patients. Combined with information from related reports, *MSI* was present in 70.3% (26/37) of breast cancer patients with *MLH1* or *MSH2* mutation, and altered MMR protein expression was noted in 72.7% (16/22) [54]. Lotsair et al. also found that the ratio of breast cancer cases with MMR protein deficiency and *MSI*-induced MMR impairment was markedly higher in MMR mutant cases than in a non-mutant group. These findings suggest that MMR dysfunction is closely related to the development of breast cancer in Lynch syndrome. However, the development pattern and onset age of breast cancer in patients with MMR mutation are similar to those in general breast cancer patients without mutation. Moreover, the frequency of MMR protein deficiency is lower than those in other Lynch syndrome-related cancers [55].

5. Epimutation and Lynch syndrome

Lynch syndrome (HNPCC) is a typical familial tumor transmitted through autosomal dominant inheritance, and is observed in about 3% of cases of colorectal cancer [56]. MMR gene aberration is involved in carcinogenesis in Lynch syndrome. Six types of MMR genes have been cloned: *MSH2, MLH1, MutS protein homolog 3 (MSH3), MutS protein homolog 6 (MSH6), Postmeiotic segregation increased 1 (PMS1),* and *Postmeiotic segregation increased 1 (PMS2)*. Mutations of 3 of these genes (*MSH2, MLH1,* and *MSH6*) in family lines with Lynch syndrome have been reported [57], with *MSH2* and *MLH1* aberrations accounting for about 90%, and *MSH6* and *PMS2* gene aberrations accounted for only 7 and 1% of cases, respectively [57]. Thus, *MLH1* and *MSH2* mutations are particularly associated with Lynch syndrome. These mutations are also predispositions to cancers in the endometrium, small intestine, and ovary [1]. Both genes encode mismatch repair proteins, and inactivation of these proteins is thought to induce MSI in tumors [27]. Since microsatellites (short-tandem repeats, STRs) are generally present in non-coding regions, mutations in STRs do not lead to abnormal protein production. However, some STRs are present in regions with important genes, such as those encoding *BCL2-associated X protein (BAX)*, which is involved in apoptosis induction, *Insulin-like growth factor 2 receptor (IGF2R)*, which is associated with inhibition of cell proliferation, and mutations in these regions are thought to be involved in cancerization of cells [1].

Typical cases of Lynch syndrome-related ovarian cancer develop early, and the tumor is FIGO cancer stage I and non-serous in many cases [58]. Grindedal et al. reported that the prognosis of Lynch syndrome-related invasive ovarian cancer is better than that of invasive cancer in patients carrying a *BRCA1/2* mutation [59]. Regarding endometrial cancer, Shih et al. investigated MMR protein deficiency in 56 women aged ≤40 years old with endometrial cancer, and found abnormal MMR in 9 cases. The families of these 9 patients had a medical history of Lynch syndrome; the mean BMIs were 23.4 and 31.2 in the patients with and without abnormal MMR, respectively; the stage was I in 80% of the cases in the patients without abnormal MMR, but ≥II in 90% of those with abnormal MMR; muscular layer and lymph vascular invasions were noted in many cases with abnormal MMR; and the 5-year/5-year exacerbation-free survival rate was 70% [60]. Many pathological aspects of familial endometrial cancer are unclear despite the high malignancy, and an effective screening method has yet to be established.

Lynch syndrome cases with epimutation of the *MLH1* or *MSH2* promoter region in blood cells without morbid MMR gene mutation have recently been discovered, showing that germline *MLH1* epimutation causes Lynch syndrome. Takahashi et al. reported that *MLH1* protein expression was deficient in Lynch syndrome patients carrying a germline mutation in the 5' splice site of *MLH1*, and that mutation of this intron of *MLH1* induced aberrant splicing, influencing the onset of Lynch syndrome [62]. In family lines with *MSH2* methylation, germline mutation of the *Epithelial cell adhesion molecule (EPCAM)* gene present upstream of *MSH2* has been reported to be the cause of epimutation. *EPCAM* is strongly expressed in epithelial tissue and cancers [63] and a defective 3'-terminal of this gene causes read-through to *MSH2*, resulting in hypermethylation of the CpG island promoter [64]. Interestingly, no *MSH2* methylation in any other cancer has been reported to date. In contrast to the allelic methylation found in many patients with constitutional methylation of *MLH1*, allelic methylation of *MSH2* occurs in only about 50%. This methylation level is also dependent on the tissues examined. Unlike *MLH1* epimutation, inheritance of *MSH2* methylation following Mendel's laws has been reported. In Lynch syndrome caused by these epimutations, methylation levels vary among epimutation carriers in the same family line and among tissues within the same patient [1]. In addition, the *MLH1* and *MSH2* mutations show racial differences. In a comparison of Asian and Western subjects based on International Society of Gastrointestinal Hereditary (InSiGHT) data, Wei et al. found differences in mutations in the regions containing *MLH1* and *MSH2*, with some mutations found to be more frequent or to be present only in Asian subjects [65]. This indicates the importance of consideration of racial differences in evaluating mutations in screening [65].

6. Conclusion

Epimutation has diverse characteristics: some epimutations are inherited or eliminated in embryogenesis, while others are inherited in patterns that do not follow Mendel's laws. Cancers associated with epimutations include Lynch syndrome (HNPCC), familial colorectal cancer, CLL, breast cancer, and ovarian cancer. Defined histological characteristics of epimutation-associated tumors have been suggested, and it is possible that the histologic type of cancers will ultimately be identifiable based on the methylation pattern detected in normal tissue, which may reduce the need for invasive tests such as tumor tissue biopsy [1]. Furthermore, elucidation of differences in the methylation pattern between healthy subjects and cancer patients may facilitate low-invasive cancer risk evaluation in healthy individuals.

To develop these techniques, it will be important to identify the causes of methylation. The extent of variation of methylation in normal somatic cell tissues within an individual is unclear, but conservation of the methylation pattern in an individual has been shown [1]. Different DNA methylation patterns in monozygotic twins have been observed, and the difference increased as the twins lived in different environments [66]. Aging-dependent methylation of non-methylated CpG islands has also been shown, and it has been suggested that metabolite ingestion can influence methyl metabolism, such as metabolism of folic acid, choline, vitamin B12, and betaine, and change the methylation pattern. In particular, the influence of environmental factors in early embryogenesis may serve as a predisposition to cancers and other diseases associated with epigenetic changes [67]. Methylation is influenced by environmental factors and aging, in addition to inheritance, as described above, and further studies on the association of these factors with epimutation are required.

Improvement of epigenetic aberration has also been attempted through induction of re-expression of tumor suppressor genes, with some success using DNA methyltransferase (DNMT) inhibitors, azacitidine and decitabine, for blood malignant tumors [68]. However, intense epigenetic therapy using a DNMT inhibitor and a histone deacetylase (HDAC) inhibitor concomitantly did not achieve complete chromosome remodeling, and stable gene re-expression was not obtained [9]. Moreover, reinhibition of re-expressed genes has occurred after suspension of epigenetic therapy in many studies. These findings indicate that there are many problems to be overcome in development of epigenetic therapy.

Acknowledgments

The authors gratefully acknowledge grant support from the Japan Society for the Promotion of Science (JSPS) through a Grant-in-Aid for Scientific Research (KAKENHI), a Grant-in-Aid for Scientific Research (B) (22390313), a Grant-in-Aid for Scientific Research (C) (22591866), and a Grant-in-Aid for Young Scientists (B) (21791573); the Ichiro Kanehara Foundation; Kobayashi Foundation for Cancer Research; and the Keio University Medical Science Fund through a Research Grant for Life Sciences and Medicine.

Author details

Kouji Banno*, Iori Kisu, Megumi Yanokura, Yuya Nogami, Kiyoko Umene, Kosuke Tsuji, Kenta Masuda, Arisa Ueki, Nobuyuki Susumu and Daisuke Aoki

*Address all correspondence to: kbanno@z7.keio.jp

Department of Obstetrics and Gynecology, School of Medicine, Keio University, Tokyo, Japan

References

[1] Banno K, Kisu I, Yanokura M, Tsuji K, Masuda K, Ueki A, Kobayashi Y, Yamagami W, Nomura H, Tominaga E, Susumu N, Aoki D. Epimutation and cancer: a new carcinogenic mechanism of Lynch syndrome (Review). International Journal of Oncology 2012;41(3) 793-797.

[2] Holliday R. The inheritance of epigenetic defects. Science 1987;238(4824) 163-170.

[3] Das OP, Messing J. Variegated phenotype and developmental methylation changes of a maize allele originating from epimutation. Genetics 1994;136(3) 1121-1141.

[4] Schofield PN, Joyce JA, Lam WK, Grandjean V, Ferguson-Smith A, Reik W, Maher ER. Genomic imprinting and cancer; new paradigms in the genetics of neoplasia. Toxicology Letters 2001;120(1-3) 151-160.

[5] Hitchins M, Williams R, Cheong K, Halani N, Lin VA, Packham D, Ku S, Buckle A, Hawkins N, Burn J, Gallinger S, Goldblatt J, Kirk J, Tomlinson I, Scott R, Spigelman A, Suter C, Martin D, Suthers G, Ward R. MLH1 germline epimutations as a factor in hereditary nonpolyposis colorectal cancer. Gastroenterology 2005;129(5) 1392-1399.

[6] Hitchins MP, Wong JJ, Suthers G, Suter CM, Martin DI, Hawkins NJ, Ward RL. Inheritance of a cancer-associated MLH1 germ-line epimutation. New England Journal of Medicine 2007;356(7) 697-705.

[7] Valle L, Carbonell P, Fernandez V, Dotor AM, Sanz M, Benitez J, Urioste M. MLH1 germline epimutations in selected patients with early-onset non-polyposis colorectal cancer. Clinical Genetics 2007;71(3) 232-237.

[8] Morak M, Schackert HK, Rahner N, Betz B, Ebert M, Walldorf C, Royer-Pokora B, Schulmann K, von Knebel-Doeberitz M, Dietmaier W, Keller G, Kerker B, Leitner G, Holinski-Feder E. Further evidence for heritability of an epimutation in one of 12 cases with MLH1 promoter methylation in blood cells clinically displaying HNPCC. European Journal of Human Genetics 2008;16(7) 804-811.

[9] Hitchins MP, Ward RL. Erasure of MLH1 methylation in spermatozoa-implications for epigenetic inheritance. Nature Genetics 2007;39(11): 1289.

[10] Buiting K, Ssitoh S, Gross S, Dittrich B, Schwartz S, Nicholls R, Horsthemke B. Inherited microdeletions in the Angelman and Prader-Willi syndromes defines an imprinting center on human chromosome 15. Nature Genetics1995;9(4) 395-400.

[11] Karin B, Stephanie G, Christina L, Gabriele G, Osman E, Bernhard H. Epimutations in Prader-willi and Angelman Syndromes: A Molecular Study of 136 Patients with an Imprinting Dfect. American Journal of Human Genetics 2003;72(3) 571-577.

[12] Cooper WN, Luharia A, Evans GA, Raza H, Haire AC, Grundy R, Bowdin SC, Riccio A, Sebastio G, Bliek J, Schofield PN, Reik W, Macdonald F, Maher ER. Molecular subtypes and phenotypic expression of Beckwith-Wiedemann syndrome. European Journal of Human Genetics 2005;13(9) 1025-1032.

[13] Schönherr N, Meyer E, Roos A, Schmidt A, Wollmann HA, Eggermann T. The centromeric 11p15 imprinting centre is also involved in Silver-Russell syndrome. Journal of Medical Genetics 2007; 44(1) 59-63.

[14] Gicquel C, Rossignol S, Cabrol A, Houang M, Steunou V, Barbu V, Danton F, Thibaud N, Merrer M, Burglen L, Bertand A, Netchine I, Bouc Y. Epimutation of the telomeric imprinting center region in chromosome 11q15 in Silver-Russell syndrome. Nature Genetics 2005; 37(9) 1003-1007.

[15] Conrad DF, Pinto D, Redon R, Feuk L, Gokcumen O, Zhang Y, Aerts J, Andrews TD, Barnes C, Campbell P, Fitzgerald T, Hu M, Ihm CH, Kristiansson K, Macarthur DG, Macdonald JR, Onyiah I, Pang AW, Robson S, Stirrups K, Valsesia A, Walter K, Wei J; Wellcome Trust Case Control Consortium, Tyler-Smith C, Carter NP, Lee C, Scherer SW, Hurles ME. Origins and functional impact of copy number variation in the human genome. Nature 2010;464(7289) 704-712.

[16] Tufarelli C, Stanley JA, Garrick D, Sharpe JA, Ayyub H, Wood WG, Higgs DR. Transcription of antisense RNA leading to gene silencing and methylation as a novel cause of human genetic disease. Nature Genetics 2003;34(2) 157-165.

[17] Friend SH, Bernards R, Rogelj S, Weinberg RA, Rapaport JM, Albert DM, Dryja TP. A human DNA segment with properties of the gene that predisposes to retinoblastoma and osteosarcoma. Nature 1986;323(6089) 643-646.

[18] Nishisho I, Nakamura Y, Miyoshi Y, Miki Y, Ando H, Horii A, Koyama K, Utsunomiya J, Baba S, Hedge P: Mutations of chromosome 5q21 genes in FAP and colorectal cancer patients. Science 1991;253(5020): 665-669.

[19] Hussussian CJ, Struewing JP, Goldstein AM, Higgins PA, Ally DS, Sheahan MD, Clark WH Jr, Tucker MA, Dracopoli NC. Germline p16 mutations in familial melanoma. Nature Genetics 1994;8(1) 15-21.

[20] Greger V, Passarge E, Höpping W, Messmer E, Horsthemke B. Epigenetic changes may contribute to the formation and spontaneous regression of retinoblastoma. Human Genetics 1989; 83(2) 155-158.

[21] Sakai T, Toguchida J, Ohtani N, Yandell DW, Rapaport JM, Dryja TP. Allele-specific hypermethylation of the retinoblastoma tumor-suppressor gene. American Journal of Human Genetics 1991; 48(5) 880-888.

[22] Herman JG, Latif F, Weng Y, Lerman MI, Zbar B, Liu S, Samid D, Duan DS, Gnarra JR, Linehan WM. Silencing of the VHL tumor-suppressor gene by DNA methylation in renal carcinoma. Proceeding of the Natlional Academy of Sciences of the United States of America 1994;91(21) 9700-9704.

[23] Kane MF, Loda M, Gaida GM, Lipman J, Mishra R, Goldman H, Jessup JM, Kolodner R. Methylation of the hMLH1 promoter correlates with lack of expression of hMLH1 in sporadic colon tumors and mismatch repair-defective human tumor cell lines. Cancer Research 1997;57(5) 808-811.

[24] Dobrovic A, Simpfendorfer D. Methylation of the BRCA1 gene in sporadic breast cancer. Cancer Research 1997;57(16) 3347-3350.

[25] Jonasch E, Futreal PA, Davis IJ, Bailey ST, Kim WY, Brugarolas J, Giaccia AJ, Kurban G, Pause A, Frydman J, Zurita AJ, Rini BI, Sharma P, Atkins MB, Walker CL, Rathmell WK. State of the Science: An Update on Renal Cell Carcinoma. Molecular Cancer Research 2012 Jun 25.

[26] Vaziri SA, Tavares EJ, Golshayan AR, Rini BI, Aydin H, Zhou M, Sercia L, Wood L, Ganapathi MK, Bukowski RM, Ganapathi R. Differing von Hippel-Lindau genotype in paired primary and metastatic tumors in patients with clear cell renal cell carcinoma. Frontiers in Oncology 2012;2 51.

[27] de la Chapelle A. Genetic predisposition to human disease: allele-specific expression and low-penetrance regulatory loci. Oncogene 2009;28(38) 3345-3348.

[28] Kawaguchi M, Banno K, Yanokura M, Kobayashi Y, Kishimi A, Ogawa S, Kisu I, Nomura H, Hirasawa A, Susumu N, Aoki D. Analysis of candidate target genes for mononucleotide repeat mutation in microsatellite instability-high (MSI-H) endometrial cancer. International Journal of Oncology 2009;35(5) 977-982.

[29] Auclair J, Vaissière T, Desseigne F, Lasset C, Bonadona V, Giraud S, Saurin JC, Joly MO, Leroux D, Faivre L, Audoynaud C, Montmain G, Ruano E, Herceg Z, Puisieux A, Wang Q. Intensity-dependent constitutional MLH1 promoter methylation leads to early onset of colorectal cancer by affecting both alleles. Genes Chromosomes & Cancer 2011;50(3) 178-185.

[30] Weisenberger DJ, Siegmund KD, Campan M, Young J, Long TI, Faasse MA, Kang GH, Widschwendter M, Weener D, Buchanan D, Koh H, Simms L, Barker M, Leggett B, Levine J, Kim M, French AJ, Thibodeau SN, Jass J, Haile R, Laird PW. CpG island methylator phenotype underlies sporadic microsatellite instability and is tightly associated with BRAF mutation in colorectal cancer. Nature Genetics 2006; 38(7) 787-793.

[31] Gazzoli I, Loda M, Garber J, Syngal S, Kolodner RD. A hereditary nonpolyposis colorectal carcinoma case associated with hypermethylation of the MLH1 gene in normal tissue and loss of heterozygosity of the unmethylated allele in the resulting microsatellite instability-high tumor. Cancer Research 2002; 62(14) 3925-3928.

[32] Suter CM, Martin DI, Ward RL. Germline epimutation of MLH1 in individuals with multiple cancerss. Nature Genetics 2004; 36(5) 497-501.

[33] Crepin M, Dieu MC, Lejeune S, Escande F, Boidin D, Porchet N, Morin G, Manouvrier S, Mathieu M, Buisine MP. Evidence of constitutional MLH1 epimutation associated to transgenerational inheritance of cancer susceptibility. Human Mutation 2012; 33(1) 180-188.

[34] Goel A, Nguyen TP, Leung HC, Nagasaka T, Rhees J, Hotchkiss E, Arnold M, Banerji P, Koi M, Kwok CT, Packham D, Lipton L, Boland CR, Ward RL, Hitchins MP. De novo constitutional MLH1 epimutations confer early-onset colorectal cancer in two new sporadic Lynch syndrome cases, with derivation of the epimutation on the paternal allele in one. International Journal of Cancer 2011;128(4) 869-878.

[35] Miyakura Y, Sugano K, Konishi F, Ichikawa A, Maekawa M, Shitoh K, Igarashi S, Kotake K, Koyama Y, Nagai H. Extensive methylation of hMLH1 promoter region predominates in proximal colon cancer with microsatellite instability. Gastroenterology 2001;121(6) 1300-1309.

[36] Miyakura Y, Sugano K, Konishi F, Fukayama N, Igarashi S, Kotake K, Matsui T, Koyama Y, Maekawa M, Nagai H. Methylation profile of the MLH1 promoter region and their relationship to colorectal carcinogenesis. Genes Chromosomes & Cancer 2003;36(1) 17-25.

[37] Miyakura Y, Sugano K, Akasu T, Yoshida T, Maekawa M, Saitoh S, Sasaki H, Nomizu T, Konishi F, Fujita S, Moriya Y, Nagai H. Extensive but hemiallelic methylation of the hMLH1 promoter region in early-onset sporadic colon cancers with microsatellite instability. Clinical Gastroenterolgy and Hepatology 2004; 2(2) 147-156.

[38] Kantelinen J, Kansikas M, Candelin S, Hampel H, Smith B, Holm L, Kariola R, Nyström M. Mismatch repair analysis of inherited MSH2 and/or MSH6 variation pairs found in cancer patients. Hum Mutation 2012May 11. doi: 10.1002/humu.22119.

[39] Borràs E, Pineda M, Brieger A, Hinrichsen I, Gómez C, Navarro M, Balmaña J, Ramón Y Cajal T, Torres A, Brunet J, Blanco I, Plotz G, Lázaro C, Capellá G. Comprehensive functional assessment of Mlh1 variants of unknown significance. Hum Mutation 2012 Jun 26. doi: 10.1002/humu.22142

[40] Wu PY, Zhang Z, Wang JM, Guo WW, Xiao N, He Q, Wang YP, Fan YM. Germline promoter hypermethylation of tumor suppressor genes in gastric cancer. World Journal of Gastroenterology 2012;18(1) 70-78.

[41] Hitchins MP, Owens SE, Kwok CT, Godsmark G, Algar UF, Ramesar RS. Identification of new cases of early-onset colorectal cancer with an MLH1 epimutation in an ethnically diverse South African cohort. Clinical Genetics 2011;80(5) 428-434.

[42] Pineda M, Mur P, Iniesta MD, Borràs E, Campos O, Vargas G, Iglesias S, Fernández A, Gruber SB, Lázaro C, Brunet J, Navarro M, Blanco I, Capellá G. MLH1 methylation screening is effective in identifying epimutation carriers. European Journal of Human Genetics 2012 Jul 4. doi: 10.1038/ejhg.2012.136.

[43] Chan TL, Yuen ST, Kong CK, Chan YW, Chan AS, Ng WF, Tsui WY, Lo MW, Tam WY, Li VS, Leung SY. Heritable germline epimutation of MSH2 in a family with hereditary nonpolyposis colorectal cancer. Nature Genetics 2006;38(10) 1178-1183.

[44] Raval A, Tanner SM, Byrd JC, Angerman EB, Perko JD, Chen SS, Hackanson B, Grever MR, Lucas DM, Matkovic JJ, Lin TS, Kipps TJ, Murray F, Weisenburger D, Sanger W, Lynch J, Watson P, Jansen M, Yoshinaga Y, Rosenquist R, de Jong PJ, Coggill P, Beck S, Lynch H, de la Chapelle A, Plass C. Downregulation of death-associated protein kinase 1 (DAPK1) in chronic lymphocytic leukemia. Cell 2007;129(5) 879-890.

[45] Reddy AN, Jiang WW, Kim M, Benoit N, Taylor R, Clinger J, Sidransky D, Califano JA. Death-associated protein kinase promoter hypermethylation in normal human lymphocytes. Cancer Research 2003;63(22) 7694-7698.

[46] Hassen S, Ali N, Chowdhury P. Molecular signaling mechanisms of apoptosis in hereditary non-polyposis colorectal cancer. World Journal of Gastrointestinal Pathophysiology 2012;3(3) 71-79.

[47] Helleman J, van Staveren IL, Dinjens WN, van Kuijk PF, Ritstier K, Ewing PC, van der Burg ME, Stoter G, Berns EM. Mismatch repair and treatment resistance in ovarian cancer. BMC Cancer 2006;6 201.

[48] Kenyon J, Fu P, Lingas K, Thomas E, Saurastri A, Santos Guasch G, Wald D, Gerson SL. Humans accumulate microsatellite instability with acquired loss of MLH1 protein in hematopoietic stem and progenitor cells as a function of age. Blood 2012 Jun 26.

[49] Foulkes WD, Stefansson IM, Chappuis PO, Bégin LR, Goffin JR, Wong N, Trudel M, Akslen LA. Germline BRCA1 mutations and a basal epithelial phenotype in breast cancer. Journal of the National Cancer Institute 2003; 95(19) 1482-1485.

[50] Esteller M, Silva JM, Dominguez G, Bonilla F, Matias-Guiu X, Lerma E, Bussaglia E, Prat J, Harkes IC, Repasky EA, Gabrielson E, Schutte M, Baylin SB, Herman JG. Promoter hypermethylation and BRCA1 inactivation in sporadic breast and ovarian tumors. Journal of the National Cancer Institute 2000; 92(7) 564-569.

[51] Catteau A, Morris JR. BRCA1 methylation: a significant role in tumour development? Catteau A, Morris JR. Semin Cancer Biology 2002;12(5) 359-371.

[52] Hedenfalk I, Duggan D, Chen Y, Radmacher M, Bittner M, Simon R, Meltzer P, Gusterson B, Esteller M, Kallioniemi OP, Wilfond B, Borg A, Trent J, Raffeld M, Yakhini

Z, Ben-Dor A, Dougherty E, Kononen J, Bubendorf L, Fehrle W, Pittaluga S, Gruvberger S, Loman N, Johannsson O, Olsson H, Sauter G. Gene-expression profiles in hereditary breast cancer. New England Journal of Medicine 2001; 344(8) 539-548.

[53] Snell C, Krypuy M, Wong EM; kConFab investigators, Loughrey MB, Dobrovic A. BRCA1 promoter methylation in peripheral blood DNA of mutation negative familial breast cancer patients with a BRCA1 tumour phenotype. Breast Cancer Research 2008;10(1) R12.

[54] Buerki N, Gautier L, Kovac M, Marra G, Buser M, Mueller H, Heinimann K. Evidence for breast cancer as an integral part of Lynch syndrome. Genes Chromosomes & Cancer 2012;51(1) 83-91.

[55] Lotsari JE, Gylling A, Abdel-Rahman WM, Nieminen TT, Aittomäki K, Friman M, Pitkänen R, Aarnio M, Järvinen HJ, Mecklin JP, Kuopio T, Peltomäki P. Breast carcinoma and Lynch syndrome: molecular analysis of tumors arising in mutation carriers, non-carriers, and sporadic cases. Breast Cancer Reserach 2012;14(3) R90.

[56] Vasen HF, Möslein G, Alonso A, Bernstein I, Bertario L, Blanco I, Burn J, Capella G, Engel C, Frayling I, Friedl W, Hes FJ, Hodgson S, Mecklin JP, Møller P, Nagengast F, Parc Y, Renkonen-Sinisalo L, Sampson JR, Stormorken A, Wijnen J. Guidelines for the clinical management of Lynch syndrome (hereditary non-polyposis cancer). Journal of Medical Genetics 2007;44(6) 353-362.

[57] Vasen HF, Stormorken A, Menko FH, Nagengast FM, Kleibeuker JH, Griffioen G, Taal BG, Moller P, Wijnen JT. MSH2 mutation carriers are at higher risk of cancer than MLH1 mutation carriers: a study of hereditary nonpolyposis colorectal cancer families. Journal of Clinical Oncology 2001;19(20) 4074-4080.

[58] Ketabi Z, Bartuma K, Bernstein I, Malander S, Grönberg H, Björck E, Holck S, Nilbert M: Ovarian cancer linked to Lynch syndrome typically presents as early-onset, nonserous epithelial tumors. Gynecologic Oncology 2011 Jun 1;121(3):462-465

[59] Grindedal EM, Renkonen-Sinisalo L, Vasen H, Evans G, Sala P, Blanco I, Gronwald J, Apold J, Eccles DM, Sánchez AA, Sampson J, Järvinen HJ, Bertario L, Crawford GC, Stormorken AT, Maehle L, Moller P. Survival in women with MMR mutations and ovarian cancer: a multicentre study in Lynch syndrome kindreds. Journal of Medical Genetics 2010;47(2) 99-102.

[60] Shih KK, Garg K, Levine DA, Kauff ND, Abu-Rustum NR, Soslow RA, Barakat RR: Clinicopathologic significance of DNA mismatch repair protein defects and endometrial cancer in women 40years of age and younger. Gynecologic Oncology 2011;123(1) 88-94.

[61] Hirata K, Kanemitsu S, Nakayama Y, Nagata N, Itoh H, Ohnishi H, Ishikawa H, Furukawa Y; HNPCC registry and genetic testing project of the Japanese Society for Cancer of the Colon and Rectum (JSCCR): A novel germline mutation of MSH2 in a hereditary nonpolyposis colorectal cancer patient with liposarcoma. American Journal of Gastroenterology 2006;101(1) 193-196.

[62] Takahashi M, Furukawa Y, Shimodaira H, Sakayori M, Moriya T, Moriya Y, Nakamura Y, Ishioka C. Aberrant splicing caused by a MLH1 splice donor site mutation found in a young Japanese patient with Lynch syndrome. Familial Cancer 2012 Jul 6.

[63] Winter MJ, Nagtegaal ID, van Krieken JH, Litvinov SV. The epithelial cell adhesion molecule (Ep-CAM) as a morphoregulatory molecule is a tool in surgical pathology. American Journal of Pathology 2003;163(6) 2139-2148.

[64] Ligtenberg MJ, Kuiper RP, Chan TL, Goossens M, Hebeda KM, Voorendt M, Lee TY, Bodmer D, Hoenselaar E, Hendriks-Cornelissen SJ, Tsui WY, Kong CK, Brunner HG, van Kessel AG, Yuen ST, van Krieken JH, Leung SY, Hoogerbrugge N. Heritable somatic methylation and inactivation of MSH2 in families with Lynch syndrome due to deletion of the 3' exons of TACSTD1. Nature Genetics 2009; 41(1) 112-117.

[65] Wei W, Liu L, Chen J, Jin K, Jiang F, Liu F, Fan R, Cheng Z, Shen M, Xue C, Cai S, Xu Y, Nan P: Racial differences in MLH1 and MSH2 mutation: an analysis of yellow race and white race based on the InSiGHT database. Journal of Bioinformatics and Computational Biology 2010;8 Suppl 1 111-125.

[66] Fraga MF, Ballestar E, Paz MF, Ropero S, Setien F, Ballestar ML, Heine-Suñer D, Cigudosa JC, Urioste M, Benitez J, Boix-Chornet M, Sanchez-Aguilera A, Ling C, Carlsson E, Poulsen P, Vaag A, Stephan Z, Spector TD, Wu YZ, Plass C, Esteller M: Epigenetic differences arise during the lifetime of monozygotic twins. Proceeding of the Natlional Academy of Sciences of the United States of America 2005; 102(30) 10604-10609.

[67] Issa JP, Ottaviano YL, Celano P, Hamilton SR, Davidson NE, Baylin SB. Methylation of the oestrogen receptor CpG island links ageing and neoplasia in human colon. Nature Genetics 1994; 7(4) 536-540.

[68] Rose MG. Hematology: Azacitidine improves survival in myelodysplastic syndromes. Nature Reviews Clinical Oncology 2009;6(9) 502-503.

Chapter 4

Evolving DNA Repair Polymerases: From Double—Strand Break Repair to Base Excision Repair and VDJ Recombination

Maria Jose Martin and Luis Blanco

Additional information is available at the end of the chapter

http://dx.doi.org/10.5772/53908

1. Introduction

Currently five polymerases have been identified in *Escherichia coli*, at least eight in *Saccharomyces cerevisiae*, nine in *Schizosaccharomyces pombe*, and fourteen in humans [1-4]. Based on the primary structure of the catalytic subunits, DNA polymerases have been classified into different families. Eukaryotic organisms have four families: A family (Polγ, Polθ and Polν), B family (Polα, Polδ, Polε and Polζ), X family (Polß, Polλ, Polμ and TdT) and Y family (Polη, Polι, Polκ and Rev1), whose members were discovered in the last decade [5], and are involved in replication through DNA lesions. Another significant development was the discovery of Polλ [6] and Polμ [7], which doubled the number of known enzymes of the X family of DNA polymerases, whose members are involved in DNA repair and generation of variability.

2. Evolution of the X family of DNA polymerases

The members of the X family are present in many organisms in all monophyletic taxa: Eukarya, Bacteria and Archaea, and even viruses with DNA genome [8]. The high degree of conservation at the structural and amino acid sequence levels between X family members suggests that they originate from a common ancestor.

Unlike viruses, prokaryotes and yeast, higher eukaryotes have more than one member of the X family. However, there are species in which no member of this family has been described, like the model organisms *Caenorhabditis elegans* and *Drosophila melanogaster* [2], so it becomes a matter of special interest to learn how they have solved the absence of these DNA polymer-

INTECH
open science | open minds

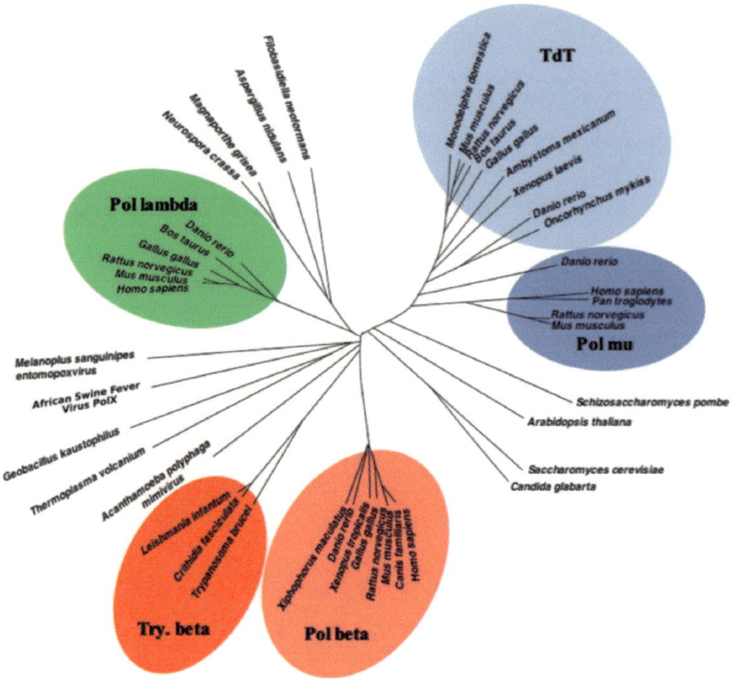

Figure 1. Evolutionary relationships between family X members. An unrooted phylogenetic tree built using a primary sequence alignment of a segment of the catalytic domain. Different enzymes are grouped (shaded areas) into the five main enzyme classes in the family: Polß, Pol λ, Polμ, TdT, and trypanosomatid (Try) Polß-like enzymes.

ases in DNA repair processes. Recent data indicate that recombination repair protein 1, the Drosophila homolog of human AP endonuclease 1 (APE1), interacts with DNA polymerase ζ [9]. It is possible that in protostomes (which include insects and nematodes), APE1-like genes are able to recruit a DNA polymerase other than an X family enzyme to AP sites on DNA. It has been proposed that protostomes evolved from organisms in the coelenterate phylum that lost a Polλ-like gene before other X family DNA polymerases were derived, since it is unlikely that multiple X family genes were lost as soon as coelenterates appeared [10].

Figure 1 shows the phylogenetic relationships between the known members of X family from different organisms. The phylogenetic tree was made using a short and highly conserved segment of the polymerization active site, in order to avoid the presence of accessory domains or small insertions or deletions that may interfere in the analysis. The results suggest that the several subfamilies that can be identified within the X family (Polß, Polλ, Polμ and TdT) have evolved from a common ancestor, perhaps to accommodate different functional requirements. The emergence of more complex organisms seems to promote the specialization of the X family members in order to increase the efficiency of the DNA synthesis processes in which they are involved. The distribution of X family DNA polymerases among different species suggests that the ancestor of the X family DNA polymerase was a Polλ-like gene, which diversified into Polß, Polμ and TdT during evolution. Polλ would have originally been involved in NHEJ to eliminate DNA damage. Subsequently, other X family DNA polymerases would have been

http://dx.doi.org/10.5772/53908

generated in some animals and fungi through gene duplications, acquiring novel roles in DNA metabolism such as in BER and V(D)J recombination. According to very recent results [11], these evolutionary forces driving creation of new polymerases are still taking place among primates: codon-based models of gene evolution yielded statistical support for the recurrent positive selection of Polλ, among other four NHEJ genes during primate evolution: XRCC4, NBS1, Artemis, and CtIP. Moreover, analysis of the mutations on the crystal structures available for XRCC4, Nbs1, and Polλ show that residues under positive selection fall exclusively on the surface of these proteins. Studies of positive local evolution on human populations show that, indeed, a single allele of Polλ has previously been reported to be under positive selection in both Asian and Sub-Sahara African populations [12]. Also, sliding-window analyses and pairwise comparisons of several strains of *Saccharomyces* indicated that several of the yeast NHEJ genes show evidence of positive selection, including POL4 [13]. A first hypothesis explaining the high level of positively selected mutations implies that as certain NHEJ components evolve, compensatory mutations may arise in other NHEJ components to re-optimize protein-protein interactions between the various partners. On the other hand, many viruses such as adenovirus, and retroviruses like HIV, interact with the proteins of the NHEJ pathway as part of their infectious life cycle [14-21]. The Corndog and Omega bacteriophages of mycobacteria have even incorporated the first gene of the bacterial NHEJ pathway, Ku, into their own genome [22]. This viral Ku now evolves under the selective pressures of the virus in order to recruit the bacterial NHEJ ligase, LigD, to circularize phage DNA. Therefore, a second hypothesis would explain the surprisingly rapid evolution of NHEJ genes as an ongoing evolutionary arms race between viruses and these critical genes.

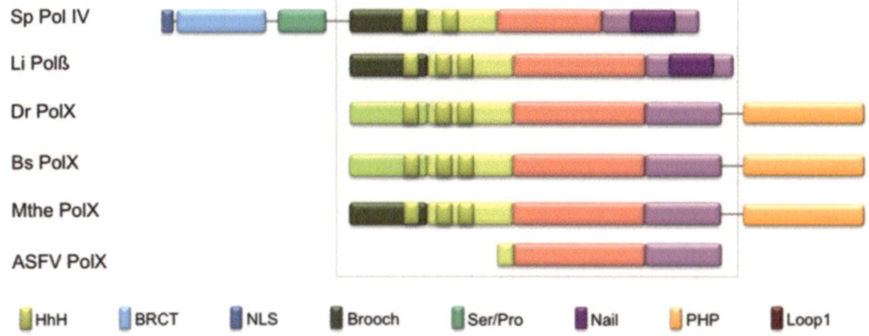

Figure 2. Modular organization of the family X polymerases. Schematic representation of the domains present in family X members from viruses to higher eukaryotes. Regarding the coloring of the 8 kDa domain, dark green represents dRP lyase-containing domains while bright green color indicates the lack of such activity. *Sc: Saccharomyces cerevisiae; Sp: Schizosaccharomyces pombe; Li: Leishmania infantum; ASFV: African swine fever virus; Bs: Bacillus subtilis; Mthe: Methanobacterium thermoautotrophicum; Dr: Deinococcus radiodurans.*

3. Comparative genomic organization of human DNA polymerases from family X

The modular organization of different members of the X family from viruses to eukaryotes indicates the existence of a conserved Polß-type core (Fig. 2), whose minimal version is the PolX from the African swine fever virus (ASFV), which contains only the palm and thumb subdomains of the polymerase domain [8]. The absence of the 8 kDa domain of both ASFV PolX and MSEV (*Melanoplus sanguinipes* entomopoxvirus) may reflect the existence of other proteins encoded by the viral genome to provide the catalytic (dRP lyase) and/or DNA binding properties residing in this domain in most of the DNA polymerases of the X family. Despite the small size of ASFV PolX, it has a second enzymatic activity: the AP-lyase, indicating a possible role in the viral BER pathway [23]. The evolutionary divergence of the members of the X family has occurred by acquisition of additional domains with regulatory properties and/or enzymatic activities. X family members from eubacteria (*Bacillus subtilis*) and Archaea (*Methanobacterium thermoautotrophicum*) have a phosphodiesterase domain (PHP, Fig. 2) fused to the Polß core domain, and thus possess polymerase and nuclease activities in the same polypeptide, a great functional benefit to carry out repair processes in the BER pathway. In eukaryotes there are members of this family from protozoa (*Leishmania infantum*) to mammals. However, there are major differences in the accessory domains that keep a very close relationship with their physiological function. The percentage of similarity at the amino acid sequence level of the Polß core between different members of this family varies from 91% between the Polß enzymes from *Crithidia* and *Leishmania* (LiPolß), and 42% between Polμ and TdT, to 19% identity between LiPolß and TdT [24]. LiPolß shows a 31% of amino-acid identity with mammalian Polß, close to the 32% between Polλ and Polß. Interestingly, both Polß enzymes from *Crithidia* and *Leishmania* present inserts within the core that allow protein-protein and protein-DNA interactions. Contrary to mammals, yeast cells have a single DNA polymerase from the X family, Pol4. Both Pol4 from *S. cerevisiae* and *S. pombe* possess two additional domains at their N-terminus: a BRCT domain followed by a regulatory Ser/Pro domain (Fig. 2). In addition, both Pol4 have a dRP-lyase activity associated with the 8 kDa domain suggesting a role in repair processes such as BER [25, 26]. Although both Pol4 enzymes share a common structural organization, they differ in terms of sequence similarity with their human counterparts. While *Sc*Pol4 is more similar in the composition of the basic Polß structure to Polλ, sharing a 25% of amino-acid identity [25], *Sp*Pol4 is closer to Polμ (27% amino-acid identity) than to Polλ (24% amino-acid identity). Based on sequence similarity one can speculate that, in yeast, *Sp*Pol4 is the orthologue of human Polμ while *Sc*Pol4 could be the orthologue of human Polλ.

The presence of BRCT domains in Pol4, Polλ, Polμ and TdT relates to the role that this domain plays in processes such as V(D)J recombination and NHEJ repair. The BRCT domain of Pol4 mediates the interaction of the polymerase with factors involved in the NHEJ pathway during repair of double-strand breaks in DNA [27, 28]. Similarly, the BRCT domains of Polλ, Polμ and TdT allow these proteins to participate in both NHEJ repair and V(D)J recombination in higher eukaryotes. It is possible that subtle differences in the amino acid sequence of the BRCT domain of each polymerase have great importance in regulating the access of each DNA polymerase to a specific substrate or protein of the route.

Finally, the eukaryotic Polß (initially thought to be exclusive of mammals) has lost some accessory domains during evolution, in a crucial step for its specialization as a housekeeping DNA repair polymerase that protects against the large amount of oxidative damage present as a result of aerobic metabolism. The conservation of the 8 kDa domain (Fig. 2), where the dRP-lyase activity resides, is central for participation in the BER pathway.

4. A BRCT domain as an ancient feature required for NHEJ

The members of the X family of polymerases are recruited to form a complex with the NHEJ core factors XRCC4/Ligase IV and Ku at the DNA break [27, 29, 30]. Recent evidence has shown that BRCT domains can be specifically involved in the interaction with phospho-serine or phospho-threonine containing motifs [31, 32], an ability that may be involved in granting access of regulated proteins to the break, even though no evidence has shown to date a phosphorylation-dependent, BRCT-mediated, interaction of NHEJ factors.

Interestingly, sequence comparisons show that the BRCT of Polμ is most similar to TdT, with 39% sequence identity that includes the residues important for NHEJ-complex formation [33]. That high level of sequence conservation is also observed at the 3D- structural level in the BRCT domains of Polμ (PDB ID: 2DUN) and TdT (PDB ID: 2COE), that in turn exhibit an a/ß motif that is similar to the BRCT found in XRCC1 (PDB ID: 1CDZ), a BER repair protein. The main differences include a shorter α -helix 2 in the TdT BRCT domain, as well as the positioning of the loop connecting α -helix 2 and ß-strand 4. The electrostatic surfaces of Polμ and TdT BRCT domains are also very similar, containing both a positively charged ridge on one face of the protein, and large negatively charged regions on the opposite faces. In the Polμ BRCT the positive ridge is formed by Arg^{44}, Arg^{52}, Arg^{85} and Arg^{86}. This positive patch has been proposed to be involved in the interaction with a phospho-modified protein [33], or most likely in the interaction with the downstream part of the DNA substrate [34]. Point mutations in several residues of the positive ridge as wells as the complete lack of the domain resulted in a diminished interaction with and activity on NHEJ substrates [34, 35]. By using the "brooch" motif (described below) to correctly orient and over-impose the crystals of the BRCT domain and the Polμ core, we found out that one of the positive patches in the BRCT domain perfectly accommodates the downstream part of the DNA substrate (Fig. 3; colored in dark blue). We then modeled the interaction of the BRCT domain of Polμ with the Ku70/Ku80 heterodimer by orienting the DNA substrate. Strikingly, the side of the BRCT domain facing the Ku heterodimer in the model was exactly the one containing the residues reported to be involved in this interaction (Fig. 3; colored in red). According to this model, the portion of the DNA substrate that would be contacted by the BRCT domain flawlessly correlates with the length of the BRCT-specific protection (6 bp) observed in our footprinting assays [34]

This DNA binding function of Polμ BRCT, independent of the core NHEJ factors, may enable a role for Polμ in the alternative NHEJ pathway, which occurs independently of Ku or Ligase IV. Polμ might bind the DNA break based on its own specificity for the 5′-P and then via the BRCT domain and using its terminal transferase activity, be in charge of the additions that

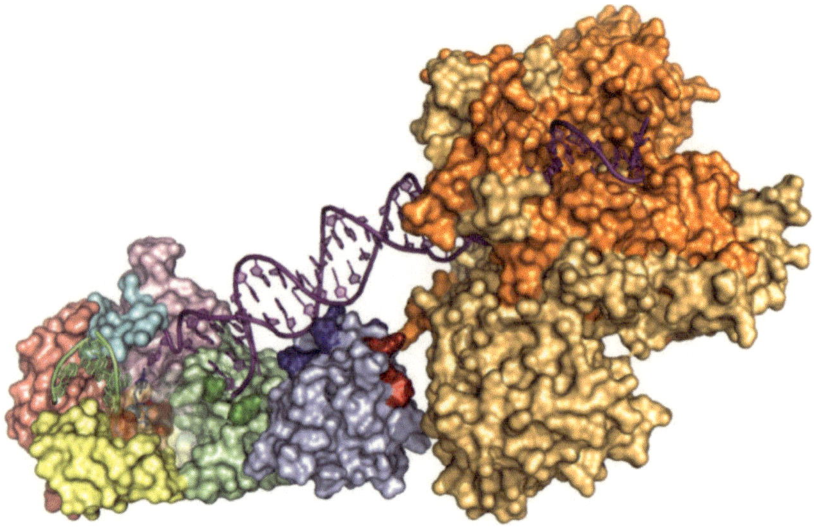

Figure 3. Model of the interaction of Polμ with the Ku heterodimer and the DNA substrate through the BRCT domain.

create the so-called polymerase-generated microhomology. In agreement with this proposed function, recent observations indicate that Polμ BRCT is atypical in the sense of not being involved in dimerization or multimerization. In fact, comparison of the structure of Polμ BRCT with other BRCT domains that effectively dimerize shows important differences, especially regarding R2 helix [36].

The sequence conservation among BRCT domains from family X polymerases is very low, with only 10 residues conserved and five of them (His^{82}, Val^{84}, Leu^{109}, Trp^{114}, and Leu^{115} in human Polλ) involved in the architecture of the domain. The other five (Gly^{54}, Arg^{57}, Gly^{69}, Thr^{81}, and Val^{125} in human Polλ) are exposed to the solvent in the surface of the protein. One of them, Arg^{43} in Polμ (Arg^{57} in Polλ), is implicated in interactions with other components of the NHEJ complex [33].

This low sequence similarity is reflected in structural variations of the family X polymerases' BRCT domains, which in turn influence the interactions established with other NHEJ factors, including an improved/preferential access of the polymerase to the DNA break. Deletion of the BRCT domain in the NHEJ-related polymerases [27, 29, 37], or point-mutagenesis of key-residues [33, 36], block the formation of complexes between the polymerase, Ku and XRCC4/LigaseIV at DNA ends.

The ability of X family polymerases to act during classical NHEJ thus relies on their interactions with other NHEJ factors through their BRCT domains, but PolXs have intrinsic capacities of gap-recognition and binding involving simultaneous recognition of both sides of the gap. As shown for Polß, the polymerase can bind both the template/primer part of the gap and also the template/downstream part, being the latter the strongest anchor point [38]. In the Polß co-crystal with a DNA gap this dual binding is clearly observable: contacts are established with the DNA backbone through a positively charged platform onto which the DNA is leaning.

http://dx.doi.org/10.5772/53908

Such a dual DNA binding is even more crucial for Polλ and Polμ, polymerases not as specialized as Polß in always confronting substrates with continuous template strands (i.e. gaps), but also in charge of bridging two separate DNA ends. The ability to independently bind and orient two DNA ends is thus closely related to their function during NHEJ, but is still found in the more recently evolved Polß as an appropriate solution for gap-filling. This tight binding to both sides of the templating base forces the formation of a sharp bend of 90° in the template strand, that has been proposed to increase nucleotide selectivity and sensitivity to mismatches, and in general is a mechanistic feature used by X polymerases to improve fidelity [39].

5. A small (8 kDa) DNA binding domain, critical for NHEJ

One of the structural features that allows polymerases from X family to bind gapped and NHEJ substrates is the 8 kDa domain (Fig. 4A), located either at the N-terminus (Polß from higher eukaryotes, bacteria and archaea), or at the N-terminal portion just after the flexible linker that contains the Ser-Pro domain (Polλ, Polμ, TdT and yeast Pol4). This 8 kDa domain is involved in contacting several parts of the DNA substrate through different motifs [40], but in some of the members of the X family bears a dRP-lyase activity, highly related to the BER pathway [41, 42].

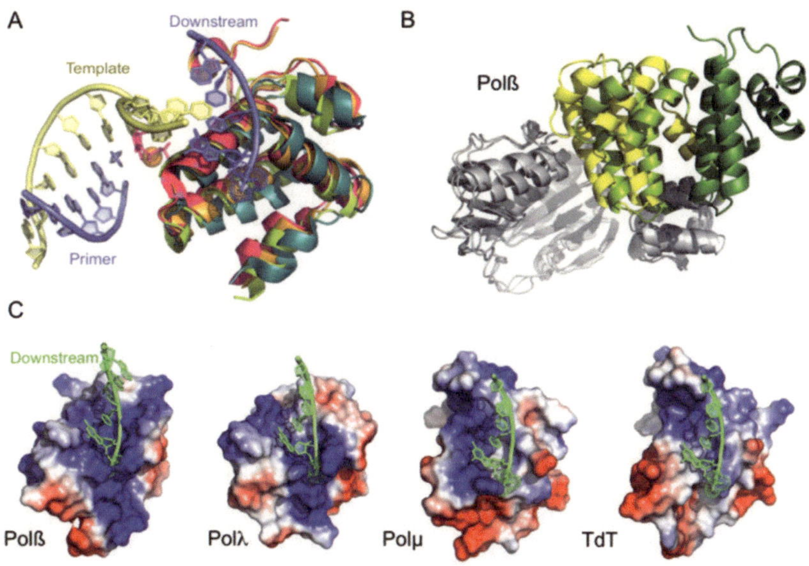

Figure 4. 8 kDa domain of the human X family members. A) Over-imposition of the 8 kDa domains of the X family members: Polß (dark pink), Polμ (orange) and Polλ (teal), shown in cartoon. B) Superimposition of the structures of Polß: apoenzyme (1BPX, dark green), binary (1BPY), light green and ternary (1BPZ, yellow) complexes. C) Electrostatic surface of the 8 kDa domain of Polß (1BPZ), TdT (1KDH), Polμ (2IHM) and Polλ (1XSN), with the downstream strand shown in green. Polμ DNA was over-imposed on the TdT structure.

With the resolution of the first crystal structures of rat and human Polß, the 8 kDa domain was found to be highly mobile (Fig. 4B), not freely, but displaying a small number of stable positions: 1) in the absence of DNA and incoming nucleotide, the 8 kDa domain is located far away from the thumb subdomain, and the polymerase is in an open conformation; 2) in the presence of a DNA gap, the 8 kDa domain moves and comes closer to the thumb through binding of the 5′-phosphate group of the downstream strand; 3) after arrival of the nucleotide, there is a further movement of the 8 kDa domain, and Polß finally adopts the closed conformation. The model proposed originally [39] explains the formation of the 90º bend in the DNA substrate in two steps: first, binding of the 8 kDa domain to the downstream part of the gap stabilizes the initial positioning of the enzyme; secondly, upon folding of the polymerase domain and binding of the primer part of the substrate, the bend of the DNA duplex is created. This bending causes the downstream part to rotate out, exposing the 3′ end of the primer.

This two-step model is confirmed by the observations derived form the solved Polλ structures, the most indicative in this matter being the co-crystal with a 2 nt gap ([43], PDB ID: 1RZT). In this case, the 5′-P is located in its correct position and bound by the 8 kDa domain, but the place of the templating base is occupied by the second template nucleotide of the gap, i.e. the one adjacent to the downstream duplex. This causes the 3′-OH of the primer to be displaced to the -1 position relative to the catalytic position, adjacent to the NTP binding site observed in the 1 nt gap co-crystal (PDB ID: 1XSN). Therefore, the location of the polymerase domain in a gap (1-nt or longer) is dictated by the binding of the 8 kDa domain to the 5′-P, and not by interactions with the primer terminus.

This conclusion has implications of great interest for the binding of the polymerase to NHEJ substrates, since 8 kDa-mediated binding would occur irrespective of the conformation of the 3′ end. The polymerase in charge for this has to be able to take advantage of micro-homologies for aligning the 3′ ends, and the 8 kDa domain provides an anchoring point for this complicated task.

5.1. Phosphate pocket

As already noted, the main function of the 8 kDa domain is the binding of the 5′-P group of the downstream strand of the DNA substrate. In fact, polymerization rates by template-instructed polymerases of the X family are greatly enhanced when the substrate contains this 5′-P group. In the case of Polß and Polλ, the processivity is also improved on long gaps (5 nt [44, 45]). In the ternary structures of Polß (PDB ID: 1BPY), Polλ (PDB ID: 1XSN) and Polμ (PDB ID: 2IHM) this 5′-P moiety is located at a positively charged pocket where binding is mediated by several hydrogen bonding interactions with basic side chains within the pocket (Fig. 4C). However, in Polμ there are fewer interactions than in Polß or Polλ, and the binding pocket is not as positively charged (Fig. 4C). There is no structure of TdT containing a downstream strand, but this enzyme still conserves the 8 kDa domain, that could be used to coordinate terminal addition of N-nucleotides with the joining of the two DNA ends generated during V(D)J recombination.

5.2. HhH domain

The 8 kDa domain contains another structural motif implicated in DNA binding, the helix-hairpin-helix (HhH) motif. These motifs bind single- or double-stranded DNA in a sequence independent manner, with the aid of a coordinated metal cation [46, 47]. In Polß, Polλ and

http://dx.doi.org/10.5772/53908

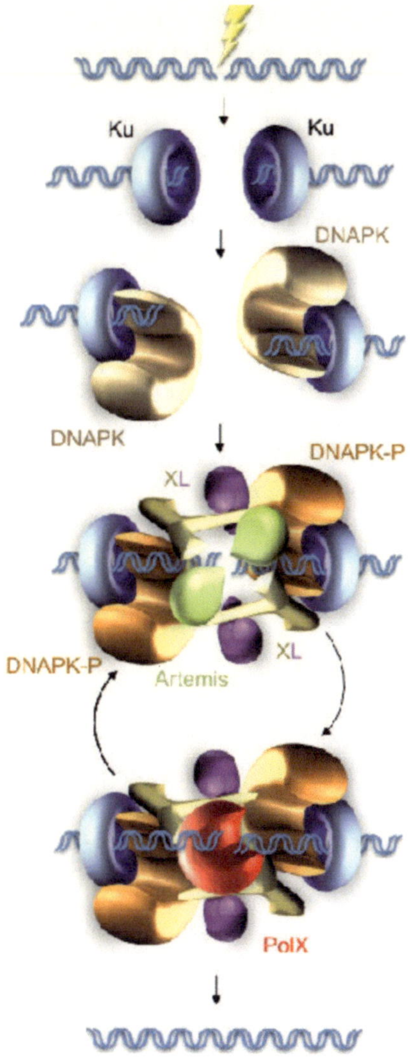

Figure 5. Non-homologous end joining pathway in eukaryotes. This pathway acts repairing damage-generated DSBs. The Ku70/80 heterodimer is the first protein factor to arrive at the site of the break and bind the DNA ends. The DNA PKcs is the recruited and forms a complex with Artemis. The phosphorylated Artemis acts as an endonuclease, generating ssDNA-protruding regions at the ends, and after this the complex dissociates from the DNA. The X family DNA polymerases are then in charge of searching for micro-homologies or generating them, and filling-in the gaps generated. Finally, the XRCC4/Ligase IV complex seals the break.

Polμ structures, this HhH interacts with the downstream part of the substrate, suggesting that its function is the stabilization of the bent DNA thereby facilitating the positioning of the two DNA ends in a NHEJ reaction.

The structures of the 8 kDa HhH motifs from the X family enzymes are not exactly the same: in Polß and Polλ this motif is similar to those found in other repair enzymes, with the GxG sequence of the hairpin and other protein residues being conserved. In Polμ and TdT, on the other hand, one of the helices is distorted, probably as a consequence of the lack of primary sequence conservation in the hairpin (CLG in TdT, HFG and YLG in mouse and human Polμ, respectively).

5.3. Polλ dRP lyase allows repair of "dirty" DSBs

The 8 kDa domains of Polß and Polλ harbor an intrinsic dRP lyase activity that is required during single-nucleotide BER to remove the residual 5′-deoxyribose-phospate moiety left by the AP-endonuclease after elimination of the nitrogenous base. This reaction proceeds through a ß-elimination mechanism *via* an Schiff base intermediate, and has been shown to be the rate-limiting step in the elimination of several DNA lesions *in vivo* [41, 48]. The studies on the structural aspects of dRP-lyase chemistry [49-51] have led to the conclusion that the amino acids serving as catalytic nucleophiles are Lys^{72} in Polß [42] and Lys^{312} in Polλ [41]. This positively charged residue is not conserved in Polμ (Val^{212}) or TdT (Val^{224}), and thus the dRP-lyase activity is not present in these enzymes.

6. Polμ: A "Jekyll & Hide" DNA polymerase at the edge between genomic stability and variability

Polμ is a DNA polymerase belonging to the X family with a strong similarity to TdT, its closest counterpart in the X family. They share 42% identity at the amino acid sequence, and also have a very similar structural organization: their N-terminal portion contains a nuclear localization sequence, followed by a BRCT domain and then the Polß-core structure already mentioned.

Regarding Polμ biochemical properties, it displays a certain terminal transferase activity [7], although it is primarily a DNA-dependent DNA polymerase [7, 52] and its activity increases strongly in the presence of a template strand of DNA. It is also known that both types of polymerization are stimulated *in vitro* in the presence of Mn^{2+} ions, the preferred metal activator, and in the presence of this cofactor Polμ exhibits a strong mutator phenotype, with a very high probability of erroneous nucleotide incorporation, being one of the most error-prone polymerases known in higher eukaryotes [7]. This strong mutator ability is based on a dislocation mechanism [53, 54] through which Polμ is capable of repositioning the template strand so that incorporation is dictated by templating bases away from the end of the primer. The mutator capacity of Polμ is further enhanced by its low sugar discrimination, being able to incorporate not only dNTPs but also NTPs [55, 56]. This may have implications in cell cycle phases in which the levels of dNTPs are very low as NTPs reserves remain high throughout the cycle.

Although the *in vivo* role of Polμ has not been clarified yet, a number of functions for the polymerase have been proposed, including its participation in the non-homologous end-joining (NHEJ) pathway, in charge of repairing the highly harmful double strand breaks in DNA. The NHEJ system relies on little or no homology between sequences to achieve repair, since the proteins involved in the process recognize the ends of DNA based on their structure

rather than its sequence (reviewed in [57]). This pathway may lead to mutagenesis, contributing to the variability of the genomes [58, 59], and is key to certain cellular processes such as antibody repertoire generation. NHEJ is the main mechanism to repair DSBs in higher eukaryotes, as it is operative throughout the cell cycle, unlike homologous recombination, a second DSB repair mechanism which is inhibited during the G0, G1 and S phases [57].
The first step of NHEJ is the binding of specific protein factors to the ends of the DNA break (Fig. 5). The Ku70/Ku80 heterodimer recognizes the ends of the break, and due to its toroidal shape accommodates the duplex DNA, preventing possible nucleolytic degradation [60]. Then, the DNA-PK kinase is recruited [61, 62], inducing a slight internalization of the Ku heterodimer [63], and allowing both sides of the break to approach through specific protein-protein interactions [64-66]. Once the ends are juxtaposed, generally cannot be directly linked, but require pre-processing. Analysis of the sequences repaired by NHEJ at the break points suggests that some of these events involve the alignment of the ends through micro-homologies (complementary sequences from 1 to 4 nt) near the site of rupture [67-69]. When there is no direct microhomology the system must generate it by certain mechanisms that involve nucleases and/or DNA polymerases [70, 71], which would be needed to process distortions, flaps or gaps that may arise as a result of the alignment of the chains (reviewed in [72]). The Ku-DNAPK complex recruits the proteins needed for processing and subsequent ligation of the ends. Artemis, an ssDNA 3'-5' exonuclease, is activated through phosphorylation by DNA-PK [71]. Polynucleotide kinase (PNK), which has kinase and phosphatase activities [73], may also intervene in end-processing [74]. If the ends at this point were compatible, the last step of the mechanism would be the recruitment of the XRCC4/LigaseIV complex by Ku, which would carry out the ligation of the ends [75-78]. If, on the contrary, the ends were not compatible, a DNA polymerase would be needed, since its activity would be critical for filling the gaps generated during the alignment of the chains of DNA [70, 79]. Polμ could even perform template-independent polymerization to create the necessary complementary sequences [80, 81]. Finally, after processing the ends, the complex formed by DNA Ligase IV/XRCC4 would be responsible for sealing the joint between the ends of the break [64, 75]. Another factor similar to the protein XRCC4 has been recently identified in mammals. It has been called XLF (XRCC4-like factor) or Cernunnos, and interacts with the DNA LigaseIV/XRCC4 complex to promote end ligation [82, 83].

On the other hand, Polμ preferential expression in lymphoid tissues, especially in the germinal centers of secondary lymphoid organs, suggests a specific role of this polymerase in processes occurring in these regions. Its resemblance to TdT at the structural level, and its ability to conduct untemplated nucleotide additions, together with the fact that TdT is not expressed in secondary lymphoid organs, allowed to propose a function for Polμ in somatic hypermutation in the germinal centers [52], which occurs in these regions as an additional mechanism for diversification of the immune response [84]. Moreover, Polμ is present also in the thymus and bone marrow, and thus may be required during the normal process of V(D)J recombination as DNA-dependent polymerase to generate palindromic sequences (P sequences) at the ends of the coding fragments, or during gap-filling reactions required for coupling N additions to the DNA ends [52]. It was recently demonstrated an *in vivo* role of Polμ in the V(D)J recombination process of the light chain (kappa) of immunoglobulins, based on the observed deletions at the junctions between these gene segments in the case of Polμ deficiency [85]. Also, recent data implicated Polμ in the DJ_H recombination in mice embryos, a stage in which TdT is still not expressed [86]. In this case, all the N-additions observed in wild type mice were completely attributable to Polμ, as shown by comparison with Polμ-KO mice. This evidence suggests a role for Polμ in the V(D)J mechanism.

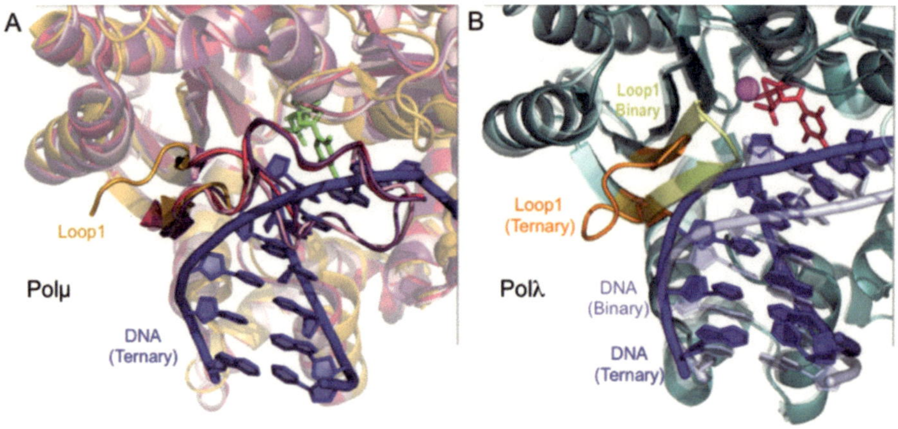

Figure 6. Loop 1 in Polμ, TdT and Polλ: movements from the binary to the ternary complexes. A) Over-imposition of the three available crystal structures of TdT (1JMS, 1KDH, 1KEJ, in light pink, dark pink and purple, respectively) and the ternary complex of Polμ (orange). B) Over-imposition of the binary (light teal) and ternary (dark teal) complexes of Polλ, shown in cartoon. Loop 1 from both structures are shown in yellow and orange, and the DNA substrates in light and dark blue, respectively.

7. A mobile loop in Polμ provides the ability to join non–homologous DNA ends

Template instruction is a general feature of most members of the X family, with the exception of TdT. TdT is the only known fully template-independent DNA polymerase, as it is able to add nucleotides to a primer DNA molecule in the absence of a template strand. This feature is crucial for its function in V(D)J recombination, where TdT adds nucleotides to the recombinational junctions of immunoglobulins and TCR receptor genes, generating variability as it creates new information [87, 88]. Interestingly, Polμ shows hybrid biochemical properties: it has an intrinsic terminal transferase activity, but it is strongly activated by a template DNA chain [7].

Understanding the structural and functional basis of the template-independence of TdT had to await the resolution of the crystal structure of the Polß-like core of TdT [89]. A loop region between ß-strands 3 and 4, referred to as Loop 1, has a similar position in all three TdT structures, and is located in a region of the DNA binding cleft that would normally be occupied by the template strand (Fig. 6A). Therefore, this loop would preclude binding of any DNA substrate possessing a template strand, thus explaining its null activity on these substrates. On that basis, and by extrapolation of the TdT structural model to Polμ, it was predicted that Loop 1, specifically present in these two enzymes, could be directly responsible for their template-independent terminal transferase activity, but in Polμ Loop 1 must be flexible enough to also allow template-directed polymerization [80]. In agreement with this prediction, when the crystal structure of Polμ bound to a gapped DNA was solved [40], Loop 1 was disordered suggesting conformational flexibility (Fig. 6A). In this structure, the DNA duplex was bound in the usual fashion within the DNA binding cleft. It was then clear that Loop 1 of Polμ cannot occupy the same position as that of TdT when a template strand is present. A comparison of the ends of the ß-strands flanking the loop shows that TdT's Loop 1 extrudes upwards, toward the DNA binding cleft, while that of Polμ appears to turn downwards, away from the cleft [40]. Although no crystal structure is available of Polμ with a single stranded or 3'-protruding DNA substrate, it is likely that Loop 1 would then be found in the same conformation as in TdT, i.e. interacting with the primer strand, somehow mimicking a template strand. The structural evidence suggested that Loop 1 in Polμ may adopt different conformations depending on the nature of the substrate: the inherent flexibility of this loop in Polμ is distinct from TdT and suggests how Polμ can accommodate different substrates. Studies including the Loop 1 chimeras on Polμ [80] and TdT [90] confirmed this hypothesis: replacement of the TdT Loop 1 with that of Polμ is sufficient to allow template-dependent additions, while the reciprocal chimera (Polμ with the TdT Loop 1) is much less inclined to perform template-dependent additions.

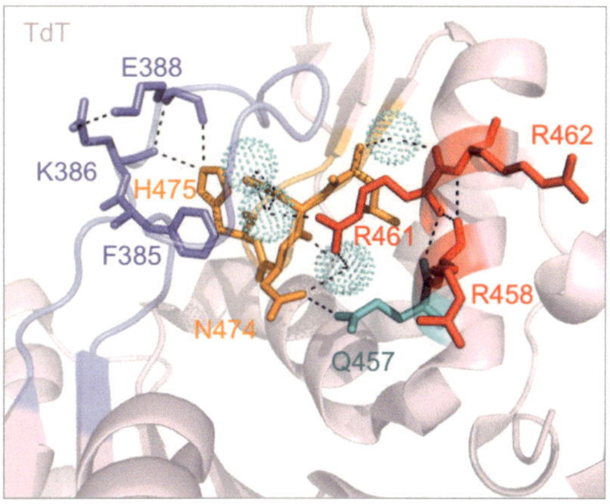

Figure 7. The Loop 1 network. Cartoon representation of the TdT apoenzyme (1JMS). Loop1 is shown in blue cartoon with selected residues involved in interactions shown in sticks, the thumb mini-loop is shown in orange with selected residues shown in sticks, arginines from the helix N are shown in red sticks, water molecules and other are shown in light teal.

The equivalent regions in Polß and Polλ would be less likely to interfere with binding of the template strand because they have a much shorter Loop 1: small enough in Polß to be described as a turn and of intermediate length in Polλ (Fig. 6B). Consistent with this idea, when Loop 1 in Polμ is shortened to a length similar to that of Polλ, the altered polymerase has higher catalytic efficiency on template-containing substrates, but is incapable of template-independent synthesis [29, 80]. Consistent with all this, Polλ has a strongly reduced ability to catalyze template-independent synthesis, but retains the ability to perform template-instructed additions. Polλ Loop 1 may be involved in a function somehow related to that in Polμ: modulation of fidelity by controlling dNTP-induced movements of the template strand and 3′-primer terminus in the transition from an inactive to an active conformation of the enzyme [91]. In fact, dNTP binding induces Polλ to transition from an inactive to an active conformation: ß-strands 3 and 4 partially unravel to form Loop 1, a nine-residue loop that repositions as the DNA template strand assumes its active conformation (Fig. 6B). Such a "fidelity checkpoint" would then be related to the energetic penalty of changing the structure of these ß-strands, that would only be overcome in the case of the formation of a correct match.

The role of Loop 1 during terminal transferase additions has been now established, but a more in depth study of how Polμ fixes and/or orients this mobile part of the protein in accordance with the substrate on which it is polymerizing is necessary. In the case of TdT, residue Phe^{401} (corresponding to Phe^{385} in Polμ), is involved in maintaining the fixed position of Loop 1 *via* a strong stacking interaction between its aromatic ring and His^{475} (His^{459} in Polμ), located in a mini-loop at the thumb subdomain (Fig. 7). Mutant F401A in TdT had a striking phenotype, turning a completely template independent enzyme into a DNA-instructed DNA polymerase [90]. This mutation clearly disrupted the network of interactions needed to maintain a fixed orientation of TdT Loop 1, that is now endowed with a greater degree of flexibility, as in Polμ, thus allowing TdT to accept a template strand. Phe^{389} is again conserved among Polμs and TdTs (Phe^{405}) of different species, and in both cases it seems to be involved in maintaining the shape and orientation of this motif. Mutation of this residue to alanine in TdT abolishes terminal transferase activity and allows templated insertion of only one nucleotide on a template/primer substrate [90]. We produced mutants in the implicated residues of Polμ and all of them lacked terminal transferase activity, indicating that the network of interactions maintaining the conformation of Loop 1 in TdT is conserved in Polμ [92]. Also, in TdT Loop 1 is interacting with another very small loop located in the thumb through His^{475} (Fig. 7), that is conserved in Polμ (His^{459}). This mini-loop is also present in the other members of the X family, but its function is different: residues from this loop directly interact with the template strand. In Polμ this mini-loop has both roles: depending on the substrate used and the desired conformation of Loop 1, the mini-loop may interact either with the template strand (through Asn^{457}) or with Loop 1 itself (through His^{459}). Accordingly, the asparagine is only needed during templated additions, and dispensable for terminal transferase activity of Polμ, while the histidine had the opposite effect [92]. We propose a regulatory function for the NSH motif in the thumb mini-loop, helping to accommodate either the template strand (as in Polß of Polλ) or Loop 1 (as in TdT) as suits best for each individual situation.

8. A single arginine in Polμ limits terminal transferase to favor fidelity during NHEJ

Having now a general idea of how these two polymerases, Polμ and TdT, are specially designed to perform this untemplated additions of nucleotide units, another question still remains: why and how the terminal transferase activity of TdT is much higher than that of Polμ? Combined structural and functional evidences for both Polμ and TdT indicate that there is one residue modulating the terminal transferase activity of both enzymes. That residue (Arg^{387} in Polμ and Lys^{403} in TdT) tunes the catalytic efficiency of the terminal transferase reaction, by regulating the rate-limiting step. Judging by the structural data available, this residue could be establishing dual and alternative interactions during the catalytic cycle of both Polμ and TdT: when the primer is bound at the unproductive position (TdT crystal 1KDH), the residue is interacting with the primer strand, while in the Polμ crystal in which the primer strand is correctly positioned in a productive complex (2IHM), the arginine is interacting with the -3 position of the template strand (Fig. 8B). In the case of Polμ, and assuming an alternative interaction as that seen in TdT, Arg^{387} acts as a brake for the necessary movement of the primer, to limit nucleotide additions before end bridging. In fact, the single change of this residue for the TdT counterpart (Polμ mutant R387K) showed an increase in untemplated additions that ranged from 10- to 100-fold, reaching levels comparable to those of TdT itself [93]. Interestingly, mutant R387K produced a very specific blockage at position +4 when continuous terminal transferase extension of a blunt end was tested [93]. This situation is such that, in a 3-protrusion of 4 nt, the second proposed protein-DNA interaction for this residue cannot occur, since the -3 position of the template strand is not available. In these substrates (ssDNA, 3′ protrusions longer than 3 nt), this residue must be adopting a new partner for this second interaction, most surely a portion of the protein that is now located in place of the template strand: Loop 1. TdT Loop 1 contains a histidine (His^{400}) that completely superimposes with the -3 position of the template strand, and this histidine is surely acting as a partner for Lys^{403} when it is not interacting with the primer (catalytically active configuration; Fig. 8A. left panel). In agreement with this, our results measuring TdT activity on substrates ranging from blunt to 11 nt 3′-protruding indicate that polymerization was inhibited when the protrusion was shorter than 3 nt (these substrates would not allow correct positioning of Loop 1 and His^{400}). A similar protein-protein interaction between Arg^{387} and Loop 1 is surely occurring in Polμ when the -3 position of the template is not available (Fig. 8B, right panel), and it is distorted when the arginine is mutated to alanine, as indicated by the completely defective terminal transferase activity of mutant R387A [92].

Interestingly, the equivalent residue in human Polλ (Lys^{472}) is also involved in regulating the catalytic cycle by means of inhibitory interactions with the primer strand [91]. Recent results suggest that Lys^{472} may help to modulate template-dependent synthesis. In the wild type Polλ binary complex (1XSL), Lys^{472} is within H-bonding distance of the 3′-O of the primer terminal nucleotide. Such hydrogen bond between Lys^{472} and the primer terminus that could stabilize the inactive conformation must be disrupted in order for the 3′-O to assume its catalytically competent position. A weakened interaction between Lys^{472} and the primer terminus would allow the 3′-O to more easily adopt a conformation that would support catalysis with an incorrect nucleotide bound, reducing the discrimination between correct and incorrect incorporation [94].

Thus, Arg^{387} plays a key role in modulating template-independent synthesis by Polμ, having a dual role: it allows terminal transferase additions to occur, but also acts as a brake that limits these additions. Substituting the homologous lysine in TdT with arginine or alanine [90] also

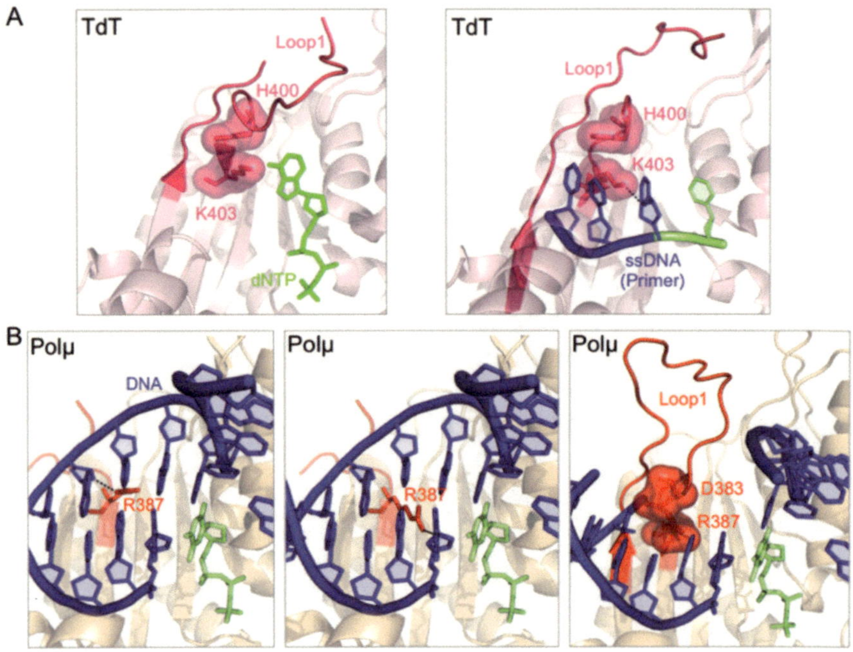

Figure 8. Arg387 triple interactions with the primer and template strands and with Loop 1. A) Cartoon representations of the binary complexes of TdT bound to dNTP (1KEJ) or ssDNA (1KDH). Loop 1 shown in dark pink and Lys403 and His400 show in sticks with semi-transparent surface. B) Cartoon representations of the ternary complex of Polμ: left panel, the original position of Arg387 contacting the template strand; middle panel, the predicted interaction with the primer; right panel, over-imposition of Loop 1 from the TdT structure (1JMS) and proposed interaction of Arg387 and Asp383.

results in loss of template-independent activity, although the properties of the two TdT mutants are not identical. In the case of TdT, residue Lys403 likely establishes a weaker interaction with the primer compared to its orthologue Arg387 in Polμ. Thus, TdT has been optimized to efficiently overcome the rate-limiting step of the terminal transferase, to exclusively perform creative synthesis.

What is the reason for this limited terminal transferase activity in Polμ? Our results indicate that when a templating base is provided *in trans* during NHEJ, the rate-limiting step is relieved. A templating base provided *in trans* by the approaching end that could be located in a proper register will stabilize the incoming (and complementary) nucleotide, thus facilitating primer translocation. As a result of this, NHEJ of many incompatible ends can be efficient and accurate. During NHEJ of this fraction of incompatible ends, an excessive terminal transferase as that displayed by mutant R387K would be disadvantageous in terms of genomic stability. On the other hand, our findings also explain the need for a mild terminal transferase activity in Polμ, not only to create connectivity in those other DNA ends that cannot be efficiently joined on a templating basis, but perhaps contributing to gain a certain degree of genome variability. Additionally, it can be inferred that TdT evolved to maximize the efficiency of the translocation mechanism in the absence of template, at the cost/benefit of introducing untemplated nucleotides, thus being devoted to generate variability at V(D)J recombination intermediates.

Is this the physiological role of the terminal transferase activity of Polμ? NHEJ of short incompatible ends can be accurate in many cases, but imprecise in others depending on both the length and sequence of each protrusion. For the latter cases, when a templating base is not in a proper register, untemplated terminal transferase addition in a NHEJ context provides a valid, although mutagenic, solution that would be conceptually similar to translesion DNA synthesis. Besides, it cannot be ruled out that Polμ's terminal transferase can extend a single short 3′-protrusion to facilitate end joining of this fraction of non-complementary ends. There is also *in vivo* evidence of untemplated insertions made by Polμ. It has been shown that mice that are TdT-/- still contain 5% of V(D)J junctions with template-independent additions, which suggested a possible role of Polμ in these reactions [95]. In agreement with that, the terminal transferase activity of Polμ has been directly implicated in variability/repair processes occurring at embryo developmental stages in which TdT is still not expressed [86].

9. From Polμ to TdT: A new variability–generation mechanism for our immune system

Polμ and TdT are the most closely related of the four members of the human X family, with a 42% identity at the level of the aminoacid sequence. Although the branch of the phylogenetic tree of the X family that contains these two enzymes appeared much sooner than that of Polß, the strict template-independent activity of TdT appears to be a recent evolutionary event that coincides with the development of V(D)J recombination in mammals (Fig. 9). TdT shares the common Polß-like core with 8 kDa, fingers, palm and thumb and also possess the C-terminal BRCT domain that allows recruitment by the Ku proteins to the site of the break. But there are some differences: even though TdT still conserves a positively charged pocket to bind a downstream 5′-P, it contains the lowest amount of positive charges of all the members of the family, and, equal to what happens in Polμ, it has lost the residues essential for the dRP-lyase activity. This first modification, together with the tightly regulated expression of TdT confined to primary lymphoid tissues including thymus and bone marrow [96-98], already indicates that TdT, even though devoted to work at DSBs, is not able to deal with damaged nucleotides and the break points must be "clean", as they are in the case of programmed breaks such as those occurring during the development of the immune response. TdT has been in fact engineered through evolution to "misbehave" and break almost every rule that can apply to a conventional DNA polymerase: it incorporates nucleotides in a template independent manner, using only single stranded DNA [99, 100] or dsDNA with a 3′-overhang longer than four nucleotides [86]. This strict preference for the DNA substrate is dictated by its long Loop 1, of about the same length as the one present in Polμ, but immobilized by several interactions not present in Polμ, such as the ones established between Loop 1 and the small thumb loop [92]. The position of Loop 1 in the crystal structure completely over-imposes with the template strand from the Polμ ternary complex, thus explaining why the length of the single stranded primer needs to be of at least 4 nucleotides for an efficient reaction to take place. This protein piece helps locate the nucleotide in place, and probably is to be blamed for the different order of substrate binding displayed by TdT in contrast with other polymerases: efficient polymerization for a template-dependent polymerase would be optimal through the strictly ordered binding of DNA substrate prior to dNTP, as the converse order of dNTP binding prior to DNA would be error-prone, being correct only once out of four times. Indeed, numerous steady-state and pre-steady state studies have validated that all template-dependent polymerases obey this mechanism [101]. The order by which TdT binds DNA and dNTP is indeed random as determined through a series of initial velocity studies [102]: TdT forms the catalytic competent ternary complex *via* binding of dNTP prior to DNA or vice versa. This scenario is similar to that observed for the *Mycobacterium* NHEJ polymerase, in which a pre-ternary complex can be formed with the nucleotide being present in the absence of a primer strand [103]. This situation could apply also to Polμ, as it would be beneficial for the efficiency of DSB repair, and could have been maintained in TdT since the ability to randomly bind substrates might play a physiological role in generating random nucleotide additions during recombination. Another feature that is present in Polμ and has been maintained in TdT during evolution is the ability to incorporate ribonucleotides. This loss of the "steric gate" probably appeared in Polμ as a collateral effect of the need for a spacious active site able to accommodate misalignments during the search for microhomology, and has been positively selected due to the optimal characteristics of the ribonucleotides as the most abundant substrates, but also due to the "length control" mechanism that the incorporation of ribonucleotides implies during un-templated addition of nucleotides: for both Polμ and TdT, further elongation of a ribonucleotide-containing primer occurs at a slower rate and the addition of more than two ribonucleotides does inhibit activity [55, 56, 104].

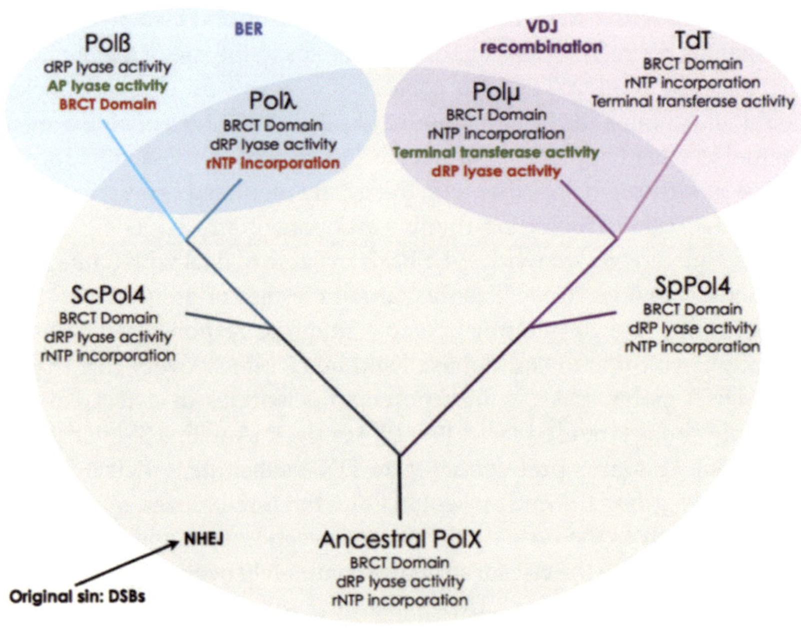

Figure 9. Evolution of family X polymerases. Red color indicates the loss of an activity or feature, green color indicates the gain of an activity or feature. See text for details.

http://dx.doi.org/10.5772/53908

Despite all the similarities between Polμ and TdT, such as the loss of the dRP-lyase activity, the ability to incorporate ribonucleotides and the presence of Loop 1, Polμ has remained preferentially a template-directed polymerase. In the first place, being a more ancient product of evolution than TdT means that its function had to be a more general one: Polμ is devoted mainly to its DNA repair function in the NHEJ pathway. The differential expression patterns of TdT and Polμ also speak in favor of this hypothesis: even though Polμ is strongly expressed in lymphoid tissues in humans, in contrast to TdT, a basal expression of Polμ is observed in a wide range of tissues, more specifically in the brain [7], that suffers from a high level of oxidative damage. Also, the structural features of Polμ support its role as a template-directed NHEJ polymerase: a flexible Loop 1, held but not constrained by several other modules in the protein (the thumb loop, the arginine helix), helps to stabilize gaps in the template strand without blocking the use of the templating base. Also, a specific arginine residue (Arg^{387}), present only in Polμ, acts as a "brake" during the terminal transferase catalytic cycle [93], limiting the number of untemplated additions and keeping the polymerase in a "stand-by" mode for a longer time, awaiting the arrival of the templating base.

Taking advantage of the Dr. Jekyll & Mr. Hyde duality of Polμ as a template-directed and also template-free polymerase, its appearance in the phylogenetic tree of the X family probably was the starter's pistol shot to the process of generating variability during development of the adaptive immune system response, without losing a DNA repair function. In fact, it has been demonstrated that Polμ still participates in the DJ_H rearrangements in mice embryos, where TdT is still not expressed [86]. Based on its DNA-dependent polymerization ability, which TdT lacks, Polμ also fills-in small sequence gaps at the coding ends and contributes to the ligation of highly processed ends, frequently found in the embryo, by pairing two internal microhomology sites. Also, Polμ is involved in V(D)J recombination at immunoglobulin k light-chain loci, after synthesis of the N-regions [85]. The lack of Polμ leads to alterations that induce a profound defect in the peripheral B cell compartment which results in an average 40% reduction in the splenic B cell fraction in Polμ knock-out mice. Polμ appears, therefore, as a key element contributing to the relative homogeneity in size of light chain CDR3 and taking part in Ig gene rearrangement at a stage where TdT is not expressed [85]. Polμ has also been shown to be up regulated in germinal centers after immunization, and although it is not a critical partner, Polμ modulates the *in vivo* somatic hypermutation (SHM) process [105]. The role of Polμ in this process was proposed some time ago [52], and further supported by studies of Polμ overexpression in a Burkitt's lymphoma cell line (with constitutive SHM), in which the SHM rate was increased [53].

10. From Polλ to Polß: Losing the BRCT and evolving base excision repair

The similarity between yeast Pol4 and Polλ, which share the same additional domains (Fig. 2), together with the extraordinary evolutionary conservation of the versions of Polλ present in various higher eukaryotes and in plants (*Arabidopsis thaliana, Wisteria max, Oryza sativa*) suggests that this is the X family member closest to the common ancestor from which all members of the family derived. This could account for the multiple functions of Polλ, since the common ancestor necessarily carried out various processes of DNA synthesis. In this sense, the presence of the Ser/Pro domain is of special relevance, as it could regulate the participation of Polλ in different processes, such as repair by BER, NHEJ and V(D)J recombination.

Members of the human X family of DNA polymerases have specialized in different processes of DNA synthesis associated with repair. Such processes are basically three: 1) base excision repair (BER), carried out mainly by Polß, although Polλ seems to have a role in specific situations; 2) non-homologous end joining (NHEJ), in which, according to the type of substrate generated, Polλ or Polμ could be involved; 3) V(D)J recombination, involving Polλ, Polμ and TdT, with different roles. Subtle differences in the biochemical properties of X family members seem to be crucial for performing one role and not other. Therefore, the members of this family have diversified to be able to carry out non-redundant tasks, achieving a high degree of specialization that has resulted in a high degree of efficiency of each polymerase on its specific function.

Polλ, as the member of the family more closely related to the common ancestor, bears many of the specific modifications needed to perform a high number of functions: it has a BRCT domain needed for interactions with the NHEJ components, and it harbors an 8 kDa domain that acts both as the main DNA binding domain through the 5′-P pocket and as the container of the dRP-lyase activity needed for an efficient performance during BER. Moreover, it contains a long *nail* motif that helps the polymerase to deal with misaligned substrates and might allow scrunching to occur. It has a brooch (WxCxQ motif) that maintains the Polß-like core in a closed conformation throughout the catalytic cycle possibly helping to correctly orient discontinuous NHEJ substrates [92], and finally it has a mid-length Loop 1 that may have a similar role to that proposed for Polμ Loop 1 during NHEJ, but with the limitation of needing some degree of complementarity between the two DNA ends, probably due to the position occupied by this loop in Polλ at the -2 to -4 positions of the template strand.

As a younger member of the family, Polß is the polymerase that has lost the majority of these features, to be focused on enhancing the efficiency of just one reaction: the filling-in of short gaps during BER. For that, it has strengthened the interactions with the DNA substrate through the 5′-P binding pocket, being the most positively charged in this region of the four human enzymes, and it has maintained the dRP-lyase activity and gained an AP-lyase activity, precious for its dedicated job as a BER polymerase. It also maintains a long *nail* that helps locating the DNA substrate on its final catalytic position, and probably helps to "count" the templating nucleotides when filling-in a long gap. It also has the capacity of changing from an "open" to a "closed conformation" since it has lost the brooch at the N-terminal portion of the core, and thus the space between the 8 kDa domain and the thumb subdomain can be expanded to accommodate the yet-to-be-copied templating nucleotides more easily. On the other hand, the loss of this "closing" motif probably meant that its role as a NHEJ polymerase was greatly impaired, together with the complete loss of the Loop 1, which is now merely a turn connecting two ß-strands. The disappearance of this flexible structure probably also led to an improvement of the polymerization on template-containing substrates such as the

http://dx.doi.org/10.5772/53908

ones produced during BER. Congruently, Polß lost the BRCT domain so it does not get recruited to DNA DSBs where it cannot act, and has in turn gained a new set of protein-protein interactions with other BER factors as XRCC1 through specific residues on the surface of its catalytic domain that are required for an efficient repair [106-108]. The Ser/Pro domain located between the BRCT and the catalytic domains in Polλ is also missing in Polß, and this, together with the total absence of CDK phosphorylation sites, unique in the human X family, indicate the lack of a cell-cycle dependent regulation that correlates with its function as a housekeeping gene. Whereas short-patch BER in mammalian cells plays an important role in the maintenance of genomic stability [109-111], it is unlikely that a similar repair pathway is present in many phylogenetically divergent organisms. Plants do not contain a homolog of DNA ligase III, which is required for mammalian short-patch BER, or a Polß homolog [112]. Additionally, the plant XRCC1 protein lacks the Polß binding domain (N-terminal domain; [113]). In contrast, all enzymes needed for long-patch BER are encoded in the genomes of *A. thaliana* and *O. sativa*, suggesting that plants utilize the long-patch BER pathway [112]. Similarly, no protostomic organism possesses the short-patch BER system [9, 114], and a short-patch BER-like pathway is present in yeast but it differs from the mammalian pathway [115]. From the data described above, we hypothesize that short-patch BER is an advanced repair pathway present only in mammals (Fig. 9). Polß, the primary DNA polymerase of this pathway, is highly expressed in brain tissue [116], and would be required mainly to minimize the accumulation of DNA damage in neuronal cells [117] that suffer from a high level of oxidative lesions [118, 119].

11. *In vivo* deficiency models for the X family polymerases: Non–redundant roles in DNA repair and immune system development

The biochemical characteristics of the four members of the X family of polymerases provide strong hints as to what physiological roles they might be performing. To obtain direct evidence of their *in vivo* functions, mouse models were developed for each of the four polymerases individually and in several combinations. In this section we will briefly recapitulate the phenotypes observed with these animals and the conclusions derived from these works.

Initially, two deficiency models were generated for Pol β. The first one eliminated the enzyme from T cells but no differences could be observed between Pol β -deficient and wild-type animals [120]. In the second case, a complete knock-out was generated but the homozygous embryos were unviable due to apoptosis of post-mitotic neurons, as a consequence of defective DNA SSB repair [117]. *In vitro* assays performed with Pol β -deficient cell extracts indicated that this polymerase bears the essential dRP-lyase activity involved in repair of oxidative base lesions [121]. The main mediator of the neuronal apoptosis observed in the Pol $\beta^{-/-}$ background is p53, as indicated by the combined deletion of both genes in the mouse [122]. However, these animals were still unviable, and the data suggested another role of Pol β in the development of certain neuronal cell types. Heterozygous mice displayed a higher risk of cancer development than wild-type mice, although no effect on the lifespan was detected [123]. These animals had normal levels of apoptosis and normal levels of BER enzymes and BER activity, except in spermatogenic cells. These results are in agreement with data showing elevated levels of mutagenesis in this compartment [124] and meiosis failure at prophase I due to defective resolution of DSBs and synapsis at this stage [125]. The sperm cells produced by these animals contained an increased level of transversion mutations. In contrast, Pol $\beta^{-/-}$ mice displayed lower levels of mutagenesis in the embryonic brain than wild-type animals [126], but this can be explained as a result of the apoptotic elimination of neurons with high levels of unrepaired DNA. Very recently, a knock-in mouse model for a natural allele of the human Pol β was reported [127]. This Y265C variant is a mutator polymerase with slower catalysis [128, 129]. The homozygous mutant mice show slower cellular proliferation and increased apoptosis, as well as deficient gap-filling during BER, with DSBs and chromosomal aberrations as a consequence. All these studies show the clear importance of Pol β in meiosis, neuronal development, DNA repair and genomic stability.

In the case of Pol λ, again two mouse models were reported at the same time. One of them showed a very dramatic phenotype of male infertility due to cilia immobility [130], which was later attributed to disruption of a neighboring gene rather than to deletion of Pol λ itself [131]. The second deficiency model was tested initially for somatic hypermutation and this process was not affected [132], but it was later shown that Pol $\lambda^{-/-}$ mice lack diversity in their antibody pools, specifically regarding the N-additions at the junctions in the heavy chain of the TCR receptors [95]. The data indicate that Pol λ might act before TdT during heavy chain rearrangement, suggesting a non-redundant role for Pol λ during V(D)J recombination. Using fibroblasts from the Pol $\lambda^{-/-}$ mice it was shown that this polymerase has a role in the BER pathway to protect cells from oxidative damage [133], and that it can act as a back-up in the absence of Pol β [134]. Moreover, Pol λ is responsible for the majority of the error-free gap-filling in the presence of the 8oxoG lesion in DNA [135].

In 1993 two independent groups published two deficiency mouse models for TdT, reaching very similar conclusions: the TCR receptors of B- and T-lymphocytes had fewer or none N-additions and thus the antibody repertoire was less diverse, maintaining the fetal phenotype in the adult animal [136, 137]. Furthermore, in the absence of TdT, homology-directed repair was detected during V(D)J recombination. Later it was shown that TdT is responsible for 90% of the diversity of the α β TCR receptor repertoire [138].

Mice deficient for Polμ have been also studied, and they are viable and fertile [132]. These mice are defective in immunoglobulin light chain rearrangements and thus development of the bone marrow and B cell differentiation are compromised [85]. A different mouse model was reported with a normal immune response but impaired centroblast development, due to defects in somatic hypermutation and V(D)J recombination [105]. These mice are hypersensitive to γ-irradiation due to a defective DSB repair also in non-hematopoietic tissues [139]. Studies of the embryonic stage, when TdT is still not expressed, indicated that Polμ is responsible for the observed N-additions at the post-gastrulation DJ_H joints during immunoglobulin gene rearrangements [86]. These results support the roles of Polμ during hematopoietic development and the processes of somatic hypermutation and class-switch recombination, during the generation of extra diversity in the immune system and, finally, its contribution to genomic stability through repair of DSBs *via* the NHEJ pathway.

http://dx.doi.org/10.5772/53908

12. A case of convergent evolution: Comparison of the characteristics shared by bacterial and eukaryotic NHEJ polymerases

Conventional replicative and lesion bypass DNA polymerases extend off dsDNA substrates, containing both primer and template strands, in a 5′ to 3′ direction. In contrast, polymerases involved in DSB repair must be capable of binding and extending off non-canonical DNA substrates, including 3′ over-hanging termini lacking continuous primer and template strands. Recent studies on the bacterial NHEJ polymerases have revealed some of the unusual activities associated with these repair enzymes that enable DNA extension under the most extreme conditions. For example, a homodimeric arrangement of the mycobacterial NHEJ polymerases can facilitate the association of two incompatible 3′-protruding DNA ends, *via* microhomology-mediated synapsis, forming a stable end-joining intermediate [140]. This synaptic complex reflects an intermediate bridging stage of the NHEJ process, prior to end processing and ligation. In this way, the polymerase restores the continuity of the dsDNA helix, catalyzing a conventional 5′-3′ extension reaction occurring on one DNA end, but templated *in trans* by a second (synapsed) DNA end. This structure showed an intrinsic difference with the eukaryotic system: working as a dimer *versus* a monomer, a two-handed *versus* a one-handed way of fixing broken DNA (Fig. 10). Despite this, and the different origins of the prokaryotic and eukaryotic NHEJ polymerases (AEP family of primases versus X family of DNA polymerases, respectively), we will discuss how these two systems share an unexpected amount of functional and structural features, making it a striking example of convergent evolution.

Mycobacterium tuberculosis PolDom is a unique polymerase with a variety of activities on different NHEJ DNA substrates, displaying terminal transferase activity on blunt and ssDNA substrates and templated polymerization: directed *in cis* on gapped and 5′-protruding substrates [22, 141, 142], and *in trans* on 3′-protruding substrates [103, 140]. The architecture of the bacterial NHEJ polymerases is different to that of the eukaryotic NHEJ polymerases from the X family, although the triad of metal-chelating aspartates is conserved and structurally over-imposable (Fig. 11A), a suggestion of the convergent evolution leading to similar catalytic mechanisms. But the convergence does not stop there: in all the activities tested, PolDom shows a marked preference for the insertion of ribonucleotides over deoxynucleotides. This preference, a consequence of the origins of PolDom from the AEP family of primases, reflects a catalytic plasticity that is maintained during evolution on other unrelated NHEJ polymerases such as Polμ [55, 56], and now serves a different purpose: to take advantage of the most abundant substrates during a laborious reaction. And, like the eukaryotic NHEJ ligase, the bacterial LigD ligates DNA containing ribonucleotides at the 3′-OH terminus [142, 143].

Another example of the common characteristics of the prokaryotic and eukaryotic NHEJ polymerases is the presence of a binding pocket for the 5′-P group of the downstream piece of DNA (Fig. 11B). This pocket, which contains residues Lys^{16} and Lys^{26}, is missing in AEPs from *Archaea* and *Eukarya,* and is the major determinant for the specific binding of PolDom to its substrates, as the interaction significantly enhances its activity [22]. While Polμ or Polλ use a specific HhH motif at the 8 kDa domain to bind the phosphate, PolDom lacks this HhH and must therefore utilize a novel structural element to facilitate this interaction.

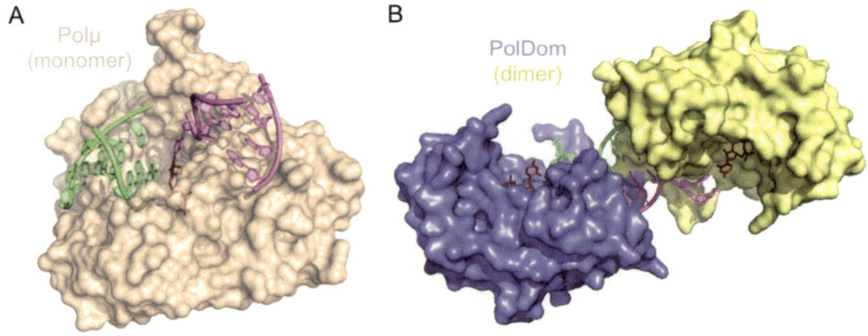

Figure 10. Different solutions for the NHEJ polymerases: monomers and dimers. A) Surface representation of a monomer of Polμ holding two pieces of DNA (green and mauve). B) Surface representation of a dimeric arrangement of *Mt*-PolDom (yellow and blue monomers) bridging two DNA ends (green and mauve).

Although recent studies have provided unique insights into polymerase-mediated orchestration of break synapsis, the order of substrate binding events and mechanism by which these NHEJ polymerases catalyze end-extension is still poorly understood. To address this question, in collaboration with Prof. Doherty (GDSC, University of Sussex), we elucidated the functional meaning of a novel crystal structure of a pre-ternary intermediate of *Mt*-PolDom bound to DNA, showing that this complex is relevant for specific DSB repair processing events [103]. This catalytically competent complex consists of a PolDom monomer, containing two metal ions and a templated nucleotide (UTP) in its active site, bound to a dsDNA end with a 3′ overhang but, significantly, lacking a primer strand. To our knowledge, this structure represents a unique example of a polymerase-DNA complex captured in a pre-ternary intermediate state, relevant for NHEJ.

Is the pre-ternary complex physiologically relevant for prokaryotic NHEJ polymerase extension reactions? Although the pre-ternary complex lacks an incoming primer strand, which provides the attacking nucleophile (3′-OH), a comparison of the positioning of the nucleotide base, phosphate tail, active site ligands and divalent metal ions to those in the active site of a polymerase ternary complex (Polλ) provides compelling evidence that the PolDom pre-ternary complex is catalytically competent (Fig. 11A). The possibility of preforming a pre-ternary complex in solution by incubating the necessary components (PolDom, DNA end, complementary nucleotide and activating metal ions) in the absence of a primer, allowed us to demonstrate its physiological relevance in accelerating NHEJ reactions, probably by providing a "ready to use" primer binding site. By testing the activity of the pre-ternary PolDom complex with different ssDNA primers, we concluded that the minimal primer utilizable by these enzymes is a dinucleotide, as PolDom was not proficient at polymerizing off a single nucleotide "primer". This fact indicates that, although PolDom is evolutionarily related to replicative AEPs, its physiological activity as a primase has effectively been lost and, instead, these polymerases have evolved to have a more restricted capacity to bind short incoming DNA termini, enabling them to perform more specialized roles in NHEJ break repair processes. The innate ability of AEPs to accept short primers may have influenced evolutionary selection of these enzymes by prokaryotes to become the NHEJ polymerase. Indeed, many

http://dx.doi.org/10.5772/53908

bacteria encode additional AEP orthologues whose physiological roles have yet to be determined. Is pre-ternary complex formation also relevant for eukaryotic NHEJ polymerases? It has been demonstrated that human Polμ can catalyze NHEJ extensions on very short and non-complementary DNA ends [29, 144], a reaction that can take advantage of a limited terminal transferase activity [93], and that can occur with both dNTPs and NTPs [145]. It is likely that formation of a Polμ pre-ternary complex, triggered by the strong recognition of a 5′-recessive phosphate and a reinforced avidity for the incoming nucleotide (both properties also intrinsic to Polμ), would be beneficial to carry out non-complementary NHEJ of minimally processed ends in eukaryotes, although this remains to be proven.

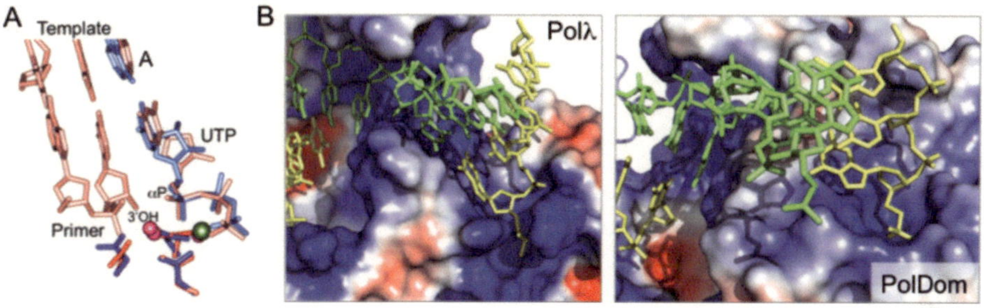

Figure 11. Similarities among the eukaryotic and prokaryotic NHEJ polymerases. A) Superimposition of the ternary complex of Polλ (1XSN) and the pre-ternary complex of Mt-PolDom (3PKY). B) Electrostatic surface of the Polλ and Mt-PolDom 5′-P binding pockets. DNA substrates are shown in green (template strand) and yellow (primer and downstream strands).

From a mechanistic point of view, our study of PolDom identified a conserved loop (loop 2), which plays a prominent role in the activation of the catalytic center. The conformation of loop 2 changes significantly, upon the templated-binding of the correct incoming nucleotide, which induces the rotation of Arg^{220} side-chain (~180°) away from the active site in the pre-ternary complex. Mutation of this invariant residue abolished the extension activity but, significantly, did not alter enzyme binding to other DNA substrates, such as gapped DNA. A comparison of the structures of the PolDom-DNA binary *versus* the pre-ternary complexes reveals the sequential movements that occur in the active site, induced by the binding of both a templating base and an incoming nucleotide. The invariant active site residue Phe^{64}, which stacks against the base of the incoming nucleotide in the PolDom-GTP binary complex, now stacks against the base of the templating nucleotide both in PolDom-DNA binary and pre-ternary complexes, orienting this base and also maintaining (together with Phe^{63}) the major kink in the template strand (~105º). In replicative DNA polymerases, aromatic tyrosine residues are commonly employed as a part of a fidelity mechanism that scrutinizes pairing of the correct incoming base with the templating base, thus acting as a molecular gatekeeper to limit the incorporation of an incorrect/mismatched base during elongation [146]. We propose that an analogous fidelity mechanism involving the two invariant phenylalanine residues also occurs in the bacterial NHEJ polymerases, but in the absence of the primer strand, thus ensuring that the correctly templated incoming base is bound in the active site prior to the encounter with the incoming end/primer providing the attacking 3′-OH.

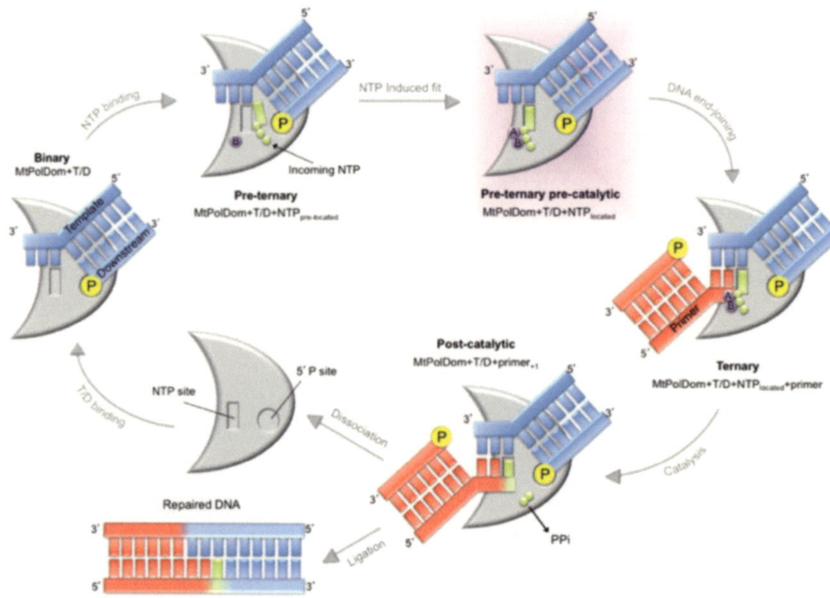

Figure 12. Catalytic Cycle of a Prokaryotic NHEJ Polymerase. Initially, a binary complex between the PolDom enzyme (gray crescent) and DNA (T/D; blue) is formed, mainly stabilized via interactions with the 5'-P. Binding of an incoming NTP (green) forms a preternary complex, still incompetent for catalysis as it lacks metal A. Upon template selection and relocation of the complementary NTP and the two metals, A and B, at the correct site (representing a primer-independent NTP induced-fit step) a preternary precatalytic complex is formed. This activated complex is ready for DNA end joining, allowing the 3'-OH of the incoming primer strand (red) to bind in the active site to form the ternary complex. Further steps of extension, PPi release, dissociation, and ligation (performed by the ligase domain of LigD), complete the DNA repair process.

This phenylalanine-mediated (Phe^{64}) stacking interaction with the templating base in the preternary complex also promotes the movement of the incoming nucleotide (UTP) into the active site and, together with the loss of specific contacts (e.g. Arg^{246}, Lys^{175}, Lys^{52}) promotes the correct repositioning of the α-phosphate group of the incoming nucleotide for catalysis. This reoriented α-phosphate moiety, together with Asp^{139}, forms a second metal binding site (A) not present in the binary structure, which is required for the two metal catalytic mechanism common to all DNA polymerases [147]. The binding of the second metal, in turn, promotes breakage of the salt bridge between Arg^{220} and Asp^{139}, repositioning this aspartate into a catalytically favorable alignment with the other catalytic aspartates, the α-phosphate group and the two bound metal ions, to form an activated pre-ternary intermediate awaiting the arrival of the nucleophile (3'-OH of the primer strand). The catalytic incompetence of the R220A mutant highlights the importance of the interaction of Arg^{220} with Asp^{139}. We propose that the maintenance of this amino acid pairing provides a significant barrier to catalysis until the enzyme becomes optimally bound to DNA, metals, and the correct incoming templated nucleotide. Once these are bound within the active site, a sequence of structural rearrangements promotes the binding of a second metal ion (A). The affinity of Asp^{139} for this second metal promotes the loss of interaction with Arg^{220}, leading to expulsion of loop 2 from the active site, which results in full activation of the catalytic center. The movement of loop 2 away from the active site, most likely, promotes this activation step in two ways. The first consequence is that breaking the salt bridge is irreversible, leading to the release of the acidic side-chain of Asp^{139}, which is involved in the binding of the second metal (A) within the active site, ensuring that it is optimally poised for catalysis. The second notable consequence, induced by the reorientation of loop 2, is a significant change in the ridge that surrounds the active site, which most likely allows the 3′-OH group of the incoming primer strand to bind in the active site and form the complete ternary complex. Further steps of catalysis, PPi release, and ligation would lead to the conclusion of the NHEJ process. A scheme of the different complexes formed during the whole NHEJ cycle is depicted in figure 12. It is remarkable how, despite the different origins of PolDom and Polß, a similar mechanism of prevention of catalysis exists in both of them: an arginine residue contacts one of the catalytic aspartates, keeping it in an unproductive conformation that does not allow catalysis until binding of the nucleotide.

We have intensively studied the loops and flexible elements in Polμ, and examined the structure and the mutagenesis studies we have performed on PolDom, reaching the conclusion that both enzymes rely on those movable pieces to perform their most specific activities. As an even more striking example of convergent evolution, PolDom possesses a prominent surface ß-hairpin structure, loop 1, which is specific to NHEJ AEPs. Conserved residues in loop 1 interact with the 3′ protrusion of NHEJ substrates and orient the synapsis of the ends [140]. Mutation of the apical residues of loop 1 to alanine did not affect binding to a primer-containing (gap) substrate, but abolished the ability of PolDom to form a synaptic complex [140] and, consequently, to catalyze trans-directed additions. Loop 1 in Polμ is also specific for binding and activity on NHEJ substrates [80, 92], through its function in the stabilization of the synapsis of two DNA ends.

13. Conclusion

In recent years, structural genomics has given rise to a vast array of knowledge, which nonetheless needs to be interpreted correctly as a range of still snapshots of a movie that, if seen, would show the highly complex and ever-moving machines that polymerases are. Helped by the biochemistry, and placed in context by the *in vivo* data, this structural approach has been used here to better understand the unique properties of each of the human DNA polymerases of the X family, and also of their bacterial counterparts. Thorough analysis of these structures has provided us with a deeper understanding of the unique abilities attributed to each polymerase.

Acknowledgements

We thank Dr. Miguel Garcia-Diaz for very interesting and insightful conversations, Dr. Antonio Bernad for providing us with up-to-date information regarding the mouse deficiency-models, Dr. Thomas Kunkel, Dr. Katharyzna Bebenek and Dr. Dale Ramsden for ten very pleasant years of parallel and coordinated research, and all the members of the Blanco lab for their dedicated work.

Author details

Maria Jose Martin and Luis Blanco*

Centro de Biología Molecular Severo Ochoa (CSIC-UAM), Madrid, Spain

References

[1] Bebenek, K, & Kunkel, T. A. *Functions of DNA polymerases.* Adv Protein Chem, (2004). , 137-165.

[2] Burgers, P. M, et al. *Eukaryotic DNA polymerases: proposal for a revised nomenclature.* J Biol Chem, (2001). , 43487-43490.

[3] Hubscher, U, Maga, G, & Spadari, S. *Eukaryotic DNA polymerases.* Annu Rev Biochem, (2002). , 133-163.

[4] Pavlov, Y. I, Shcherbakova, P. V, & Rogozin, I. B. *Roles of DNA polymerases in replication, repair, and recombination in eukaryotes.* Int Rev Cytol, (2006). , 41-132.

[5] Ohmori, H, et al. *The Y-family of DNA polymerases.* Mol Cell, (2001). , 7-8.

[6] Garcia-diaz, M, et al. *DNA polymerase lambda (Pol lambda), a novel eukaryotic DNA polymerase with a potential role in meiosis.* J Mol Biol, (2000). , 851-867.

[7] Dominguez, O, et al. *DNA polymerase mu (Pol mu), homologous to TdT, could act as a DNA mutator in eukaryotic cells.* EMBO J, (2000). , 1731-1742.

[8] Oliveros, M, et al. *Characterization of an African swine fever virus 20-kDa DNA polymerase involved in DNA repair.* J Biol Chem, (1997). , 30899-30910.

[9] Takeuchi, R, et al. *Drosophila DNA polymerase zeta interacts with recombination repair protein 1, the Drosophila homologue of human abasic endonuclease 1.* J Biol Chem, (2006). , 11577-11585.

[10] Uchiyama, Y, et al. *Distribution and roles of X-family DNA polymerases in eukaryotes.* Biochimie, (2009). , 165-170.

[11] Demogines, A, et al. *Ancient and recent adaptive evolution of primate non-homologous end joining genes.* PLoS Genet, (2010). , e1001169.

[12] Kelley, J. L, et al. *Targeted resequencing of two genes, RAGE and POLL, confirms findings from a genome-wide scan for adaptive evolution and provides evidence for positive selection in additional populations.* Hum Mol Genet, (2009). , 779-784.

[13] Sawyer, S. L, & Malik, H. S. *Positive selection of yeast nonhomologous end-joining genes and a retrotransposon conflict hypothesis.* Proc Natl Acad Sci U S A, (2006). , 17614-17619.

[14] Bruton, R. K, et al. *C-terminal-binding protein interacting protein binds directly to adenovirus early region 1A through its N-terminal region and conserved region 3.* Oncogene, (2007). , 7467-7479.

[15] Evans, J. D, & Hearing, P. *Relocalization of the Mre11-Rad50-Nbs1 complex by the adenovirus E4 ORF3 protein is required for viral replication.* J Virol, (2005). , 6207-6215.

[16] Jayaram, S, et al. *E1B 55k-independent dissociation of the DNA ligase IV/XRCC4 complex by E4 34k during adenovirus infection.* Virology, (2008). , 163-170.

[17] Kilzer, J. M, et al. *Roles of host cell factors in circularization of retroviral dna.* Virology, (2003). , 460-467.

[18] Li, L, et al. *Role of the non-homologous DNA end joining pathway in the early steps of retroviral infection.* EMBO J, (2001). , 3272-3281.

[19] Lin, C. W, & Engelman, A. *The barrier-to-autointegration factor is a component of functional human immunodeficiency virus type 1 preintegration complexes.* J Virol, (2003). , 5030-5036.

[20] Stracker, T. H, Carson, C. T, & Weitzman, M. D. *Adenovirus oncoproteins inactivate the Mre11-Rad50-NBS1 DNA repair complex.* Nature, (2002). , 348-352.

[21] Weitzman, M. D, et al. *Interactions of viruses with the cellular DNA repair machinery.* DNA Repair (Amst), (2004). , 1165-1173.

[22] Pitcher, R. S, et al. *Structure and function of a mycobacterial NHEJ DNA repair polymerase.* J Mol Biol, (2007). , 391-405.

[23] Garcia-escudero, R, et al. *DNA polymerase X of African swine fever virus: insertion fidelity on gapped DNA substrates and AP lyase activity support a role in base excision repair of viral DNA.* J Mol Biol, (2003). , 1403-1412.

[24] Taladriz, S, et al. *Nuclear DNA polymerase beta from Leishmania infantum. Cloning, molecular analysis and developmental regulation.* Nucleic Acids Res, (2001). , 3822-3834.

[25] Bebenek, K, et al. *Biochemical properties of Saccharomyces cerevisiae DNA polymerase IV.* J Biol Chem, (2005). , 20051-20058.

[26] Gonzalez-barrera, S, et al. *Characterization of SpPol4, a unique X-family DNA polymerase in Schizosaccharomyces pombe.* Nucleic Acids Res, (2005). , 4762-4774.

[27] Tseng, H. M, & Tomkinson, A. E. *A physical and functional interaction between yeast Pol4 and Dnl4-Lif1 links DNA synthesis and ligation in nonhomologous end joining.* J Biol Chem, (2002)., 45630-45637.

[28] Tseng, H. M, & Tomkinson, A. E. *Processing and joining of DNA ends coordinated by interactions among Dnl4/Lif1, Pol4, and FEN-1.* J Biol Chem, (2004)., 47580-47588.

[29] Nick McElhinnyS.A., et al., *A gradient of template dependence defines distinct biological roles for family X polymerases in nonhomologous end joining.* Mol Cell, (2005)., 357-366.

[30] Lee, J. W, et al. *Implication of DNA polymerase lambda in alignment-based gap filling for nonhomologous DNA end joining in human nuclear extracts.* J Biol Chem, (2004)., 805-811.

[31] Manke, I. A, et al. *BRCT repeats as phosphopeptide-binding modules involved in protein targeting.* Science, (2003)., 636-639.

[32] Yu, X, et al. *The BRCT domain is a phospho-protein binding domain.* Science, (2003)., 639-642.

[33] Derose, E. F, et al. *Solution structure of polymerase mu's BRCT Domain reveals an element essential for its role in nonhomologous end joining.* Biochemistry, (2007)., 12100-12110.

[34] Martin, M. J, Juarez, R, & Blanco, L. *DNA-binding determinants promoting NHEJ by human Polmu.* Nucleic Acids Res, (2012)., 11389-11403.

[35] Matsumoto, T, et al. *BRCT domain of DNA polymerase mu has DNA-binding activity and promotes the DNA polymerization activity.* Genes Cells, (2012)., 790-806.

[36] Mueller, G. A, et al. *A comparison of BRCT domains involved in nonhomologous end-joining: introducing the solution structure of the BRCT domain of polymerase lambda.* DNA Repair (Amst), (2008)., 1340-1351.

[37] Fan, W, & Wu, X. *DNA polymerase lambda can elongate on DNA substrates mimicking non-homologous end joining and interact with XRCC4-ligase IV complex.* Biochem Biophys Res Commun, (2004)., 1328-1333.

[38] Prasad, R, Beard, W. A, & Wilson, S. H. *Studies of gapped DNA substrate binding by mammalian DNA polymerase beta. Dependence on 5'-phosphate group.* J Biol Chem, (1994)., 18096-18101.

[39] Pelletier, H, et al. *Crystal structures of human DNA polymerase beta complexed with DNA: implications for catalytic mechanism, processivity, and fidelity.* Biochemistry, (1996)., 12742-12761.

[40] Moon, A. F, et al. *Structural insight into the substrate specificity of DNA Polymerase mu.* Nat Struct Mol Biol, (2007)., 45-53.

[41] Garcia-diaz, M, et al. *Identification of an intrinsic 5′-deoxyribose-5-phosphate lyase activity in human DNA polymerase lambda: a possible role in base excision repair.* J Biol Chem, (2001). , 34659-34663.

[42] Prasad, R, et al. *Human DNA polymerase beta deoxyribose phosphate lyase. Substrate specificity and catalytic mechanism.* J Biol Chem, (1998). , 15263-15270.

[43] Garcia-diaz, M, et al. *A structural solution for the DNA polymerase lambda-dependent repair of DNA gaps with minimal homology.* Mol Cell, (2004). , 561-572.

[44] Singhal, R. K, & Wilson, S. H. *Short gap-filling synthesis by DNA polymerase beta is processive.* J Biol Chem, (1993). , 15906-15911.

[45] Garcia-diaz, M, et al. *DNA polymerase lambda, a novel DNA repair enzyme in human cells.* J Biol Chem, (2002). , 13184-13191.

[46] Doherty, A. J, Serpell, L. C, & Ponting, C. P. *The helix-hairpin-helix DNA-binding motif: a structural basis for non-sequence-specific recognition of DNA.* Nucleic Acids Res, (1996). , 2488-2497.

[47] Mullen, G. P, & Wilson, S. H. *DNA polymerase beta in abasic site repair: a structurally conserved helix-hairpin-helix motif in lesion detection by base excision repair enzymes.* Biochemistry, (1997). , 4713-4717.

[48] Sobol, R. W, et al. *The lyase activity of the DNA repair protein beta-polymerase protects from DNA-damage-induced cytotoxicity.* Nature, (2000). , 807-810.

[49] Beard, W. A, & Wilson, S. H. *Structure and mechanism of DNA polymerase Beta.* Chem Rev, (2006). , 361-382.

[50] Garcia-diaz, M, et al. *Structure-function studies of DNA polymerase lambda.* DNA Repair (Amst), (2005). , 1358-1367.

[51] Prasad, R, et al. *Structural insight into the DNA polymerase beta deoxyribose phosphate lyase mechanism.* DNA Repair (Amst), (2005). , 1347-1357.

[52] Ruiz, J. F, et al. *DNA polymerase mu, a candidate hypermutase?* Philos Trans R Soc Lond B Biol Sci, (2001). , 99-109.

[53] Ruiz, J. F, et al. *Overexpression of human DNA polymerase mu (Pol mu) in a Burkitt's lymphoma cell line affects the somatic hypermutation rate.* Nucleic Acids Res, (2004). , 5861-5873.

[54] Zhang, Y, et al. *Highly frequent frameshift DNA synthesis by human DNA polymerase mu.* Mol Cell Biol, (2001). , 7995-8006.

[55] Nick McElhinnyS.A. and D.A. Ramsden, *Polymerase mu is a DNA-directed DNA/RNA polymerase.* Mol Cell Biol, (2003). , 2309-2315.

[56] Ruiz, J. F, et al. *Lack of sugar discrimination by human Pol mu requires a single glycine residue.* Nucleic Acids Res, (2003). , 4441-4449.

[57] Lieber, M. R, et al. *The mechanism of vertebrate nonhomologous DNA end joining and its role in V(D)J recombination.* DNA Repair (Amst), (2004). , 817-826.

[58] Ferguson, D. O, et al. *The nonhomologous end-joining pathway of DNA repair is required for genomic stability and the suppression of translocations.* Proc Natl Acad Sci U S A, (2000). , 6630-6633.

[59] Heidenreich, E, et al. *Non-homologous end joining as an important mutagenic process in cell cycle-arrested cells.* EMBO J, (2003). , 2274-2283.

[60] Walker, J. R, Corpina, R. A, & Goldberg, J. *Structure of the Ku heterodimer bound to DNA and its implications for double-strand break repair.* Nature, (2001). , 607-614.

[61] Dvir, A, et al. *Ku autoantigen is the regulatory component of a template-associated protein kinase that phosphorylates RNA polymerase II.* Proc Natl Acad Sci U S A, (1992). , 11920-11924.

[62] Gottlieb, T. M, & Jackson, S. P. *The DNA-dependent protein kinase: requirement for DNA ends and association with Ku antigen.* Cell, (1993). , 131-142.

[63] Dynan, W. S, & Yoo, S. *Interaction of Ku protein and DNA-dependent protein kinase catalytic subunit with nucleic acids.* Nucleic Acids Res, (1998). , 1551-1559.

[64] Chen, L, et al. *Interactions of the DNA ligase IV-XRCC4 complex with DNA ends and the DNA-dependent protein kinase.* J Biol Chem, (2000). , 26196-26205.

[65] Defazio, L. G, et al. *Synapsis of DNA ends by DNA-dependent protein kinase.* EMBO J, (2002). , 3192-3200.

[66] Yaneva, M, Kowalewski, T, & Lieber, M. R. *Interaction of DNA-dependent protein kinase with DNA and with Ku: biochemical and atomic-force microscopy studies.* EMBO J, (1997). , 5098-5112.

[67] Kramer, K. M, et al. *Two different types of double-strand breaks in Saccharomyces cerevisiae are repaired by similar RAD52-independent, nonhomologous recombination events.* Mol Cell Biol, (1994). , 1293-1301.

[68] Moore, J. K, & Haber, J. E. *Cell cycle and genetic requirements of two pathways of nonhomologous end-joining repair of double-strand breaks in Saccharomyces cerevisiae.* Mol Cell Biol, (1996). , 2164-2173.

[69] Roth, D. B, & Wilson, J. H. *Nonhomologous recombination in mammalian cells: role for short sequence homologies in the joining reaction.* Mol Cell Biol, (1986). , 4295-4304.

[70] Wilson, T. E, & Lieber, M. R. *Efficient processing of DNA ends during yeast nonhomologous end joining. Evidence for a DNA polymerase beta (Pol4)-dependent pathway.* J Biol Chem, (1999). , 23599-23609.

[71] Ma, Y, et al. *Hairpin opening and overhang processing by an Artemis/DNA-dependent protein kinase complex in nonhomologous end joining and V(D)J recombination.* Cell, (2002). , 781-794.

[72] Hefferin, M. L, & Tomkinson, A. E. *Mechanism of DNA double-strand break repair by non-homologous end joining.* DNA Repair (Amst), (2005). , 639-648.

[73] Karimi-busheri, F, et al. *Molecular characterization of a human DNA kinase.* J Biol Chem, (1999). , 24187-24194.

[74] Chappell, C, et al. *Involvement of human polynucleotide kinase in double-strand break repair by non-homologous end joining.* EMBO J, (2002). , 2827-2832.

[75] Grawunder, U, et al. *Activity of DNA ligase IV stimulated by complex formation with XRCC4 protein in mammalian cells.* Nature, (1997). , 492-495.

[76] Schar, P, et al. *A newly identified DNA ligase of Saccharomyces cerevisiae involved in RAD52-independent repair of DNA double-strand breaks.* Genes Dev, (1997). , 1912-1924.

[77] Teo, S. H, & Jackson, S. P. *Identification of Saccharomyces cerevisiae DNA ligase IV: involvement in DNA double-strand break repair.* EMBO J, (1997). , 4788-4795.

[78] Wilson, T. E, Grawunder, U, & Lieber, M. R. *Yeast DNA ligase IV mediates non-homologous DNA end joining.* Nature, (1997). , 495-498.

[79] Ramsden, D. A. *Polymerases in nonhomologous end joining: building a bridge over broken chromosomes.* Antioxid Redox Signal, (2011). , 2509-2519.

[80] Juarez, R, et al. *A specific loop in human DNA polymerase mu allows switching between creative and DNA-instructed synthesis.* Nucleic Acids Res, (2006). , 4572-4582.

[81] Ma, Y, et al. *A biochemically defined system for mammalian nonhomologous DNA end joining.* Mol Cell, (2004). , 701-713.

[82] Ahnesorg, P, Smith, P, & Jackson, S. P. *XLF interacts with the XRCC4-DNA ligase IV complex to promote DNA nonhomologous end-joining.* Cell, (2006). , 301-313.

[83] Hentges, P, et al. *Evolutionary and functional conservation of the DNA non-homologous end-joining protein, XLF/Cernunnos.* J Biol Chem, (2006). , 37517-37526.

[84] Papavasiliou, F, et al. *V(D)J recombination in mature B cells: a mechanism for altering antibody responses.* Science, (1997). , 298-301.

[85] Bertocci, B, et al. *Immunoglobulin kappa light chain gene rearrangement is impaired in mice deficient for DNA polymerase mu.* Immunity, (2003). , 203-211.

[86] Gozalbo-lopez, B, et al. *A role for DNA polymerase mu in the emerging DJH rearrangements of the postgastrulation mouse embryo.* Mol Cell Biol, (2009). , 1266-1275.

[87] Bentolila, L. A, et al. *The two isoforms of mouse terminal deoxynucleotidyl transferase differ in both the ability to add N regions and subcellular localization.* EMBO J, (1995). , 4221-4229.

[88] Bentolila, L. A, et al. *Extensive junctional diversity in Ig light chain genes from early B cell progenitors of mu MT mice.* J Immunol, (1999). , 2123-2128.

[89] Delarue, M, et al. *Crystal structures of a template-independent DNA polymerase: murine terminal deoxynucleotidyltransferase.* EMBO J, (2002). , 427-439.

[90] Romain, F, et al. *Conferring a template-dependent polymerase activity to terminal deoxynucleotidyltransferase by mutations in the Loop1 region.* Nucleic Acids Res, (2009). , 4642-4656.

[91] Bebenek, K, et al. *Loop 1 modulates the fidelity of DNA polymerase lambda.* Nucleic Acids Res, (2010). , 5419-5431.

[92] Martin, M. J. *Exclusive Polymerases Repairing Double Strand Breaks. The same magics from bacteria to man.*, (2011). Universidad Autonoma de Madrid.

[93] Andrade, P, et al. *Limited terminal transferase in human DNA polymerase mu defines the required balance between accuracy and efficiency in NHEJ.* Proc Natl Acad Sci U S A, (2009). , 16203-16208.

[94] Bebenek, K, et al. *The frameshift infidelity of human DNA polymerase lambda. Implications for function.* J Biol Chem, (2003). , 34685-34690.

[95] Bertocci, B, et al. *Nonoverlapping functions of DNA polymerases mu, lambda, and terminal deoxynucleotidyltransferase during immunoglobulin V(D)J recombination in vivo.* Immunity, (2006). , 31-41.

[96] Bollum, F. J. *Terminal deoxynucleotidyl transferase as a hematopoietic cell marker.* Blood, (1979). , 1203-1215.

[97] Coleman, M. S, Hutton, J. J, & Bollum, F. J. *Terminal riboadenylate transferase in human lymphocytes.* Nature, (1974). , 407-409.

[98] Kunkel, T. A, et al. *Rearrangements of DNA mediated by terminal transferase.* Proc Natl Acad Sci U S A, (1986). , 1867-1871.

[99] Bollum, F. J. *Mammalian enzymes of desoxyribonucleic acid synthesis.* Ann N Y Acad Sci, (1959). , 792-793.

[100] Bollum, F. J. *Chemically Defined Templates and Initiators for Deoxypolynucleotide Synthesis.* Science, (1964). , 560.

[101] Benkovic, S. J, & Cameron, C. E. *Kinetic analysis of nucleotide incorporation and misincorporation by Klenow fragment of Escherichia coli DNA polymerase I.* Methods Enzymol, (1995). , 257-269.

[102] Deibel, M. R, & Jr, M. S. Coleman, *Biochemical properties of purified human terminal deoxynucleotidyltransferase.* J Biol Chem, (1980)., 4206-4212.

[103] Brissett, N. C, et al. *Structure of a preternary complex involving a prokaryotic NHEJ DNA polymerase.* Mol Cell, (2011)., 221-231.

[104] Roychoudhury, R. *Enzymic synthesis of polynucleotides. Oligodeoxynucleotides with one 3'-terminal ribonucleotide as primers for polydeoxynucleotide synthesis.* J Biol Chem, (1972)., 3910-3917.

[105] Lucas, D, et al. *Polymerase mu is up-regulated during the T cell-dependent immune response and its deficiency alters developmental dynamics of spleen centroblasts.* Eur J Immunol, (2005)., 1601-1611.

[106] Dianova, I. I, et al. *XRCC1-DNA polymerase beta interaction is required for efficient base excision repair.* Nucleic Acids Res, (2004)., 2550-2555.

[107] Gryk, M. R, et al. *Mapping of the interaction interface of DNA polymerase beta with XRCC1.* Structure, (2002)., 1709-1720.

[108] Marintchev, A, et al. *Domain specific interaction in the XRCC1-DNA polymerase beta complex.* Nucleic Acids Res, (2000)., 2049-2059.

[109] Fortini, P, et al. *Different DNA polymerases are involved in the short- and long-patch base excision repair in mammalian cells.* Biochemistry, (1998)., 3575-3580.

[110] Sobol, R. W, et al. *Requirement of mammalian DNA polymerase-beta in base-excision repair.* Nature, (1996)., 183-186.

[111] Sobol, R. W, & Wilson, S. H. *Mammalian DNA beta-polymerase in base excision repair of alkylation damage.* Prog Nucleic Acid Res Mol Biol, (2001)., 57-74.

[112] Kimura, S, & Sakaguchi, K. *DNA repair in plants.* Chem Rev, (2006)., 753-766.

[113] Uchiyama, Y, Suzuki, Y, & Sakaguchi, K. *Characterization of plant XRCC1 and its interaction with proliferating cell nuclear antigen.* Planta, (2008)., 1233-1241.

[114] Radford, S. J, et al. *Heteroduplex DNA in meiotic recombination in Drosophila mei-9 mutants.* Genetics, (2007)., 63-72.

[115] Alseth, I, et al. *Biochemical characterization and DNA repair pathway interactions of Mag1-mediated base excision repair in Schizosaccharomyces pombe.* Nucleic Acids Res, (2005)., 1123-1131.

[116] Hirose, F, et al. *Difference in the expression level of DNA polymerase beta among mouse tissues: high expression in the pachytene spermatocyte.* Exp Cell Res, (1989)., 169-180.

[117] Sugo, N, et al. *Neonatal lethality with abnormal neurogenesis in mice deficient in DNA polymerase beta.* EMBO J, (2000)., 1397-1404.

[118] Nakamura, J, & Swenberg, J. A. *Endogenous apurinic/apyrimidinic sites in genomic DNA of mammalian tissues.* Cancer Res, (1999). , 2522-2526.

[119] Wilson, D. M, & Rd, D. R. McNeill, *Base excision repair and the central nervous system.* Neuroscience, (2007). , 1187-1200.

[120] Gu, H, et al. *Deletion of a DNA polymerase beta gene segment in T cells using cell type-specific gene targeting.* Science, (1994). , 103-106.

[121] Allinson, S. L, Dianova, I. I, & Dianov, G. L. *DNA polymerase beta is the major dRP lyase involved in repair of oxidative base lesions in DNA by mammalian cell extracts.* EMBO J, (2001). , 6919-6926.

[122] Sugo, N, et al. *p53 deficiency rescues neuronal apoptosis but not differentiation in DNA polymerase beta-deficient mice.* Mol Cell Biol, (2004). p. 9470-7.

[123] Cabelof, D. C, et al. *Haploinsufficiency in DNA polymerase beta increases cancer risk with age and alters mortality rate.* Cancer Res, (2006). , 7460-7465.

[124] Allen, D, et al. *Mutagenesis is elevated in male germ cells obtained from DNA polymerase-beta heterozygous mice.* Biol Reprod, (2008). , 824-831.

[125] Kidane, D, et al. *DNA polymerase beta is critical for genomic stability of sperm cells.* DNA Repair (Amst), (2011). , 390-397.

[126] Niimi, N, et al. *Decreased mutant frequency in embryonic brain of DNA polymerase beta null mice.* Mutagenesis, (2006). , 55-59.

[127] Senejani, A. G, et al. *Y265C DNA polymerase beta knockin mice survive past birth and accumulate base excision repair intermediate substrates.* Proc Natl Acad Sci U S A, (2012). , 6632-6637.

[128] Washington, S. L, et al. *A genetic system to identify DNA polymerase beta mutator mutants.* Proc Natl Acad Sci U S A, (1997). , 1321-1326.

[129] Opresko, P. L, Sweasy, J. B, & Eckert, K. A. *The mutator form of polymerase beta with amino acid substitution at tyrosine 265 in the hinge region displays an increase in both base substitution and frame shift errors.* Biochemistry, (1998). , 2111-2119.

[130] Kobayashi, Y, et al. *Hydrocephalus, situs inversus, chronic sinusitis, and male infertility in DNA polymerase lambda-deficient mice: possible implication for the pathogenesis of immotile cilia syndrome.* Mol Cell Biol, (2002). , 2769-2776.

[131] Zariwala, M, et al. *Investigation of the possible role of a novel gene, DPCD, in primary ciliary dyskinesia.* Am J Respir Cell Mol Biol, (2004). , 428-434.

[132] Bertocci, B, et al. *Cutting edge: DNA polymerases mu and lambda are dispensable for Ig gene hypermutation.* J Immunol, (2002). , 3702-3706.

[133] Braithwaite, E. K, et al. *DNA polymerase lambda protects mouse fibroblasts against oxidative DNA damage and is recruited to sites of DNA damage/repair.* J Biol Chem, (2005). , 31641-31647.

[134] Braithwaite, E. K, et al. *DNA polymerase lambda mediates a back-up base excision repair activity in extracts of mouse embryonic fibroblasts.* J Biol Chem, (2005). , 18469-18475.

[135] Maga, G, et al. *Replication protein A and proliferating cell nuclear antigen coordinate DNA polymerase selection in 8-oxo-guanine repair.* Proc Natl Acad Sci U S A, (2008). , 20689-20694.

[136] Gilfillan, S, et al. *Mice lacking TdT: mature animals with an immature lymphocyte repertoire.* Science, (1993). , 1175-1178.

[137] Komori, T, et al. *Lack of N regions in antigen receptor variable region genes of TdT-deficient lymphocytes.* Science, (1993). , 1171-1175.

[138] Cabaniols, J. P, et al. *Most alpha/beta T cell receptor diversity is due to terminal deoxynucleotidyl transferase.* J Exp Med, (2001). , 1385-1390.

[139] Lucas, D, et al. *Altered hematopoiesis in mice lacking DNA polymerase mu is due to inefficient double-strand break repair.* PLoS Genet, (2009). , e1000389.

[140] Brissett, N. C, et al. *Structure of a NHEJ polymerase-mediated DNA synaptic complex.* Science, (2007). , 456-459.

[141] Zhu, H, & Shuman, S. *Substrate specificity and structure-function analysis of the 3'-phosphoesterase component of the bacterial NHEJ protein, DNA ligase D.* J Biol Chem, (2006). , 13873-13881.

[142] Della, M, et al. *Mycobacterial Ku and ligase proteins constitute a two-component NHEJ repair machine.* Science, (2004). , 683-685.

[143] Yakovleva, L, & Shuman, S. *Nucleotide misincorporation, 3'-mismatch extension, and responses to abasic sites and DNA adducts by the polymerase component of bacterial DNA ligase D.* J Biol Chem, (2006). , 25026-25040.

[144] Davis, B. J, Havener, J. M, & Ramsden, D. A. *End-bridging is required for pol mu to efficiently promote repair of noncomplementary ends by nonhomologous end joining.* Nucleic Acids Res, (2008). , 3085-3094.

[145] Martin, M. J, et al. *Ribonucleotides and manganese ions improve non-homologous end joining by human Polmu.* Nucleic Acids Res, (2012).

[146] Johnson, K. A. *The kinetic and chemical mechanism of high-fidelity DNA polymerases.* Biochim Biophys Acta, (2010). , 1041-1048.

[147] Brautigam, C. A, & Steitz, T. A. *Structural and functional insights provided by crystal structures of DNA polymerases and their substrate complexes.* Curr Opin Struct Biol, (1998). , 54-63.

Chapter 5

Direct Repair in Mammalian Cells

Stephanie L. Nay and Timothy R. O'Connor

Additional information is available at the end of the chapter

http://dx.doi.org/10.5772/54449

1. Introduction

Direct repair is defined as the elimination of DNA and RNA damage using chemical reversion that does not require a nucleotide template, breakage of the phosphodiester backbone or DNA synthesis. As such, the process of direct repair is completely error-free, granting a major advantage in preservation of genetic information. In mammalian cells, direct repair is utilized to repair specific types of DNA and RNA damage caused by ubiquitous alkylating agents. Only two major types of proteins conduct direct repair in mammalian cells, O6-methylguanine-DNA methyltransferase (MGMT or AGT) and ALKBH family Fe(II)/α-keto-glutarate dioxygenases (FeKGDs). In humans and mice, a single direct repair methyltransferase protein exists, MGMT. In contrast, ALKBH FeKGDs represent a family of nine homologs with conserved active site domains. Although the biochemical function of a number of ALKBH proteins and their biological roles require further investigation, several directly repair alkylation damage in DNA and RNA at base-pairing sites.

2. Direct repair substrates—DNA and RNA alkylation damage

Exposure to alkylating agents is major cause of DNA and RNA damage, generating adducts that can compromise genomic integrity. As a result, repair of alkylation adducts is mediated by a variety of DNA repair pathways, some with overlapping substrate specificity. However, direct DNA repair proteins utilize unique mechanisms to specifically eliminate damage at base-pairing sites. The frequency and site of DNA and RNA damage occurrence is dependent on the source and type of alkylating agent exposure, as discussed in this section.

3. Sources of alkylation damage

Alkylating agents are present environmentally and also generated within the cell via oxidative metabolism. They modify DNA and RNA, forming adducts that disrupt replication and transcription, trigger cell cycle checkpoints, and/or initiate apoptosis. If left unrepaired, some adducts formed by alkylation damage can be cytotoxic and/or mutagenic [1-3].

Environmental alkylating agents fall into two primary groups, nitrosoureas that generate primarily O-alkylations and methanesulfonates that cause mostly N-alkylations [1, 3] (Figure 1). These exogenous alkylating agents are present in air, water, plants and food, in the form of nitrosamines, chloro- and bromomethane gases, myosamines and halocarbons [4]. There are also industrially produced alkylating agents, including various chemotherapeutic agents [5, 6].

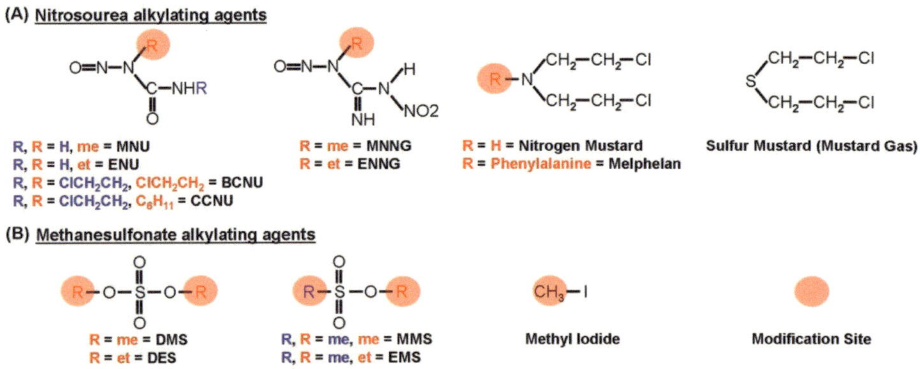

Figure 1. Examples of nitrosourea and methanesulfonate alkylating agents. (A) Nitrosourea, S_N1, alkylating agents. Abbrevations are as follows: methylnitrosourea (MNU); ethylnitrosourea (ENU); 1,3-bis (2chloroethyl)-1-nitrosourea (BCNU); N-(2-chloroethyl)-N-cyclohexyl-N-nitrosourea- (CCNU); N-methyl-N-nitro-N-nitrosoguanidine (MNNG); N-ethyl-N-nitro-N-nitrosoguanidine (ENNG). (B) Methanesulfonate, S_N2, alkylating agents. Abbrevations are as follows: dimethylsufate (DMS); diethylsulfate (DES); methylmethanesulfonate (MMS); ethylmethanesulfonate (EMS). [14]

Enzymes involved in cellular metabolism are responsible for the majority of endogenous alkylating agent damage. Nitrosating agents are generated, resulting in amine nitrosation, and reactive oxygen species (ROS), which cause lipoperoxidation [7]. Additionally, a family of S-adenosyl methionine (SAM) methyltransferase enzymes is involved in more than 40 metabolic reactions using SAM as a methyl donor to modify nucleic acids, proteins and lipids [8, 9]. Four of those SAM methyltransferase enzymes participate in DNA and RNA modification in mammalian cells. DNMT1, DNMT3A, and DNMT3B catalyze methyl group transfer at the C5 position of cytosine in DNA CpG sequences [10], whereas TRDMT1 (DNMT2) methylates the C5 position of cytosine 38 in aspartic acid tRNA [11].

3.1. Types of alkylating agents

Alkylating agents can be categorized by their method of activation. Some alkylating agents react directly with DNA and do not require any activation, whereas many alkylating agents, including many carcinogens, must undergo metabolic activation by the cytochrome P450 system to generate reactive species capable of modifying DNA [3, 12, 13]. In addition, alkylating agents are electrophilic compounds that possess either one or two reactive groups that can interact with the nucleophilic centers of DNA and RNA bases. Alkylating agents that can only react with one nucleophilic center are mono-functional, whereas bi-functional agents can react with two sites in DNA or RNA [1, 13]. Alkylating agents that are mono-functional primarily transfer alkyl groups to ring nitrogens, while agents that react in a bi-functional manner not only react with ring nitrogens, but can form cyclized DNA bases, by reacting with exocylic nitrogen and oxygen groups [13] (Figure 2). In addition to methylating agents, larger alkylating agents also modify nucleic acids—bi-functional ethylating agents can form exocyclic ethano and etheno adducts at nitrogen and oxygen molecules in all DNA and RNA bases. Additionally, bi-functional alkylating agents can produce DNA inter- and/or intrastrand cross-links [13]. Some alkylating agents also react at phosphate residues to generate phosphotriesters, leading to potential single-strand breaks [13] (Figure 2). Two main pathways, characterized as S_N1 or S_N2, are defined based on the kinetics of the alkylation reaction, leading to the above mentioned modifications of DNA and RNA bases [2].

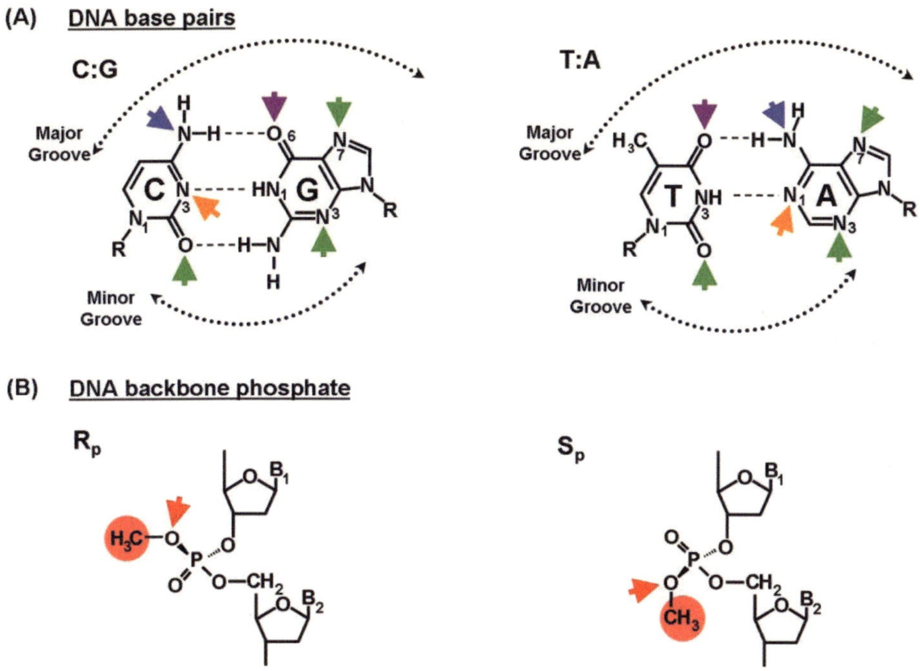

Figure 2. (A) Purple arrows indicate sites in DNA most often methylated by S_N1 alkylating agents. Green arrows indicate sites commonly modified by S_N2 alkylating agents, orange arrows indicate sites in single-stranded DNA. Blue arrows indicate exocyclic amino groups important in formation of cyclized DNA adducts. The location of the major and minor grooves in DNA are indicated. "R" is the attachment of the base to the deoxyribose and phosphodiester backbone. (B) Modified phosphodiester isoforms in the DNA backbone. S_N1 alkylating agents generally form more phosphotriester products than S_N2 agents. [2,14]

S_N1 agents act via a two step reaction involving a unimolecular nucleophilic substitution with a rate-limiting step that generates an intermediate carbonium ion electrophile that reacts with nucleophilic DNA sites. Thus, the reaction kinetics depend only on the formation of the carbonium ion intermediate (first-order). The triganol planar conformation of the *sp*^{2} hybridized carbon generated in the carbocation intermediate permits nucleophilic attack from either side, yielding a racemic mixture of reaction products at chiral centers [13] (Figure 3). Though agents that react via an S_N1 mechanism produce both N- and O-alkylations, increased amounts of modified oxygens are generated, compared to agents that react via an S_N2 mechanism.

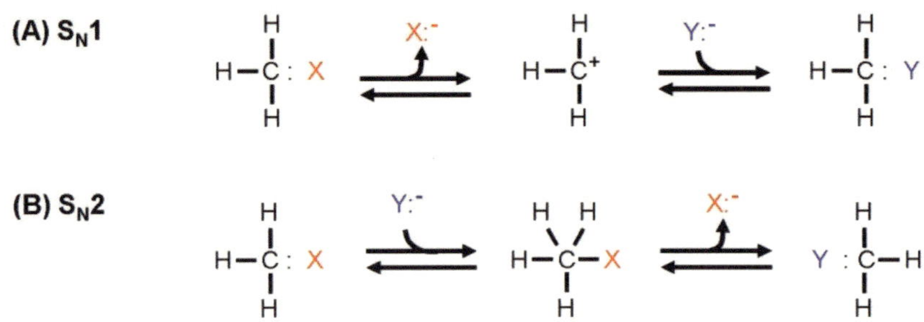

Figure 3. S_N1 and S_N2 nucleophilic substitution reactions. (A) Example of an S_N1 reaction. S_N1 reactions are dependent on formation of a carbonium ion intermediate that rate-limiting. Product chiral centres are a racemic mixture because the intermediate can be attacked by either side. (B) Example of an S_N2 reaction. Both reactants are required and there is direct attack by the nuclephile in S_N2 reactions. Chirality is maintained since a transition state is formed with the chiral center. [2,14]

In contrast, S_N2 reaction mechanisms depend on both the alkylating agent and its target to define the kinetics (second-order). Using a one step reaction where both the electrophile and nucleophile are involved in the transition state, S_N2 alkylating agents proceed with direct attack by the nucleophile on an electron deficient center. The nucleophile attacks from the back of the electrophile, forming the carbon-nucleophile bond and breaking the carbon-leaving group bond. Simultaneous backside, nucleophilic attack and leaving group departure cause the incoming group to replace the leaving group. Because a transition state is formed with the chiral center, chirality is maintained, leading to a stereocenter (inversion) configuration [13] (Figure 3). Alkylating agents that react via an S_N2 mechanism cause primarily N-alkylations.

3.2. DNA and RNA alkylation damage

Modification sites of DNA bases are the same for all alkylating agents and include all the exocyclic nitrogens and oxygens, as well as ring nitrogens without hydrogen. Though all DNA nucleobase oxygen or nitrogen atoms can be alkylated, the type and frequency of specific damage varies depending on the type of alkylating agent, the structure of the substrate, and the position of the damage site [13] (Table 1). Generally, alkylation damage at nitrogen

http://dx.doi.org/10.5772/54449

molecules is less mutagenic than oxygen, though both types of alkylation damage are cytotoxic and genotoxic [14].

Common alkylations generated by exogenous alkylating agents include O[6]-alkylguanine and O[4]-alkylthymine adducts, as well as N7-alkylguanine, N3-alkyladenine, N1-alkyladenine, and N3-alkylcytosine [13] (Figure 1). Moreover, the frequency of each adduct type depends on whether the DNA and RNA substrates are single- or double-stranded [13] (Table 1). For instance, nitrogen molecules involved in DNA base-pairing are less vulnerable to alkylation damage than the same base nitrogens in a single-stranded region arising during replication and transcription.

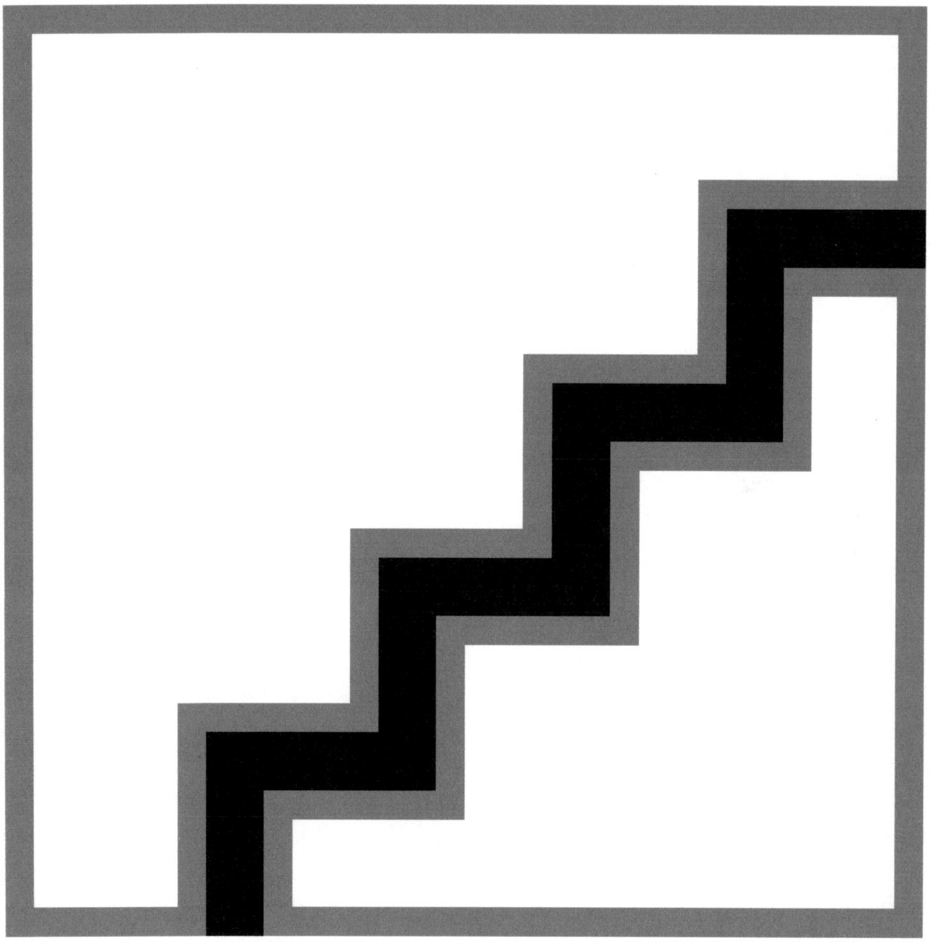

Table 1. % of Total DNA alkylation adduct formation in single- and double-strand DNA. Modifications following S_N2 alkylating agent methylmethanesulfonate (MMS) or S_N1 alkylating agent treatments methylnitrosourea (MNU) or ethylnitrosourea (ENU). Sites where % alkylation is undetermined are indicated as (--) [13].

4. Direct repair proteins

Numerous cellular mechanisms have evolved to deal with various types of DNA damage and each DNA repair pathway is important to maintain genomic integrity. However, most repair mechanisms require DNA synthesis and therefore an intrinsic risk of causing mutation in executing the repair. In contrast, direct repair proteins, MGMT and ALKBH family proteins employ direct reversal mechanisms that result in complete restoration of DNA bases and are thus error-free mechanisms. Moreover, MGMT, ALKBH2, and ALKBH3 repair endogenous and exogenous DNA and RNA alkylation damage at critical base-pairing sites, facilitating proper replication of genetic information or transcription. This section will discuss each of these direct DNA repair enzymes in detail.

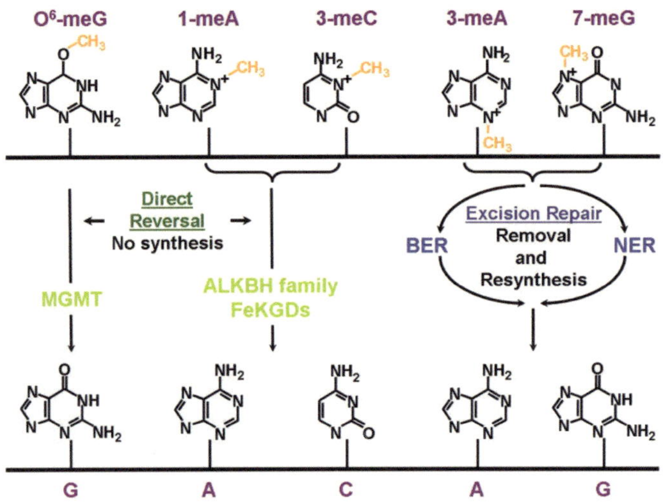

Figure 4. Major mechanisms of alkylation adduct repair. Direct repair pathways are indicated in green. Base and nucleotide excision repair pathways are indicated in blue [2,14].

4.1. Mechanisms of alkylation repair

Multiple mechanisms are employed to rid the genome of alkyl adducts, thereby preventing detrimental effects within the cell (Figure 4). Mismatch repair (MMR), base excision repair (BER) and nucleotide excision repair (NER) and direct repair (DR) pathways all participate in alkylation damage repair [15-24]. Specifically, BER and NER repair small alkylated base damage including 7-methylguanine (7-meG) and 3-methyladenine (3-meA) DNA adducts [25]. Although BER repairs the majority of small alkylated base damage (methyl and ethyl adducts) the NER system can also remove small, as well as bulky adducts larger than ethylated bases [24, 26]. As an alternative to NER, incomplete BER repair intermediates can be processed by homologous recombination (HR) [27]. However, BER, NER and HR repair pathways generate strand breaks during repair of alkyl adducts and could introduce mutations or rearrangements [28]. On the contrary, DR mechanisms, provided by methyltransferase MGMT and ALKBH homologs, eliminate alkylation damage at DNA base-pairing sites, including O^6-methylguanine (O^6-meG), 1-methyladenine (1-meA) and 3-methylcytosine (3-meC) and do not require a nucleotide template, result in phosphodiester backbone breakage, nor do they require DNA synthesis.

4.2. Methyl Guanine Methyl Transferase (MGMT) proteins

In mammals, methylguanine DNA methyltransferase (MGMT or AGT), can repair two types of DNA adducts: O^6-methylguanine (O^6-meG) and O^4-methylthymine (O^4-meT). O^6-meG adducts in DNA are extremely mutagenic [29, 30] and also block DNA polymerase extension, which is generally associated with cytotoxicity [31, 32]. The primary mutations observed when there is a failure to repair O^6-meG adducts prior to replication are G:C ▪ A:T transitions, whereas a failure to repair O^4-meT results primarily in T:A ▪ C:G transition mutations [29]. In mammals, elimination of O^6-meG by MGMT is preferred over O^4-meT, but the respective efficiency of each type of reversion is species dependent [29, 33-37].

Removal of O^6-meG and O^4-meT modifications are achieved via a one-step methyltransferase reaction, wherein MGMT accepts the alkyl adduct from the modified oxygen molecule, onto an internal residue, directly restoring the DNA base and inactivating the protein [38] (Figure 5). In addition to methyl groups, several other alkyl-adducts can also be transferred from guanine to MGMT, including ethyl-, propyl- butyl-, benzyl- and 2-chloroethyl-. However, the efficiency of the reaction is decreased for alkyl adducts greater than methylated bases [39]. Once modified, the protein is targeted for elimination via the proteasome [40].

4.2.1. Protein structure/active site organization

Alkyltransferase proteins are found in eukaryotic and prokaryotic organisms and have been identified in as many as 100 organisms [41]. Though sequences are not highly conserved between human MGMT and Eubacterial, Archea, and Eukaryotic DNA methyltransferase enzymes, structural domains and active site residues are almost identical [42-46].

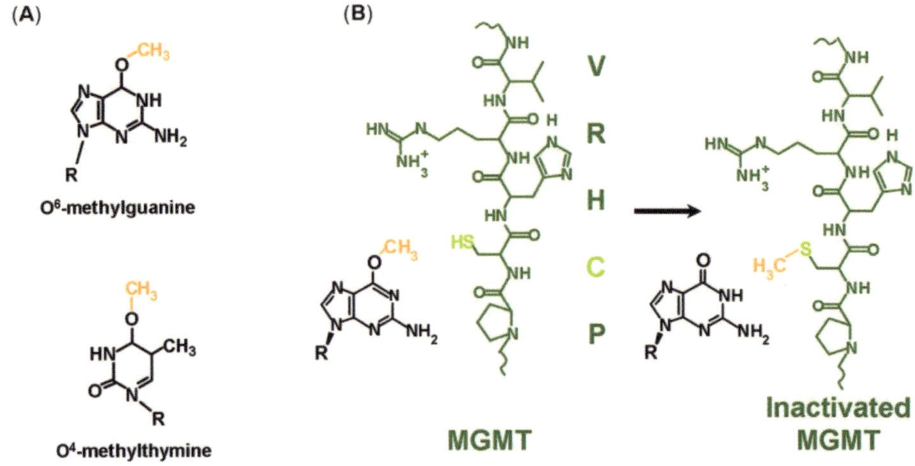

Figure 5. Methylguanine methyltransferase (MGMT) activity. (A) MGMT DNA repair substrates (B) MGMT repair reaction. Transfer of the methyl group (orange) from the damaged DNA base to the internal Cys145 (light green) is a suicide reaction, inactivating MGMT. [14]

In human MGMT, a conserved α/β roll structure, containing a three-stranded, anti-parallel β-sheet, followed by two helices, make up the N-terminus (residues 1-85). The MGMT C-terminus (residues 86-207) contains a short, two-stranded, parallel β-sheet, four α-helices and a 3_{10} helix [42, 47]. Found only in humans, a zinc ion stabilizes the interface between the N- and C-termini, binding Cys5, Cys24, His29 and His85 in a tetrahedral conformation to bridge three strands of the N-terminal β-sheet with the coil preceding the 3_{10} helix in the C-terminus [47].

The conserved active site cysteine motif (-PCHR-) is located in the C-terminus contained within the DNA binding channel, and the helix-turn-helix (HTH) DNA binding motif. Residues Try114-Ala121 form the first helix of the HTH motif and residues Ala127-Gly136 form the second, "recognition" helix, which interacts with DNA. Linked by an Asn-hinge (Asn137) that stabilizes the over-lapping turns by binding Val139, Ille143 and the Cys145 thiol, the -PHCR- active site is located near the "recognition" helix [42, 47, 48].

The active site of human MGMT is composed of at least ten residues that participate in substrate binding, enzyme structure and alkyl transfer. Residues Val155-Gly160 and Met134 generate a hydrophobic cleft in the active site loop, while residues Tyr114, His146, Val148, Ser159, and Glu172 participate in active site coordination and alkyl group transfer to residue Cys145. Not unexpectedly, mutation of residue Cys145 results in elimination of alkyl group transfer, however substrate binding is unaffected [49] (Figure 6).

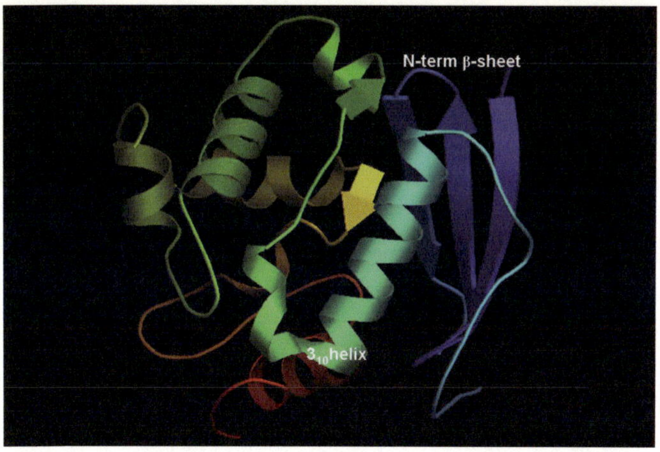

Figure 6. Structure of human MGMT (PDBid1QNT). The N-termianl p-sheet and C-terminal 3_{10} helix of the α/β roll structure, conserved in AGT proteins are indicated. In humans, a zinc ion stabilizes interaction of MGMT N-and C-termini [46].

4.2.2. Substrate recognition/repair mechanism

In repair, MGMT is unique in that one molecule is responsible for the removal of one O^6-meG or O^4-meT adduct. Unlike most enzymes with the capacity to catalyze multiple reactions, MGMT catalyzed reactions are stoichiometric and capable of only a single repair reaction [50]. As a result, removal of O^6-meG and O^4-meT alkyl adducts is dependent on both MGMT and the substrate concentrations (second-order reaction).

The recognition of guanine and thymine base methylation is accomplished by a highly conserved amino acid structure. The hydrophobic cleft of the active site loop and -PCHR- motif within the binding channel allow MGMT to bind to the minor-groove of DNA using residues Ala126, Ala127, Ala129, Gly131, and Gly132, of the HTH "recognition" helix [51, 52], which is followed by necessary conformational changes to orient the damaged base within the active site.

Identified based on bacterial Ada homology and human MGMT structures, following substrate recognition, the target base is repaired using a base flipping mechanism [53-58]. In the MGMT repair reaction, the damaged base undergoes a residue Tyr114-mediated, sterically enforced 3′ phosphate rotation into the active-site pocket. The hydrophobic cleft formed by the active site loop easily accepts the extra-helical base, causing the DNA minor groove to widen [51]. The arginine finger residue, Arg128, intercalates between the DNA bases and interacts with the unpaired cytosine, via a charged hydrogen bond [55], maintaining an appropriate DNA duplex conformation (Figure 6).

Once bound within the MGMT active site, numerous residues participate in the methyltransferase reaction. A hydrogen bond network, conserved in AGTs, is formed between Glu172, His146, water and Cys145. His146 acts as a water-mediated base that deprotonates Cys145, converting Cys145 to a cystine thiolate anion and generating an imidazolium ion that is stabilized by Glu172 [35, 59]. Residues, Val148 and Cys145 carbonyls accept guanine exocyclic amine hydrogen bonds and nitrogen atoms of residues Tyr114 and Ser159 donate protons to N3 and O^6 of O^6-meG, respectively. The deprotonated Tyr114 residue abstracts a proton from Lys165, simultaneously transferring the alkyl group from the O^6 position of guanine to the thiolate anion of the Cys145 residue [35]. Transfer of the alkyl group generates a thioether, S-alkylcysteine, and results in complete restoration of the guanine base, as well as irreversible inactivation of the methyltransferase enzyme (Figure 5). While many DNA repair proteins have a specific requirement for double-stranded DNA, MGMT can also bind to single-stranded DNA [60].

4.2.3. Gene expression/protein regulation

Removal of O^6-meG modifications by MGMT has a major role in cell cycle checkpoint control, proliferation, and differentiation [61]. As a result, *MGMT* is a house-keeping gene that is expressed in all tissues; though expression varies depending on cell type [62]. *MGMT* expression in an individual cell or tissue type is dependent on a variety of factors, including numerous types of stimuli and promoter regulator elements. However, the relationship between factors that mediate *MGMT* expression and the regulation of its function is not well-understood. The lack of understanding regarding the consequences of *MGMT* regulation is illustrated by the fact that *MGMT* expression is silenced in some cancers, but expression is up-regulated in others [62, 63].

MGMT is a single gene on chromosome 10q26, spanning approximately 300kb [64]. The gene has five exons, but the first is non-coding [65, 66]. The promoter of *MGMT* is a non-TATA-box promoter that contains a GC-rich CpG island of 780 bp that includes 97 CpG dinucleotides [67]. CpG islands are commonly associated with promoter regions of constitutively expressed genes, from which transcription is initiated from a single promoter site [68-70]. Additionally, the promoter contains six transcription consensus binding sites (SP1, AP1, and AP2), three upstream and three downstream of the transcription start site, a glucocorticoid-responsive element, and a 3′ enhancer element [62, 67, 69, 71]. Though unmethylated in normal cells, promoter CpG island methylation-induced silencing of *MGMT* is found in various cancer types and MGMT-deficient cell lines and is one mechanism that regulates *MGMT* expression [72-76]. However, whether *MGMT* promoter methylation disables transcription factor binding or contributes to chromatin reorganization remains uncertain [71, 75].

In addition to numerous transcription factor binding sites that surround the *MGMT* promoter transcription start site, the *MGMT* promoter CpG islands exhibit a chromatin structure that mediates interaction with transcription factors. The *MGMT* gene is organized around five or more nucleosomes in a manner that positions 300 bp region of the promoter sequence, which contains known *MGMT* transcription factor binding sites, so that it does not lie within the nucleosomes, and therefore does not maintain a higher-order chromatin structure [62, 72, 77]. Such nucleosomal positioning facilitates an "open" stretch of DNA that enables constitutive interaction of transcription factors with the promoter.

Methylation of the CpG island surrounding the transcription factor binding sites contributes to lack of transcription factor binding, but could also effect nucleosomal positioning of the *MGMT* promoter [62, 71], suggested by histone H3 Lys9 (H3K9) di-methylation, exhibited in relationship to *MGMT* silencing [78, 79]. Further, deacetylation of histones H3 and H4 could also be associated nucleosome organization that is more condensed, resulting in transcription inactivation. Therefore, the chromatin structure of the *MGMT* promoter, as well as CpG island methylation, mediate transcription factor access to the promoter and are important for *MGMT* expression.

4.2.4. Protein localization and cell type dependence

Immunofluorescence studies indicate MGMT nuclear localization at discrete nuclear regions [80]. Although a nuclear localization signal (NLS) for MGMT has not been identified, the small size of MGMT, 23 kDa, may not require an active translocation signal to traverse nuclear pores [53]. However, a –PKAAR- sequence within the DNA binding domain of MGMT is necessary for DNA interactions to facilitate nuclear retention [81]. The highest MGMT expression levels are found in the liver, where high levels of endogenous nitrosating agents are present, but MGMT is also expressed at high levels in the lung, kidney and colon. MGMT expression is heterogeneous in the brain and the lowest levels are observed in the pancreas, hematopoietic cells, lymphoid tissues [62, 67, 82-86].

4.2.5. Post-translational modification

Once MGMT has transferred a methyl group to its Cys145 residue, no further reactions are catalyzed, so the protein must be eliminated. The degradation of MGMT is an ubiquitination-dependent process that has been evaluated using inactivation of the protein by O^6-BzG, BCNU, or NO-generating agents at position Cys145 [40, 87, 88]. Conformational changes in the protein structure after alkyl group transfer target MGMT for ubiquitination and proteasomal degradation [40, 89]. Two sites within MGMT, Lys125 and Lys178, have been identified as ubiquitination targets in B lymphocyte (NCI-H929) or 293T, and myeloid (MV4-11) cells, respectively. Additionally, examination of potential MGMT modification sites using predictive software also identifies Lys104 as an ubiquitination target. Furthermore, predictions also indicate post-translational modification sites for methylation (Arg128, Arg135), acetylation (Lys8, 125, 178, 193), and sumoylation (Lys75, 205, 18, 107), as well as numerous phosphorylation sites (Ser36, 56, 130, 182, 202, 206, 208; Thr37; Tyr91, 115) [90-93], which all merit further consideration. Notably, phosphorylation of residues Thr10 and Thr11 was also noted in HeLa cells [92], and phosphorylation of Ser201 is observed in B lymphocyte cells (DG75 and GM00130), KGI myeloid cells, and HeLa cervical cancer cells. Importantly, crystallographic data suggests that modification of Ser201 could disrupt interaction with DNA [48, 51, 55].

4.3. Alkbh Fe(II)/α-ketoglutarate-dependent dioxygenases

In mammals, repair of cytosine and adenine base methylation at base-pairing positions is specifically associated with the AlkB family dioxygenase proteins [92, 94-96]. Discovered first in *Escherichia coli* (*E. coli*) in 1983 [96] alkylation protein B (AlkB) belongs to a superfamily of Fe(II)/α-ketoglutarate-dependent dioxygenases (FeKGDs), with roles in histone demethylation [97-99], proline hydroxylation [95] and in the case of AlkB, the ability to directly remove alkyl adducts generated in DNA residues as a result of exposure to S_N2 alkylating agents [94, 100]. Originally predicted to act on 1-methyladenine (1-meA) and 3-methylcytosine (3-meC), bacterial AlkB has been shown to repair a variety of DNA and RNA adducts, including 1-meA, 3-meC, 1-meG, 3-meT, 1-etA, as well as aromatic ethyl, 3-etC, and etheno adducts, 1,N^6-ethenoadenine (εA) and 3,N^4-ethenocytosine (εC) [94, 100-108] (Figure 7).

Using bioinformatics, nine human ALKBH family enzymes, ALKBH1-8 and FTO, were identified, of which only four have been reported to have DNA repair activity, ALKBH1 – ALKBH3 and FTO [109, 110]. Though all of the ALKBH homologs contain conserved catalytic domain residues, none entirely encompass the enzymatic activity of AlkB [15, 103, 104, 111-114]. Removal of alkyl adducts from DNA is only accomplished by three ALKBH proteins, ALKBH1-3, known to remove 1-meA and 3-meC adducts. However, ALKBH1 is reportedly a mitochondrial protein [115], therefore in the nucleus ALKBH2 and ALKBH3 proteins are employed to remove specific adducts in single- or double-stranded DNA or in RNA [104]. Lesions that are repaired by ALKBH proteins generally interfere with base-pairing and block replication and transcription, triggering cell cycle checkpoints and apoptosis [92, 95, 96, 110, 115]. In *E. coli* AlkB mutants, as well as in Alkbh2- or Alkbh3-deficient mouse embryonic fibroblasts, cells exhibit increased sensitivity to alkylating agents, particularly the S_N2 type, and increased mutant frequency [101, 116-119].

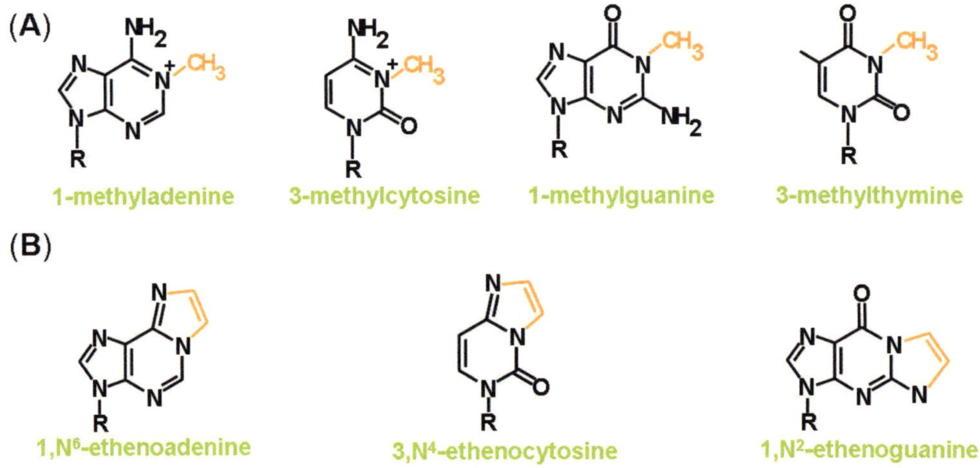

Figure 7. ALKBH protein substrates. (A) DNA methyl adducts repaired by ALKBH proteins. (B) DNA etheno adducts repaired by ALKHB proteins.

4.3.1. *Protein structure/active site organization*

Similar to MGMT, the sequences of human ALKBH proteins do not contain a high percentage of sequence homology in regions other than active sites and conserved domains, but do have conserved secondary structures [109, 110, 114, 120-122]. In AlkB family proteins, the catalytic core is composed of three major components, the double-stranded β-helix (DSBH), the nucleotide recognition lid (NRL) and the N-terminal extension (NTE) (Figure 8). The DSBH is comprised of eight β-strands in the C-terminal portion that form two β-sheets to create a central core jelly-roll fold. Within the major and minor β-sheets of the DSBH lie conserved catalytic residues RxxxxxR and $HxDx_nH$, respectively [120, 121, 123]. The HxD dyad is near the amino terminal end and is located in a flexible loop that follows the first strand, stacking with the minor β-sheet. The carboxy-terminal histidine of the conserved $HxDx_nH$ residues is associated with the beginning of the sixth strand and together these residues coordinate iron (His171, Asp173 and His236—Alkbh2; His191, Asp193 and His258—Alkbh3) [114, 120, 121, 123, 124]. The histidine and aspartic acid residues (Asp248 and Asp254—ALKBH2; Asp269 and Asp275—ALKBH3), conserved in the DSBH minor β-sheet, coordinate Fe(II), α-ketoglutarate and the DNA or RNA repair substrate within the catalytic core. A conserved Arg residue in the C-terminal β-strand (Arg254—ALKBH2 and Arg275—ALKBH3) sets AlkB family proteins apart from other α-ketoglutarate-dependent dioxygenases within the Fe(II)/α-ketoglutarate dioxygenase superfamily, forming the base of the substrate binding pocket [110, 120, 121, 123].

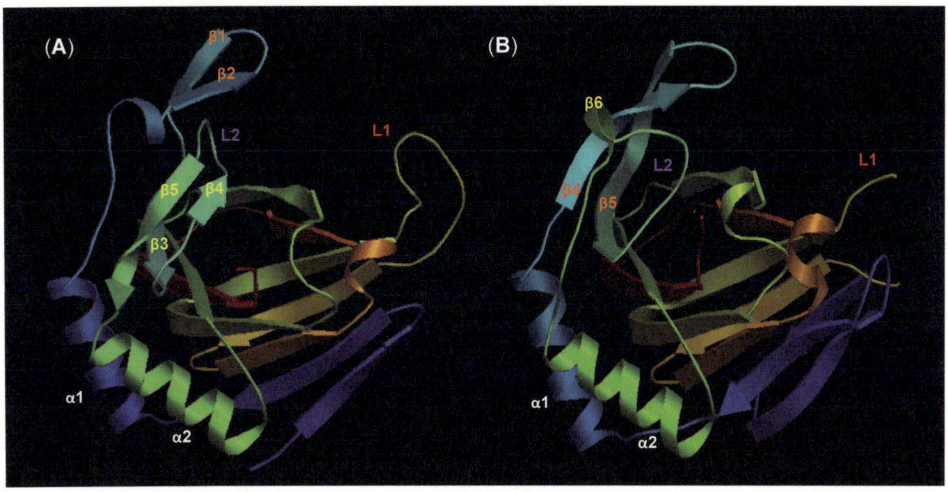

Figure 8. Structure of human AlkB homolog DNA repair proteins. Two looped structures (flip1 and flip2) generated by anti-parallel β-sheets create the nucleotide recognition lid (NRL) and are involved in DNA base flipping. (A) Structure of ALKBH2 (PDBid3BTX). ALKBH2 double-strand DNA substrate specificity is facilitated by residues in loops L1 and L2. (B) Structure of ALKBH3 (PDBid2IUW). β -sheets 4 and 5 form the β-hairpin motif in ALKBH3. Part of loop 1, involved in ALKBH substrate specificity, was omitted due to electron density problems. [121]

The N-terminal extension (NTE) and Nucleotide Recognition Lid (NRL) are formed by the β-hairpin motifs that extend from the DSBH jelly-roll, forming a substrate binding groove that covers the active site until bound. Ninety residues are contained within two looped structures, forming "flips" that lie between a single β-sheet and two α-helices in the N-terminal portion of the catalytic core [120, 121]. Secondary structures are of similar size, but possess different characteristics important for substrate specificity and DNA activity. In ALKBH2, the first flip is 20 residues that make up a β-hairpin and short α-helix, creating a hydrophobic binding groove. In contrast, the first flip in ALKBH3 is a β-hairpin made up of 17 residues that form a hydrophilic, positively charged binding groove, more suitable for single-stranded DNA or RNA substrates [15, 120]. The characteristics of the second flip are also unique. Flip two of ALKBH2 spans 24 residues that is made up of three β-sheets, with numerous sites for DNA substrate interaction. The orientation of the three β-sheets, which fold back towards the C-terminal end of the first α-helix, is also unique only to ALKBH2 [114, 121]. However, flip 2 of ALKBH3 is only 12 residues and contains a single β-sheet [114]. The N-terminal regions of each ALKBH homolog are more variable and hypothesized to play roles in sub-cellular sorting and protein-protein interactions [114, 115] (Figure 8).

In addition to the conserved catalytic dioxygenase residues, some human ALKBH proteins also contain additional catalytic residues and domains [104, 109, 110, 113, 125] (Figure 9). Structural analysis of bacterial AlkB and human ALKBH homologs provides insight into substrate preferences and repair capabilities. For instance, ALKBH2 contains three unique motifs that facilitate enhanced activity on double-stranded DNA [121]. A long, flexible β-sheet hairpin loop that contains DNA binding residues Arg198, Gly204 and Lys205, a short loop that contains the RKK motif (Arg241-Lys243) and an aromatic finger residue (Phe102) are used to make contacts with both DNA strands, rotate and take the place of the damaged base in duplex DNA molecules. On the other hand, the number and organization of the catalytic domains in ALKBH3 result in differential manipulation of the DNA backbone, explaining the preference for single-strand substrates. Lack of an aromatic finger residue and RKK motif in ALKBH3, the damaged base is squeezed on either side, forcing it to rotate, and the immediate 5′ and 3′ bases to stack against one another. However, structural analysis of ALKBH3 has identified residue Arg122, specifically the arginine side chain length, as important for double-stranded DNA substrate activity, possibly mimicking the base-flipping and stacking activities of ALKBH2 residue Phe102 [114, 121].

Unfortunately, extensive biochemical analysis or structural studies have not been conducted on ALKBH homologs 4-8. However, it is apparent that differences in the number and organization of catalytic residues, as well as secondary structures play a large role in the diversity of ALKBH family protein substrate specificities and enzymatic activities [113]. For instance, although single- or double-strand DNA repair activity has not been established for ALKBH8, the presence of RNA binding and methyltransferase domains in ALKBH8 (Figure 9) suggested that this homolog plays a role in maintenance of methylation patterns. Investigation of such activities led to the identification of ALKBH8 tRNA methyltransferase activity, necessary in the biogenesis of wobble uridine modifications utilized in translational decoding [126, 127].

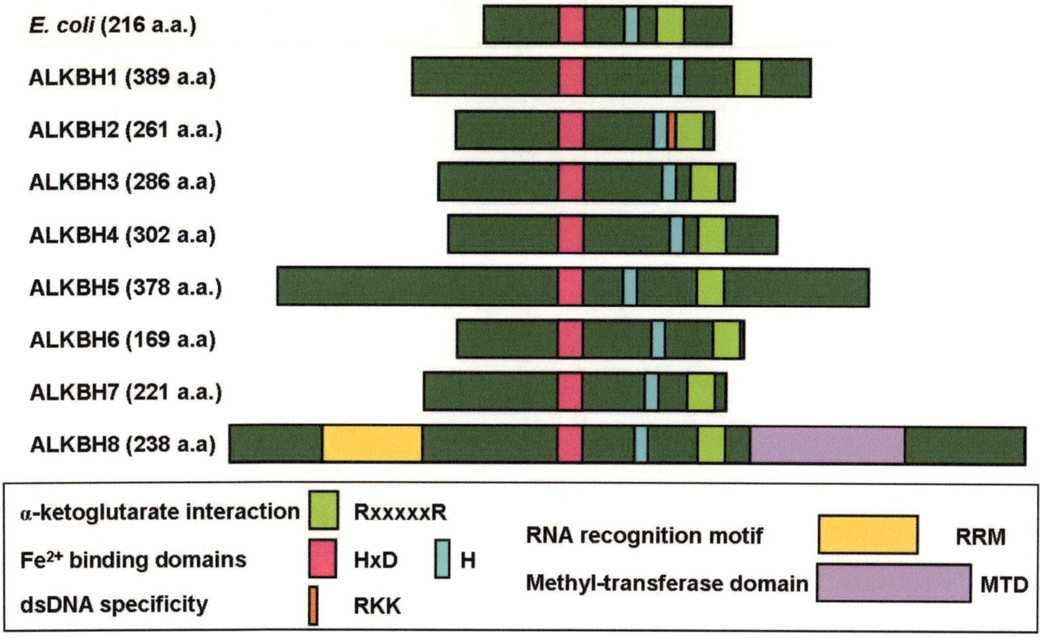

Figure 9. AlkB family protein domain alignment. Conserved amino acid sequences and domain function are indicated. The total number of amino acids is indicated to the right of each homolog. [110,113,125]

4.3.2. *Substrate recognition/repair mechanism*

Initially, it was predicted that AlkB family proteins directly repaired alkylation adducts by hydroxylating methyl groups and removing the resultant hydroxymethyl groups via an oxidative reaction that directly restores the undamaged base [94, 109, 112, 124, 128, 129]. However, specific investigation of the AlkB family dealkylation mechanism [130] determined that the direct repair reaction mediated by AlkB family proteins involves several intermediate steps that had not yet been identified. Regardless, dealkylation catalyzed by AlkB and its human homologs occurs via transformation of α-ketoglutarate into succinate, formaldehyde release, and restoration of the undamaged base [94, 100, 111, 130, 131] (Figure 10).

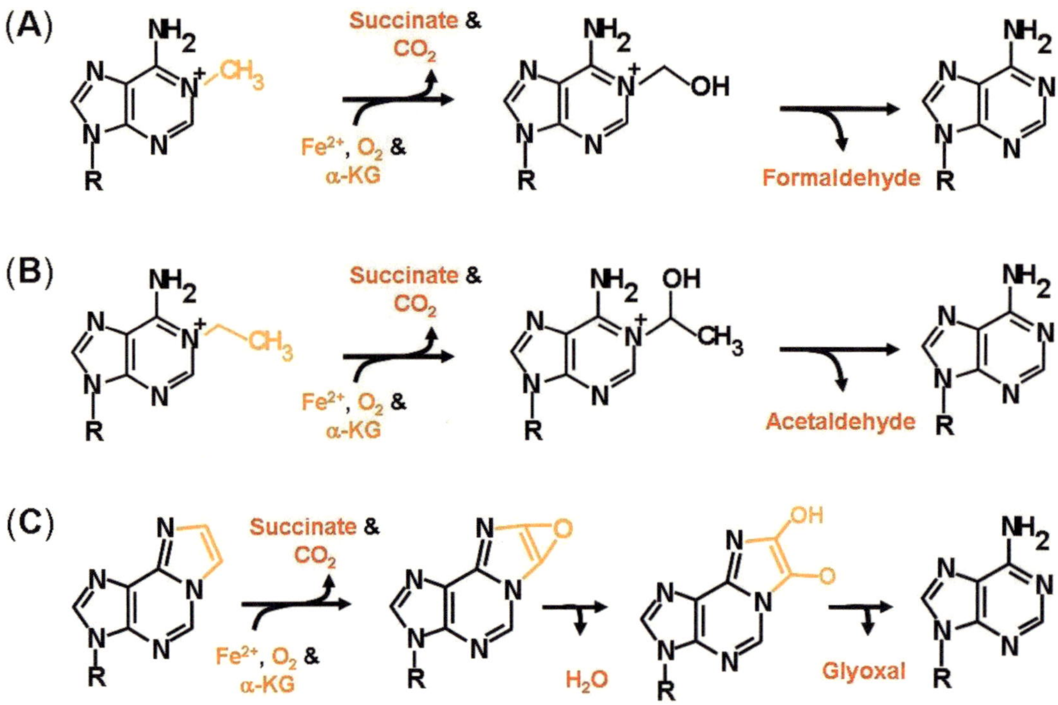

Figure 10. ALKBH protein repair reactions. (A) ALKBH methyl adduct repair reaction. (B) ALKBH ethyl adduct repair reaction. (C) ALKBH etheno adduct repair reaction. Repair of ethyl and etheno adducts requires the same co-factors, but displaces acetaldehyde or water and glyoxal as byproducts of the repair reaction, respectively, instead of formaldehyde [100,102,103]

First, Fe(II) and three water molecules must be coordinated within the conserved catalytic core, stimulating α-ketoglutarate (KG) binding in the catalytic pocket. Binding of α-KG into the catalytic pocket chelates Fe(II) by displacing two water molecules to create the Fe(II)/α-KG active-site complex. Ligation of dioxygen to the Fe(II) molecule displaces the remaining water molecule, generating a ferric-superoxido species that undergoes self-redox and nucleophilic attack on the α-keto group. This nucleophilic attack is necessary to decarboxylate α-KG, releasing succinate and generating a ferryl-oxo intermediate. Reorientation of this intermediate facilitates removal of a hydrogen atom from the methyl adduct. Finally, radical rebound hydroxylation of the methylene group results in decomposition of the hydroxymethyl nucleobase, yielding formaldehyde and the repaired nucleobase. Though two co-factors were noted initially, α-ketoglutarate and Fe(II), ascorbate also plays a role, helping to convert the Fe(III) to Fe(II), thereby regenerating the original oxidative state of iron in the Alkbh proteins that permits enzymatic cycling [94, 111, 112, 122, 124, 130].

The major methylated bases repaired by ALKBH proteins are 1-methyladenine (1-meA) and 3-methylcytosine (3-meC), however homologs have also been reported to repair ethylated, and some etheno and exocyclic bases [102-105, 107, 131, 132]. Similar mechanisms are proposed for repair of ethano and exocyclic etheno (ε) adducts, though the final steps of these reactions result in release of acetylaldehyde and glycol, respectively [130] (Figure 10). However, additional biochemical studies are needed to confirm these mechanisms in similar detail to removal of methyl adducts from DNA.

4.3.3. Gene expression/protein regulation

Human AlkB DNA repair homologs, *ALKBH2* and *ALKBH3* are single genes on chromosomes 12q24 and 11p11, respectively. Expression of human AlkB homologs has been reported in a variety of normal tissue samples, including ALKBH homologs 4-8, despite the lack of DNA repair activity in the literature [133]. Expression of ALKBH family proteins varies depending on cell types. Protein expression levels in the various tissue types vary depending on the homolog evaluated. Little is known of ALKBH protein regulation mechanisms and is an area in need of further study.

4.3.4. Protein localization and cell type dependence

Differences amongst AlkB homolog proteins in their biological roles are partially ascribed to their sub-cellular localizations. ALKBH2 and ALKBH3 homolog proteins are expressed at the highest levels in the testis and ovary, however detectable expression of all AlkB homolog proteins is exhibited in the spleen, pancreas, lung, kidney, prostate and brain [133]. Although ALKBH1 activity is confined to mitochondria [115], immunofluorescence imaging indicates that the protein is cytoplasmic and nuclear [133]. Similarly, AlkB homolog proteins ALKBH3, 4, 6, and 7 are also present in the nucleus and cytoplasm [133], though ALKBH3 is the only homolog reported to possess repair activity [1, 104, 111]. Localization of ALKBH3 in both the nucleus and cytoplasm are consistent with identified interactions with helicase enzymes to facilitate DNA repair [134] and roles in mRNA repair [131]. ALKBH2 is present only in the nucleus and exhibits diffuse as well as localized, punctate staining, supporting pre-established co-localization with PCNA at replication foci during S phase [111, 131, 133], suggesting a role in replication- and transcription-related repair, as well as genome maintenance. On the contrary, AlkB homolog proteins ALKBH5 and 8 are present only in the cytoplasm [133], which supports known ALKBH8 tRNA methyltransferase activity [126, 127].

4.3.5. Post-translational modification

Unlike MGMT, ALKBH proteins are not suicide enzymes and a single protein can catalyze multiple direct repair reactions, requiring only ascorbate to regenerate the Fe(II) active site center [135]. Therefore, immediate degradation of ALKBH proteins following repair is not required, as it is for MGMT. Other possible post-translational modifications in ALKBH2 and ALKBH3 include candidate sites for phosphorylation and acetylation. Mass-spectrometric analysis of a curated database of cell lines revealed that both ALKBH2 and ALKBH3 proteins undergo post-translational modification of specific residues present in various cancer types [92].

Post-translational modifications curated for ALKBH2 include acetylation of residue Lys34 and Lys104 in various colorectal cancer cell types (HCT116, HT29, XY3-92-T and XY3-68-T), as well as phosphorylation of residue Thr252 in esophageal cancer cell line XY2-E111N [92]. Though the exact effects of these modifications are unknown, it is important to state that Lys34 is within the variable region of the N-terminus that is thought to provide protein specificity. Similarly, Lys104 is between two residues that make contact with the complimentary DNA strand during double-strand DNA repair and Thr230 is a residue in the most C-terminal α-helix of the active site [92]. Examination of potential ALKBH2 modification sites using predictive software shows possible post-translational modification sites for methylation (Arg128, 135), sumoylation (Lys75, 205), and ubiquitination (Lys104), along with other possible phosphorylation sites (Ser36, 56, 130, 182, 202, 206, 208; Thr37; Tyr91, 115) [90-93]. All of those possible post-translational modifications merit further consideration.

Post-translational modifications were also present in ALKBH3, corresponding to various disease states. Phosphorylation of Thr126 and Tyr127 residues in the β-hairpin of the NRL, as well as residue Try229 in the ALKBH3 active site, was present in acute myelogenous, chronic myelogenous and/or T-cell leukemia [92]. Additionally, phosphorylation of Tyr127 was exhibited in lung and non-small cell lung cancer cell lines. Phosphorylation of residue Tyr143, which precedes the first residue of the second β-hairpin in the NRL, was also noted in the gastric carcinoma cell line MKN-45, as well as phosphorylation of residues T212 and T214, within the ALKBH3 active site, was found in liver cancer tissue samples [92]. Examination of potential ALKBH3 modification sites using predictive software shows possible post-translational modification sites for acetylation (Lys43, 116, 219, 220), and sumoylation (Lys57, 236), along with other possible phosphorylation sites (Ser32, 50, 187, 192, 208, 265; Thr29, 41; Tyr78, 127, 229) [90-93]. All of those possible post-translational modifications merit further consideration.

5. Biological significance of direct repair in mammalian cells

Normal cells depend on direct repair to eliminate damage that is possibly cytotoxic or mutagenic. Our knowledge of the biological significance of direct repair proteins in mammalian cells is based on the evaluation of effects on cell cytotoxicity, replication, transcription and subsequent mutagenic consequences observed in the absence of each protein of interest. Recent investigations performed in model system organisms, most prominently in mice, to assess the impact of the absence of Mgmt or Alkbh family proteins will be highlighted in this section. These studies also provide insight into the function and importance of direct repair proteins in humans.

5.1. Knock-out animal models

It is important to remember that a number of DNA repair systems are implicated in the elimination of DNA lesions formed by exposure to alkylating agents. Therefore, dysfunction of repair systems can lead to pathologies that include cancer development. However, without use of a model organism to assay the effects, the consequences to the organism as a whole cannot be assessed. Knock-out animal models are a valuable tool for understanding the overall physiological effects of genes on an organism, and provide insight into disease research and therapeutic development.

Murine Mgmt models have been studied by multiple groups to evaluate sensitivity to alkylating agents commonly used in chemotherapeutics [5, 6, 82, 86, 136-139]. Though Mgmt repairs DNA damage that is known to be mutagenic, Mgmt-deficient mice surprisingly lack any overt phenotype. However, these mice are significantly more sensitive to treatment with N-methyl-N-nitrosourea (MNU), 1,3-bis(2-chloroethyl)-1-nitrosourea (BCNU), 1-(4-amino-2-methyl-5-pyrimidinyl)methyl-3-(2-chloroethyl)3-nitrosourea (ACNU), streptozotocin, temozolomide, and dacarbazine alkylating agents [5, 136, 137, 139-142]. Mgmt knock-out mice treated with various chemotherapeutic agents also show ablation of hematopoietic tissues at the stem cell level [38, 141, 143] and are prone to development of thymic lymphomas [144]and lung adenomas [82, 138, 144, 145]. Similarly, mouse embryonic stem (ES), embryonic fibroblasts (MEFs) and bone marrow cells deficient in Mgmt also exhibit a significant increase in sensitivity (~10-fold) to MNU and BCNU [83, 141, 146]. However, mice heterozygous for *Mgmt* do not display a significant reduction in survival following treatment with nitrosoureas or increased tumorigenesis, compared to their wild-type counterparts.

Although *in vitro* DNA repair activity has been established for ALKBH1, studies conducted in murine models lacking Alkbh1 suggest roles involved in transcription. Mice deficient in Alkbh1 exhibit apoptosis in adult testis, sex-ratio distortion and unilaterial eye defects, as well as impaired differentiation of specific trophoblast lineages in the developing placenta [147, 148]. Though the specific activity and function of ALKBH1 remains to be determined, ALKBH1 biological roles seem linked to spermatogenesis and embryonic development.

On the other hand, Alkbh2- and/or Alkbh3-deficient murine models do not manifest any obvious phenotype or histopathological changes [116, 119, 132]. However, over time mice lacking Alkbh2 accumulate significant levels of 1-meA, confirming a role in removing endogenous DNA alkyl adducts. In a recent study, *Alkbh2,Alkbh3,Aag* knock-out mice (Aag also known as Mpg, a DNA glycosylase in the BER pathway) were viable, but underwent rapid death when exposed to a chemically-induced colitis treatment [119]. Similarly, primary mouse embryonic fibroblasts (MEFs) derived from mice lacking functional Alkbh2 exhibited significantly increased cytotoxicity and mutagenesis following exposure to the S_N2 alkylating agent methyl methanesulfonate (MMS) [116, 118, 119]. Survival of Alkbh3-deficient MEFs exposed to MMS was reduced by ~50% compared to wild type MEF sensitivity, though mutant frequency did not significantly increase [116].

5.2. Replication and transcription defects

Though not all lesions generated by exposure to alkylating agents cause defects in replication and transcription, DNA and RNA adducts that are specifically removed via a direct repair mechanism interfere with replication and transcription machinery. The presence of O^6-meG in DNA impedes polymerization by DNA and RNA polymerases [31, 32, 149, 150]. Polymerase beta (β), involved in base excision repair (BER) of alkylation adducts, is completely blocked by O^6-meG adducts [150]. Polymerase delta (δ) is able to replicate past, but insertion of the correct base opposite O^6-methylguanine is very inefficient. However, these adducts can be bypassed using polymerase eta (η) [149], a member of the Y-family DNA translesion synthesis (TLS) polymerases, but TLS polymerases are notorious for being error-prone. Interestingly, when replicating past O^6-meG DNA adducts, TLS polymerase, Polη is twice as efficient at inserting cytosines opposite O^6-meG as replicative polymerase, Pol δ [32].

1-meA and 3-meC lesions that are repaired by Alkbh2 and Alkbh3 are at DNA base-pairing positions and hinder proper base insertion [101]. During replication, this can lead to arrest of nucleotide synthesis, resulting in replication fork collapse [151]. Similarly, 1-meA and 3-meC adducts can also cause stalling of transcription. Correspondingly, Alkbh2 co-localizes with replication foci during S-phase [111, 131, 133] and Alkbh3 has a role in removal of alkyl adducts from mRNA [1, 15, 108, 115, 131, 152]. However, a TLS polymerase that is linked to 1-meA and/or 3-meC DNA adduct bypass has not been identified.

5.3. Cell cytotoxicity

Treatment with alkylating agents introduces a variety of adducts into DNA and RNA (Figure 2, Table 1). In the absence of direct repair proteins, those lesions can lead to cell death or damage tolerance, which allows for cell survival, but can introduce mutations into the genome that could have detrimental effects [101, 116, 142, 153]. As exhibited in Mgmt- and Alkbh-deficient murine models, lack of direct repair proteins correlates with a significant increase in cell death following treatment with S_N1 or S_N2 alkylating agents, respectively [116, 118, 140, 141].

5.4. Mutagenesis

When a modified nucleoside can form at least two hydrogen bonds, transcription and replication templates and translation of messengers are active [13]. O^6-meG, 1-meA, and 3-meC are all involved in DNA base-pairing. Modification at O^6-meG and 3-meC still allow for formation of two hydrogen bonds, while 1-meA results in only a single hydrogen bond between paired bases [13]. However, the exocyclic amino group of 1-meA can rotate so that both amino group hydrogen molecules can generate the necessary base-pairing bonds, though a slight distortion of the double-strand DNA helix does occur [13]. The addition of a methyl group to O^6-G, N1-A, or N3-C interferes with normal replication, and could recruit DNA translesion synthesis (TLS) polymerases to bypass the DNA adducts. The size and organization of the Y-family TLS polymerase active sites is variable and allows for accommodation of numerous adducts. However, not only are TLS polymerases inherently error-prone [154, 155], the number and type of hydrogen bonds that can be made with the modified bases has been altered. Those factors can produce insertion of an erroneous base during bypass that accompanies replication or transcription.

O^6-meG mutagenicity has been established in bacterial and mammalian systems [29, 30]. O^6-meG is mutagenic and primarily gives rise to G:C→A:T mutations. A mis-insertion of thymine is thought to occur due to mis-identification of O^6-meG as adenine, as hydrogen bonding can occur with the N1 and exocyclic amino group of O^6-meG [13].

Unfortunately, studies evaluating the mutagenicity of a site-specific 1-meA, 3-meC, 1-meG, or 3-meT adducts have not been conducted in mammalian systems, but studies in *E. coli*, show that 1-meA adducts are only slightly mutagenic, whereas 3-meC, 1-meG, and 3-meT adducts are much more mutagenic [101]. Work evaluating the anti-mutagenic role of Alkbh2 and Alkbh3 in a murine model showed increased mutant frequency, specifically for mouse embryonic fibroblast (MEF) cells deficient in either Alkbh2 or Alkbh3 [116]. Those Alkbh-deficient cells exhibited increased amounts of C:G→A:T C:G→T:A mutations, respectively. Additionally, when treated with MMS, Alkbh2-deficient MEFs displayed an increased frequency of C:G→T:A and T:A→A:T mutations. Similarly, Alkbh3-deficient MEFs also exhibited an increased frequency of T:A→A:T mutations, as well as an increased frequency of A:T→G:C mutations, in response to MMS treatment. Like O^6-meG, misidentification of the modified DNA bases due to the presence of two sites for hydrogen bond formation could arise if 1-meG or 3-meC is recognized as thymine and an adenine is paired with the two remaining hydrogen bond acceptors. Furthermore, T:A→A:T mutations could arise if 3-meT becomes recognized as adenine and a thymine is paired via hydrogen bonds between thymine O^4 and O^2 and adenine N-3 exocyclic amino group nitrogen. It is likely that 1-meA is rarely mutagenic in *E. coli*, deficient in AlkB, because 1-meA can utilize the C6 exocyclic amine and N7 as an alternative binding site providing two sites for hydrogen bond formation with thymine N-7 and O^4 molecules, using Hoogsteen base-pairing [156].

6. Medical significance of direct repair proteins in humans

Genetic and epigenetic controls that regulate *MGMT*, *ALKBH2*, and *ALKBH3* gene expression and influence how these proteins directly repair DNA are critical factors that can lead to a better understanding of cancer development. In addition, comprehension of factors that cause variations in the direct DNA repair activities of cancer cells will provide important progress toward formulating cancer therapeutics that target MGMT or ALKBH proteins. Understanding the impact of direct DNA repair proteins will eventually result in treatments that can be tailored to achieve better therapeutic results or to predict treatment and/or disease outcomes.

6.1. Epigenetic and transcriptional regulation

Epigenetic modifications are stable alterations of DNA that are heritable in the short term, but do not involve mutations of the DNA itself, and are mediated by DNA methylation and histone modifications. The stable alterations that are involved in epigenetics have a major role in exerting control on gene expression. Endogenous cell signaling as well as external influences, including diet and other life style choices, can alter gene expression mediated by changes in epigenetic modifications [157, 158]. Methylation of cytosines at transcription factor recognition sites can interfere with binding and/or function and repress transcription of that gene [159, 160]. Alternatively, protein recruitment that binds methyl CpG islands can block transcription machinery or alter chromatin structure [161, 162]. Transcriptional silencing also is connected to histone deacetylation [163, 164]. Methyl CpG binding domain

(MBD) family proteins direct histone deacetylases to remove acetyl groups from lysines in the amino terminal histone tails, stabilizing DNA-histone interactions, and condensing chromatin so that transcription factor binding sites are inaccessible.

Though unmethylated in normal cells, transcriptional silencing of *MGMT*, associated with promoter CpG island methylation has been reported in a variety of cancer cell types and MGMT-deficient cell lines [82, 138]. Additionally, in a glioma mouse model a subpopulation of glioma cells with stem cell properties were identified [165] that are capable of re-establishing tumor growth following temozolomide treatment. Although *Mgmt* promoter CpG methylation or protein levels were not determined in that study, when *MGMT* transcript levels were evaluated in glioma patients [166], those with *MGMT* CpG promoter methylation had increased response to temozolomide, but also maintained a subset of glioma cells with stem cell-like character and *MGMT* promoter methylation. Interestingly, mRNA levels of *DNMT1* and *DNMT3b* methyltransferases are increased in a number of human glioma patients, but there does not appear to be a link to *MGMT* expression levels [167]. Moreover, *MGMT* promoter CpG methylation levels and DNA methyltransferase levels alone do not account for patient response to alkylating agent therapy. However, whether *MGMT* promoter methylation disables transcription factor binding or contributes to chromatin reorganization remains uncertain [71, 72, 74]. Therefore, regulation of *MGMT* expression is still unclear and merits intense scrutiny.

The inability to establish direct connections among *MGMT* expression, CpG methylation, and response to alkylating agent therapy indicates that other mechanisms contribute in regulating MGMT levels. Studies evaluating *MGMT* expression and microRNAs in patient samples have established a modest inverse correlation between the levels of *MGMT* transcript and miR-181d [168]. Moreover, expression of mi-181d in A1207 glioblastoma cells, results in abnormal sensitivity to temozolomide. However, expression of *MGMT* cDNA, restores the survival to levels close to that of the A1207 parental line. These results suggest that identification of other miRNAs involved in regulating *MGMT* expression will help elucidate the mechanisms that control the gene transcript levels.

In addition to control at the DNA and transcript levels, histone modifications can also control the epigenetic state and direct expression. Acetylated histone H3 and H4 levels also increase in cell lines expressing MGMT, compared to cell lines deficient in MGMT [169], which would facilitate nucleosomal positioning that enables transcription factor interactions. Further, binding of MBD proteins in the *MGMT* promoter of was greater in *MGMT*-silenced cells, implicating MBD proteins in recruitment of histone deactylases that remove lysine acetylation from the amino-terminal tails of histones H3 and H4, resulting in more condensed chromatin and transcription inactivation [73, 79, 170]. Therefore, epigenetic and/or enzymatic CpG island methylation at the *MGMT* promoter influences transcription factor access, as well as chromatin structure that are important for *MGMT* expression.

ALKBH2 and *ALKBH3* both have CpG islands in their promoters, but epigenetic regulation and/or gene silencing has not been reported for either homolog. However, mutations that alter protein expression have been observed [171], but it is likely that methylation of CpG islands near any of the seven transcription factor binding sites in the promoter of ALKBH2 or the single transcription factor binding sites within the promoter region of ALKBH3, would repress transcription factor binding and possibly gene expression. Because data on the function of ALKBH promoters are less abundant compared to those available for the MGMT promoter, examination of the promoter function for those genes is an area that would benefit from further investigation.

6.2. Links to cancer

Dysregulation of numerous DNA repair pathways are involved in tumor development, progression, diagnosis, treatment and prognosis, including direct DNA repair proteins [82, 159, 172-179]. Over-expression of direct repair proteins is generally associated with a protective effect against cell death that would otherwise be induced by alkylating agent treatment. However, down-regulation or silencing of direct repair protein expression is associated with increased mutagenesis that precedes tumorgenesis. Therefore expression profiles could be used to predict potential resistance or enhanced sensitivity to therapeutics.

MGMT has been implicated in many types of human tumors. Numerous *MGMT* polymorphisms have risk associations with breast, lung, colon, and head and neck cancers [63, 82, 180-186]. Decreased *MGMT* expression is also found in glioma, lymphoma, retinoblastoma, breast (including triple-negative breast cancer) and prostate cancer [82, 138, 187] [188]. Moreover, lack of MGMT is associated with enhanced outcomes using alkylating agent therapies [5, 62, 67, 82, 86, 138, 139, 180, 181, 183, 189]. Though *MGMT* silencing occurs in a variety of tumor types, increased levels have also been observed in non-Hodgkin lymphoma, myeloma and glioma, as well as in some colon, pancreatic, breast, and lung cancers [63, 183, 184].

Mutations in *ALKBH2* and *3* have been associated with an enhanced expression of these proteins in glioma cells and pediatric brain tumors [171, 190]. Similarly, over-expression of *ALKBH3* has been associated with human rectal carcinoma [191] and prostate cancer, as well as, lung adenocarcinoma and non-small-cell lung cancer [134] [192]. On the contrary, down regulation of *ALKBH2* has been observed in gastric cancer, promoting growth of gastric cancer cells [193]. Although down regulation of *ALKBH2* in gastric cancer cells caused increased proliferation, *ALKBH2* silencing in H1299 lung cancer cells had the opposite effect, increasing cisplatin sensitivity. Similarly, *ALKBH3* silencing induced senescence and sensitivity to alkylating agents in human adenocarcinoma and prostate cancer cells [134, 193]. Therefore, further study of the role of ALKBH2 and 3 in both normal and tumor cells is necessary to elucidate their biological role(s).

6.3. Therapeutic targets

Understanding the mechanism of proteins involved in various DNA repair pathways is crucial for developing new chemotherapeutic targets and eventually new drugs. DNA alkylating agents and ionizing radiation (IR) are often used as chemotherapeutic treatments because of ability to control the dose administered and area of treatment, as well as the major cytotoxic effects of both agents at high doses. However, in addition to generation of cytotoxic adducts that cause apoptosis, alkylating agents and IR also form adducts that can be mutagenic and as a result can cause initiation of secondary cancers. Although DNA repair deficiencies are associated with increased cancer risk and formation, cancer cells proficient in DNA repair can reduce therapeutic efficacy. Currently, combination cancer treatment regimens are being explored that utilize chemotherapy or IR and target specific DNA repair proteins with pharmacological agents to enhance treatment efficacy and eliminate resistance to treatment regimens exhibited in some patients [189].

6.3.1. MGMT

Chemotherapeutic drugs such as temozolamide (TMZ) and bis-(2-chloroethyl)-nitrosourea (BCNU) generate some lesions repaired via the direct methyltransferase mechanism. Combination treatment with MGMT inhibitors prevents repair and resistance to methylating and chloroethylating agents [1, 38, 137] and has also been shown to reverse cisplatin drug resistance [194].

Understanding cellular regulation of *MGMT* expression will allow for selective down regulation and sensitization of tumors to alkylating agent chemotherapies. Studies have evaluated manipulation of *MGMT* expression and protein levels. Initial experiments evaluating MGMT inhibitors identified O^6-benzyl guanine (BG) as an efficacious inhibitor of MGMT activity, a single, micromolar dose depleting greater than 99% of MGMT activity in human cells for 24-hours following drug removal [195]. Moreover, treatment with BG lacks any mutagenic or cytotoxic effects [195-197]. Clinical trials combining BG and BCNU treatment have been conducted in colon cancer, sarcoma, melanoma and myeloma, as well as studies evaluating combination of BG and TMZ [138]. Since synthesis of BG, additional BG-like inhibitors have been developed [196], including O^6-(4-bromothenyl) guanine, which has been evaluated in patients with glioma [187]. Similarly, targeting of MGMT along with combination of platinum drugs, including cis- and carboplatinum [198], as well as topoisomerase I inhibitors has been investigated in various clinical trials [86].

Another approach to regulate MGMT that holds great, essentially untapped therapeutic potential is strategies utilizing RNA interference-mediated gene silencing to target MGMT [168, 199, 200]. For instance, if anti-sense molecules can specifically target MGMT mRNA translation, and degradation is also inhibited, depletion of MGMT is sustainable for long periods of time [62]. As seen in glioblastoma patients, expression levels of various miRNA markers correlate with prognosis [168, 199, 200]. Therefore, one potential new treatment could use miRNAs, such as miR-181d, to decrease MGMT levels, thus increasing sensitivity to alkylating agents [168]. Similarly, targeting regions of the MGMT promoter that is accessible to transcription factors could interfere with binding and down-regulate *MGMT* transcription. However, non-specific targeting of MGMT inhibitors in all cells increases chemotherapeutic toxicity. Therefore, mutant forms of MGMT that are resistant to BG-like inhibitors are also being evaluated to limit myelosuppression, affording hematopoietic progenitor cells protection from BG and BCNU or temozolomide treatment [201-204].

http://dx.doi.org/10.5772/54449

6.3.2. Alkbh homologs

Similar to MGMT, the role of ALKBH2 and ALKBH3 in repair of DNA alkylation damage at base-pairing sites is anti-carcinogenic. However, investigations indicate that over-expression of ALKBH proteins in various cancer cell lines shields those cells against methylating agent toxicity and would thereby protect against some chemotherapeutic treatments [134, 171, 192]. Additionally, because loss of ALKBH2 and/or ALKBH3 leads to disruption of replication, inhibition of ALKBH2 and/or ALKBH3 is a strong target for the development of novel chemotherapeutic agents. Some specific inhibitors of these proteins have already been identified [135, 205, 206], as well as generic α-KG/dioxygenase inhibitors including dimethyl oxalylglycine (DMOG) and α-ketoglutarate derivatives such as oxoglutarate. Studies have addressed the application of DNA aptamers as inhibitors of ALKBH proteins [207]. However, to date no studies have been conducted in mammalian models that evaluate the combination of ALKBH inhibitors with chemotherapeutic alkylating agents.

7. Summary

Direct repair proteins represent a unique class of enzymes that remove DNA damage without a dependence on DNA synthesis. In the future, better comprehension of how these proteins function and are produced in cells will lead to understanding their roles in formation of mutations that cause cancer. Eventually, that knowledge will foster the development of drugs to target these proteins and/or to regulate their expression to improve patient outcomes.

Author details

Stephanie L. Nay[1,2] and Timothy R. O'Connor[2]

1 Irell and Manella Graduate School of Biological Sciences, USA

2 Department of Cancer Biology, Beckman Research Institute, Duarte, CA, USA

References

[1] Drablos F, Feyzi E, Aas PA, Vaagbo CB, Kavli B, Bratlie MS, et al. Alkylation damage in DNA and RNA--repair mechanisms and medical significance. DNA Repair (Amst). 2004;3(11):1389-407.

[2] Sedgwick B. Repairing DNA-methylation damage. Nat Rev Mol Cell Biol. 2004;5(2): 148-57.

[3] Hecht SS. DNA adduct formation from tobacco-specific N-nitrosamines. Mutat Res. 1999;424(1-2):127-42.

[4] Ballschmiter K. Pattern and sources of naturally produced organohalogens in the marine environment: biogenic formation of organohalogens. Chemosphere. 2003;52(2): 313-24.

[5] Sanada M, Takagi Y, Ito R, Sekiguchi M. Killing and mutagenic actions of dacarbazine, a chemotherapeutic alkylating agent, on human and mouse cells: effects of Mgmt and Mlh1 mutations. DNA Repair (Amst). 2004;3(4):413-20.

[6] Shiraishi A, Sakumi K, Sekiguchi M. Increased susceptibility to chemotherapeutic alkylating agents of mice deficient in DNA repair methyltransferase. Carcinogenesis. 2000;21(10):1879-83.

[7] Taverna P, Sedgwick B. Generation of an endogenous DNA-methylating agent by nitrosation in Escherichia coli. J Bacteriol. 1996;178(17):5105-11.

[8] Cantoni GL. The nature of the active methyldonor formed enzymatically from L-methionine and adenosinetriphosphate.. J Am Chem Soc. 1952;74(11):2942-3.

[9] Cantoni GL, Scarano E. The formation of S-adenosylhomocysteine in enzymatic transmethylation reactions. J Am Chem Soc. 1954;76(18):4744-.

[10] Kumar S, Cheng X, Klimasauskas S, Mi S, Posfai J, Roberts RJ, et al. The DNA (cytosine-5) methyltransferases. Nucleic Acids Res. 1994;22(1):1-10.

[11] Goll MG, Kirpekar F, Maggert KA, Yoder JA, Hsieh CL, Zhang X, et al. Methylation of tRNAAsp by the DNA methyltransferase homolog Dnmt2. Science. 2006;311(5759):395-8.

[12] Patterson LH, Murray GI. Tumour cytochrome P450 and drug activation. Curr Pharm Des. 2002;8(15):1335-47.

[13] Singer B, Grunberger D, editors. Molecular Biology of Mutagens and Carcinogens. 1 ed. New York: Plenum; 1983.

[14] Friedberg EC, Walker GC, Siede W. DNA Repair and mutagenesis. Washington DC: ASM Press; 1995.

[15] Aas PA, Otterlei M, Falnes PO, Vagbo CB, Skorpen F, Akbari M, et al. Human and bacterial oxidative demethylases repair alkylation damage in both RNA and DNA. Nature. 2003;421(6925):859-63.

[16] Fu D, Calvo JA, Samson LD. Balancing repair and tolerance of DNA damage caused by alkylating agents. Nat Rev Cancer. 2012;12(2):104-20.

[17] Mishina Y, Duguid EM, He C. Direct Reversal of DNA Alkylation Damage. Chem Rev. 2006;106(2):215-32.

[18] Baker DJ, Wuenschell G, Xia L, Termini J, Bates SE, Riggs AD, et al. Nucleotide excision repair eliminates unique DNA-protein cross-links from mammalian cells. J Biol Chem. 2007;282(31):22592-604.

[19] Bjelland S, Bjoras M, Seeberg E. Excision of 3-methylguanine from alkylated DNA by 3-methyladenine DNA glycosylase I of Escherichia coli. Nucleic Acids Res. 1993;21(9):2045-9.

[20] Jones LE, Jr., Ying L, Hofseth AB, Jelezcova E, Sobol RW, Ambs S, et al. Differential effects of reactive nitrogen species on DNA base excision repair initiated by the alkyladenine DNA glycosylase. Carcinogenesis. 2009;30(12):2123-9.

[21] Fortini P, Dogliotti E. Base damage and single-strand break repair: mechanisms and functional significance of short- and long-patch repair subpathways. DNA Repair (Amst). 2007;6(4):398-409.

[22] Houtgraaf JH, Versmissen J, van der Giessen WJ. A concise review of DNA damage checkpoints and repair in mammalian cells. Cardiovasc Revasc Med. 2006;7(3): 165-72.

[23] Samson L, Han S, Marquis JC, Rasmussen LJ. Mammalian DNA repair methyltransferases shield O4MeT from nucleotide excision repair. Carcinogenesis. 1997;18(5): 919-24.

[24] Ziemba A, Derosier LC, Methvin R, Song CY, Clary E, Kahn W, et al. Repair of triplex-directed DNA alkylation by nucleotide excision repair. Nucleic Acids Res. 2001;29(21):4257-63.

[25] Ye N, Holmquist GP, O'Connor TR. Heterogeneous repair of N-methylpurines at the nucleotide level in normal human cells. J Mol Biol. 1998;284(2):269-85.

[26] Kondo N, Takahashi A, Ono K, Ohnishi T. DNA damage induced by alkylating agents and repair pathways. Journal of nucleic acids. 2010;2010:543531. Epub 2010/11/30.

[27] Sobol RW, Kartalou M, Almeida KH, Joyce DF, Engelward BP, Horton JK, et al. Base excision repair intermediates induce p53-independent cytotoxic and genotoxic responses. J Biol Chem. 2003;278(41):39951-9.

[28] Hoeijmakers JH. Genome Maintenance Mechanisms for Preventing Cancer. Nature. 2001(411):366 - 74.

[29] Dosanjh MK, Singer B, Essigmann JM. Comparative mutagenesis of O6-methylguanine and O4-methylthymine in Escherichia coli. Biochemistry. 1991;30(28):7027-33. Epub 1991/07/16.

[30] Ellison KS, Dogliotti E, Connors TD, Basu AK, Essigmann JM. Site-specific mutagenesis by O6-alkylguanines located in the chromosomes of mammalian cells: influence of the mammalian O6-alkylguanine-DNA alkyltransferase. Proc Natl Acad Sci U S A. 1989;86(22):8620-4.

[31] Reha-Krantz LJ, Nonay RL, Day RS, Wilson SH. Replication of O6-methylguanine-containing DNA by repair and replicative DNA polymerases. J Biol Chem. 1996;271(33):20088-95.

[32] Voigt JM, Topal MD. O6-methylguanine-induced replication blocks. Carcinogenesis. 1995;16(8):1775-82.

[33] Fang Q, Noronha AM, Murphy SP, Wilds CJ, Tubbs JL, Tainer JA, et al. Repair of O6-G-alkyl-O6-G interstrand cross-links by human O6-alkylguanine-DNA. Biochemistry. 2008;47(41):10892-903.

[34] Graves RJ, Li BF, Swann PF. Repair of O6-methylguanine, O6-ethylguanine, O6-isopropylguanine and. Carcinogenesis. 1989;10(4):661-6.

[35] Jena NR, Shukla PK, Jena HS, Mishra PC, Suhai S. O6-methylguanine repair by O6-alkylguanine-DNA alkyltransferase. J Phys Chem B. 2009;113(51):16285-90.

[36] Kawate H, Ihara K, Kohda K, Sakumi K, Sekiguchi M. Mouse methyltransferase for repair of O6-methylguanine and O4-methylthymine in. Carcinogenesis. 1995;16(7): 1595-602.

[37] Swann PF. Why do O6-alkylguanine and O4-alkylthymine miscode? The relationship between the. Mutat Res. 1990;233(1-2):81-94.

[38] Verbeek B, Southgate TD, Gilham DE, Margison GP. O6-Methylguanine-DNA methyltransferase inactivation and chemotherapy. Br Med Bull. 2008;85:17-33.

[39] Parkinson JF, Wheeler HT, McDonald KL. Contribution of DNA repair mechanisms to determining chemotherapy response in high-grade glioma. J Clin Neurosci. 2008;15(1):1-8.

[40] Srivenugopal KS, Yuan XH, Friedman HS, Ali-Osman F. Ubiquitination-dependent proteolysis of O6-methylguanine-DNA methyltransferase in human and murine tumor cells following inactivation with O6-benzylguanine or 1,3-bis(2-chloroethyl)-1-nitrosourea. Biochemistry. 1996;35(4):1328-34. Epub 1996/01/30.

[41] Fang Q, Kanugula S, Pegg AE. Function of domains of human O6-alkylguanine-DNA alkyltransferase. Biochemistry. 2005;44(46):15396-405.

[42] Daniels DS, Tainer JA. Conserved structural motifs governing the stoichiometric repair of alkylated DNA. Mutat Res. 2000;460(3-4):151-63.

[43] Hashimoto H, Inoue T, Nishioka M, Fujiwara S, Takagi M, Imanaka T, et al. Hyperthermostable protein structure maintained by intra and inter-helix ion-pairs. J Mol Biol. 1999;292(3):707-16.

[44] Moore MH, Gulbis JM, Dodson EJ, Demple B, Moody PC. Crystal structure of a suicidal DNA repair protein: the Ada O6-methylguanine-DNA. Embo J. 1994;13(7): 1495-501.

[45] Roberts A, Pelton JG, Wemmer DE. Structural studies of MJ1529, an O6-methylguanine-DNA methyltransferase. Magn Reson Chem. 2006;44 Spec No:S71-82.

[46] Wibley JE, Pegg AE, Moody PC. Crystal structure of the human O(6)-alkylguanine-DNA alkyltransferase. Nucleic Acids Res. 2000;28(2):393-401.

[47] Rasimas JJ, Kanugula S, Dalessio PM, Ropson IJ, Fried MG, Pegg AE, et al. Effects of zinc occupancy on human O6-alkylguanine-DNA alkyltransferase. Biochemistry. 2003;42(4):980-90.

[48] Daniels DS, Mol CD, Arvai AS, Kanugula S, Pegg AE, Tainer JA. Active and alkylated human AGT structures: a novel zinc site, inhibitor and extrahelical base binding. Embo J. 2000;19(7):1719-30.

[49] Crone TM, Pegg AE. A single amino acid change in human O6-alkylguanine-DNA alkyltransferase decreasing sensitivity to inactivation by O6-benzylguanine. Cancer Res. 1993;53(20):4750-3.

[50] Lindahl T, Demple B, Robins P. Suicide inactivation of the E. coli O6-methylguanine-DNA methyltransferase. Embo J. 1982;1(11):1359-63.

[51] Daniels DS, Woo TT, Luu KX, Noll DM, Clarke ND, Pegg AE, et al. DNA binding and nucleotide flipping by the human DNA repair protein AGT. Nat Struct Mol Biol. 2004;11(8):714-20.

[52] Duguid EM-, Rice PA, He C. The structure of the human AGT protein bound to DNA and its implications for. J Mol Biol. 2005;350(4):657-66.

[53] Pegg AE. Repair of O(6)-alkylguanine by alkyltransferases. Mutat Res. 2000;462(2-3): 83-100.

[54] Tubbs JL, Latypov V, Kanugula S, Butt A, Melikishvili M, Kraehenbuehl R, et al. Alkylated DNA damage flipping bridges base and nucleotide excision repair. Nature. 2009;459(7248):808-13.

[55] Tubbs JL, Pegg AE, Tainer JA. DNA binding, nucleotide flipping, and the helix-turn-helix motif in base repair. DNA Repair (Amst). 2007;6(8):1100-15.

[56] Verdemato PE, Brannigan JA, Damblon C, Zuccotto F, Moody PC, Lian LY. DNA-binding mechanism of the Escherichia coli Ada O(6)-alkylguanine-DNA alkyltransferase. Nucleic Acids Res. 2000;28(19):3710-8.

[57] Yang CG, Garcia K, He C. Damage Detection and Base Flipping in Direct DNA Alkylation Repair. Chembiochem. 2009.

[58] Zak P, Kleibl K, Laval F. Repair of O(6)-alkylguanine by alkyltransferases. J Biol Chem. 2000;462(2-3):83-100.

[59] Yarosh DB, Rice M, Day RS, 3rd, Foote RS, Mitra S. O6-Methylguanine-DNA methyltransferase in human cells. Mutat Res. 1984;131(1):27-36.

[60] Fried MG, Kanugula S, Bromberg JL, Pegg AE. The modified human DNA repair enzyme O(6)-methylguanine-DNA methyltransferase is a negative regulator of estrogen receptor-mediated transcription upon alkylation DNA damage. Biochemistry. 2001;21(20):7105-14.

[61] Groth P, Auslander S, Majumder MM, Schultz N, Johansson F, Petermann E, et al. Methylated DNA causes a physical block to replication forks independently of damage signalling, O(6)-methylguanine or DNA single-strand breaks and results in DNA damage. J Mol Biol. 2010;402(1):70-82.

[62] Pieper RO. Understanding and manipulating O6-methylguanine-DNA methyltransferase expression. Pharmacol Ther. 1997;74(3):285-97.

[63] Matsukura S, Miyazaki K, Yakushiji H, Ogawa A, Harimaya K, Nakabeppu Y, et al. Expression and prognostic significance of O6-methylguanine-DNA methyltransferase. Ann Surg Oncol. 2001;8(10):807-16.

[64] Natarajan AT, Vermeulen S, Darroudi F, Valentine MB, Brent TP, Mitra S, et al. Chromosomal localization of human O6-methylguanine-DNA methyltransferase (MGMT). Mutagenesis. 1992;7(1):83-5.

[65] Nakatsu Y, Hattori K, Hayakawa H, Shimizu K, Sekiguchi M. Organization and expression of the human gene for O6-methylguanine-DNA. Mutat Res. 1993;293(2): 119-32.

[66] Tano K, Shiota S, Collier J, Foote RS, Mitra S. Isolation and structural characterization of a cDNA clone encoding the human DNA. Proc Natl Acad Sci U S A. 1990;87(2): 686-90.

[67] Soejima H, Zhao W, Mukai T. Epigenetic silencing of the MGMT gene in cancer. Biochem Cell Biol. 2005;83(4):429-37.

[68] Gardiner-Garden M, Frommer M. CpG islands in vertebrate genomes. J Mol Biol. 1987;196(2):261-82.

[69] Harris LC, Potter PM, Tano K, Shiota S, Mitra S, Brent TP. Characterization of the promoter region of the human O6-methylguanine-DNA. Nucleic Acids Res. 1991;19(22):6163-7.

[70] Takai D, Jones PA. Comprehensive analysis of CpG islands in human chromosomes 21 and 22. Proc Natl Acad Sci U S A. 2002;99(6):3740-5.

[71] Pieper RO, Patel S, Ting SA, Futscher BW, Costello JF. Methylation of CpG island transcription factor binding sites is unnecessary for. J Biol Chem. 1996;271(23): 13916-24.

[72] Costello JF, Futscher BW, Kroes RA, Pieper RO. Methylation-related chromatin structure is associated with exclusion of. Mol Cell Biol. 1994;14(10):6515-21.

[73] Pieper RO, Costello JF-, Kroes RA, Futscher BW, Marathi U, Erickson LC. Direct correlation between methylation status and expression of the human. Cancer Commun. 1991;3(8):241-53.

[74] Costello JF, Futscher BW, Tano K, Graunke DM, Pieper RO. Graded methylation in the promoter and body of the O6-methylguanine DNA. J Biol Chem. 1994;269(25): 17228-37.

[75] Qian X, von Wronski MA, Brent TP. Localization of methylation sites in the human O6-methylguanine-DNA. Carcinogenesis. 1995;16(6):1385-90.

[76] Silber JR, Blank A, Bobola MS, Mueller BA, Kolstoe DD, Ojemann GA, et al. Lack of the DNA repair protein O6-methylguanine-DNA methyltransferase in. Proc Natl Acad Sci U S A. 1996;93(14):6941-6.

[77] Patel SA, Graunke DM, Pieper RO. Aberrant silencing of the CpG island-containing human O6-methylguanine DNA methyltransferase gene is associated with the loss of nucleosome-like positioning. Mol Cell Biol. 1997;17(10):5813-22. Epub 1997/10/07.

[78] Nakagawachi T, Soejima H, Urano T, Zhao W, Higashimoto K, Satoh Y, et al. Silencing effect of CpG island hypermethylation and histone modifications on O6-methylguanine-DNA methyltransferase (MGMT) gene expression in human cancer. Oncogene. 2003;22(55):8835-44.

[79] Zhao W, Soejima H, Higashimoto K, Nakagawachi T, Urano T, Kudo S, et al. The essential role of histone H3 Lys9 di-methylation and MeCP2 binding in MGMT. J Biochem. 2005;137(3):431-40.

[80] Ali RB, Teo AK, Oh HK, Chuang LS, Ayi TC, Li BF. Implication of localization of human DNA repair enzyme O6-methylguanine-DNA. Mol Cell Biol. 1998;18(3):1660-9.

[81] Lim A, Li BF. The nuclear targeting and nuclear retention properties of a human DNA repair. Embo J. 1996;15(15):4050-60.

[82] Gerson SL. MGMT: its role in cancer aetiology and cancer therapeutics. Nat Rev Cancer. 2004;4(4):296-307.

[83] Kaina B, Christmann M, Naumann S, Roos WP. MGMT: key node in the battle against genotoxicity, carcinogenicity and apoptosis. DNA Repair (Amst). 2007;6(8): 1079-99.

[84] Liu L, Gerson SL. Targeted modulation of MGMT: clinical implications. Clin Cancer Res. 2006;12(2):328-31.

[85] Pegg AE, Fang Q, Loktionova NA. Human variants of O6-alkylguanine-DNA alkyltransferase. DNA Repair (Amst). 2007;6(8):1071-8.

[86] Sabharwal A, Middleton MR. Exploiting the role of O6-methylguanine-DNA-methyltransferase (MGMT) in cancer therapy. Curr Opin Pharmacol. 2006;6(4):355-63.

[87] Srivenugopal KS, Yuan XH, Friedman HS, Ali-Osman F. Inhibition by nitric oxide of the repair protein, O6-methylguanine-DNA-methyltransferase. Biochemistry. 1994;15(3):443-7.

[88] Hwang CS, Shemorry A, Varshavsky A. Two proteolytic pathways regulate DNA repair by cotargeting the Mgt1 alkylguanine. Proc Natl Acad Sci U S A. 2009;106(7): 2142-7.

[89] Srivenugopal KS, Ali-Osman F. The DNA repair protein, O(6)-methylguanine-DNA methyltransferase is a proteolytic. Oncogene. 2002;21(38):5940-5.

[90] Li T, Du Y, Wang L, Huang L, Li W, Lu M, et al. Characterization and prediction of lysine (K)-acetyl-transferase specific acetylation sites. Molecular & cellular proteomics : MCP. 2012;11(1):M111 011080. Epub 2011/10/04.

[91] Artimo P, Jonnalagedda M, Arnold K, Baratin D, Csardi G, de Castro E, et al. ExPASy: SIB bioinformatics resource portal. Nucleic Acids Res. 2012;40(Web Server issue):W597-603. Epub 2012/06/05.

[92] Hornbeck PV, Kornhauser JM, Tkachev S, Zhang B, Skrzypek E, Murray B, et al. PhosphoSitePlus: a comprehensive resource for investigating the structure and function of experimentally determined post-translational modifications in man and mouse. Nucleic Acids Res. 2012;40(Database issue):D261-70. Epub 2011/12/03.

[93] Shi SP, Qiu JD, Sun XY, Suo SB, Huang SY, Liang RP. PMeS: prediction of methylation sites based on enhanced feature encoding scheme. PLoS ONE. 2012;7(6):e38772. Epub 2012/06/22.

[94] Begley TJ, Samson LD. AlkB mystery solved: oxidative demethylation of N1-methyladenine and N3-methylcytosine adducts by a direct reversal mechanism. Trends Biochem Sci. 2003;28(1):2-5.

[95] Flashman E, Davies SL, Yeoh KK, Schofield CJ. Investigating the dependence of the hypoxia-inducible factor hydroxylases (factor inhibiting HIF and prolyl hydroxylase domain 2) on ascorbate and other reducing agents. Biochem J. 2010;427(1):135-42.

[96] Kataoka H, Yamamoto Y, Sekiguchi M. A new gene (alkB) of Escherichia coli that controls sensitivity to methyl methane sulfonate. J Bacteriol. 1983;153(3):1301-7.

[97] Schneider J, Shilatifard A. Histone demethylation by hydroxylation: chemistry in action. ACS Chem Biol. 2006;1(2):75-81.

[98] Tsukada Y, Fang J, Erdjument-Bromage H, Warren ME, Borchers CH, Tempst P, et al. Histone demethylation by a family of JmjC domain-containing proteins. Nature. 2006;439(7078):811-6.

[99] Yamane K, Toumazou C, Tsukada Y, Erdjument-Bromage H, Tempst P, Wong J, et al. JHDM2A, a JmjC-containing H3K9 demethylase, facilitates transcription activation by androgen receptor. Cell. 2006;125(3):483-95.

[100] Trewick SC, Henshaw TF, Hausinger RP, Lindahl T, Sedgwick B. Oxidative demethylation by Escherichia coli AlkB directly reverts DNA base damage. Nature. 2002;419(6903):174-8.

[101] Delaney JC, Essigmann JM. Mutagenesis, genotoxicity, and repair of 1-methyladenine, 3-alkylcytosines, 1-methylguanine, and 3-methylthymine in alkB Escherichia coli. Proc Natl Acad Sci U S A. 2004;101(39):14051-6. Epub 2004/09/24.

[102] Delaney JC, Smeester L, Wong C, Frick LE, Taghizadeh K, Wishnok JS, et al. AlkB reverses etheno DNA lesions caused by lipid oxidation in vitro and in vivo. Nat Struct Mol Biol. 2005;12(10):855-60.

[103] Falnes PO. Repair of 3-methylthymine and 1-methylguanine lesions by bacterial and human AlkB proteins. Nucleic Acids Res. 2004;32(21):6260-7.

[104] Falnes PO, Bjoras M, Aas PA, Sundheim O, Seeberg E. Substrate specificities of bacterial and human AlkB proteins. Nucleic Acids Res. 2004;32(11):3456-61.

[105] Frick LE, Delaney JC, Wong C, Drennan CL, Essigmann JM. Alleviation of 1,N6-ethanoadenine genotoxicity by the Escherichia coli adaptive response protein AlkB. Proc Natl Acad Sci U S A. 2007;104(3):755-60.

[106] Koivisto P, Robins P, Lindahl T, Sedgwick B. Demethylation of 3-methylthymine in DNA by bacterial and human DNA dioxygenases. J Biol Chem. 2004;279(39):40470-4.

[107] Mishina Y, Yang CG, He C. Direct repair of the exocyclic DNA adduct 1,N6-ethenoadenine by the DNA repair AlkB proteins. J Am Chem Soc. 2005;127(42):14594-5.

[108] Ougland R, Zhang CM, Liiv A, Johansen RF, Seeberg E, Hou YM, et al. AlkB restores the biological function of mRNA and tRNA inactivated by chemical methylation. Mol Cell. 2004;16(1):107-16.

[109] Aravind L, Koonin EV. The DNA-repair protein AlkB, EGL-9, and leprecan define new families of 2-oxoglutarate- and iron-dependent dioxygenases. Genome Biol. 2001;2(3):RESEARCH0007.

[110] Kurowski MA, Bhagwat AS, Papaj G, Bujnicki JM. Phylogenomic identification of five new human homologs of the DNA repair enzyme AlkB. BMC Genomics. 2003;4(1):48.

[111] Duncan T, Trewick SC, Koivisto P, Bates PA, Lindahl T, Sedgwick B. Reversal of DNA alkylation damage by two human dioxygenases. Proc Natl Acad Sci U S A. 2002;99(26):16660-5.

[112] Mishina Y, He C. Oxidative dealkylation DNA repair mediated by the mononuclear non-heme iron AlkB proteins. J Inorg Biochem. 2006;100(4):670-8.

[113] Sedgwick B, Robins P, Lindahl T. Direct removal of alkylation damage from DNA by AlkB and related DNA dioxygenases. Methods Enzymol. 2006;408:108-20.

[114] Sundheim O, Talstad VA, Vagbo CB, Slupphaug G, Krokan HE. AlkB demethylases flip out in different ways. DNA Repair (Amst). 2008;7(11):1916-23.

[115] Westbye MP, Feyzi E, Aas PA, Vagbo CB, Talstad VA, Kavli B, et al. Human AlkB homolog 1 is a mitochondrial protein that demethylates 3-methylcytosine in DNA and RNA. J Biol Chem. 2008;283(36):25046-56.

[116] Nay SL, Lee DH, Bates SE, O'Connor TR. Alkbh2 protects against lethality and mutation in primary mouse embryonic. DNA Repair (Amst). 2012;11(5):502-10.

[117] Nieminuszczy J, Mielecki D, Sikora A, Wrzesinski M, Chojnacka A, Krwawicz J, et al. Mutagenic potency of MMS-induced 1meA/3meC lesions in E. coli. Environ Mol Mutagen. 2009;50(9):791-9.

[118] Ringvoll J, Nordstrand LM, Vagbo CB, Talstad V, Reite K, Aas PA, et al. Repair deficient mice reveal mABH2 as the primary oxidative demethylase for repairing 1meA and 3meC lesions in DNA. EMBO J. 2006;25(10):2189-98.

[119] Calvo JA, Meira LB, Lee CYI, Erkul CA, Abolhassani N, Taghizadeh K, et al. DNA repair is indispensable for survival after acute inflammation. J Clin Invest. 2012;122(7):2680-9.

[120] Sundheim O, Vagbo CB, Bjoras M, Sousa MM, Talstad V, Aas PA, et al. Human ABH3 structure and key residues for oxidative demethylation to reverse DNA/RNA damage. EMBO J. 2006;25(14):3389-97.

[121] Yang CG, Yi C, Duguid EM, Sullivan CT, Jian X, Rice PA, et al. Crystal structures of DNA/RNA repair enzymes AlkB and ABH2 bound to dsDNA. Nature. 2008;452(7190):961-5.

[122] Yi C, Yang CG, He C. A Non-Heme Iron-Mediated Chemical Demethylation in DNA and RNA. Acc Chem Res. 2009;42(4):519-29.

[123] Yu B, Edstrom WC, Benach J, Hamuro Y, Weber PC, Gibney BR, et al. Crystal structures of catalytic complexes of the oxidative DNA/RNA repair enzyme AlkB. Nature. 2006;439(7078):879-84.

[124] Bleijlevens B, Shivarattan T, Flashman E, Yang Y, Simpson PJ, Koivisto P, et al. Dynamic states of the DNA repair enzyme AlkB regulate product release. EMBO Rep. 2008;9(9):872-7.

[125] Sedgwick B, Bates PA, Paik J, Jacobs SC, Lindahl T. Repair of alkylated DNA: recent advances. DNA Repair (Amst). 2007;6(4):429-42.

[126] Shimada K, Nakamura M, Anai S, De Velasco M, Tanaka M, Tsujikawa K, et al. A novel human AlkB homologue, ALKBH8, contributes to human bladder cancer progression. Cancer Res. 2009;69(7):3157-64.

[127] Songe-Moller L, van den Born E, Leihne V, Vagbo CB, Kristoffersen T, Krokan HE, et al. Mammalian ALKBH8 possesses tRNA methyltransferase activity required for the

biogenesis of multiple wobble uridine modifications implicated in translational decoding. Mol Cell Biol. 2010;30(7):1814-27.

[128] Falnes PO, Johansen RF, Seeberg E. AlkB-mediated oxidative demethylation reverses DNA damage in Escherichia coli. Nature. 2002;419(6903):178-82.

[129] Kataoka H, Sekiguchi M. Molecular cloning and characterization of the alkB gene of Escherichia coli. Mol Gen Genet. 1985;198(2):263-9.

[130] Liu H, Llano J, Gauld JW. A DFT study of nucleobase dealkylation by the DNA repair enzyme AlkB. J Phys Chem B. 2009;113(14):4887-98.

[131] Lee DH, Jin SG, Cai S, Chen Y, Pfeifer GP, O'Connor TR. Repair of methylation damage in DNA and RNA by mammalian AlkB homologues. J Biol Chem. 2005;280(47): 39448-59.

[132] Ringvoll J, Moen MN, Nordstrand LM, Meira LB, Pang B, Bekkelund A, et al. AlkB homologue 2-mediated repair of ethenoadenine lesions in mammalian DNA. Cancer Res. 2008;68(11):4142-9.

[133] Tsujikawa K, Koike K, Kitae K, Shinkawa A, Arima H, Suzuki T, et al. Expression and sub-cellular localization of human ABH family molecules. J Cell Mol Med. 2007;11(5):1105-16.

[134] Dango S, Mosammaparast N, Sowa M, Xiong L, Wu F, Park K, et al. DNA Unwinding by ASCC3 Helicase Is Coupled to ALKBH3-Dependent DNA Alkylation Repair and Cancer Cell Proliferation. Molecular Cell. 2011(44):373–84.

[135] Welford RW, Schlemminger I, McNeill LA, Hewitson KS, Schofield CJ. The selectivity and inhibition of AlkB. J Biol Chem. 2003;278(12):10157-61.

[136] Tsuzuki T, Sakumi K, Shiraishi A, Kawate H, Igarashi H, Iwakuma T, et al. Targeted disruption of the DNA repair methyltransferase gene renders mice hypersensitive to alkylating agent. Carcinogenesis. 1996;17(6):1215-20.

[137] D'Atri S, Graziani G, Lacal PM, Nistico V, Gilberti S, Faraoni I, et al. Attenuation of O(6)-methylguanine-DNA methyltransferase activity and mRNA levels by cisplatin and temozolomide in jurkat cells. J Pharmacol Exp Ther. 2000;294(2):664-71.

[138] Gerson SL. Clinical relevance of MGMT in the treatment of cancer. J Clin Oncol. 2002;20(9):2388-99.

[139] Hansen RJ, Ludeman SM, Paikoff SJ, Pegg AE, Dolan ME. Role of MGMT in Protecting against Cyclophosphamide-Induced Toxicity in Cells and. DNA Repair (Amst). 2007;6(8):1145-54.

[140] Glassner BJ, Weeda G, Allan JM, Broekhof JL, Carls NH, Donker I, et al. DNA repair methyltransferase (Mgmt) knockout mice are sensitive to the lethal. Mutagenesis. 1999;14(3):339-47.

[141] Roos WP, Christmann M, Fraser ST, Kaina B. Mouse embryonic stem cells are hypersensitive to apoptosis triggered by the DNA damage O(6)-methylguanine due to high E2F1 regulated mismatch repair. Cell Death Differ. 2007;14(8):1422-32.

[142] Sakumi K, Shiraishi A, Shimizu S, Tsuzuki T, Ishikawa T, Sekiguchi M. Methylnitrosourea-induced tumorigenesis in MGMT gene knockout mice. Cancer Res. 1997;57(12):2415-8.

[143] Bobola MS, Blank A, Berger MS, Silber JR. O6-methylguanine-DNA methyltransferase deficiency in developing brain. DNA Repair (Amst). 2007;6(8):1127-33.

[144] Dumenco Ll, Allay E, Norton K, Gerson SL. The prevention of thymic lymphomas in transgenic mice by human. Science. 1993;259(5092):219-22.

[145] Horsfield JA, Anagnostou SH, Hu JK, Cho KH, Geisler R, Lieschke G, et al. Cohesin-dependent regulation of Runx genes. Development. 2007;134(14):2639-49.

[146] Tominaga Y, Tsuzuki T, Shiraishi A, Kawate H, Sekiguchi M. Alkylation-induced apoptosis of embryonic stem cells in which the gene for DNA-repair, methyltransferase, had been disrupted by gene targeting. Carcinogenesis. 1997;18(5):889-96.

[147] Nordstrand L, Svard J, Larsen E, Nilsen A, Ougland R, Furu K, et al. Mice lacking Alkbh1 display sex-ratio distortion and unilateral eye defects. PLoS Biol. 2010;5(11).

[148] Pan Z, Sikandar S, Witherspoon M, Dizon D, Nguyen T, Benirschke K, et al. Impaired placental trophoblast lineage differentiation in Alkbh1(-/-) mice. Dev Dyn. 2008;237(2):316-27.

[149] Haracska L, Prakash S, Prakash L. Replication past O(6)-methylguanine by yeast and human DNA polymerase eta. Mol Cell Biol. 2000;20(21):8001-7.

[150] Singh J, Su L, Snow ET. Replication across O6-methylguanine by human DNA polymerase beta in vitro. Insights into the futile cytotoxic repair and mutagenesis of O6-methylguanine. J Biol Chem. 1996;271(45):28391-8.

[151] Andreassen PR, Ho GP, D'Andrea AD. DNA damage responses and their many interactions with the replication fork. Carcinogenesis. 2006;27(5):883-92.

[152] Feyzi E, Sundheim O, Westbye MP, Aas PA, Vagbo CB, Otterlei M, et al. RNA base damage and repair. Curr Pharm Biotechnol. 2007;8(6):326-31.

[153] Loechler EL, Green CL, Essigmann JM. In vivo mutagenesis by O6-methylguanine built into a unique site in a viral genome. Proc Natl Acad Sci U S A. 1984;81(20):6271-5.

[154] McCulloch SD, Kunkel TA. The fidelity of DNA synthesis by eukaryotic replicative and translesion synthesis. Cell Res. 2008;18(1):148-61.

[155] Prakash S, Johnson RE, Prakash L. Eukaryotic translesion synthesis DNA polymerases: specificity of structure and. Annu Rev Biochem. 2005;74:317-53.

[156] Yang H, Lam SL. Effect of 1-methyladenine on thermodynamic stabilities of double-helical DNA structures. FEBS Lett. 2009;583(9):1548-53.

[157] Rodenhiser D, Mann M. Epigenetics and human disease: translating basic biology into clinical applications. Cmaj. 2006;174(3):341-8.

[158] Laird PW, Jaenisch R. The role of DNA methylation in cancer genetic and epigenetics. Annu Rev Genet. 1996;30:441-64.

[159] Wang Z, Cummins JM, Shen D, Cahill DP, Jallepalli PV, Wang TL, et al. Three classes of genes mutated in colorectal cancers with chromosomal instability. Cancer Res. 2004;64(9):2998-3001. Epub 2004/05/06.

[160] Wiseman H, Halliwell B. Damage to DNA by reactive oxygen and nitrogen species: role in inflammatory disease and progression to cancer. Biochem J. 1996;313 (Pt 1): 17-29.

[161] Bird AP, Wolffe AP. Methylation-induced repression--belts, braces, and chromatin. Cell. 1999;99(5):451-4.

[162] Hendrich B, Bird A. Identification and characterization of a family of mammalian methyl-CpG binding. Mol Cell Biol. 1998;18(11):6538-47.

[163] Jones PL, Veenstra GJ, Wade PA, Vermaak D, Kass SU, Landsberger N, et al. Methylated DNA and MeCP2 recruit histone deacetylase to repress transcription. Nat Genet. 1998;19(2):187-91.

[164] Nan X, Ng HH, Johnson CA, Laherty CD, Turner BM, Eisenman RN, et al. Transcriptional repression by the methyl-CpG-binding protein MeCP2 involves a. Nature. 1998;393(6683):386-9.

[165] Chen J, Li Y, Yu TS, McKay RM, Burns DK, Kernie SG, et al. A restricted cell population propagates glioblastoma growth after chemotherapy. Nature. 2012;488(7412): 522-6. Epub 2012/08/03.

[166] Villalva C, Cortes U, Wager M, Tourani JM, Rivet P, Marquant C, et al. O6-Methylguanine-Methyltransferase (MGMT) Promoter Methylation Status in Glioma Stem-Like Cells is Correlated to Temozolomide Sensitivity Under Differentiation-Promoting Conditions. Int J Mol Sci. 2012;13(6):6983-94. Epub 2012/07/28.

[167] Kreth S, Thon N, Eigenbrod S, Lutz J, Ledderose C, Egensperger R, et al. O-methylguanine-DNA methyltransferase (MGMT) mRNA expression predicts outcome in malignant glioma independent of MGMT promoter methylation. PLoS ONE. 2011;6(2):e17156. Epub 2011/03/03.

[168] Zhang W, Zhang J, Hoadley K, Kushwaha D, Ramakrishnan V, Li S, et al. miR-181d: a predictive glioblastoma biomarker that downregulates MGMT expression. Neuro Oncol. 2012;14(6):712-9.

[169] Danam RP, Howell SR, Brent TP, Harris LC. Epigenetic regulation of O6-methylguanine-DNA methyltransferase gene expression. Mol Cancer Ther. 2005;4(1):61-9.

[170] Sansom OJ, Maddison K, Clarke AR. Mechanisms of disease: methyl-binding domain proteins as potential therapeutic targets in cancer. Nat Clin Pract Oncol. 2007;4(5): 305-15.

[171] Cetica V, Genitori L, Giunti L, Sanzo M, Bernini G, Massimino M, et al. Pediatric brain tumors: mutations of two dioxygenases (hABH2 and hABH3) that directly repair alkylation damage. J Neurooncol. 2009;94(2):195-201. Epub 2009/03/18.

[172] Caldecott KW. Single-strand break repair and genetic disease. Nat Rev Genet. 2008;9(8):619-31.

[173] Chen S, Tang D, Xue K, Xu L, Ma G, Hsu Y, et al. DNA repair gene XRCC1 and XPD polymorphisms and risk of lung cancer in a Chinese population. Carcinogenesis. 2002;23(8):1321-5.

[174] Gangawar R, Ahirwar D, Mandhani A, Mittal RD. Impact of nucleotide excision repair ERCC2 and base excision repair APEX1 genes polymorphism and its association with recurrence after adjuvant BCG immunotherapy in bladder cancer patients of North India. Med Oncol. 2010;27(2):159-66. Epub 2009/02/27.

[175] Karran P, Offman J, Bignami M. Human mismatch repair, drug-induced DNA damage, and secondary cancer. Biochimie. 2003;85(11):1149-60.

[176] Khanna KK, Jackson SP. DNA double-strand breaks: signaling, repair and the cancer connection. Nat Genet. 2001;27(3):247-54.

[177] Li X, Heyer WD. Homologous recombination in DNA repair and DNA damage tolerance. Cell Res. 2008;18(1):99-113.

[178] Thompson D, Easton DF. Cancer Incidence in BRCA1 mutation carriers. J Natl Cancer Inst. 2002;94(18):1358-65.

[179] Wiseman H, Kaur H, Halliwell B. DNA damage and cancer: measurement and mechanism. Cancer Lett. 1995;93(1):113-20.

[180] Esteller M, Garcia-Foncillas J, Andion E, Goodman SN, Hidalgo OF, Vanaclocha V, et al. Inactivation of the DNA-repair gene MGMT and the clinical response of gliomas to. N Engl J Med. 2000;343(19):1350-4.

[181] Esteller M, Hamilton SR, Burger PC, Baylin SB, Herman JG. Inactivation of the DNA repair gene O6-methylguanine-DNA methyltransferase by. Cancer Res. 1999;59(4): 793-7.

[182] Kitajima Y, Miyazaki K, Matsukura S, Tanaka M, Sekiguchi M. Loss of expression of DNA repair enzymes MGMT, hMLH1, and hMSH2 during tumor progression in gastric cancer. Gastric Cancer. 2003;6(2):86-95.

[183] Sharma S, Salehi F, Scheithauer BW, Rotondo F, Syro LV, Kovacs K. Role of MGMT in tumor development, progression, diagnosis, treatment and. Anticancer Res. 2009;29(10):3759-68.

[184] Shen L, Kondo Y, Rosner GL, Xiao L, Hernandez NS, Vilaythong J, et al. MGMT promoter methylation and field defect in sporadic colorectal cancer. J Natl Cancer Inst. 2005;97(18):1330-8.

[185] Silber JR, Bobola MS, Ghatan S, Blank A, Kolstoe DD, Berger MS. O6-methylguanine-DNA methyltransferase activity in adult gliomas: relation to. Cancer Res. 1998;58(5): 1068-73.

[186] Zuo C, Ai L, Ratliff P, Suen JY, Hanna E, Brent TP, et al. O6-methylguanine-DNA methyltransferase gene: epigenetic silencing and prognostic value in head and neck squamous cell carcinoma. Cancer Epidemiol Biomarkers Prev. 2004;13(6):967-75.

[187] Hegi ME, Liu L, Herman JG, Stupp R, Wick W, Weller M, et al. Correlation of O6-methylguanine methyltransferase (MGMT) promoter methylation. J Clin Oncol. 2008;26(25):4189-99.

[188] Fumagalli C, Pruneri G, Possanzini P, Manzotti M, Barile M, Feroce I, et al. Methylation of O6-methylguanine-DNA methyltransferase (MGMT) promoter gene in triple-negative breast cancer patients. Breast Cancer Res Treat. 2012;134(1):131-7. Epub 2012/01/10.

[189] Sanchez-Perez I. DNA repair inhibitors in cancer treatment. Clin Transl Oncol. 2006;8(9):642-6.

[190] Lee SY, Luk SK, Chuang CP, Yip SP, To SST, Yung YM. TP53 regulates human AlkB homologue 2 expression in glioma resistance to. Br J Cancer. 2010;103(3):362-9.

[191] Choi SY, Jang JH, Kim KR. Analysis of differentially expressed genes in human rectal carcinoma using. Clin Exp Med. 2011;11(4):219-26.

[192] Tasaki M, Shimada K, Kimura H, Tsujikawa K, Konishi N. ALKBH3, a human AlkB homologue, contributes to cell survival in human non-small-cell lung cancer. British Journal of Cancer. 2011:1-7.

[193] Wu SS, Xu W, Liu S, Chen B, Wang XL, Wang Y, et al. Down-regulation of ALKBH2 increases cisplatin sensitivity in H1299 lung cancer cells. Acta Pharmacologica Sinica. 2011:1-6.

[194] Qiu YY, Mirkin BL, Dwivedi RS. Inhibition of DNA methyltransferase reverses cisplatin induced drug resistance in murine neuroblastoma cells. Cancer Detect Prev. 2005;29(5):456-63.

[195] Dolan ME, Mitchell RB, Mummert C, Moschel RC, Pegg AE. Effect of O6-benzylguanine analogues on sensitivity of human tumor cells to the. Cancer Res. 1991;51(13): 3367-72.

[196] Chae MY, Swenn K, Kanugula S, Dolan ME, Pegg AE, Moschel RC. 8-Substituted O6-benzylguanine, substituted 6(4)-(benzyloxy)pyrimidine, and. J Med Chem. 1995;38(2):359-65.

[197] Dolan ME, Pegg AE, Dumenco LL, Moschel RC, Gerson SL. Comparison of the inactivation of mammalian and bacterial O6-alkylguanine-DNA. Carcinogenesis. 1991;12(12):2305-9.

[198] Sato K, Kitajima Y, Nakagawachi T, Soejima H, Miyoshi A, Koga Y, et al. Cisplatin represses transcriptional activity from the minimal promoter of the. Oncol Rep. 2005;13(5):899-906.

[199] Lakomy R, Sana J, Hankeova S, Fadrus P, Kren L, Lzicarova E, et al. MiR-195, miR-196b, miR-181c, miR-21 expression levels and O-6-methylguanine-DNA methyltransferase methylation status are associated with clinical outcome in glioblastoma patients. Cancer Sci. 2011;102(12):2186-90.

[200] Zinn P, Sathyan P, Mahajan B, Bruyere J, Hegi ME, Majumder S, et al. A Novel Volume-Age-KPS (VAK) Glioblastoma Classification Identifies a Prognostic Cognate microRNA-Gene Signature. PLoS One. 2012;7(8):e41522.

[201] Chinnasamy N, Rafferty JA, Hickson I, Lashford LS, Longhurst SJ, Thatcher N, et al. Chemoprotective gene transfer II: multilineage in vivo protection of haemopoiesis. Gene Ther. 1998;5(6):842-7.

[202] Hickson I, Fairbairn LJ, Chinnasamy N, Lashford LS, Thatcher N, Margison GP, et al. Chemoprotective gene transfer I: transduction of human haemopoietic progenitors. Gene Ther. 1998;5(6):835-41.

[203] Koc ON, Reese JS, Davis BM, Liu L, Majczenko KJ, Gerson SL. DeltaMGMT-transduced bone marrow infusion increases tolerance to O6-benzylguanine. Hum Gene Ther. 1999;10(6):1021-30.

[204] Reese JS, Koc ON, Lee KM, Liu L, Allay JA, Phillips WP, Jr., et al. Retroviral transduction of a mutant methylguanine DNA methyltransferase gene into. Proc Natl Acad Sci U S A. 1996;93(24):14088-93.

[205] Karkhanina AA, Mecinovic J, Musheev MU, Krylova SM, Petrov AP, Hewitson KS, et al. Direct analysis of enzyme-catalyzed DNA demethylation. Anal Chem. 2009;81(14):5871-5.

[206] Woon EC, Demetriades M, Bagg EAL, Aik WS, Krylova SM, Ma JHY, et al. Dynamic combinatorial mass spectrometry leads to inhibitors of a. J Med Chem. 2012;55(5): 2173-84.

[207] Krylova SM, Koshkin V, Bagg E, Schofield CJ, Krylov SN. Mechanistic studies on the application of DNA aptamers as inhibitors of. J Med Chem. 2012;55(7):3546-52.

Chapter 6

Chromatin Remodeling in Nucleotide Excision Repair in Mammalian Cells

Wilner Martínez-López, Leticia Méndez-Acuña, Verónica Bervejillo, Jonatan Valencia-Payan and Dayana Moreno-Ortega

Additional information is available at the end of the chapter

http://dx.doi.org/10.5772/54709

1. Introduction

The chromatin basic structure named nucleosome contains 147 DNA base pairs wounded 1.65 times around an octamer of histone proteins which consist of two copies of H2A, H2B, H3, and H4, separated by linker regions of 20-110 nucleotides. Nucleosome assembly in the nucleus proceeds in two stages. At first, hetero-tetramer H3/H4 integrates into the DNA and at the second stage the heterodimer H2A/H2B is added. Nucleosomes are further condensed into 30 nm fibers through the incorporation of histone H1, located in the linker regions, achieving an additional 250-fold structural compaction in metaphase chromosomes. Nucleosome packaging restricts protein binding and obstructs DNA-templated reactions. Therefore, local modulation of DNA accessibility is necessary for the fundamental processes of transcription, replication and DNA repair to occur. In this sense, chromatin structure is not static but subject to changes at every level of its hierarchy. Nucleosomes are considered dynamic and instructive particles that are involved in practically all chromosomal processes, being subjected to highly ordered changes considered as epigenetic information, which modulates DNA accessibility [1, 2]. Nucleosomes exhibit three dynamic properties: a) covalent histone post-translational modifications, b) change of composition due to removal of histones and c) movement along DNA. The latter two are carried out by ATP-dependent chromatin remodeling complexes [3]. Histone post-translational modifications (PTMs) such as the addition of acetyl, methyl, phosphate, ubiquitin, and sumo groups change the properties of histones, modifying histone-DNA or histone-histone interactions [4]. Modifying complexes add or remove covalent modifications on particular residues of the N- and C-terminal domains of histone proteins, altering the structure of chromatin and creating "flags" which can be recognized by different regulatory proteins. Many chromatin-associated proteins contain protein domains that bind these moieties such as the bromodomain that recognizes acetylated residues and chromodomains, Tudor, Plant Homeo Domain (PHD) fingers, Malignant brain tumor (MBT) domains that bind to methylated lysines or arginines [5].

In the regulation of gene expression a "code of histones" has been determined, where different PTMs allow the recruitment of different factors specifying determined functions on chromatin [2]. Certain histone modifications can even induce or inhibit the appearance of other modifications in adjacent aminoacidic residues [6]. ATP-dependent chromatin remodeling factors use ATP hydrolysis to slide or unwrap DNA. These multi-subunit complexes can also catalyze eviction of histone octamers to promote histone variant replacement [7]. Eukaryotic cells also contain alternative versions of the canonical histones, differing in the aminoacidic sequences. One of these isoforms is histone H2AX, which differs from the canonical H2A histone by the presence of a short C-terminal tail. Nucleosomes containing canonical histones are formed during replication, and non-canonical histones replace canonical ones in the course of DNA metabolic processes not associated with replication, such as transcription and repair. Other protein complexes participating in the process of nucleosome assembly/disassembly such as histones chaperones like the chromatin assembly factor 1 (CAF-1), composed by three subunits: p150, p60 and p48, which has been suggested to play a pivotal role in chromatin assembly after DNA replication and repair [8]. During DNA replication, CAF-1 complex binds to newly synthesized histone H3 and H4 and deposits the histone tetramers onto replicating DNA to form the chromatin precursor in a PCNA-dependent manner. The replicated precursor then serves as the template for deposition of either old or new histone H2A and H2B.

In response to both DNA damage and replication stress, a signal transduction cascade known as the checkpoint response is activated. This phenomenon is also referred to as the DNA damage response. It is becoming clear that DNA damage sensors can recognize the chromatin-associated signals of DNA damage. This information is then transmitted via signal transducers, including diffusible protein kinases, to effector molecules such as the checkpoint kinases that mediate the physiological response of the cell to DNA damage, which ultimately promotes efficient repair and cell survival. The primary target of this pathway is the arrest or slowing of the cell cycle, providing time for DNA repair to take place. Depending on the type of DNA damage induced, different repair mechanisms can be activated, such as non-homologous end joining and homologous recombination in case of double strand breaks induction and excision repair mechanisms in case of nucleotide or base damage. As for DNA transcription, a regulatory role of the epigenetic code in DNA repair has been proposed [3, 4, 9, 10]. Chromatin remodeling processes not only influence access to DNA but also serves as a docking site for repair and signaling proteins [7, 10-12]. Chromatin plays a pivotal role in regulating DNA-associated processes and it is itself subject of regulation by the DNA-damage response. In this chapter, we summarize the current knowledge on the involvement of chromatin remodeling processes in nucleotide excision repair in mammalian cells.

2. Chromatin structure after UVC-induced DNA damage

Endogenous and exogenous DNA damaging agents modify DNA. One of the most common environmental stresses that produce lesions in DNA is UV light. UVC irradiation induces cyclobutane pyrimidine dimers (CPDs) and pyrimidine 6-4 pyrimidone photoproducts (6-4PP) which result in an abnormal DNA structure that signals the lesion [7], [13-15]. However, they can be distributed differently along the chromatin structure. CPDs are mainly found in the minor groove of DNA facing away from the histone surface and 6-4PPs are preferentially formed in linker DNA but can also be seen throughout the histone core region. This indicates that nucleosomes can actually confer partial protection against this type of DNA damage. Moreover, an *in vitro* study in specific sites with mono-nucleosomes showed that elimination of UVC-induced lesions is highly inhibited by nucleosomes [16, 17]. Chromatin plays a role not only in the spectrum of DNA damage formation but also in the repair of these lesions. In this respect, it has been shown that chromatin structure has an inhibitory effect on the repair of both CPDs and 6–4PPs [18]. For instance, excision activity in the nucleosome core center is nearly sevenfold lower than that in free DNA [15].

Access to these lesions in chromatin can be achieved mainly by the action of ATP-dependent chromatin remodeling factors and the addition of post-translational modifications on histones [19], which could facilitate their removal. However, like DNA repair enzymes, both chromatin remodeling proteins and histone modification factors require initial localization to damaged sites, but the mechanism by which UVC-damaged DNA in chromatin is recognized by these factors and how damaged from undamaged chromatin can be distinguished remain unclear. A recent study using reconstituted nucleosomes containing DNA with CPDs or 6–4PPs showed that the presence of these lesions does not affect the reconstitution of nucleosomes *in vitro*, but the dynamic equilibrium of DNA unwrapping-rewrapping around the nucleosome switches toward the unwrapped state. These *in vitro* experiments suggest that intrinsic nucleosome dynamics, specially increased unwrapping of the DNA around damaged nucleosomes, facilitate the access of factors involved in recognizing damage and/or those involved in chromatin remodeling. Therefore, once remodeling factors are recruited to the damaged nucleosomes, disruption of local chromatin structure could initiate the recruitment of the multiple repair proteins [14]. Nevertheless, it is important to take into account that *in vivo*, in the context of all chromatin factors, the recognition step of the photolesions may be more complex. Apart from the DNA distortion, other factors also actively contribute to reveal and mark lesion sites for recruitment of the repair machinery.

3. Nucleotide excision repair in chromatin

Nucleotide excision repair (NER) system is more efficient in naked DNA than in chromatin and it is inhibited by the presence of nucleosomes and heterochromatin, which limit the access of repair proteins to DNA [20]. Thus, for NER to recognize, excise and repair DNA damage efficiently, chromatin needs to be adapted [21]. Therefore, a chromatin rearrangement is a necessary step in the access of repair proteins to DNA damage sites and led to the "access, repair, restore" model of NER in chromatin. This model suggests that early chromatin remodeling steps and/or intrinsic dynamic changes in chromatin may allow the access of repair complexes to damaged sites, followed by restoration of the original nucleosomal organization after DNA repair [1, 22]. In NER, lesions that are located in linker regions are more accessible for binding by the recognizing proteins. A plausible scenario for DNA repair implies that the lesion is recognized and eliminated in the most accessible sites for repair proteins. Therefore, nucleosome modification and initiation of chromatin relaxation around the repair site start at considerable distances from the initiation point of DNA repair. As a result, other lesions, particularly those in the core of nucleosomes, become more accessible. Thus, proteins responsible for recognizing UVC-induced DNA lesions can recognize and bind them even if they are located in the core of the nucleosome [23, 24].

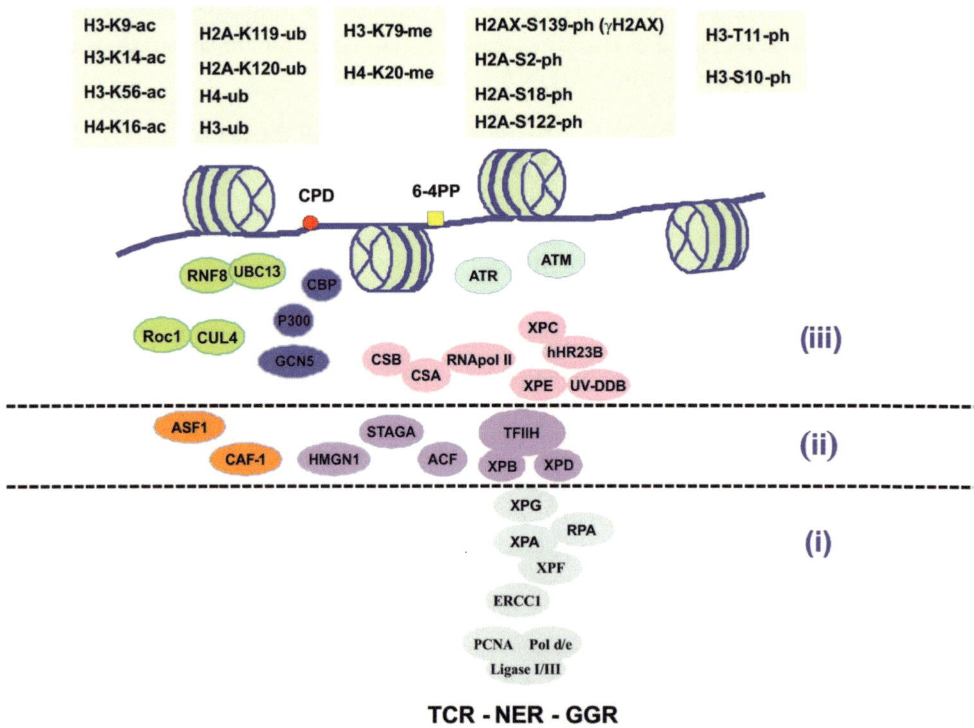

Figure 1. Nucleotide excision repair in the chromatin context. Nucleotide damage induced by UVC (CPDs and 6-4-PPs) is represented on a 11 nm chromatin fiber. Main proteins acting during the cellular response to UVC-induced damage are presented: (i) key proteins implicated in nucleotide excision repair (NER) (TCR and GGR) in mammalian cells (grey); (ii) chromatin assembly or remodeling factors recruited by chromatin modifications (violet) and histone chaperons involved in NER (orange); (iii) sensor proteins belonging to TCR (CSA, CSB, RNApolII) or GGR (XPC-HHR23B, XPE-UV-DDB) (pink); and histone modifying enzymes responsible for post-translational covalent modifications (PTMs): histone acetyl transferases (HATs) (blue), enzymes that conjugate ubiquitin moieties (green) and kinases (light-blue). Known PTMs appearing in response to UVC-induced damage are highlighted in green on top of the figure. See text for more details concerning the activities of every protein. Ac: acetylation, Ph: Phosphorylation, Ub: ubiquitylation, K: lysine, S: serine, T: threonine.

NER removes a wide range of bulky DNA adducts that distort the double helix of DNA, including those induced by UVC. NER system can be divided into two pathways: transcriptional coupled repair (TCR) pathway, that repairs lesions that occur in transcriptionally active genes and global genome repair (GGR) that acts into lesions in non transcribed DNA [1, 25, 26]. Both pathways involves the action of about 20-30 proteins (Figure 1) in a "cut-and-paste-like" mechanism [26, 27] divided in five steps: a) lesion detection; b) recruitment of TFIIH-XPB-XPD complex, which directs DNA unwinding around the damaged nucleotide; c) recruitment of ERCC1- XPF, XPG, XPA and RPA that induce 5′ and 3′ breaks around the lesion and remove the damaged nucleotide; d) DNA synthesis directed by DNA polymerase δ/ε, PCNA and other accessory factors and e) strand ligation (ligase I/III) [1, 26]. Both pathways use the same cellular machinery in all steps except from lesion recognition. At this initial step, in TCR CSA and CSB direct the basic repair machinery to RNA polymerase II stalled at the lesion [28]. On the other hand, in GGR damage site recognition is carried out by XPC-hHR23B and UV-DDB/XPE complexes [13, 25, 29-31]. The defect in one of the NER proteins is the consequence of three rare recessive syndromes: Xeroderma pigmentosum (XP), Cockayne syndrome (CS) and the photosensitive brittle hair disorder trichothiodystrophy (TTD) [26, 31, 32].

Apart from ATP-dependent chromatin remodeling factors and histone modifications, repair factors themselves could cause chromatin rearrangements. Particularly good candidates for this type of function in the NER system are the transcription-coupled repair factor CSB, which has homology to SWI/SNF chromatin remodeling proteins, and the TFIIH complex that contains the helicase subunits XPD and XPB [33]. However, a non-mutually exclusive suggestion is that global chromatin relaxation increases accessibility over the whole genome in response to damage in order to expose the individual damage sites for recognition [34]. After removal of the DNA lesion and completion of new DNA synthesis by DNA polymerase and DNA ligase, the original structure of chromatin is restored by the action of CAF-1 [22, 31]. The recruitment of mammalian CAF-1 is restricted to damaged sites and depends on NER, binding concomitantly with repair synthesis [8]. Chromatin restoration does not simply recycle histones, but also incorporate new histones and histones with distinct post-translational modifications into chromatin. For example, new histone H3.1, deposited during DNA replication, is incorporated into chromatin as a marker of sites of UVC-induced DNA damage repaired by NER [35].

4. Histone covalent modifications in NER

One of the most important chromatin remodeling processes that occur during NER is histone covalent modification, which constitutes a reversible process. The most frequent histone tail modification is the histone acetylation/deacetylation process, which is controlled by histone acetyltransferases (HAT) and histone deacetylases (HDAC), determining either gene activation or inactivation, respectively. Meanwhile, histone methylation is carried out by histone methyl-transferases (HMT) and histone demethylases (HDM) are used for the reverse reaction.

Finally, kinases like ATR are responsible for histone phosphorylation, and histone ubiquitination is driven by histone ubiquitin ligases.

4.1. Histone acetylation

The acetylation of the ε-amino group of lysine (K) side chains is a major histone modification involved in numerous cellular processes, such as transcription and DNA repair. Acetylation neutralizes the lysines positive charge and this action may consequently weaken the electrostatic interactions between histones and DNA. Thus, acetylated histones could enhance chromatin accessibility by reducing the attractive force between the nucleosome core and negatively charged DNA. For this reason, histone acetylation is often associated with a more "open" chromatin conformation. UVC irradiation induces global and local changes in chromatin structure in order to increase accessibility for repair proteins and hence a proper NER occurs [34]. Early studies demonstrated that acetylated nucleosomes enhance NER efficiency [36]. In this respect, UVC-induced acetylation of H3 K9 and H4 K16 has been observed [37, 38]. H3 K9 acetylation after UVC irradiation requires the recruitment of the transcription factor E2F1, which interacts with the HAT GCN5. In fact, inactivation of GCN5 in human cells decreases recruitment of NER factors to damaged sites, which demonstrates that GCN5 is important for a timely and efficient NER [38]. Besides, UV-DDB complex (DDB1–DDB2) recruits two HATs, such as CBP/p300 and STAGA (a SAGA-like complex containing GCN5L) [39, 40], whose activities induce chromatin remodeling to allow recruitment of the repair complexes at the UVC-induced damage sites. By the same token, it has also been observed that p33ING2, a member of the inhibitor of growth (ING) family proteins, enhances NER in a p53-dependent manner by inducing chromatin relaxation following UVC irradiation, increased acetylation of histone H4 and recruitment of NER factors to sites of damage [41]. Actually, it has also been observed that CBP/p300 is recruited to UVC damaged sites in a p53-dependent manner via its interaction with CSB, accompanied by an increase in H3 acetylation [34, 42]. Hence, increased histone acetylation at the NER site is likely to contribute to the p53-induced chromatin relaxation that is induced by DNA damage, suggesting that the function of UVC-induced histone acetylation is to promote opening up on the chromatin to facilitate repair. However, employing the *in situ* nick translation technique, we have observed that chromatin decondensation is also induced in p53 mutant Chinese hamster (CHO) cell lines, either proficient or deficient in TCR (simile Cockayne's Syndrome B or CSB cells), and that this chromatin decondensation process is related to histone acetylation (data not published yet). Actually, it seems that the extent and type of histone acetylation may vary depending on the structure of chromatin associated with repair sites and the type of NER pathway (GGR or TCR). On the other hand, we have demonstrated in Chinese hamster chromosomes that acetylated histone H4 regions are preferred sites for radiation- and endonucleases-induced chromosome lesions [43, 44]. Altogether, these results could indicate that certain chromatin modifications can take place independently of NER, acting as a signal for the recruitment of chromatin remodeling factors. Moreover, it has been proposed that H3 K56 deacetylation is an early event triggered by DNA damage upon UVC irradiation in mammalian cells [45]. According to this, DNA damage results in the prompt deacetylation of H3 K56, which contribute to the recruitment of different factors including chromatin remodelers to relax the chromatin structure for allowing easy access to the NER complex and cell cycle checkpoints. Upon successful completion of DNA repair, the histone chaperone anti-silencing function1A (ASF1A) is recruited in an ATM-dependent manner, facilitating the recruitment of HATs needed for the restoration of native H3 K56 acetylation status, but the molecular mechanism of ASF1A recruitment is not clear yet [45]. Finally, High mobility group protein B1 (HMGB1), a multifunctional protein that, influences chromatin structure and remodeling by binding to the internucleosomal linker regions in chromatin [46] and facilitating nucleosome sliding [47], has been shown to affect DNA damage-induced chromatin remodeling. It was observed that after UVC irradiation of the HMGB1 knockout MEFs cells, their ability to remove UVC-induced DNA damage and the increasing of histone acetylation was significantly affected [48]. This distortion may assist the NER system in recognizing the damage [49] and facilitating repair of the lesion. HMGB1 also affects chromatin remodeling after DNA damage, so its binding to the lesion could increase the accessibility of repair factors to the site of DNA damage.

4.2. Histone phosphorylation

The phosphorylation of serine (S), threonine (T), and tyrosine (Y) residues has been documented on all core and most variant histones. Phosphorylation alters the charge of the protein, affecting its ionic properties and influencing the overall structure and function of the local chromatin environment [50]. Although there is no evidence that PI3K enzymes could be activated by DNA lesions repaired by NER, when DNA replication fork is stalled, NER protein foci are formed, creating single strand breaks (SSBs) which can be covered by RPA/ATRIP and activate the kinase activity of ATR [51]. However, these NER intermediates (SSBs arising from excised lesions) can activate ATR, even outside S-phase [52]. Several histone phosphorylation changes after UVC irradiation have been observed, such as H2AX histone variant which is phosphorylated at S139 (named gamma-H2AX) [52]. H2AX phosphorylation upon UVC in non-S-phase cells depends on ATR and active processing of the lesion by the NER machinery [53], suggesting that NER-intermediates trigger this response. The notion that gamma-H2AX formation occurs in response to NER and that NER is proficient in H2AX-deficient cells, suggests that this modification mainly plays a role in checkpoint activation during the repair of UVC lesion. Besides, S2, S18 and S122 H2A residues play important roles in survival following UVC exposure [54]. Two aminoacidic residues of histone H3, S10 and T11, appear to be a target of differential phosphorylation during NER. H3 S10 and H3 T11 in mouse are dephosphorylated by UVC irradiation and rephosphorylated after DNA damage repair. Hypophosphorylation of H3 S10 and H3 T11 are associated with transcription repression, and this histone modification might be one of the mechanisms that cells employ to inhibit transcription at UVC-damaged sites [25].

4.3. Histone methylation

Histone methylation is carried out by a group of enzymes called histone methyltransferases HMT, which covalently modify the lysine and arginine (R) residues of histones by transferring one, two or three methyl groups to the ε-amino group of lysine residues or to the guanidino group of arginine residues [6]. Methylation, unlike acetylation and phosphorylation, does not alter the overall charge of histones. Histone methylation in combination with acetylation creates specific modification signatures which can influence transcription [55, 56]. Lysine methylation has a different impact on transcription, depending on the positions and degree of methylation (mono-, di-, tri-methylation). Methylation of H3 lysine (H3 K4 and 36) is associated with transcribed domains, whereas methylation of H3 K9, H3 K27 and H4 K20 appears to correlate with transcriptional repression. Human Chd1 binds to methylated H3 K4 through its tandem chromodomains, linking the recognition of histone modifications to non-covalent chromatin remodeling [57]. In contrast, methylated H3 K9 and H3 K27 are recognized by heterochromatin protein 1 (HP1) and polycomb repressive complexes (PRC). Different from histone acetylation, which has been known to be implicated in NER for a long time, histone methylation was found to be implicated in NER recently [58, 59]. The knockdown of the best known methyltransferase of histone H3 K79 (called Dot1 in yeast or DOT1L in mammals), results in complete loss of methylation on this site either in yeast [60], flies [61] or mice [62]. In mammaliam cells, several enzymes target histone H4 K20 methylation. Mouse cells lacking the Suv4-20h histone methyltransferase have only mono-methylated but essentially no di- and tri-methylated H4 K20. These mutant mouse cells are sensitive to DNA damaging agents, including UV and defective in repair of DSBs [63]. However, if methylation of histone H4 K20 also plays a role in NER is unknown. Moreover, there is not much knowledge about its role in DNA repair in mammalian cells. Finally, it has not been determined yet if global histone methylation levels change in response to DNA damage, although it is well known that they affect cell cycle checkpoints through interactions with checkpoint components.

4.4. Histone ubiquitination

All of the previously described histone modifications result in relatively small molecular changes in the aminoacid side chains. In contrast, ubiquitination results in a much larger covalent modification. Ubiquitin itself is a 76-amino acid polypeptide that is attached to histone lysines via the sequential action of three enzymes, E1-activating, E2-conjugating and E3-ligating enzymes [6]. Histones H2B, H3 and H4 are constitutively ubiquitinated, but at very low levels (0.3% of the total H3, 0.1% for H4) [64]. In an effort to purify and characterize histone ubiquitin ligases, it was found an ubiquitin ligase activity capable of ubiquitinating all histones *in vitro* [65]. The ligase was later characterized as CUL4–DDB–ROC1 complex, an enzyme that is known for ubiquitinating DDB2 and XPC at UVC damaged sites [66, 67]. A small fraction of histone H3 and H4 (0.3% and 0.1%, respectively) is found ubiquitinated *in vivo* and siRNA mediated knockdown of CUL4A, B and DDB1 decreases the H3 and H4 ubiquitination levels. In addition, the dynamics of CUL4–DDB–ROC1-mediated H3 and H4 ubiquitination is similar to that of XPC. Actually, further biochemical studies indicate that the H3 and H4 ubiquitination weakens the interaction between histones and DNA, and facilitates the recruitment of XPC repair factor to damaged DNA [65]. These studies point out the role of H3 and H4 ubiquitination in chromatin disassembly at the sites of UVC lesions. However Takedachi et al. [68] found that ubiquitination of H3 and H2B by the CUL4A complex was not sufficient to destabilize the nucleosome and proposed that ubiquitination around damaged sites functions as a signal that enhances the recruitment of XPA repair protein to lesions. Moreover, as well as H2B, H3 and H4, H2A displays some constitutive ubiquitination being the primary targets

K119 and K120. H2A ubiquitination by UBC13/RNF8 ubiquitin ligase complex also occurs at the sites of UVC-induced DNA damage [69]. Depletion of these enzymes causes UVC hypersensitivity, without affecting NER, suggesting that UBC13 and RNF8 are involved in the UVC-induced DNA damage response. It has also been reported the recruitment of uH2A to sites of DNA damage as a post-excision repair event, in which transiently disrupted chromatin is restored through repair synthesis-coupled chromatin assembly [31], showing that the formation of uH2A foci do not involve pre-incision events mediated by Cul4A-DDB ubiquitin ligase, but require successful NER through either GGR or TCR subpathway. In this respect, it was recently shown that monoubiquitination of H2A K119 and K120 by DDB1-CUL4B^{DDB2} is critical for destabilization of the photolesion-containing nucleosomes, leading to eviction of H2A from the nucleosome, and that the partial eviction of H3 from the nucleosomes also depends on ubiquitinated H2A K119/K120. Furthermore, nucleosomal structure has consequences for the binding of E3 ligase complex; polyubiquitinated DDB2 is only released from the destabilized nucleosome, presumably releasing space around the lesion to load the NER pre-incision complex and proceed with repair. These results reveal how post-translational modification of H2A at the site of a photolesion initiates the repair process, which affects the stability of the genome [70].

5. ATP-dependent chromatin remodeling during NER

Chromatin remodeling complexes (CRCs) in contrast to PTMs utilize the energy of ATP to disrupt nucleosome DNA contacts, move nucleosomes along DNA and remove or exchange nucleosomes [71]. Thus, they make DNA/chromatin available to proteins that need to access DNA or histones during cellular processes [72]. A large array of different chromatin-remodeling complexes has been identified, which play important roles in controlling gene expression by regulating recruitment and access of transcription factors [73]. ATP-dependent chromatin remodelers belong to the SWI2/SNF2 (switching/sucrose non fermenting) superfamily and can be divided into several subfamilies on the basis of their ATPase domain structure and protein motifs outside the ATPase domain [74]. Among the different complexes identified in different species, four structurally related families have been described: SWI/SNF (switching defective/sucrose non fermenting), INO80 (inositol requiring 80), CHD (chromodomain, helicase, DNA binding) and ISWI (imitation SWI). Each family is defined by its characteristic catalytic ATPase core enzyme from the SWI2/SNF2 [5]. The essential role of these enzymes is reflected in the fact that many of them are required for diverse but specific aspects of embryonic development including pluripotency, cardiac development, dendritic morphogenesis and self-renewal of neural stem cells. However, in adults, deletion or mutation of these proteins often leads to apoptosis or tumorigenesis as a consequence of dysregulated cell cycle control. In recent years, it has become clear that ATP-dependent chromatin remodeling factors not only are involved in transcription regulation, but also play an important role in a number of DNA repair pathways including double strand break repair, base excision repair as well as nucleotide excision repair (NER) [71]. UVC damage itself enhances unwrapping of nucleosomes, which normally exist in a dynamic equilibrium between wrapping and unwrapping [75]. This enhanced "DNA breathing" may assist the repair of lesions in chromatin by increasing the time window for repair factor access and their binding to lesions might further unwrap the DNA [14]. ATP-dependent chromatin remodeling may play a role in opening the chromatin structure for access during DNA damage repair, facilitating the early step of NER in the recognition of the damage [76]. In this respect, three SWI2/SNF2 subfamilies have been implicated in the cell response to UVC radiation as it is shown in Table 1 [71, 77]. Several factors have been implicated on stimulating the repair of UVC-induced DNA damage by increasing chromatin accessibility. Numerous studies showed that there is an association between histone hyperacetylation and chromatin relaxation in response to UVC-irradiation that enhances NER [76]. GCN5-mediated acetylation of histone H3 contribute to the recruitment of the SWI/SNF chromatin remodeling complex via the bromodomains of BRG1 or hBRM [38]. CSB/ERCC6, one of the major TCR proteins, contains a SWI2/SNF2 ATPase domain, which is essential for recruitment of the protein to chromatin [78]. CSB is able to remodel chromatin *in vitro* in an ATP-dependent manner and is required for the recruitment of NER factors to sites of TCR [42, 79], suggesting that repair enzymes and remodeling complexes may work in concert to allow access of DNA lesions to the repair machinery.

FAMILY	COMPLEX	ATPase	ROLE IN NER
SWI/SNF	BAF	SMARCA4/BRG1, SMARCA2/BRM	Stimulates the removal of 6–4PPs and CPDs in a UVC-dependent histone H3 hyperacetylation manner [71]
	PBAF	SMARCA4/BRG1, SMARCA2/BRM	
INO80	INO80	INO80	Promotes the removal of UVC lesions (CPDs,6–4PPs) by NER in not transcribed regions [71]
	TRRAP/Tip601	EP400/p400	
ISWI	ACF	SMARCA5/hSNF2H	Not fully understood [71]
	CHRAC	SMARCA5/hSNF2H	
	WICH	SMARCA5/hSNF2H	
	NURF	SMARCA1/hSNF2L	
OTHER	ERCC6/CSB		Remodels chromatin *in vitro* in an ATP-dependent manner. Required for the recruitment of NER factors to sites of TCR [73]

Table 1. Mammalian ATP-dependent chromatin remodeling complexes identified as taking part in nucleotide excision repair.

5.1. SWI/SNF

The SWI/SNF chromatin-remodeling complex plays essential roles in a variety of cellular processes including differentiation, proliferation and DNA repair. Loss of SWI/SNF subunits has been reported in a number of malignant cell lines and tumors, and a large number of experimental observations suggest that this complex functions as a tumor suppressor [80]. Interestingly, inactivation of the SWI/SNF-like BRG1/BRM-associated factors (BAF) complexes renders human cells sensitive to DNA damaging agents, such as UVC and ionizing radiation [81]. The mammalian SWI/SNF complexes contain either of two ATPase subunits, BRM (brahma) or BRG1 (Brahma Related Gene). Both of them form a discrete complex by interacting with other BAFs and may have distinct roles in cellular processes [65, 81].

Several studies have indicated that the SWI/SNF complex plays an essential role in the removal of UVC-damage by NER [82]. In mammals, the SWI/SNF ATPase subunit BRG1/SMARCA4 stimulates efficient repair of CPDs but not of 6-4PPs. For Example, BRG1 interacts with XPC and it is recruited to an UVC lesion in a DDB2 [83] and XPC [76] dependent manner. BRG1, in turn, modulates UVC-induced chromatin remodeling and XPC stability and subsequently promotes damage excision and repair synthesis by facilitating the recruitment of XPG and PCNA to the damage site [76], suggesting the essential role of Brg1 in prompt elimination of UVC-induced DNA damage by NER in mammalian cells. Finally, BRG1 may also transcriptionally regulate the UVC-induced G1/S checkpoint, as loss of BRG1 leads to increased UVC-induced apoptosis [81]. Besides BRG1, the mammalian SWI/SNF subunit SNF5/SMARCB1 also interacts with XPC. Inactivation of SNF5 causes UVC hypersensitivity and inefficient CPD removal [82]. Intriguingly, BRG1/BRM, but none of the other subunits, is also important to the UVC response in germ cells, suggesting that the involvement of individual SWI/SNF subunits may differ between cell types. Interestingly, UVC hypersensitivity resulting from BRG1 inactivation depends on the presence of the checkpoint protein TP53, extending the complexity of the involvement of BRG1 in UVC-induced DNA damage response [83]. Several lines of evidence suggest that recruitment of factors like SWI/SNF and their functional participation help to recruit downstream factors for processing DNA damage.

5.2. INO80

The INO80 family of CRCs function in a diverse array of cellular processes, including DNA repair, cell cycle checkpoint and telomeric stability [84, 85]. The INO80 complex also contains three actin-related proteins (ARPs). ARP5 and ARP8 are specific to the INO80 complex. Deletion of either INO80-specific ARP compromises the ATPase activity of the remaining complex and gives rise to DNA-damage-sensitive phenotypes indistinguishable to the INO80 null mutant [86]. Purification of human INO80 revealed a complex with virtually identical core components and a role in transcription [87, 88], indicating that the INO80 complex is highly conserved within eukaryotes [89]. The role for various remodeling activities is likely to promote the timely repair of lesions, rather than being an essential component for lesion removal. For example, some observations suggest that loss of remodeling activity leads to attenuation of photolesion repair, but not a complete impairment. Thus, it supports the idea that INO80 carry out an important chromatin remodeling activity for an efficient NER [74].

The link between INO80 and NER function may reflect the underlying mechanism for the UVC hypersensitivity of INO80 mutant cells and the broadening connections between chromatin remodeling and DNA repair in general [89]. The mammalian INO80 complex functions during earlier NER steps facilitating the recruitment of early NER factors such as XPC and XPA and, in contrast to yeast, it localizes to DNA damage independently of XPC [89]. Furthermore, INO80 facilitates efficient 6-4PPs and CPDs removal and together with the Arp5/ ACTR5 subunit, interacts with the NER initiation factor DDB1, but not with XPC. These discrepancies may reflect interspecies differences, but may also point out multiple functions of INO80 chromatin remodeling during NER that are experimentally difficult to dissect. INO80 may function to facilitate damage detection as well as to restore chromatin after damage has been repaired [5]. A recent study shows that the INO80 complex plays an important role in facilitating NER by providing access to lesion processing factors, suggesting a functional connection between INO80-dependent chromatin remodeling and NER [89].

5.3. ISWI

ISWI complexes are a second major category of ATP-dependent chromatin remodeling complexes. In mammals, two ISWI-homologs, named SNF2H and SNF2L, have been described. While most of the complexes contain SNFH; up to now, SNF2L has only been found in the human NURF complex [90, 91]. Subunits related to ACF1 are similar to these ISWI-containing remodeling complexes, which contain PHD and bromodomains [92]. Snf2h is a gene essential for the early development of mammalian embryos, suggesting that ISWI complexes [93] may be required for cell proliferation [94]. Besides, ISWI cooperates with histone chaperones in the assembly and remodeling of chromatin [95]. These complexes accumulate at sites of heterochromatin concomitant with their replication, suggesting a role for ISWI chromatin remodeling functions in replication of DNA in highly condensed chromatin [96]. ISWI complexes also may have a role in facilitating repair and recombination of DNA in chromatin. Several experiments have suggested that ISWI-mediated chromatin remodeling also functions to regulate NER, although its precise role remains unknown [5]. Moreover, SNF2H interacts with CSB [97], and the ACF1 subunit is recruited to UVC-induced DNA damage [98]. Knockdown of the mammalian ISWI ATPase SNF2H/SMARCA5 or its auxiliary factor ACF1/BAZ1A also leads to mild UVC sensitivity [99]. However, further experimental evidence is required to understand how ISWI chromatin remodeling functions in the UVC-DNA damage response.

6. Discussion and perspectives

When DNA is damaged, the chromatin, far from acting as an inhibitory barrier to lesion removal, can actively signal its presence, promoting the overall physiological response of the cell to damage, which stimulates the removal of the DNA damage itself. By the same token, the most challenging step in NER is the recognition of DNA lesions in their chromatin context. Nucleosomes on damaged DNA inhibit efficient NER and a functional connection between chromatin remodeling and the initiation steps of NER has been described [18].

In this respect, the relevance of the histone acetylation balance and some ATP-dependent chromatin remodeling complexes to facilitate the early damage-recognition step of NER has been demonstrated, since changes in chromatin conformation could interfere with the correct interactions between repair proteins and DNA lesions which are immersed in a dynamic chromatin structure [38, 76, 100]. Besides, neuronal survival has been related to the balance between HAT and HDAC activities [101]. For example, it has been shown that in the presence of histone deacetylase inhibitors, normal neuron cells increase the frequency of apoptosis. Moreover, in transgenic mice, carrying neurodegeneration diseases characterized by histone hypoacetylation, their neurodegeneration phenotypes can be diminished in the presence of HDAC inhibitors [102, 103]. By the same token, alterations in the acetylation/deacetylation balance by changes in HATs or HDACs activities have been associated with the development of different cancers [104].

Another interesting issue in favor of the relevance of chromatin remodeling is the fact that transcription coupled repair (TCR) seems not to be responsible for the higher UVC sensitivity evidenced through the increased frequency of chromosomal aberrations observed in Cockayne's Syndrome (CS) simile cells exposed to UVC [105]. In this respect, we have found that chromosome breakpoints were distributed more random in CS simile cells than in normal ones instead of being concentrated on the transcribed chromosome regions as expected [106]. Since DNA accessibility for DNA repair proteins is limited in nucleosomes [16, 75], different chromatin organization after UVC exposure in CS simile cells could influence the distribution of CPDs in eu- and heterochromatic regions as well as their removal by TCR, leading to increased frequencies of chromosomal aberrations in these cells.

Although many of the chromatin remodeling factors observed in yeast have also been found in mammals, different functions have been attributed to some of them (i.e. H3K56 acetylation and INO80 mentioned previously), indicating that in spite of being quite well evolutionary conserved, they could have another function in mammals. Moreover, due to the multifunctional role of chromatin remodeling complexes become still very difficult to arise questions such as by which mechanism the damage is sensed or how the cell is able to choose a particular repair pathway, by which mechanisms chromatin remodelers are directed to a specific repair pathway or by which mechanisms chromatin reassembly takes place. Therefore, it is clear that we just begin to understand the DNA repair in the context of chromatin and, therefore, further work it is needed to elucidate either the individual functions or the coordinated activities of chromatin remodeling in all DNA repair pathways.

Abbreviations and acronyms

6-4PP	Pyrimidine 6-4 pyrimidone photoproducts
ARPs	Actin-related proteins
ASF1A	Histone chaperone anti-silencing function1A
ATM	Ataxia telangiectasia mutated

ATR	Ataxia-telangiectasia Rad3-related
ATRIP	ATR interacting protein
BAF	BRG1/BRM-associated factors
BRG1	Brahma Related Gene
BRM	Brahma
CAF-1	Chromatin assembly factor 1
CBP	Creb-binding protein
CPDs	Cyclobutane pyrimidine dimers
CRCs	Chromatin remodeling complexes
CS	Cockayne syndrome
CSB	Cockayne syndrome group B protein
CUL4–DDB–ROC1	Culin 4- DNA damage-binding protein- RING finger protein
CHD	Chromodomain
CHO	Chinese hamster cell lines
E2F1	Transcription factor
ERCC1	Excision repair cross complementing 1
ERCC6	Excision repair cross complementing 6
GCN5	General control non-derepressible 5
GGR	Global genome repair
HAT	Histone acetyltransferases
HDAC	Histone deacetylases
HDM	Histone demethylases
hHR23B	Human homologue of the yeast protein RAD23
HMGB1	High mobility group protein B1
HMT	Histone methyl-transferases
HP1	Heterochromatin protein 1
ING	Inhibitor of growth
INO80	Inositol requiring 80
ISWI	Imitation SWI
K	Lysine
MBT	Malignant brain tumor
NER	Nucleotide excision repair
NURF	Nucleosome remodeling factor
p300	Histone acetyltransferase named p300
p53	Tumor supressor p53 gene
PCNA	Proliferating cell nuclear antigen
PHD	Plant Homeo Domain
PI3K	Phosphoinositide 3-kinase
PTMs	Histone post-translational modifications
R	Arginine
RNF8	Ring finger protein 8
RPA	Replication protein A
S	Serine
SMARCA4	Transcription activator BRG1

http://dx.doi.org/10.5772/54709

SNF2H and SNF2L	ISWI-homologs
SNF5/SMARCB1	Mammalian SWI/SNF subunit
SSBs	Single strand breaks
STAGA	SAGA-like complex containing GCN5L
SWI/SNF	Switching defective/sucrose non fermenting
SWI2/SNF2	Switching/sucrose non fermenting
T	Threonine
TCR	Transcriptional coupled repair
TFIIH	Transcription factor II H
TP53	Tumor suppressor protein 53
TTD	Trichothiodystrophy
UBC13	Ubiquitin-conjugating enzyme
UVC	Ultraviolet light C
UV-DDB	UV-damaged DNA binding protein consisting of two subunits (DDB1 and DDB2)
XP	Xeroderma pigmentosum
XPA	Xeroderma Pigmentosum group A
XPB	Xeroderma Pigmentosum group B
XPC	Xeroderma Pigmentosum group C
XPD	Xeroderma Pigmentosum group D
XPE	Xeroderma Pigmentosum group E
XPF	Xeroderma Pigmentosum group F
XPG	Xeroderma Pigmentosum group G
Y	Tyrosine

Acknowledgements

This work was partially supported by the Program of Development of the Basic Sciences (PEDECIBA) from Uruguay. W M-L was supported by a Marie Curie Fellowship from the Frame Program Seven (EC-FP7) of the European Community. L M-A was supported by a Post-graduate fellowship of the National Agency of Research and Innovation (ANII) from Uruguay.

Author details

Wilner Martínez-López*, Leticia Méndez-Acuña, Verónica Bervejillo, Jonatan Valencia-Payan and Dayana Moreno-Ortega

*Address all correspondence to: wlopez@iibce.edu.uy

Epigenetics and Genomics Instability Laboratory, Instituto de Investigaciones Biológicas Clemente Estable (IIBCE), Montevideo, Uruguay

References

[1] Nag R, Smerdon MJ. Altering the chromatin landscape for nucleotide excision repair. *Mutation research* 2009; 682(1):13-20.

[2] Strahl BD, Allis CD. The language of covalent histone modifications. *Nature* 2000; 403(6765):41-45.

[3] Hassa PO, Hottiger MO. An epigenetic code for DNA damage repair pathways? *Biochemistry and cell biology* 2005; 83(3):270-285.

[4] Loizou JI, Murr R, Finkbeiner MG, Sawan C, Wang ZQ, Herceg Z. Epigenetic information in chromatin: the code of entry for DNA repair. *Cell Cycle* 2006; 5(7):696-701.

[5] Lans H, Marteijn JA, Vermeulen W. ATP-dependent chromatin remodeling in the DNA-damage response. *Epigenetics & chromatin* 2012; 5:4.

[6] Bannister AJ, Kouzarides T. Regulation of chromatin by histone modifications. *Cell research* 2011; 21(3):381-395.

[7] Ataian Y, Krebs JE. Five repair pathways in one context: chromatin modification during DNA repair. *Biochemistry and cell biology* 2006; 84(4):490-494.

[8] Green CM, Almouzni G. Local action of the chromatin assembly factor CAF-1 at sites of nucleotide excision repair in vivo. *The EMBO journal* 2003; 22(19):5163-5174.

[9] Karagiannis TC, El-Osta A. Chromatin modifications and DNA double-strand breaks: the current state of play. *Leukemia* 2007; 21(2):195-200.

[10] Escargueil AE, Soares DG, Salvador M, Larsen AK, Henriques JA. What histone code for DNA repair? *Mutation research* 2008; 658(3):259-270.

[11] Méndez-Acuña L, Di Tomaso M, Palitti F, Martínez-López W. Histone post-translational modifications in DNA damage response. *Cytogenetic and genome research* 2010; 128(1-3):28-36.

[12] Tjeertes JV, Miller KM, Jackson SP. Screen for DNA-damage-responsive histone modifications identifies H3K9Ac and H3K56Ac in human cells. *The EMBO journal* 2009; 28(13):1878-1889.

[13] Farrell AW, Halliday GM, Lyons JG. Chromatin Structure Following UV-Induced DNA Damage-Repair or Death? *Int J Mol Sci* 2011; 12(11):8063-8085.

[14] Duan MR, Smerdon MJ. UV damage in DNA promotes nucleosome unwrapping. *J Biol Chem* 2010; 285(34):26295-26303.

[15] Korolev V. Chromatin and DNA damage repair. *Russian Journal of Genetics* 2011; 47(4): 394-403.

[16] Thoma F. Light and dark in chromatin repair: repair of UV-induced DNA lesions by photolyase and nucleotide excision repair. *EMBO J* 1999; 18(23):6585-6598.

[17] Hara R, Mo J, Sancar A. DNA damage in the nucleosome core is refractory to repair by human excision nuclease. *Mol Cell Biol* 2000; 20(24):9173-9181.

[18] Ura K, Araki M, Saeki H, Masutani C, Ito T, Iwai S, Mizukoshi T, Kaneda Y, Hanaoka F. ATP-dependent chromatin remodeling facilitates nucleotide excision repair of UV-induced DNA lesions in synthetic dinucleosomes. *EMBO J* 2001; 20(8):2004-2014.

[19] Allis CD. Epigenetics. Cold Spring Harbor, N. Y.: CSHL Press; 2007.

[20] Gong F, Kwon Y, Smerdon MJ. Nucleotide excision repair in chromatin and the right of entry. *DNA Repair (Amst)* 2005; 4(8):884-896.

[21] Reed SH. Nucleotide excision repair in chromatin: damage removal at the drop of a HAT. *DNA Repair (Amst)* 2011; 10(7):734-742.

[22] Green CM, Almouzni G. When repair meets chromatin. First in series on chromatin dynamics. *EMBO reports* 2002; 3(1):28-33.

[23] Ura K, Hayes JJ. Nucleotide excision repair and chromatin remodeling. *Eur J Biochem* 2002; 269(9):2288-2293.

[24] Gong F, Fahy D, Smerdon MJ. Rad4-Rad23 interaction with SWI/SNF links ATP-dependent chromatin remodeling with nucleotide excision repair. *Nat Struct Mol Biol* 2006; 13(10):902-907.

[25] Dinant C, Houtsmuller AB, Vermeulen W. Chromatin structure and DNA damage repair. *Epigenetics & chromatin* 2008; 1(1):9.

[26] de Boer J, Hoeijmakers JH. Nucleotide excision repair and human syndromes. *Carcinogenesis* 2000; 21(3):453-460.

[27] Nouspikel T. DNA repair in mammalian cells : Nucleotide excision repair: variations on versatility. *Cellular and molecular life sciences : CMLS* 2009; 66(6):994-1009.

[28] Mitchell JR, Hoeijmakers JH, Niedernhofer LJ. Divide and conquer: nucleotide excision repair battles cancer and ageing. *Curr Opin Cell Biol* 2003; 15(2):232-240.

[29] Volker M, Moné MJ, Karmakar P, van Hoffen A, Schul W, Vermeulen W, Hoeijmakers JHJ, van Driel R, van Zeeland AA, Mullenders LHF. Sequential assembly of the nucleotide excision repair factors in vivo. *Molecular cell* 2001; 8(1):213-224.

[30] Giglia-Mari G, Zotter A, Vermeulen W. DNA damage response. *Cold Spring Harb Perspect Biol* 2011; 3(1):a000745.

[31] Zhu Q, Wani G, Arab HH, El-Mahdy MA, Ray A, Wani AA. Chromatin restoration following nucleotide excision repair involves the incorporation of ubiquitinated H2A at damaged genomic sites. *DNA repair* 2009; 8(2):262-273.

[32] Cleaver JE, Lam ET, Revet I. Disorders of nucleotide excision repair: the genetic and molecular basis of heterogeneity. *Nature Reviews Genetics* 2009; 10(11):756-768.

[33] Moné MJ, Bernas T, Dinant C, Goedvree FA, Manders EMM, Volker M, Houtsmuller AB, Hoeijmakers JHJ, Vermeulen W, Van Driel R. In vivo dynamics of chromatin-

associated complex formation in mammalian nucleotide excision repair. *Proceedings of the National Academy of Sciences of the United States of America* 2004; 101(45):15933.

[34] Rubbi CP, Milner J. p53 is a chromatin accessibility factor for nucleotide excision repair of DNA damage. *EMBO J* 2003; 22(4):975-986.

[35] Polo SE, Roche D, Almouzni G. New histone incorporation marks sites of UV repair in human cells. *Cell* 2006; 127(3):481-493.

[36] Ramanathan B, Smerdon MJ. Enhanced DNA repair synthesis in hyperacetylated nucleosomes. *The Journal of biological chemistry* 1989; 264(19):11026-11034.

[37] Yu Y, Teng Y, Liu H, Reed SH, Waters R. UV irradiation stimulates histone acetylation and chromatin remodeling at a repressed yeast locus. *Proc Natl Acad Sci U S A* 2005; 102(24):8650-8655.

[38] Guo R, Chen J, Mitchell DL, Johnson DG. GCN5 and E2F1 stimulate nucleotide excision repair by promoting H3K9 acetylation at sites of damage. *Nucleic Acids Res* 2011; 39(4): 1390-1397.

[39] Datta A, Bagchi S, Nag A, Shiyanov P, Adami GR, Yoon T, Raychaudhuri P. The p48 subunit of the damaged-DNA binding protein DDB associates with the CBP/p300 family of histone acetyltransferase. *Mutation Research/DNA Repair* 2001; 486(2):89-97.

[40] Martinez E, Palhan VB, Tjernberg A, Lymar ES, Gamper AM, Kundu TK, Chait BT, Roeder RG. Human STAGA complex is a chromatin-acetylating transcription coactivator that interacts with pre-mRNA splicing and DNA damage-binding factors in vivo. *Molecular and cellular biology* 2001; 21(20):6782-6795.

[41] Wang J, Chin MY, Li G. The novel tumor suppressor p33ING2 enhances nucleotide excision repair via inducement of histone H4 acetylation and chromatin relaxation. *Cancer research* 2006; 66(4):1906-1911.

[42] Fousteri M, Vermeulen W, van Zeeland AA, Mullenders LH. Cockayne syndrome A and B proteins differentially regulate recruitment of chromatin remodeling and repair factors to stalled RNA polymerase II in vivo. *Mol Cell* 2006; 23(4):471-482.

[43] Martínez-López W, Folle G, Obe G, Jeppesen P. Chromosome regions enriched in hyperacetylated histone H4 are preferred sites for endonuclease-and radiation-induced breakpoints. *Chromosome Research* 2001; 9(1):69-75.

[44] Martínez-López W, Di Tomaso M. Chromatin remodelling and chromosome damage distribution. *Human & experimental toxicology* 2006; 25(9):539-545.

[45] Battu A, Ray A, Wani AA. ASF1A and ATM regulate H3K56-mediated cell-cycle checkpoint recovery in response to UV irradiation. *Nucleic Acids Research* 2011; 39(18): 7931-7945.

[46] Nightingale K, Dimitrov S, Reeves R, Wolffe AP. Evidence for a shared structural role for HMG1 and linker histones B4 and H1 in organizing chromatin. *The EMBO journal* 1996; 15(3):548-561.

[47] Bonaldi T, Längst G, Strohner R, Becker PB, Bianchi ME. The DNA chaperone HMGB1 facilitates ACF/CHRAC-dependent nucleosome sliding. *The EMBO journal* 2002; 21(24): 6865-6873.

[48] Lange SS, Mitchell DL, Vasquez KM. High mobility group protein B1 enhances DNA repair and chromatin modification after DNA damage. *Proceedings of the National Academy of Sciences of the United States of America* 2008; 105(30):10320-10325.

[49] Reddy MC, Christensen J, Vasquez KM. Interplay between human high mobility group protein 1 and replication protein A on psoralen-cross-linked DNA. *Biochemistry* 2005; 44(11):4188-4195.

[50] Dawson MA, Kouzarides T. Cancer epigenetics: from mechanism to therapy. *Cell* 2012; 150(1):12-27.

[51] Jeggo P, Lobrich M. Radiation-induced DNA damage responses. *Radiation protection dosimetry* 2006; 122(1-4):124-127.

[52] Hanasoge S, Ljungman M. H2AX phosphorylation after UV irradiation is triggered by DNA repair intermediates and is mediated by the ATR kinase. *Carcinogenesis* 2007; 28(11):2298-2304.

[53] Marti TM, Hefner E, Feeney L, Natale V, Cleaver JE. H2AX phosphorylation within the G1 phase after UV irradiation depends on nucleotide excision repair and not DNA double-strand breaks. *Proc Natl Acad Sci U S A* 2006; 103(26):9891-9896.

[54] Moore JD, Yazgan O, Ataian Y, Krebs JE. Diverse roles for histone H2A modifications in DNA damage response pathways in yeast. *Genetics* 2007; 176(1):15-25.

[55] Kouzarides T. Chromatin modifications and their function. *Cell* 2007; 128(4):693-705.

[56] Ehrenhofer-Murray AE. Chromatin dynamics at DNA replication, transcription and repair. *Eur J Biochem* 2004; 271(12):2335-2349.

[57] Sims III RJ, Chen CF, Santos-Rosa H, Kouzarides T, Patel SS, Reinberg D. Human but not yeast CHD1 binds directly and selectively to histone H3 methylated at lysine 4 via its tandem chromodomains. *Journal of Biological Chemistry* 2005; 280(51):41789-41792.

[58] Nguyen AT, Zhang Y. The diverse functions of Dot1 and H3K79 methylation. *Genes & development* 2011; 25(13):1345-1358.

[59] Li S. Implication of Posttranslational Histone Modifications in Nucleotide Excision Repair. *International Journal of Molecular Sciences* 2012; 13(10):12461-12486.

[60] van Leeuwen F, Gafken PR, Gottschling DE. Dot1p modulates silencing in yeast by methylation of the nucleosome core. *Cell* 2002; 109(6):745-756.

[61] Shanower GA, Muller M, Blanton JL, Honti V, Gyurkovics H, Schedl P. Characterization of the grappa gene, the Drosophila histone H3 lysine 79 methyltransferase. *Genetics* 2005; 169(1):173-184.

[62] Jones B, Su H, Bhat A, Lei H, Bajko J, Hevi S, Baltus GA, Kadam S, Zhai H, Valdez R *et al*. The histone H3K79 methyltransferase Dot1L is essential for mammalian development and heterochromatin structure. *PLoS genetics* 2008; 4(9):e1000190.

[63] Schotta G, Sengupta R, Kubicek S, Malin S, Kauer M, Callen E, Celeste A, Pagani M, Opravil S, De La Rosa-Velazquez IA *et al*. A chromatin-wide transition to H4K20 monomethylation impairs genome integrity and programmed DNA rearrangements in the mouse. *Genes & development* 2008; 22(15):2048-2061.

[64] Nouspikel T. Multiple roles of ubiquitination in the control of nucleotide excision repair. *Mechanisms of ageing and development* 2011; 132(8-9):355-365.

[65] Wang H, Zhai L, Xu J, Joo HY, Jackson S, Erdjument-Bromage H, Tempst P, Xiong Y, Zhang Y. Histone H3 and H4 ubiquitylation by the CUL4-DDB-ROC1 ubiquitin ligase facilitates cellular response to DNA damage. *Mol Cell* 2006; 22(3):383-394.

[66] Sugasawa K, Okuda Y, Saijo M, Nishi R, Matsuda N, Chu G, Mori T, Iwai S, Tanaka K, Hanaoka F. UV-induced ubiquitylation of XPC protein mediated by UV-DDB-ubiquitin ligase complex. *Cell* 2005; 121(3):387-400.

[67] El-Mahdy MA, Zhu Q, Wang QE, Wani G, Praetorius-Ibba M, Wani AA. Cullin 4A-mediated proteolysis of DDB2 protein at DNA damage sites regulates in vivo lesion recognition by XPC. *The Journal of biological chemistry* 2006; 281(19):13404-13411.

[68] Takedachi A, Saijo M, Tanaka K. DDB2 complex-mediated ubiquitylation around DNA damage is oppositely regulated by XPC and Ku and contributes to the recruitment of XPA. *Molecular and cellular biology* 2010; 30(11):2708-2723.

[69] Marteijn JA, Bekker-Jensen S, Mailand N, Lans H, Schwertman P, Gourdin AM, Dantuma NP, Lukas J, Vermeulen W. Nucleotide excision repair-induced H2A ubiquitination is dependent on MDC1 and RNF8 and reveals a universal DNA damage response. *The Journal of cell biology* 2009; 186(6):835-847.

[70] Lan L, Nakajima S, Kapetanaki MG, Hsieh CL, Fagerburg M, Thickman K, Rodriguez-Collazo P, Leuba SH, Levine AS, Rapic-Otrin V. Monoubiquitinated histone H2A destabilizes photolesion-containing nucleosomes with concomitant release of UV-damaged DNA-binding protein E3 ligase. *The Journal of biological chemistry* 2012; 287(15):12036-12049.

[71] Hargreaves DC, Crabtree GR. ATP-dependent chromatin remodeling: genetics, genomics and mechanisms. *Cell research* 2011; 21(3):396-420.

[72] Clapier CR, Cairns BR. The biology of chromatin remodeling complexes. *Annu Rev Biochem* 2009; 78:273-304.

[73] Bell O, Tiwari VK, Thoma NH, Schubeler D. Determinants and dynamics of genome accessibility. *Nature reviews Genetics* 2011; 12(8):554-564.

[74] Udugama M, Sabri A, Bartholomew B. The INO80 ATP-dependent chromatin remodeling complex is a nucleosome spacing factor. *Mol Cell Biol* 2011; 31(4):662-673.

[75] Thoma F. Repair of UV lesions in nucleosomes--intrinsic properties and remodeling. *DNA Repair (Amst)* 2005; 4(8):855-869.

[76] Zhao Q, Wang QE, Ray A, Wani G, Han C, Milum K, Wani AA. Modulation of nucleotide excision repair by mammalian SWI/SNF chromatin-remodeling complex. *J Biol Chem* 2009; 284(44):30424-30432.

[77] Vignali M, Hassan AH, Neely KE, Workman JL. ATP-dependent chromatin-remodeling complexes. *Mol Cell Biol* 2000; 20(6):1899-1910.

[78] Lake RJ, Geyko A, Hemashettar G, Zhao Y, Fan HY. UV-induced association of the CSB remodeling protein with chromatin requires ATP-dependent relief of N-terminal autorepression. *Molecular cell* 2010; 37(2):235-246.

[79] Citterio E, Van Den Boom V, Schnitzler G, Kanaar R, Bonte E, Kingston RE, Hoeijmakers JH, Vermeulen W. ATP-dependent chromatin remodeling by the Cockayne syndrome B DNA repair-transcription-coupling factor. *Mol Cell Biol* 2000; 20(20):7643-7653.

[80] Reisman D, Glaros S, Thompson E. The SWI/SNF complex and cancer. *Oncogene* 2009; 28(14):1653-1668.

[81] Gong F, Fahy D, Liu H, Wang W, Smerdon MJ. Role of the mammalian SWI/SNF chromatin remodeling complex in the cellular response to UV damage. *Cell Cycle* 2008; 7(8):1067-1074.

[82] Ray A, Mir SN, Wani G, Zhao Q, Battu A, Zhu Q, Wang QE, Wani AA. Human SNF5/INI1, a component of the human SWI/SNF chromatin remodeling complex, promotes nucleotide excision repair by influencing ATM recruitment and downstream H2AX phosphorylation. *Mol Cell Biol* 2009; 29(23):6206-6219.

[83] Zhang L, Zhang Q, Jones K, Patel M, Gong F. The chromatin remodeling factor BRG1 stimulates nucleotide excision repair by facilitating recruitment of XPC to sites of DNA damage. *Cell Cycle* 2009; 8(23):3953-3959.

[84] Vincent JA, Kwong TJ, Tsukiyama T. ATP-dependent chromatin remodeling shapes the DNA replication landscape. *Nat Struct Mol Biol* 2008; 15(5):477-484.

[85] Pisano S, Leoni D, Galati A, Rhodes D, Savino M, Cacchione S. The human telomeric protein hTRF1 induces telomere-specific nucleosome mobility. *Nucleic Acids Research* 2010; 38(7):2247-2255.

[86] Shen X, Ranallo R, Choi E, Wu C. Involvement of actin-related proteins in ATP-dependent chromatin remodeling. *Molecular cell* 2003; 12(1):147-155.

[87] Cai Y, Jin J, Yao T, Gottschalk AJ, Swanson SK, Wu S, Shi Y, Washburn MP, Florens L, Conaway RC. YY1 functions with INO80 to activate transcription. *Nature structural & molecular biology* 2007; 14(9):872-874.

[88] Jin J, Cai Y, Yao T, Gottschalk AJ, Florens L, Swanson SK, Gutiérrez JL, Coleman MK, Workman JL, Mushegian A. A mammalian chromatin remodeling complex with

similarities to the yeast INO80 complex. *Journal of Biological Chemistry* 2005; 280(50): 41207-41212.

[89] Jiang Y, Wang X, Bao S, Guo R, Johnson DG, Shen X, Li L. INO80 chromatin remodeling complex promotes the removal of UV lesions by the nucleotide excision repair pathway. *Proceedings of the National Academy of Sciences* 2010; 107(40):17274-17279.

[90] Barak O, Lazzaro MA, Lane WS, Speicher DW, Picketts DJ, Shiekhattar R. Isolation of human NURF: a regulator of Engrailed gene expression. *The EMBO journal* 2003; 22(22): 6089-6100.

[91] Bozhenok L, Wade PA, Varga-Weisz P. WSTF–ISWI chromatin remodeling complex targets heterochromatic replication foci. *The EMBO journal* 2002; 21(9):2231-2241.

[92] Längst G, Becker PB. Nucleosome mobilization and positioning by ISWI-containing chromatin-remodeling factors. *Journal of cell science* 2001; 114(14):2561.

[93] Strohner R, Nemeth A, Jansa P, Hofmann-Rohrer U, Santoro R, Längst G, Grummt I. NoRC—a novel member of mammalian ISWI-containing chromatin remodeling machines. *The EMBO journal* 2001; 20(17):4892-4900.

[94] Stopka T, Skoultchi AI. The ISWI ATPase Snf2h is required for early mouse development. *Proceedings of the National Academy of Sciences of the United States of America* 2003; 100(24):14097.

[95] Emelyanov AV, Vershilova E, Ignatyeva MA, Pokrovsky DK, Lu X, Konev AY, Fyodorov DV. Identification and characterization of ToRC, a novel ISWI-containing ATP-dependent chromatin assembly complex. *Genes & development* 2012; 26(6):603-614.

[96] Eberharter A, Becker PB. ATP-dependent nucleosome remodelling: factors and functions. *J Cell Sci* 2004; 117(Pt 17):3707-3711.

[97] Cavellan E, Asp P, Percipalle P, Farrants AK. The WSTF-SNF2h chromatin remodeling complex interacts with several nuclear proteins in transcription. *J Biol Chem* 2006; 281(24):16264-16271.

[98] Luijsterburg MS, Dinant C, Lans H, Stap J, Wiernasz E, Lagerwerf S, Warmerdam DO, Lindh M, Brink MC, Dobrucki JW *et al.* Heterochromatin protein 1 is recruited to various types of DNA damage. *The Journal of cell biology* 2009; 185(4):577-586.

[99] Sanchez-Molina S, Mortusewicz O, Bieber B, Auer S, Eckey M, Leonhardt H, Friedl AA, Becker PB. Role for hACF1 in the G2/M damage checkpoint. *Nucleic Acids Res* 2011; 39(19):8445-8456.

[100] Fousteri M, Mullenders LH. Transcription-coupled nucleotide excision repair in mammalian cells: molecular mechanisms and biological effects. *Cell research* 2008; 18(1): 73-84.

[101] Rouaux C, Loeffler JP, Boutillier AL. Targeting CREB-binding protein (CBP) loss of function as a therapeutic strategy in neurological disorders. *Biochemical pharmacology* 2004; 68(6):1157-1164.

[102] Minamiyama M, Katsuno M, Adachi H, Waza M, Sang C, Kobayashi Y, Tanaka F, Doyu M, Inukai A, Sobue G. Sodium butyrate ameliorates phenotypic expression in a transgenic mouse model of spinal and bulbar muscular atrophy. *Human molecular genetics* 2004; 13(11):1183-1192.

[103] Ryu H, Smith K, Camelo SI, Carreras I, Lee J, Iglesias AH, Dangond F, Cormier KA, Cudkowicz ME, H Brown Jr R. Sodium phenylbutyrate prolongs survival and regulates expression of anti-apoptotic genes in transgenic amyotrophic lateral sclerosis mice. *Journal of neurochemistry* 2005; 93(5):1087-1098.

[104] Lafon-Hughes L, Di Tomaso MV, Méndez-Acuña L, Martínez-López W. Chromatin-remodelling mechanisms in cancer. *Mutation Research/Reviews in Mutation Research* 2008; 658(3):191-214.

[105] De Santis LP, Garcia CL, Balajee AS, Brea Calvo GT, Bassi L, Palitti F. Transcription coupled repair deficiency results in increased chromosomal aberrations and apoptotic death in the UV61 cell line, the Chinese hamster homologue of Cockayne's syndrome B. *Mutation Research/DNA Repair* 2001; 485(2):121-132.

[106] Martínez-López W, Marotta E, Di Tomaso M, Méndez-Acuña L, Palitti F. Distribution of UVC-induced chromosome aberrations along the X chromosome of TCR deficient and proficient Chinese hamster cell lines. *Mutation Research/Genetic Toxicology and Environmental Mutagenesis* 2010; 701(1):98-102.

Chapter 7

Emerging Features of DNA Double-Strand Break Repair in Humans

Hyun Suk Kim, Robert Hromas and Suk-Hee Lee

Additional information is available at the end of the chapter

http://dx.doi.org/10.5772/53811

1. Introduction

Ionizing radiation (IR) and various cytotoxic chemicals including reactive oxygen species (ROS) induce DNA double-strand breaks (DSBs) when they attack the phosphate backbones of the two DNA strands simultaneously. DSBs, once generated, not only cause a discontinuity in the genetic code, but also are vulnerable to further loss of DNA from a nuclease attack or the formation of abnormal DNA structures from chromosomal translocation, all of which can significantly increase genomic instability leading to cancer. Repair of DSB damage is therefore crucial for maintaining the physical and genetic integrity of the genome.

DNA damage sensors are the first responder to various types of DNA damages. Upon DSB damage, Mre11–Rad50–Nbs1 (MRN) complex initially recognizes DNA damage, and recruits and activates the ataxia-telangiectasia mutated (ATM) through protein interaction with Nbs1 (Fig. 1) [1, 2]. ATM is a member of the phosphoinositide 3-kinase (PI3K)-related protein kinase (PIKK) family of serine/threonine protein kinases that phosphorylates a number of target proteins containing conserved phosphorylation motif (SQ/TQ) in response to DNA damage [3] that include MRN complex, a histone variant, H2AX, a checkpoint mediator, MDC1, a checkpoint kinase, CHK2 and p53 [4]. Phosphorylations of MRN complex, H2AX and MDC1 are necessary for recruitment of the factors involved in signal transduction and homologous recombination (HR) to facilitate the repair process [5-9]. A marginal repair defect was observed in AT cells, which could be due to the reduced efficiency of homologous recombination [10]. Damage-induced phosphorylation of CHK2 and activation of p53 also induce the cell cycle arrest at the G1 phase [6, 11, 12].

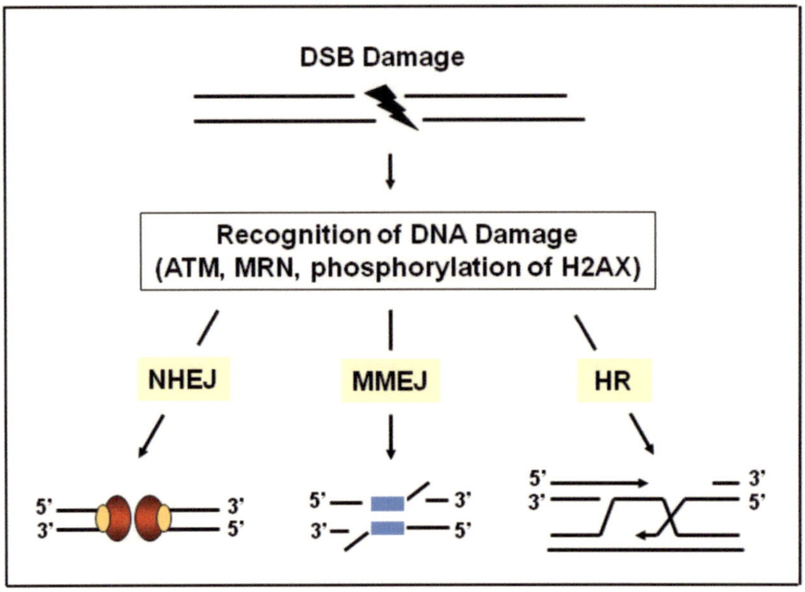

Figure 1. *Three major DSB repair pathways in mammals.* Following recognition of DSB damage by MRN complex and ATM, leading to phosphorylation of H2AX, DSB repair can occur through nonhomologous end joining (NHEJ), homologous recombination (HR), or microhomology-mediated end joining (MMEJ) repair pathways. The error-free pathway of HR in the late S- and G2-phases of the cell cycle requires a sister chromatid to restore broken DNA to its original sequence, whereas the error-prone pathway of NHEJ often processes the DNA by adding or deleting nucleotides before joining the ends. In some circumstances one or more of the broken ends is refractory to Ku mediated NHEJ. In this case, MMEJ can proceed by nucleolytic processing and resection of the 3'-end until a short region of complimentary bases is revealed. Pairing of this microhomology stabilizes the broken ends, displaced flaps are removed and ligation can occur. Although many of the proteins involved in these major DSB repair pathways have been identified, the precise mechanisms involved remain poorly understood.

In mammals, DSB damages are largely repaired by non-homologous end joining (NHEJ) pathway throughout the cell cycle that directly ligates the break ends without the need for a homologous template (Fig. 1), so NHEJ is an error-prone repair pathway. Microhomology-mediated end joining (MMEJ) shares the repair proteins with NHEJ pathway, except that it uses a short patch (5-25 base pairs) of homologous sequences to align the broken strands before joining (Fig. 1). When a break occurs a homology of 5-25 complementary base pairs on both strands is identified and used as a basis for which to align the strands with mismatched ends. Once aligned, any overhang or mismatched bases on both strands are removed and any missing nucleotides are inserted. MMEJ works by ligating the mismatched hanging strands of DNA, removing overhanging nucleotides and filling in the missing base pairs. MMEJ repair occurs during the S-phase of the cell cycle, as opposed to the G0/G1 and early S phases in NHEJ. MMEJ ligates the DNA strands without checking for consistency and causes deletions, since it removes base pairs (flaps) on the strand in order to align the two pieces; it is an error-prone repair pathway and results in deletion mutations. In most cases, a cell uses MMEJ only when the NHEJ repair is not available or unsuitable due to the disadvantage posed by introducing deletions into the genetic code. When a sister chromatid is available during late S- and G2-phases of the cell cycle, DSB damage can also be repaired by homology-directed repair, called homologous recombination (HR) (Fig. 1). This requires extensive 5′-3′ resection of DNA to generate a 3′ single-stranded tail. This is then displaced by the RAD51 recombinase, which forms a nucleoprotein filament which invades a homologous DNA duplex. This process named strand exchange forms a DNA crossover or Holliday junction which provides a primer to initiate new DNA synthesis. At this point there can be several outcomes. In synthesis dependent strand annealing the newly synthesized DNA reverts back to its original partner where it can be used as a template to complete repair. Alternatively for homologous recombination, the Holliday junction migrates away from the initial point of exchange (branch migration) until the junction is resolved by nucleolytic cleavage of either the crossed strands or non-crossed strands of the junction. Resolution of the two Holliday junctions in different orientations results in the exchange of flanking markers (crossover), whereas resolution in the same orientation does not result in exchange of flanking markers (non-crossover).

Since NHEJ repair involves a direct rejoining of the separated DNA ends, it requires the coordinated assembly of damage-responsive proteins at the damage site. DSB repair through NHEJ is initiated by binding Ku70-Ku80 complex to the DSB ends (Fig. 2). The Ku70/80 complex first binds to the DNA ends and recruits DNA-dependent protein kinase catalytic subunit (DNA-PKcs), a 465-kDa ser/thr kinase that mediates synapsis of the ends and then undergoes activation of its kinase. DNA-PKcs is a member of PIKK family [13], but its contribution to checkpoint response is insignificant. Kinase activity is required for NHEJ, but its function remains unclear. Rather, it phosphorylates multiple proteins involved in NHEJ [14]. Artemis, a nuclease, and PNK, a kinase/phosphatase, process the ends [15-17], and DNA ligase IV, a complex with XRCC4, ligates two DSB ends (Fig. 2) [18, 19]. The recruitment of the XRCC4-DNA ligase IV (Lig4) complex is essential for the final step of ligation. XLF (also known as Cernunnos) is known to stimulate Lig4 *in vitro* through its interaction with XRCC4. Although DNA end joining systems in mammals are dependent on above-mentioned factors (Ku70/80, DNA-PKcs, and XRCC4/Lig4), additional factors are required for end processing during NHEJ. Artemis exists in a complex with DNA-PKcs and has nuclease activity. Mre11 and Artemis possess 3′-5′ and 5′-3′ exonuclease, respectively, both of which may be involved in promoting the joining of noncomplementary ends via utilizing microhomologies near the ends of the DSB. The Werner syndrome protein (WRN) with its DNA cleavage activity stimulated by Ku complex is also a potential player in DNA end processing. Others implicated in DNA end processing include FEN-1, PNK, and DNA polymerases μ and λ. In addition, DNA polymerase(s) are also likely involved in the gap filling of NHEJ reaction. Metnase (also known as SETMAR) is a new comer in DSB repair pathways that not only methylates histone H3 lysine 36 at DSB sites but also plays several other roles in the joining of DSB damages. Although this review discussed current issues on DSB repair in general, it mainly focuses on the emerging roles of Metnase in DSB repair pathway.

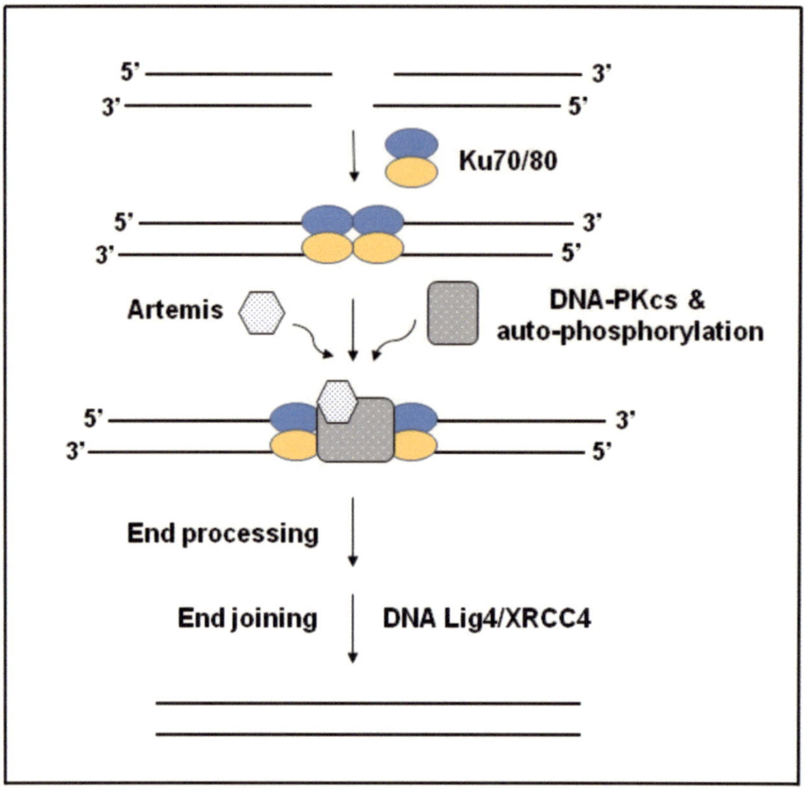

Figure 2. *Nonhomologous end joining (NHEJ) repair pathway in mammals.* When a DSB is introduced, Ku binds to the DNA because of its high affinity for DNA ends. The binding of Ku elicits conformational changes that allow it to bind DNA-PKcs. Ku may also serve as an alignment factor for the accuracy of NHEJ. Upon the assembly of DNA-PK on DNA breaks, this DNA repair complex activates its serine/threonine protein kinase activity and phosphorylates target substrates such as Artemis that colocalize at the ends of broken DNA prior to end processing and end joining events.

2. Human SET-Transposase chimeric protein in DSB repair

Transposases mediate DNA movement by recognizing both ends of transposon to excise the element from one site and insert it at other location in the genome, a process which can be repeated multiple times for a given segment [20-25]. It is likely that the ends are brought together and form a synaptic complex comprising two transposase molecules and the two ends of the corresponding element [25-28]. While transposase has played an important evolutionary role accounting for half of the present organization of the human genome [29], transposase activity was thought to be extinct in humans because unregulated DNA mobility could be highly deleterious in a long lived organism. To date, only one example of an intact copy of the Hsmar1 transposase domain has been identified within the human genome [30]. The Hsmar1 transposon, a class II transposable element, is an ancient element within the human genome introduced at least 50 million years ago in ancestral primates [23]. This "functional" Hsmar1 transposase domain exists as a chimeric fusion protein, Metnase (also known as SETMAR), which resulted from an insertion of the Hsmar1 transposon downstream of a SET gene (suppressor of variegation 3-9, enhancer-of-zeste, trithorax)1 encoding a histone lysine methyltransferase (HLMT), generating the SET and transposase fusion protein [23, 30]. Metnase is not found in prosimian monkeys or other mammals. Presumably this fusion event has conferred some evolutionary advantage to anthropoid primates as the activities of both the SET domain and transposase domain have largely been retained.

The Metnase-SET domain comprises pre-SET (aa 14-118), SET (aa 120-256), and post-SET (aa 273-302) domains (Fig. 3). The pre-SET domain contains a cysteine- and histidine-rich putative Zn^{++} binding motif, and the SET domain has the conserved the histone lysine methyltransferase motif shared with other SET proteins in humans [31, 32]. On the other hand, the Metnase-Transposase domain contains the conserved DNA binding and the catalytic motifs (Fig. 3). Potential DNA-binding motifs in the Metnase transposase were identified by comparative sequence analysis. These include a Nuclease-associated modular DNA-binding 1 (NUMOD1) motif, residues 417-434 representing a DNA binding helix-turn-helix based on its similarity to other families [33, 34], and a helix-turn-helix (HTH) motif, residues 347-381 (Fig. 3). Although Metnase cannot perform transposition, it has been shown to retain a number of activities associated with transposases including 5′-terminal inverted repeats (TIR)-specific DNA binding [23, 35-37], DNA looping activity [25], 5′-end processing activity [25, 35, 37], and promotion of integration at a TA dinucleotide target site [25, 38]. Recent structural analysis of the Metnase transposase domain has revealed features within the catalytic site that are distinct from those of related transposases and yet were likely present within the ancestral *Hsmar1* transposase. However, Metnase's DNA cleavage activity, unlike other functionally active transposases, is not coupled to its TIR-specific DNA binding [35, 37].

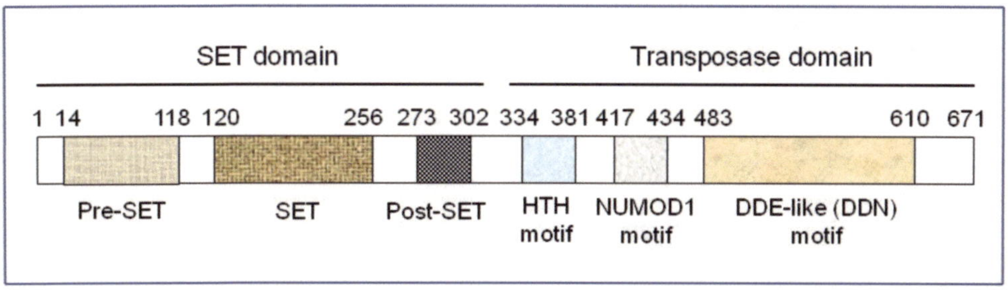

Figure 3. *Schematic diagram of human Metnase (SETMAR).* The Pre-SET domain contains cysteine- and histidine-rich putative Zn^{++} binding motif. The SET domain has the HLMT motif; transposase domain contains DNA binding motifs [helix-turn-helix (HTH) and NUMOD1] and a conserved DNA cleavage (DDE-like) motif.

Metnase is widely expressed in human tissues promotes NHEJ repair and mediates genomic integration of foreign DNA [32, 35, 39]. Metnase's involvement in NHEJ repair came from an in vivo study showing that overexpression of Metnase increased NHEJ repair, while it did not produce any significant changes in HR repair [32]. Similarly, cells treated with Metnase-specific siRNA showed a significant reduction in NHEJ repair activity in vivo. Metnase overexpression resulted in a 3-fold survival advantage after IR treatment compared to a vector control [32], further evidence of a role for Metnase in NHEJ. Metnase is also involved in genomic integration of foreign DNA [40, 41] that depends on some of the other NHEJ factors [42, 43]. Earlier study showed that a deletion of either SET or the transposase domain abrogated Metnase's function in DNA repair, indicating that both domains are required for this function [40]. Upon DNA damage, Metnase colocalizes with other DSB repair factors and has been shown to directly interact with Pso4 [34, 36], a human homolog of the 55-kDa protein encoded by the PSO4/PRP19 gene in *Saccharomyces cerevisiae* that has pleiotropic functions in DNA recombination and error-prone repair [44-47]. Metnase-mediated stimulation of DNA end joining in vivo requires both histone methyltransferase and transposase-associated activities [32], indicating that it has multiple functions in NHEJ repair. The SET-transposase fusion protein not only promotes DSB repair, but also physically interacts with Topo IIα and enhances Topo II-mediated chromosomal decatenation [24, 39], both of which are crucial for controlling DSB damage. Metnase is widely expressed, and is located at chromosome 3p26, a region of frequent abnormalities in various cancers [23, 32]. Metnase is the only known example of a protein involved in DNA repair that includes a SET domain as well as the only intact and functional *Hsmar1* transposase within the human genome.

3. Histone H3 dimethylation of Lys36 at DSB sites

DSB damage induces post-translational modification of histone proteins at the DNA damage sites, which not only is necessary for DNA damage sensing but also promotes DNA repair [48-57]. H2AX, a member of the histone H2A family, is rapidly phosphorylated in response to ionizing radiation and DNA damaging drug, generating γH2AX [50, 53, 55-57]. Phosphorylation of the histone variant H2AX occurs at the conserved C-terminal phosphatidylinositol 3-OH-kinase-related kinase (PI3KK) motif, and likely play a key role in DDR and is required for the assembly of DNA repair proteins at the sites containing damaged chromatin as well as for activation of checkpoints proteins which arrest the cell cycle progression [58-61]. DSB damage also induces non-proteolytic ubiquitylation near DNA damage site on the chromatin. DSB-induced ubiquitination is mediated by the RNF8/RNF168 ubiquitin ligase cascade [60], and has emerged as a key mechanism for restoration of genome integrity by licensing the DSB-modified chromatin to recruit genome caretaker proteins such as 53BP1 and BRCA1 near the lesions. In parallel, Sumoylation of upstream DSB regulators is also required for execution of this ubiquitin-dependent chromatin response, although its molecular basis is not clear.

Histone methylation plays a key role in and as such regulates transcription, replication, cell differentiation, genome stability, and apoptosis [62-66]. Mounting evidence points to a role for histone lysine methylation in DSB repair [67-72]. In mammalian cells, H3K79 methylation is crucial for 53BP1 localization at DSB sites and interaction with p53 in damage checkpoint activation [73]. In *S. cerevisiae*, loss of H3K79 methylation inhibits Rad9-dependent activation of the checkpoint kinase Rad53 following DSB damage [74, 75], and in fission yeast controls the recruitment of the damage checkpoint adaptor protein, Crb2 [76-78]. A recent study showed that DSB damage induces dimethylation of histone H3 at lysine 36 (H3K36me2) in human cells [31, 32]. Chromatin immunoprecipitation (ChIP) and immunoblot analyses indicated that H3K36me2 is actually formed at DSB sites [31]. H3-K36 is associated with chromatin opening [79-84], which may also be a part of its DSB localization via chromatin modulation. In fact, mutations at known conserved SET domain amino acids (N210S, alteration at the NHSC at 210-213 to AAAA, and the YDY at 247-249 to AAA) significantly lowered DNA end joining [32]. Two conserved amino acid sequences (210-NHSCXPN-216 and 242-EEELXXXY-249) in the Metnase-SET domain are likely responsible for the interaction with SAM since a mutation at these sites failed to interact with ^{3}H-labeled SAM [85-88]. Levels of DSB-induced H3K36me2 strongly correlate with Metnase expression and that the mutant (D248S) lacking HLMT activity fails to generate H3K36me2, suggesting that Metnase is responsible for the induction of H3K36me2 at DSB site [32]. Considering that the D248S mutant of Metnase fails to promote NHEJ repair, dimethylation of H3K36 is likely a major function of Metnase in promoting chromosomal DSB repair. Although the mechanism by which H3K36me2 promotes DSB repair is not clear, H3K36 methylation has been linked to chromatin opening accessible to transcription regulators and DNA repair proteins [89]. H3K36me2, once formed at DSB site, may create docking sites for other repair proteins, recruiting them for transcription and DNA repair. For example, H3K36 methylation attracts the histone deacetylase Rpd3S, which compact chromatin in the middle of transcribed genes, and inhibits false initiation of transcription during the elongation phase [90]. The methyltransferase Setd2 (also known as Set2) mediates trimethylation of H3K36me3 (H3K36me3), and it binds the phosphorylated tail of RNA polymerase II, implicating a role for H3K36me3 in transcription [49, 51, 91]. Setd2 mediates H3k36me3 in mammalian cells, but not di- or mono-methylation [92], raising a possibility that Metnase or other H3K36 dimethyltransferases may be necessary to generate H3K36me2 before Setd2 acts. In *Drosophila*, dimethylation of H3K36 peaks adjacent to promoters and requires distinct methyltransferases than those that mediate H3K36me3 [93]. The formation of H3K36me2 might also facilitate histone eviction at the DSB site, which then facilitates an access of the repair machineries to DNA damage site. This is supported by an observation that H3K36me2 enhances the presence of MRN complex and Ku70 at the DSB site [31]. These DNA repair proteins show an increased interaction with H3K36me2 after IR, and their presence at an induced DSB also correlated with Metnase expression levels. In addition, the chromatin immunoprecipitation study revealed that H3K36me2 not only enhances the rate of association of these repair proteins with the DSB but decreases their disassociation rates as well [31]. Because the MRN and Ku complexes can bind free DNA ends at a DSB in nonchromatinized DNA, the decreased rates of disassociation are likely the more important role of H3K36me2. This implies that the main benefit of H3K36me2 in DSB repair is more likely to stabilize the repair components at the DSB than to enhance their recruitment. It is possible that dimethylation of H3K36 at DSBs was an epiphenomenon and was not responsible for enhanced localization of early DSB repair components. On the other hand, when a point mutation at H3-K36 (K36R or K36A) caused a marked decrease in both the recruitment of NBS1 and Ku70 to the DSB and in DSB repair [31], indicating that H3K36me2 is required for efficient assembly and retention of repair components at DSBs and for optimum DSB repair. The identification of dimethylated H3K36 as a chromatin modification that enhances DSB repair by NHEJ places this modification alongside and ubiquitylated H2A as DNA damage-induced histone modifications that recruit repair components to DSBs and enhance repair [31, 94, 95]. In this regard, H3K36me2 by Metnase is consistent with an NHEJ histone code, as defined in the original histone code hypothesis for transcriptional regulation as histone modifications, acting in a combinatorial fashion on histones, which specify unique downstream functions [56]. Previous reports indicate that histone methylation may be important in DNA DSB repair by homologous recombination: The DSB repair component 53BP1, which is required for proper homologous recombination, is recruited to sites of damage by methylated histone H3 lysine 79 (H3K79) and histone H4 lysine 20 (H4K20) [76, 78, 96]. However, neither H3K79 nor H4K20 methylation is induced by DNA damage [96]. H3K36me2 is likely reserved for NHEJ repair pathway, because Ku70 and Metnase are involved in DSB repair by NHEJ rather than HR repair and because the latter requires complete histone eviction adjacent to the DSB. Human cancer cells that express Metnase at high levels display enhanced resistance to treatment with radiation or chemotherapy [32, 131, 132]. The resistance mediated by Metnase could reflect improved stabilization of the assembly of DSB repair components at DSB sites due to the generation of H3K36me2 at these sites. If so, a targeting of Metnase's HLMT activity may improve the efficacy of common cancer therapies based on DNA damaging agents.

4. DNA endonuclease activity in the joining of DSB damage

IR induces DNA double strand breaks with different ends, most of which are not directly ligatable. Therefore, they need to be processed before end joining event in all three major DSB repair pathways, with the exception of adding nucleotides opposite to 5′-overhang by DNA polymerase [97-100]. DNA end processing can be divided into two types: ssDNA cleavage that removes either a 5′- or 3′-overhang to leave a blunt end, and nuclease activity producing a deletion that is consistent with alignment of the DNA ends by base pairing in region(s) of microhomology [17, 97, 99, 101]. Several endonucleases and their binding partners have been shown to participate in end processing during DSB repair. Mre11 and Artemis possess 3′-5′ exonuclease activity and ssDNA-specific 5′-3′ exonuclease, respectively, both of which may be involved in promoting the joining of noncomplementary ends via utilizing microhomologies near the ends of the DSB [17, 100, 102-106]. MRN's exonuclease activity is for mismatched DNA ends and pauses at sites of microhomology [100], while its endonuclease is to open fully paired hairpin DNA [105]. Artemis possesses an endonuclease activity specific for hairpins and 5′- or 3′-overhangs following phosphorylation by DNA-PKcs [17, 106], suggesting that it plays a role in V(D)J recombination repair and perhaps in removing the 5′- and 3′-overhangs of non-compatible ends during NHEJ repair. Human CtIP physically and functionally interacting with MRN is another player in DNA end processing [107]. CtIP was originally identified as a binding partner for CtBP11 and the tumor suppressor proteins RB1 [108] and BRCA1 [86, 109], and is recruited to DNA damage and complexes with BRCA1 to control the G2/M DNA-damage checkpoint [110-112]. CtIP and the MRN complex promote ATR activation and HR through mediating DSB resection [107]. The Werner syndrome protein (WRN), a RecQ-like DNA helicase also possesses 3′-5′ exonuclease activity [42, 43, 113]. Considering that WRN is phosphorylated by DNA-PKcs [113], and its DNA cleavage activity is stimulated by Ku complex [114], WRN could play a role in DNA end processing. Other DNA helicases such as Bloom (BLM) and DNA2 may also play a role in DNA end processing [85]. These two DNA helicases physically interact to each other to resect DNA in a process that is ATP-dependent and requires BLM helicase and DNA2 nuclease functions [85]. RPA is essential for both DNA unwinding by BLM and enforcing 5′-3′ resection polarity by DNA2. MRN accelerates processing by recruiting BLM to the end. In the other, EXO1 resects the DNA and is stimulated by BLM, MRN, and RPA. BLM increases the affinity of EXO1 for ends, and MRN recruits and enhances the processivity of EXO1 [85].

Metnase possesses a unique endonuclease activity that preferentially acts on ssDNA overhang of a partial duplex DNA [35]. Cell extracts lacking Metnase exhibited significantly lowered end joining activity comparable to those seen in extracts lacking DNA-PKcs or Ku80 [35], whereas cell extracts over-expressing Metnase not only stimulated DNA end joining but also showed an enhanced end processing of non-compatible ends based on DNA sequencing analysis of end joining products [32, 35, 37]. Metnase has no hairpin or loop opening activity [35], indicating that it does not play a role in V(D)J recombination. Given that DNA end processing facilitates end joining by increasing the chance for partial annealing between two non-compatible ends, Metnase's endonuclease activity may play a direct role in stimulating DNA end joining through processing of non-compatible ends. While Metnase contributes to DNA end joining through an enhanced processing of non-compatible ends, its DNA cleavage activity cannot explain Metnase's stimulatory role in the joining of compatible ends [32, 35, 37]. Similar to DNA-PK- and Ku80-defective cells, cell extracts lacking Metnase failed to support joining of compatible ends [32], suggesting that Metnase also has a role in the joining of compatible ends, perhaps by promoting recruitment of the XRCC4-DNA ligase 4 (Lig4) complex [115], an essential player in the ligation step through a physical interaction upon DNA damage. The DNA binding property of Metnase may assist in the localization of DNA Lig4 at the free DNA ends. In this case, Metnase is epistatically above end-processing and subsequent joining, but perhaps below free end recognition and protection, in the NHEJ cascade.

One intriguing thing is how a transposase possesses ssDNA overhang cleavage activity in the absence of TIR sequence. The Metnase-transposase domain has a conserved DDE-like motif (D483, D575, and N610) that is crucial for DNA cleavage activity (Fig. 3) [35, 37, 116]. The function of residues in the DDE-motif includes coordination of a metal ion required for catalysis in other transposases. In addition to these residues, several other residues potentially play a role in the catalytic activity of the transposase domain [116]. Based on the crystal structure of the Metnase-transposase, the active sites of the two subunits that make up the dimer are distinctly different [116]; one subunit has bound metal in the active site and the other does not [116]. Metal is bound to the active site of one molecule comprising the dimer coordinated to Asp 483 and Asp 575. Residues K445, R578, and H580 within the catalytic pocket adopt different conformations in the metal-bound vs. non-metal bound active site structures and may also play important catalytic functions in ss-overhang cleavage activity. A loop within the active site of Metnase adopts two very different conformations resulting in a translation of a full residue when superimposed such that Arg 578 is located within the active site hydrogen-bonded to Glu 484 in the non-metal bound conformation and flipped out of the active site in the metal bound conformation. Similarly, the position of His 580 is quite different in each of the two different conformations in our structure. Interestingly, each conformation of His 580 is hydrogen-bonded to Glu 484. It remains to be seen what unique feature(s) of the catalytic domain with Metnase is directly linked to its role in DNA repair and replication fork arrest as compared to traditional transposase function.

5. Metnase binding partners in DSB repair

Metnase is a DNA repair factor colocalized with MRN complex and other repair factors at the DNA damage sites [36]. On the other hand, it is a transposase that has a capacity to interact with thousands of potential binding sites (TIR) in human chromosomes [23, 25, 37]. Metnase binds to a specific 19 bp sequence within the consensus Hsmar1 TIR [23, 30, 38, 117]. Similar to other Mariner transposases, the Metnase Helix-Turn-Helix (HTH) motif accounts for this binding; specifically the R432 residue within the HTH region is essential for this binding [37]. In human genomes there are a large number of miniature inverted-repeat transposable elements (MITES). If the solo TIRs are added to the number of MITES, there are approximately 7,000 potential Metnase binding sites in human genome. How does a transposase with a sequence-specific DNA binding activity get localized at the DSB sites? A recent study identified Pso4 as a Metnase binding partner that seems to play a role in Metnase localization at DSB sites [36]. Although Pso4 is Metnase's binding partner, coimmunoprecipitation of Metnase and Pso4 also pulled down the human homolog of Spf27, a member of the Prp19 core complex involved in pre-mRNA splicing [36]. Given that Pso4 is a part of the pre-mRNA splicing complex consisting of Pso4, Cdc5L, Plrg1, and Spf27 [118], the Metnase-Pso4 complex may be a part of the bigger complex including other members of the pre-mRNA splicing complex *in vivo*. Although the physiologic role of the Metnase-Pso4 interaction is still unclear, cells lacking Pso4 failed to show Metnase localization at the DSB sites [36], suggesting that Pso4 play a role in the recruitment of Metnase to the DSB sites. Upon DNA damage, Pso4 is induced [46] and formed a stable complex with Metnase [36]. A recent biochemical analysis suggested several interesting implications for the architecture of the Metnase-Pso4 complex on DNA. First, Metnase dimer forms a 1:1 stoichiometric complex with Pso4 on dsDNA [35, 36]. Although both Metnase and Pso4 can independently interact with TIR DNA, Pso4 is solely responsible for binding to dsDNA once the two proteins form a stable complex [35]. This claim is based on the findings that 1) the Metnase-Pso4 complex interacted with same stoichiometric amount of non-TIR DNA as the TIR DNA, 2) the Metnase-Pso4 complex interacted with same number of TIR molecules as Metnase or Pso4 alone did, and 3) formation of the Metnase-TIR complex was significantly inhibited by excess of TIR and not by non-TIR, whereas the Metnase-Pso4-TIR complexes were equally inhibited by both TIR and non-TIR DNA [35]. It is possible that Pso4, once forming a complex with Metnase, may directly interfere with Metnase's DNA binding domain (helix-turn-helix motif) [37]. This notion is supported by findings that Metnase bound to TIR DNA went through a conformational change and was less effective than free Metnase in interacting with Pso4 [35]. Pso4 has 6 C-terminal WD-40 repeats [119], a module that is known to interact with post-translationally modified histone 3, including dimethylated-K4 [120]. Given that Metnase HLMT activity targets H3-K4 as well as H3-K36 [32], it is possible that chromatin association of Pso4 may occur via Metnase-mediated H3-K4 methylation, while Metnase requires Pso4 for its DSB localization. Since Pso4 is induced following IR treatment *in vivo* [36, 46, 121], formation of a stable Metnase-Pso4 complex likely occurs in response to DNA damage. The Pso4 also undergoes structural alterations in response to DNA damage [121]. The Metnase-Pso4 complex, once formed, likely goes to nonTIR sites such as DSB sites [36], since Pso4 is solely responsible for binding to DNA in forming the Metnase-Pso4-DNA complex. It would be interesting to see whether Pso4 also affects Metnase's other biochemical functions such as DNA cleavage activity and HLMT activity. Further structural study would be necessary to clarify this intriguing issue.

Metnase also physically interacts with DNA ligase IV (Lig4), an essential DSB repair factor involved in the final end joining step in response to DNA damage [24], which supports the observations that Metnase promoted joining of both compatible and non-compatible ends [32, 35]. It remains to be seen whether Metnase plays a direct role in the recruitment of the XRCC4- Lig4 complex via its interaction with Lig4.

6. Metnase's role in the replication fork arrest

DNA double-strand breaks can be generated at the replication forks when the replication machinery encounters a single-strand break (SSB) or other types of DNA adducts. Attempted replication past a SSB can generate one-sided DSB which topologically differs from DSBs introduced by IR (Fig. 4). One-sided DSB is not a natural substrate for NHEJ, so these breaks can be repaired by homologous recombination repair pathway. Otherwise, it will remain unrepaired generating chromatid breaks, or it may ligate with a DSB in a different chromosome producing radial chromosomes. Stalled replication forks can also regress to generate a chicken-foot structure with a double stranded end (Fig. 4). Such a structure is topologically distinct from IR-induced DSBs in that it encompasses a single double-strand end rather than two double-strand ends.

Metnase possesses a distinct yet undefined role in the replication stress response [122]. Its role appears to be limited to restart of stalled and/or collapsed replication forks. DNA replication analyses indicated that Metnase promotes cell survival only when cells are subjected to replication stress such as hydroxyurea (HU), camptothecin (CT), or UV treatment [122].

Interestingly, when Metnase knockdown cells were treated with HU, the percentage of stopped forks greatly increased and there was a corresponding large decrease in the percentage of continuing forks, while new forks were extremely rare in both HU treated and untreated Metnase knockdown cells [122], indicating that Metnase plays a critical role in restarting stalled replication forks. It also suggests that Metnase may regulate new origin firing when cells experience replication stress. Metnase also regulates the efficiency of replication fork restart, and possibly initiation after replication stress, but it has no effect on the speed of ongoing forks [122].

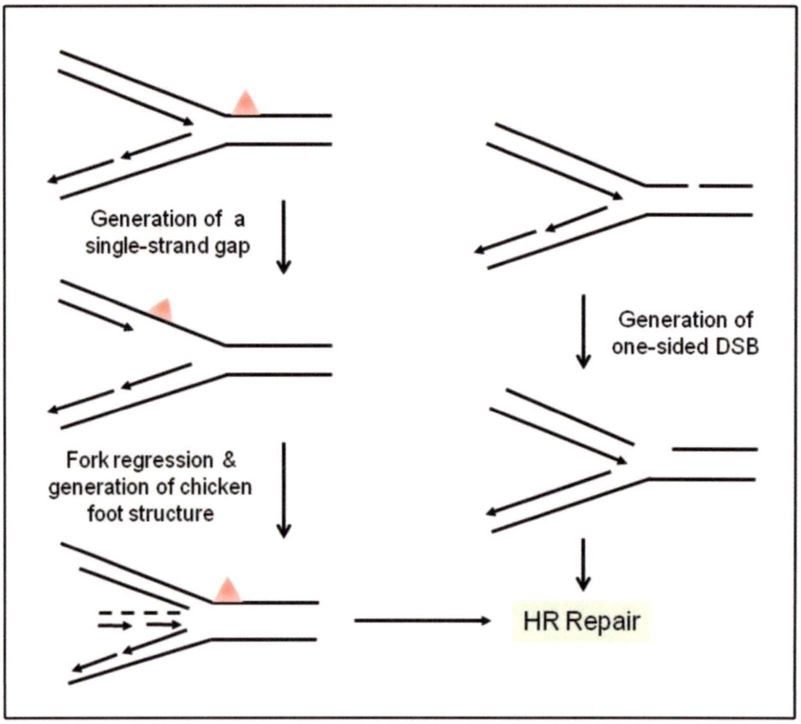

Figure 4. *Generation of DSB damage and its repair during replication.* Replication forks frequently encounter blocks to their progression including lesions such as single strand breaks. Structures such as a one sided DSB or a chicken-foot structure generated by fork regression can arise as a consequence of such replication stalling and the available evidence suggests a major function of HR is to repair or resolve such lesions.

Interestingly, a recent study with poly ADP-ribose polymerase 1 (PARP-1) revealed that it recruits MRE11 to stalled replication forks [123]. MRE11 with its endonuclease activity may play a role in processing stalled forks leading to RPA recruitment and eventual restart through HR . It is possible that Metnase promotes replication fork restart by promoting NHEJ [124]. NHEJ factors involved in NHEJ are known to promote cell survival after replication stress perhaps by facilitating rejoining of DSEs at collapsed forks [125, 126]. Since each collapsed fork produces only a single broken end that is not a natural substrate for NHEJ, however, it would be highly inaccurate producing radial chromosomes. Another possibility would be that NHEJ factors promote replication fork restart indirectly through interactions with HR factors [127]. When replication fork stalls, the initial cellular response is to stabilize the replisome to prevent fork collapse. Metnase does not appear to play a role in fork stabilization as similar fractions of cells with collapsed forks were observed regardless of Metnase expression level [122]. Another mechanism by which Metnase could promote fork restart is through its interactions with replisome factors including PCNA and RAD9. Although it is not yet known whether Metnase interacts directly with these proteins, the fact that the Metnase SET domain has a conserved PIP box is highly suggestive of direct interactions. Regardless, our results clearly place Metnase at stalled replication fork. The Metnase SET domain encodes a protein methylase, and Metnase is known to methylate histone H3 and itself [124, 128]. Metnase could regulate PCNA and/or RAD9 function through transmethylation, or it could have a more general effect through chromatin modification. In particular, Metnase targets histone H3 lysines 4 and 36, which are associated with chromatin opening, these modifications could enhance repair factor recruitment to stalled or collapsed forks. Given the well-established role of RAD9 in the intra-S checkpoint response [129], Metnase could promote fork restart by influencing checkpoint activation or downstream checkpoint-dependent processes such as inhibition of origin firing. In addition, Metnase could affect replication fork restart through its direct interaction with Topoisomerase IIα (TopoIIα). TopoIIα is proposed to relax positive supercoils that form ahead of replication forks [130]. Currently there is no information about whether supercoils persist in front of stalled forks. However, when one of the replicative polymerases encounters a blocking lesion, the other polymerase can become uncoupled and progress for a distance, producing a single-stranded gap that is bound by RPA, triggering the intra-S checkpoint [129]. This uncoupled synthesis depends on continued DNA unwinding by the MCM helicase complex, thus positive supercoils will continue to accumulate. By promoting TopoIIα-dependent relaxation of these supercoils, Metnase could help create a favorable topological state that assists in fork restart. Conceivably, this could involve restart of stalled forks that are processed to a chicken-foot structure since the resolution of such structures is likely dependent on the topological context of the stalled fork. Alternatively, at collapsed forks, the required HR-mediated invasion of the DSE into the unbroken sister chromatid, require unwinding of the sister duplex and could similarly be affected by the local topological state. Metnase may play different roles depending on the particular state of the stalled or collapsed replication fork.

7. Abnormal expression of Metnase in tumor specimens

The Metnase gene has three exons spread over 13.8 kB located at 3p26, a region of frequent abnormalities in non-Hodgkin's lymphoma, acute and chronic lymphocytic leukemia, myeloma, myelodysplasia, hereditary prostate cancer, and breast cancer (http://cgap.nci.nih.gov/Chromosomes/Mitelman). Metnase is expressed in all human tissues tested to various extents (32), with the highest expression in placenta and ovary and the lowest expression in skeletal muscle, which is reminiscent of expression patterns of other DNA repair proteins (131). Interestingly, different transcript variants were found in both normal and cancerous tissues (23), suggesting that Metnase is broadly expressed and has an important function in human. Metnase is frequently overexpressed in leukemia and breast cancer cell lines, and importantly, downregulating Metnase greatly enhances tumor cell sensitivity to common chemotherapeutics including epididophylotoxins and anthracyclines [132, 133]. Although the precise mechanism(s) by which Metnase promotes restart of the replication fork, Metnase may be a reasonable target for the therapeutic strategies that block DNA synthesis or take advantage of inherent defects of tumor cells in replication fork restart [134, 135].

8. Concluding remarks

While transposase accounts for half of the present organization of the human genome, transposase activity was thought to be extinct in humans probably because unregulated transposition would directly affect genomic stability, resulting in an unacceptably high rate of apoptosis or malignancy [29]. For this reason, transposase functions have been selected against the mammalian organisms [29], which lead to a generation of the SET-Transposase chimeric protein termed Metnase with novel functions in DSB repair, replication fork arrest, and chromosome decatenation that could actually defend the genome against improper DNA movement or DSB damage (Fig. 5).

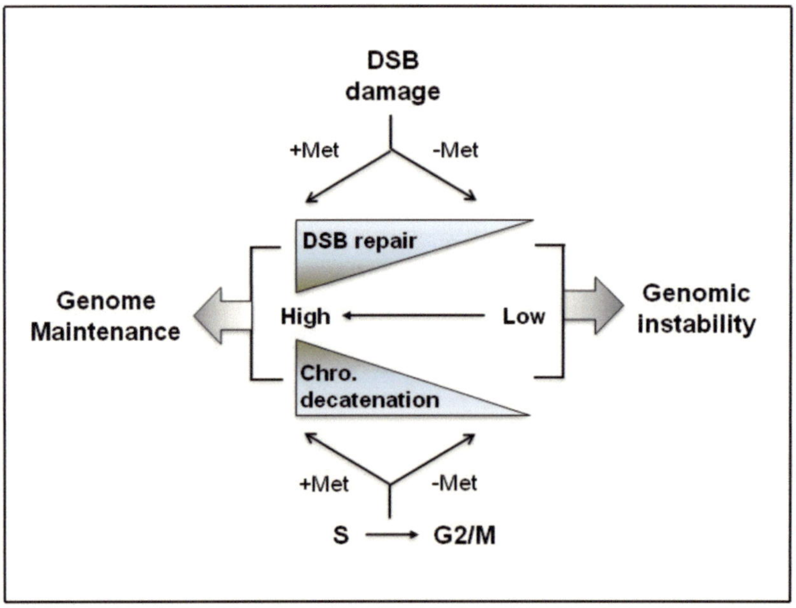

Figure 5. Metnase contributes to genome maintenance by promoting DSB repair and chromosome decatenation.

It should be pointed out that there are no other DNA repair proteins in which the DNA cleavage and histone lysine methyltransferase activities reside within the same protein.

http://dx.doi.org/10.5772/53811

Although the role(s) of Metnase in DSB repair and other DNA metabolism are yet to be defined, a deletion of either the SET or the transposase domain abrogated its function in DNA repair [32], indicating that both domains are essential for this function. Histone lysine methyltransferases (HLMT) is a critical participant in chromatin integrity as evidenced by the number of human diseases including cancers associated with the aberrant expression of its family members [136]. Although the underlying mechanisms of tumorigenesis are still largely unknown, Metnase HLMT targeting of H3K36 dimethylation at DSB damage sites is not only crucial for damage recognition and the early stage of DSB repair, but is also of our interest in tumorigenesis [31]. Metnase may thus be a viable anticancer target for a wide variety of tumor types. Given that altered expression of Metnase affect joining of both compatible- and non-compatible ends [24, 32, 35, 37], Metnase likely have two separate functions in the joining of DSB damage: 1) the Metnase-Lig4 interaction [24] for joining of compatible ends by promoting recruitment of Lig4 complex to DSB sites, and 2) Metnase's structure-specific endonuclease for joining of non-compatible ends by promoting end processing (Fig. 6). Further structure-function studies would be necessary to understand how a transposase becomes an endonuclease with ss-overhang cleavage in a TIR-independent manner.

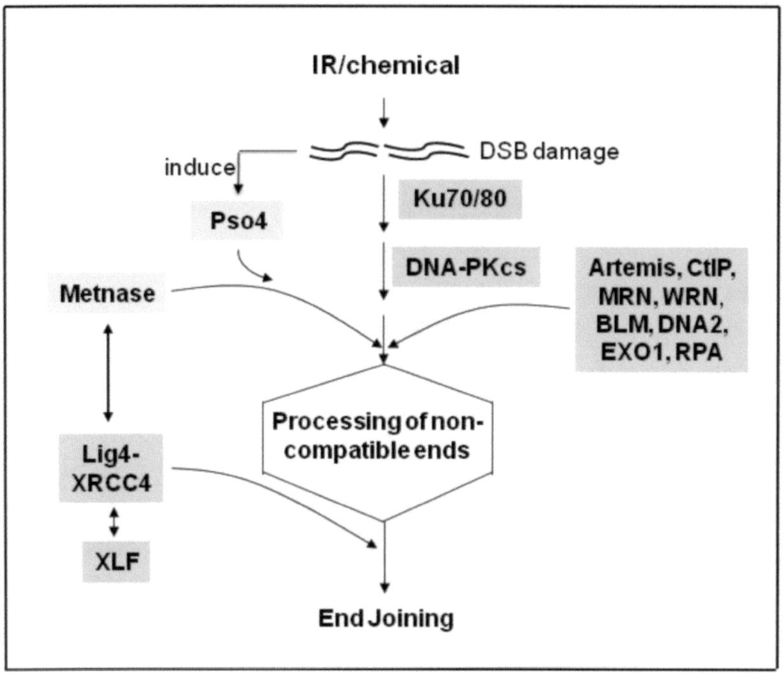

Figure 6. *Proposed role(s) for Metnase in DSB repair and chromosome decatenation.* Upon DSB damage, the Ku complex first binds to the DNA ends and recruits DNA-PKcs. Metnase binding partner, Pso4 is induced upon DSB damage, which, along with the Ku70/80, likely plays a crucial role in Metnase localization at DSB sites. Metnase's interaction with Lig4 is also induced upon DSB damage, which promotes joining of compatible ends, while Metnase's nuclease activity plays a role in joining of non-compatible ends.

Acknowledgments

This research was supported by grants from NIH (CA151367 and CA140422).

Author details

Hyun Suk Kim[1], Robert Hromas[2] and Suk-Hee Lee[1*]

1 Department of Biochemistry & Molecular Biology, Indiana University School of Medicine, Indianapolis, Indiana, USA

2 Department of Medicine, University of Florida and Shands Health Care System, Gainesville, FL, USA

References

[1] Carney JP, et al. The hMre11/hRad50 protein complex and Nijmegen breakage syndrome: linkage of double-strand break repair to the cellular DNA damage response. Cell 1998;93(3) 477-486.

[2] Falck J, Coates J, and Jackson SP. Conserved modes of recruitment of ATM, ATR and DNA-PKcs to sites of DNA damage. Nature 2005;434(7033) 605-611.

[3] Savitsky K, et al. A single ataxia telangiectasia gene with a product similar to PI-3 kinase. Science 1995;268(5218) 1749-1753.

[4] Matsuoka S, et al. ATM and ATR substrate analysis reveals extensive protein networks responsive to DNA damage. Science 2007;316(5828) 1160-1166.

[5] Stewart GS, et al. MDC1 is a mediator of the mammalian DNA damage checkpoint. Nature 2003;421(6926) 961-966.

[6] Lou Z, et al. MDC1 is coupled to activated CHK2 in mammalian DNA damage response pathways. Nature 2003;421(6926) 957-961.

[7] Costanzo V, et al. Mre11 protein complex prevents double-strand break accumulation during chromosomal DNA replication. Mol Cell 2001;8(1) 137-147.

[8] Burma S, et al. ATM phosphorylates histone H2AX in response to DNA double-strand breaks. J Biol Chem 2001;276(45) 42462-42467.

[9] Goldberg M, et al. MDC1 is required for the intra-S-phase DNA damage checkpoint. Nature 2003;421(6926) 952-956.

[10] Jeggo PA, Carr AM, and Lehmann AR. Splitting the ATM: distinct repair and checkpoint defects in ataxia-telangiectasia. Trends Genet 1998;14(8) 312-316.

[11] Canman CE, et al. Activation of the ATM kinase by ionizing radiation and phosphorylation of p53. Science 1998;281(5383) 1677-1679.

[12] Kang J, et al. Functional interaction of H2AX, NBS1, and p53 in ATM-dependent DNA damage responses and tumor suppression. Mol Cell Biol 2005;25(2) 661-670.

[13] Hartley KO, et al. DNA-dependent protein kinase catalytic subunit: a relative of phosphatidylinositol 3-kinase and the ataxia telangiectasia gene product. Cell 1995;82(5) 849-856.

[14] Dobbs TA, Tainer JA, and Lees-Miller SP. A structural model for regulation of NHEJ by DNA-PKcs autophosphorylation. DNA Repair (Amst) 2010;9(12) 1307-1314.

[15] Caldecott KW. Single-strand break repair and genetic disease. Nat Rev Genet 2008;9(8) 619-631.

[16] Pannicke U, et al. Functional and biochemical dissection of the structure-specific nuclease ARTEMIS. EMBO J 2004;23(9) 1987-1997.

[17] Ma Y, Schwarz K, and Lieber MR. The Artemis:DNA-PKcs endonuclease cleaves DNA loops, flaps, and gaps. DNA Repair (Amst) 2005;4(7) 845-851.

[18] Grawunder U, et al. Activity of DNA ligase IV stimulated by complex formation with XRCC4 protein in mammalian cells. Nature 1997;388(6641) 492-495.

[19] Critchlow SE, Bowater RP, and Jackson SP. Mammalian DNA double-strand break repair protein XRCC4 interacts with DNA ligase IV. Curr Biol 1997;7(8) 588-598.

[20] Ivics Z, et al. The Sleeping Beauty transposable element: evolution, regulation and genetic applications. Curr Issues Mol Biol 2004;6(1) 43-55.

[21] Miskey C, et al. DNA transposons in vertebrate functional genomics. Cell Mol Life Sci 2005;62(6) 629-641.

[22] Brillet B, Bigot Y, and Auge-Gouillou C. Assembly of the Tc1 and mariner transposition initiation complexes depends on the origins of their transposase DNA binding domains. Genetica 2007;130(2) 105-120.

[23] Cordaux R, et al. Birth of a chimeric primate gene by capture of the transposase gene from a mobile element. Proc Natl Acad Sci U S A 2006;103(21) 8101-8106.

[24] Hromas R, et al. The human set and transposase domain protein Metnase interacts with DNA Ligase IV and enhances the efficiency and accuracy of non-homologous end-joining. DNA Repair (Amst) 2008;7(12) 1927-1937.

[25] Liu D, et al. The human SETMAR protein preserves most of the activities of the ancestral Hsmar1 transposase. Mol Cell Biol 2007;27(3) 1125-1132.

[26] Adams CD, et al. Tn5 transposase loops DNA in the absence of Tn5 transposon end sequences. Mol Microbiol 2006;62(6) 1558-1568.

[27] Richardson JM, et al. Mechanism of Mos1 transposition: insights from structural analysis. EMBO J 2006;25(6) 1324-1334.

[28] Crellin P, Sewitz S, and Chalmers R. DNA looping and catalysis; the IHF-folded arm of Tn10 promotes conformational changes and hairpin resolution. Mol Cell 2004;13(4) 537-547.

[29] Lander ES, et al. Initial sequencing and analysis of the human genome. Nature 2001;409(6822) 860-921.

[30] Robertson HM, Zumpano KL. Molecular evolution of an ancient mariner transposon, Hsmar1, in the human genome. Gene 1997;205(1-2) 203-217.

[31] Fnu S, et al. Methylation of histone H3 lysine 36 enhances DNA repair by nonhomologous end- joining. Proc Natl Acad Sci U S A 2011;108(2) 540-545.

[32] Lee SH, et al. The SET domain protein Metnase mediates foreign DNA integration and links integration to nonhomologous end-joining repair. Proc Natl Acad Sci U S A 2005;102(50) 18075-18080.

[33] Sitbon E, and Pietrokovski S. New types of conserved sequence domains in DNA-binding regions of homing endonucleases. Trends Biochem Sci 2003;28(9) 473-477.

[34] Beck BD, et al. Regulation of Metnase's TIR binding activity by its binding partner, Pso4. Arch Biochem Biophys 2010;498(2) 89-94.

[35] Beck BD, et al. Biochemical Characterization of Metnase's Endonuclease Activity and Its Role in NHEJ Repair. Biochemistry 2011;50(20) 4360-4370.

[36] Beck BD, et al. Human Pso4 is a metnase (SETMAR)-binding partner that regulates metnase function in DNA repair. J Biol Chem 2008;283(14) 9023-9030.

[37] Roman Y, et al. Biochemical characterization of a SET and transposase fusion protein, Metnase: its DNA binding and DNA cleavage activity. Biochemistry 2007;46(40) 11369-11376.

[38] Miskey C, et al. The ancient mariner sails again: transposition of the human Hsmar1 element by a reconstructed transposase and activities of the SETMAR protein on transposon ends. Mol Cell Biol 2007;27(12) 4589-4600.

[39] Williamson EA, et al. The SET and transposase domain protein Metnase enhances chromosome decatenation: regulation by automethylation. Nucleic Acids Res 2008;36(18) 5822-5831.

[40] Sekiguchi JM, and Ferguson DO. DNA double-strand break repair: a relentless hunt uncovers new prey. Cell 2006;124(2) 260-262.

[41] Paull TT, and Gellert M. The 3' to 5' exonuclease activity of Mre 11 facilitates repair of DNA double-strand breaks. Mol Cell 1998;1(7) 969-979.

[42] Kamath-Loeb AS, et al. Werner syndrome protein. II. Characterization of the integral 3'-5' DNA exonuclease. J Biol Chem 1998;273(51) 34145-34150.

[43] Shen JC, et al. Werner syndrome protein. I. DNA helicase and dna exonuclease reside on the same polypeptide. J Biol Chem 1998;273(51) 34139-34144.

[44] da Silva KV, de Morais Junior MA, and Henriques JA. The PSO4 gene of S. cerevisiae is important for sporulation and the meiotic DNA repair of photoactivated psoralen lesions. Curr Genet 1995;27(3) 207-212.

[45] Henriques JA, et al. PSO4: a novel gene involved in error-prone repair in Saccharomyces cerevisiae. Mutat Res 1989;218(2) 111-124.

[46] Mahajan KN, and Mitchell BS. Role of human Pso4 in mammalian DNA repair and association with terminal deoxynucleotidyl transferase. Proc Natl Acad Sci U S A 2003;100(19) 10746-10751.

[47] Zhang N, et al. The Pso4 mRNA splicing and DNA repair complex interacts with WRN for processing of DNA interstrand cross-links. J Biol Chem 2005;280(49) 40559-40567.

[48] Wang H, et al. mAM facilitates conversion by ESET of dimethyl to trimethyl lysine 9 of histone H3 to cause transcriptional repression. Mol Cell 2003;12(2) 475-487.

[49] Sun J, and Li R. Human negative elongation factor activates transcription and regulates alternative transcription initiation. J Biol Chem 2010;285(9) 6443-6452.

[50] Buro LJ, Chipumuro E, and Henriksen MA. Menin and RNF20 recruitment is associated with dynamic histone modifications that regulate signal transducer and activator of transcription 1 (STAT1)-activated transcription of the interferon regulatory factor 1 gene (IRF1). Epigenetics Chromatin 2010;3(1) 16.

[51] Schwartz S, Meshorer E, and Ast G. Chromatin organization marks exon-intron structure. Nat Struct Mol Biol 2009;16(9) 990-995.

[52] Yoh SM, Lucas JS, and Jones KA. The Iws1:Spt6:CTD complex controls cotranscriptional mRNA biosynthesis and HYPB/Setd2-mediated histone H3K36 methylation. Genes Dev 2008;22(24) 3422-3434.

[53] Ahmad A, Zhang Y, and Cao XF. Decoding the epigenetic language of plant development. Mol Plant 2010;3(4) 719-728.

[54] Hake SB, Xiao A. and Allis CD. Linking the epigenetic 'language' of covalent histone modifications to cancer. Br J Cancer 2007;96 Suppl R31-39.

[55] Stucki M, and Jackson SP. gammaH2AX and MDC1: anchoring the DNA-damage-response machinery to broken chromosomes. DNA Repair (Amst) 2006;5(5) 534-543.

[56] Strahl BD, and Allis CD. The language of covalent histone modifications. Nature 2000;403(6765) 41-45.

[57] Fernandez-Capetillo O, et al. H2AX: the histone guardian of the genome. DNA Repair (Amst) 2004;3(8-9) 959-967.

[58] Podhorecka M, Skladanowski A, and Bozko P. H2AX Phosphorylation: Its Role in DNA Damage Response and Cancer Therapy. J Nucleic Acids 2010;2010 1-9

[59] Moon SH, et al. Dephosphorylation of gamma-H2AX by WIP1: an important homeostatic regulatory event in DNA repair and cell cycle control. Cell Cycle 2010;9(11) 2092-2096.

[60] Yan J, and Jetten AM. RAP80 and RNF8, key players in the recruitment of repair proteins to DNA damage sites. Cancer Lett 2008;271(2) 179-190.

[61] Downs JA. Chromatin structure and DNA double-strand break responses in cancer progression and therapy. Oncogene 2007;26(56) 7765-7772.

[62] Hayashi M, Chin GM, and Villeneuve AM. C. elegans germ cells switch between distinct modes of double-strand break repair during meiotic prophase progression. PLoS Genet 2007;3(11) e191.

[63] Reardon JT, Cheng Y, and Sancar A. Repair of DNA-protein cross-links in mammalian cells. Cell Cycle 2006;5(13) 1366-1370.

[64] Pasierbek P, et al. A Caenorhabditis elegans cohesion protein with functions in meiotic chromosome pairing and disjunction. Genes Dev 2001;15(11) 1349-1360.

[65] Moens PB, et al. Meiosis in a temperature-sensitive DNA-synthesis mutant and in an apomictic yeast strain (Saccharomyces cerevisiae). Philos Trans R Soc Lond B Biol Sci 1977;277(955) 351-358.

[66] Rhodes MC, et al. Assessing a Theoretical Risk of Dolutegravir-Induced Developmental Immunotoxicity in Juvenile Rats. Toxicol Sci 2012.

[67] Kassmeier MD, et al. VprBP binds full-length RAG1 and is required for B-cell development and V(D)J recombination fidelity. EMBO J 2012;31(4) 945-958.

[68] Dalal I, et al. Novel mutations in RAG1/2 and ADA genes in Israeli patients presenting with T-B-SCID or Omenn syndrome. Clin Immunol 2011;140(3) 284-290.

[69] Grundy GJ, Yang W, and Gellert M. Autoinhibition of DNA cleavage mediated by RAG1 and RAG2 is overcome by an epigenetic signal in V(D)J recombination. Proc Natl Acad Sci U S A 2010;107(52) 22487-22492.

[70] Arnal SM, et al. Non-consensus heptamer sequences destabilize the RAG post-cleavage complex, making ends available to alternative DNA repair pathways. Nucleic Acids Res 2010;38(9) 2944-2954.

[71] Grundy GJ, et al. Initial stages of V(D)J recombination: the organization of RAG1/2 and RSS DNA in the postcleavage complex. Mol Cell 2009;35(2) 217-227.

[72] Zhang M, and Swanson PC. HMGB1/2 can target DNA for illegitimate cleavage by the RAG1/2 complex. BMC Mol Biol 2009;10 24.

[73] Tsuji H, et al. Rag-dependent and Rag-independent mechanisms of Notch1 rearrangement in thymic lymphomas of Atm(-/-) and scid mice. Mutat Res 2009;660(1-2) 22-32.

[74] Pavlicek JW, Lyubchenko YL, and Chang Y. Quantitative analyses of RAG-RSS interactions and conformations revealed by atomic force microscopy. Biochemistry 2008;47(43) 11204-11211.

[75] Kriatchko AN, Bergeron S, and Swanson PC. HMG-box domain stimulation of RAG1/2 cleavage activity is metal ion dependent. BMC Mol Biol 2008;9 32.

[76] Botuyan MV, et al. Structural basis for the methylation state-specific recognition of histone H4-K20 by 53BP1 and Crb2 in DNA repair. Cell 2006;127(7) 1361-1373.

[77] Drejer-Teel AH, Fugmann SD, and Schatz DG. The beyond 12/23 restriction is imposed at the nicking and pairing steps of DNA cleavage during V(D)J recombination. Mol Cell Biol 2007;27(18) 6288-6299.

[78] Sanders SL, et al. Methylation of histone H4 lysine 20 controls recruitment of Crb2 to sites of DNA damage. Cell 2004;119(5) 603-614.

[79] Hah YS, Lee JH, and Kim DR. DNA-dependent protein kinase mediates V(D)J recombination via RAG2 phosphorylation. J Biochem Mol Biol 2007;40(3) 432-438.

[80] Kato M, et al. Omenn syndrome--review of several phenotypes of Omenn syndrome and RAG1/RAG2 mutations in Japan. Allergol Int 2006;55(2) 115-119.

[81] Messier TL, et al. In vivo transposition mediated by V(D)J recombinase in human T lymphocytes. EMBO J 2003;22(6) 1381-1388.

[82] Ciubotaru M, et al. RAG1-DNA binding in V(D)J recombination. Specificity and DNA-induced conformational changes revealed by fluorescence and CD spectroscopy. J Biol Chem 2003;278(8) 5584-5596.

[83] Jones JM, and Gellert M. Intermediates in V(D)J recombination: a stable RAG1/2 complex sequesters cleaved RSS ends. Proc Natl Acad Sci U S A 2001;98(23) 12926-12931.

[84] Harfst E, et al. Normal V(D)J recombination in cells from patients with Nijmegen breakage syndrome. Mol Immunol 2000;37(15) 915-929.

[85] Lin Y, et al. Detecting S-adenosyl-L-methionine-induced conformational change of a histone methyltransferase using a homogeneous time-resolved fluorescence-based binding assay. Anal Biochem 2012;423(1) 171-177.

[86] Foreman KW, et al. Structural and functional profiling of the human histone methyltransferase SMYD3. PLoS One 2011;6(7) e22290.

[87] Manzur KL, et al. A dimeric viral SET domain methyltransferase specific to Lys27 of histone H3. Nat Struct Biol 2003;10(3) 187-196.

[88] Min J, et al. Structure of the SET domain histone lysine methyltransferase Clr4. Nat Struct Biol 2002;9(11) 828-832.

[89] Bernstein BE, et al. Methylation of histone H3 Lys 4 in coding regions of active genes. Proc Natl Acad Sci U S A 2002;99(13) 8695-8700.

[90] Carrozza MJ, et al. Histone H3 methylation by Set2 directs deacetylation of coding regions by Rpd3S to suppress spurious intragenic transcription. Cell 2005;123(4) 581-592.

[91] Zentner GE, Tesar PJ, and Scacheri PC. Epigenetic signatures distinguish multiple classes of enhancers with distinct cellular functions. Genome Res 2011;21(8) 1273-1283.

[92] Edmunds JW, Mahadevan LC, and Clayton AL. Dynamic histone H3 methylation during gene induction: HYPB/Setd2 mediates all H3K36 trimethylation. EMBO J 2008;27(2) 406-420.

[93] Bell O, et al. Localized H3K36 methylation states define histone H4K16 acetylation during transcriptional elongation in Drosophila. EMBO J 2007;26(24) 4974-4984.

[94] Paull TT, et al. A critical role for histone H2AX in recruitment of repair factors to nuclear foci after DNA damage. Curr Biol 2000;10(15) 886-895.

[95] Bergink S, et al. DNA damage triggers nucleotide excision repair-dependent monoubiquitylation of histone H2A. Genes Dev 2006;20(10) 1343-1352.

[96] Huyen Y, et al. Methylated lysine 79 of histone H3 targets 53BP1 to DNA double-strand breaks. Nature 2004;432(7015) 406-411.

[97] Budman J. and Chu G. Processing of DNA for nonhomologous end-joining by cell-free extract. EMBO J 2005;24(4) 849-860.

[98] Gellert M. V(D)J recombination: RAG proteins, repair factors, and regulation. Annu Rev Biochem 2002;71 101-132.

[99] Lieber MR, et al. Mechanism and regulation of human non-homologous DNA end-joining. Nat Rev Mol Cell Biol 2003;4(9) 712-720.

[100] Paull TT, and Gellert M. A mechanistic basis for Mre11-directed DNA joining at microhomologies. Proc Natl Acad Sci U S A 2000;97(12) 6409-6414.

[101] Lieber MR, et al. The mechanism of vertebrate nonhomologous DNA end joining and its role in V(D)J recombination. DNA Repair (Amst) 2004;3(8-9) 817-826.

[102] Maser RS, et al. Mre11 complex and DNA replication: linkage to E2F and sites of DNA synthesis. Mol Cell Biol 2001;21(17) 6006-6016.

[103] Mirzoeva OK, Kawaguchi T, and Pieper RO. The Mre11/Rad50/Nbs1 complex interacts with the mismatch repair system and contributes to temozolomide-induced G2 arrest and cytotoxicity. Mol Cancer Ther 2006;5(11) 2757-2766.

[104] Mirzoeva OK, and Petrini JH. DNA damage-dependent nuclear dynamics of the Mre11 complex. Mol Cell Biol 2001;21(1) 281-288.

[105] Paull TT, and Gellert M. Nbs1 potentiates ATP-driven DNA unwinding and endonuclease cleavage by the Mre11/Rad50 complex. Genes Dev 1999;13(10) 1276-1288.

[106] Ma Y, et al. Hairpin opening and overhang processing by an Artemis/DNA-dependent protein kinase complex in nonhomologous end joining and V(D)J recombination. Cell 2002;108(6) 781-794.

[107] Li J, Wei H, and Zhou MM. Structure-guided design of a methyl donor cofactor that controls a viral histone H3 lysine 27 methyltransferase activity. J Med Chem 2011;54(21) 7734-7738.

[108] Wang R, et al. Formulating a fluorogenic assay to evaluate S-adenosyl-L-methionine analogues as protein methyltransferase cofactors. Mol Biosyst 2011;7(11) 2970-2981.

[109] Islam K, et al. Expanding cofactor repertoire of protein lysine methyltransferase for substrate labeling. ACS Chem Biol 2011;6(7) 679-684.

[110] Binda O, et al. A chemical method for labeling lysine methyltransferase substrates. Chembiochem 2011;12(2) 330-334.

[111] Cao F, et al. An Ash2L/RbBP5 heterodimer stimulates the MLL1 methyltransferase activity through coordinated substrate interactions with the MLL1 SET domain. PLoS One 2010;5(11) e14102.

[112] Chen NC, et al. Regulation of homocysteine metabolism and methylation in human and mouse tissues. FASEB J 2010;24(8) 2804-2817.

[113] Yannone SM, et al. Werner syndrome protein is regulated and phosphorylated by DNA-dependent protein kinase. J Biol Chem 2001;276(41) 38242-38248.

[114] Cooper MP, et al. Ku complex interacts with and stimulates the Werner protein. Genes Dev 2000;14(8) 907-912.

[115] Hromas R, et al. The human set and transposase domain protein Metnase interacts with DNA Ligase IV and enhances the efficiency and accuracy of non-homologous end-joining. DNA Repair (Amst) 2008;7(12) 1927-1937

[116] Goodwin KD, et al. Crystal structure of the human Hsmar1-derived transposase domain in the DNA repair enzyme Metnase. Biochemistry 2010;49(27) 5705-5713.

[117] Jordan IK. Evolutionary tinkering with transposable elements. Proc Natl Acad Sci U S A 2006;103(21) 7941-7942.

[118] Ajuh P, et al. Functional analysis of the human CDC5L complex and identification of its components by mass spectrometry. EMBO J 2000;19(23) 6569-6581.

[119] Vander Kooi CW, et al. The Prp19 U-box crystal structure suggests a common dimeric architecture for a class of oligomeric E3 ubiquitin ligases. Biochemistry 2006;45(1) 121-130.

[120] Taverna SD, et al. How chromatin-binding modules interpret histone modifications: lessons from professional pocket pickers. Nat Struct Mol Biol 2007;14(11) 1025-1040.

[121] Lu X, and Legerski RJ. The Prp19/Pso4 core complex undergoes ubiquitylation and structural alterations in response to DNA damage. Biochem Biophys Res Commun 2007;354(4) 968-974.

[122] De Haro LP, et al. Metnase promotes restart and repair of stalled and collapsed replication forks. Nucleic Acids Res 2010;38(17) 5681-5691.

[123] Bryant HE, et al. PARP is activated at stalled forks to mediate Mre11-dependent replication restart and recombination. EMBO J 2009;28(17) 2601-2615.

[124] Lee SH, et al. The SET domain protein Metnase mediates foreign DNA integration and links integration to nonhomologous end-joining repair. Proc Natl Acad Sci U S A 2005;102(50) 18075-18080.

[125] Lundin C, et al. Different roles for nonhomologous end joining and homologous recombination following replication arrest in mammalian cells. Mol Cell Biol 2002;22(16) 5869-5878.

[126] Arnaudeau C, Lundin C, and Helleday T. DNA double-strand breaks associated with replication forks are predominantly repaired by homologous recombination involving an exchange mechanism in mammalian cells. J Mol Biol 2001;307(5) 1235-1245.

[127] Shrivastav M, et al. DNA-PKcs and ATM co-regulate DNA double-strand break repair. DNA Repair (Amst) 2009;8(8) 920-929.

[128] Williamson EA, et al. The SET and transposase domain protein Metnase enhances chromosome decatenation: regulation by automethylation. Nucleic Acids Res 2008;36(18) 5822-5831.

[129] Budzowska M, and Kanaar R. Mechanisms of dealing with DNA damage-induced replication problems. Cell Biochem Biophys 2009;53(1) 17-31.

[130] McClendon AK, Rodriguez AC, and Osheroff N. Human topoisomerase IIalpha rapidly relaxes positively supercoiled DNA: implications for enzyme action ahead of replication forks. J Biol Chem 2005;280(47) 39337-39345.

[131] Moll U, et al. DNA-PK, the DNA-activated protein kinase, is differentially expressed in normal and malignant human tissues. Oncogene 1999;18(20) 3114–3126.

[132] Wray J, et al. Metnase mediates resistance to topoisomerase II inhibitors in breast cancer cells. PLoS One 2009;4(4) e5323.

[133] Wray J, et al. Metnase mediates chromosome decatenation in acute leukemia cells. Blood 2009;114(9) 1852-1858.

[134] Bryant HE, et al. Specific killing of BRCA2-deficient tumours with inhibitors of poly(ADP-ribose) polymerase. Nature 2005;434(7035) 913-917.

[135] Farmer H, et al. Targeting the DNA repair defect in BRCA mutant cells as a therapeutic strategy. Nature 2005;434(7035) 917-921.

[136] Sims RJ 3rd, Nishioka K, and Reinberg D. Histone lysine methylation: a signature for chromatin function. Trends Genet 2003;19(11) 629-639.

Chapter 8

Regulation of DNA Repair Process by the Pro-Inflammatory NF-κB Pathway

Simarna Kaur, Thierry Oddos,
Samantha Tucker-Samaras and Michael D. Southall

Additional information is available at the end of the chapter

http://dx.doi.org/10.5772/54341

1. Introduction

Skin is the largest organ of the body. It is organized into three main layers, epidermis, dermis and subcutaneous layer. The epidermis, an outermost avascular layer, is formed by keratinocytes at the epidermal basal layer that differentiate into corneocytes at the outer layer of the epidermis. The dermis lies below the epidermis separated by a basement membrane and is composed mainly of fibroblasts. The primary function of skin is to constitute an efficient barrier to protect the organism both from water evaporation and from external aggressions. Skin is an excellent organ system to study DNA damage and repair since skin is routinely exposed to external and internal aggressors which can induce DNA damage. Sunlight is the primary environmental inducer of damage in the skin. In particular ultraviolet radiations (UVR) are known to induce damage on DNA bases by direct absorption of photons. Typical damages from the direct effect of UVR are the cyclobutane pyrimidine dimers (CPD) or the 6-4 photoproducts formation both created by dimerization of contiguous pyrimidines on the DNA [1]. Sunlight also induces significant damage to skin cells through the generation of Reactive Oxygen Species (ROS) which damage DNA nucleobases and the sugar phosphate backbone. Depending on the attacking ROS (singlet oxygen and hydroxyl radicals through the formation of superoxide radicals), different modifications are generated to DNA such as bulky (8-oxo- guanosine, as guanine is the most easily oxidized base, thymidine and cytosine glycol) and non bulky (cyclo purine and etheno adducts) base modifications, spontaneous hydrolysis of a normal or damaged nucleobase leading to an abasic site, (See review [2]). Finally ROS may also generate other forms of DNA damage such as single strand breaks (SSB) or double strand breaks (DSB) when the free radical attack is located on the poly- deoxy- ribose chain. Other external aggressors, such as cigarette smoke and pollution, may favor DNA damage onset by depleting intracellular anti-oxidant molecules such as glutathione and thus shifting the oxidative balance to favor oxidation by ROS. In addition to external aggression, cells are also subjected to internal aggression from ROS generated by oxidative metabolism or respiration as well as to the attack of genotoxic or photo-sensitizers coming from the diet.

DNA integrity being one of the key parameters to maintain a healthy organism, living cells have developed strategies not only to prevent DNA damage but also to efficiently repair any damaged DNA. In human cells, DNA is repaired by different mechanisms: Base Excision Repair (BER), Nucleotide Excision Repair (NER), Single and Double stranded Breaks Repair (SSBR and DSBR), Homologous Recombination (HR) and Mismatched repair. Basically, DNA alterations without strand breaks are repaired mainly by excision repair mechanisms where the damaged bases are removed from the DNA molecule by excision and then replaced with the right bases. In the case of the Nucleotide Excision Repair (NER) an oligonucleotide fragment of approximately 25-30 nucleotides is removed around the damaged DNA and the gap generated in the DNA duplex is filled by DNA synthesis using the opposite, normal DNA strand as a template. To complete the process of NER, the last nucleotide incorporated is covalently joined to the extent DNA by ligation [3]. BER consists of four to five steps in which specific enzymes play a role: excision of the damaged base by a glycosylase, incision of the resulting abasic site, processing of the generated termini at the strand break, DNA synthesis and ligation [4, 5]. A third mechanism called mismatched repair occurs when only one nucleotide mismatch appears in the DNA double chain. This mechanism is particularly effective for the repair of DNA error arising during replication due to the limited fidelity of the replicative machinery. Finally, DNA double strand breaks can be repaired by a specific process called homologous recombination and non homologous end joining [6].

The importance of the DNA repair process and its relevance in skin aging and skin cancer has been highlighted by genetic disorders affecting genes responsible for DNA repair. For example the genetic diseases Xeroderma Pigmentosum (XP), Cockayne syndrome (CS) and Ataxia telangiectasia (AT) are rare autosomal recessive pathologies where different and specific enzymes of the NER and BER pathways are deficient due to inactivating mutation in their genes [7, 8]. These diseases are characterized at the level of the skin by extreme sensitivity to sunlight, resulting in sunburn, pigmentation changes, an early onset of the appearance of skin aging signs and a greatly elevated incidence of skin cancers in particular for XP disorder [9]. These changes can be explained by long lasting DNA damages that induces prolonged cellular inflammation through the activation of the NF-κB pathway [10-13] and an acquired immune deficiency [14] as well as rapid accumulation of mutation leading to cell apoptosis, senescence and cell tumorigenesis [15, 16][17, 18].

2. Inflammation and DNA repair

During tissue damage and the subsequent inflammation, a number of mediators are released which have been shown to modulate DNA repair. The activation of the Melanocortin

Receptor 1 (MCR1) by either its natural ligand, the α-Melanocyte stimulating Hormone αMSH or synthetic analogs [17, 18] can enhance the DNA repair activity in cells. Also two interleukins (IL), IL12 and IL23, known to display anti-tumor activity [19-22], have been shown to accelerate the repair of UVB induced CPDs. Activation of detoxifying mechanisms such as the NRf2 pathway may enhance also DNA repair [23]. Finally mono- and poly-ubiquitilation as well as sumoylation play an important role in the regulation of DNA repair (see review by[24]). Thus inflammatory mediators can directly affect the DNA repair process and therefore could be regulatory factors either enhancing or repressing DNA repair. Recent studies have identified that the NF-kB pathway, which is a key regulator in the expression of inflammatory proteins, may be an important mediator in DNA damage and the subsequent repair.

3. NF-κB signal transduction

NF-κB was first described in 1986 as a nuclear factor essential for immunoglobulin κ light chain transcription in B cells [25]. Since that initial discovery, NF-κB has been found to be a primary mediator involved in regulating immune responses, apoptosis and cellular growth, as well as being present in inflammatory diseases such as arthritis and asthma, [26]. The NF-κB family of transcription factors shares a high-conserved sequence of amino acids within their *amino terminus,* which contains a nuclear localization sequence that is involved in the dimerization with sequence-specific DNA binding and with the inhibitory IκB proteins.

In unstimulated cells, NF-κB-family proteins exists as heterodimers or homodimers that are sequestred in the cytoplasm in an inactive form by virtue of their association with a member of the IκB family of inhibitory proteins, most notably IκBα, IκBβ and IκBγ [27, 28]. About 200 extracellular signals can lead to activation through the dissociation of NF-κB from the IκB proteins. These activating signals include viral and bacterial products, oxidative stress, pro-inflammatory cytokines including IL-1 and TNF-α, and phorbol esters [29-33]. Ultraviolet (UV) radiation from sunlight induces IL-1 and TNF-α and creates reactive oxygen species that then leads to NF-κB-mediated inflammation [34, 35]. The kinase activity of IκK phosphorylates two serine residues (Ser32 and Ser36) on IκB proteins, which results in the ubiquitination and degradation of IκB by the proteasome. The degradation of IκB reveals the nuclear localization sequence of NF-κB [27, 28]. Free NF-κB can then translocate to the nucleus and bind to a NF-κB *consensus* sequence present within the promoter region of target genes, thereby upregulating the expression of hundreds of genes, including cytokines (Interleukin-1, -2, -6, etc.), TNF-α, immunoreceptors (immunoglobin kappa light chain, MHC class I, etc.), cellular adhesion molecules (ICAM-1, VCAM-1, ELAM-1), and many others [33].

4. NF-κB and DNA damage

The NF-κB pathway has been shown to be regulated by ionizing radiation at both the mRNA and protein levels by Brach et al., who demonstrated that NF-κB transcripts were transiently increased after irradiation, which was preceded by enhanced DNA binding activity of this transcription factor [36]. The causal role of NF-κB in DNA damage has been hypothesized since suppression of the NF-κB pathway by a pharmacological inhibitor resulted in a significant reduction in DNA damage as determined by T-T dimer formation in skin cells (Figure 1). Nuclear DNA double strand breaks (DSBs) are one of the most potent DNA damage signals to activate NF-κB. This process can occur within 1–2 h after break induction through activation of the canonical inhibitor of κB (IκB) kinase (IKK) complex and IκBa degradation [12]. NF-κB can be activated by Topoisomerase inhibitors (such as camptothecin) potentially via the generation of double strand breaks as well [13]. Furthermore activation of IKK following treatment with topoisomerase inhibitors was described to be dependent on the zinc finger domain in NF-κB essential modulator (NEMO) [24]. DSBs can trigger two independent signaling cascades that eventually lead to the induction of NF-κB via NEMO [35]. In one case, DSBs can activate ATM, which in turn can bind to and phosphorylate NEMO. In a parallel cascade, the p53-induced protein with a death domain (PIDD) translocates to the nucleus leading to the SUMOylation of NEMO. Consequently, the resulting activation of NF-κB favors cell survival by turning on the transcription of several anti-apoptotic genes. In response to DSB, PIDD as well as ATM are capable of initiating cascades leading to pro- or antiapoptotic signals, NF-κB presumably being a part of the pro-survival cascade [35]. Miyamoto et al., have summarized this model of NF-κB activation by DNA damage as a 'two signal' model as it requires coincident NEMO SUMOylation and ATM activation by double strand breaks to permit robust NF-κB activation [12]. Taken together these findings suggest that NF-κB may be both have both causal and effector roles in the development of DNA damage.

5. NF-κB and the DNA repair process

Although the mechanisms by which NF-κB affects DNA damage are not fully established, one possibility is that NF-κB may either directly or indirectly regulate DNA repair processes in cells. Protecting cells from apoptotic cell death following DNA damage is one of the major ways that NF-κB activation regulates the DNA repair process. Wang et al., have demonstrated that NF-κB functions as a positive modulator of cellular senescence, an intrinsic tumor suppression mechanism, by showing that human fibroblasts lacking NF-κB activity prematurely exit from senescence [37]. Others have shown that skin cells devoid of NF-κB activity exhibit deregulated growth correlating with impaired cell-cycle control [38, 39]. It has been proposed that the role of NF-κB in cellular senescence could be cell type specific, differentially initiating senescence or acting further downstream in the DNA repair process to maintain the senescent state [37]. DNA damage caused by chemical genotoxic agents, such as camptothecin, has been described to activate the Ataxia Telangiectasia-Mutated (ATM) kinase and NEMO (IκB kinase), leading to the inducing of NF-κB p50/p65 heterodimer [40]. In a parallel signaling pathway, ROS can be generated by genotoxic agents in sufficient quantities to activate the NF-κB pathway. ROS can also act as signaling molecules in immune responses, cell death and inflammation, where NF-κB is involved [40]. Depending on the relative degree of DNA damage, multiple mechanisms of NF-κB activation are engaged. Physical genotoxic agents such as UVA or hydrogen peroxide lead to extensive oxidative damage within the cytoplasm which can signal the activation of NF-κB pathway in the absence of DNA damage.

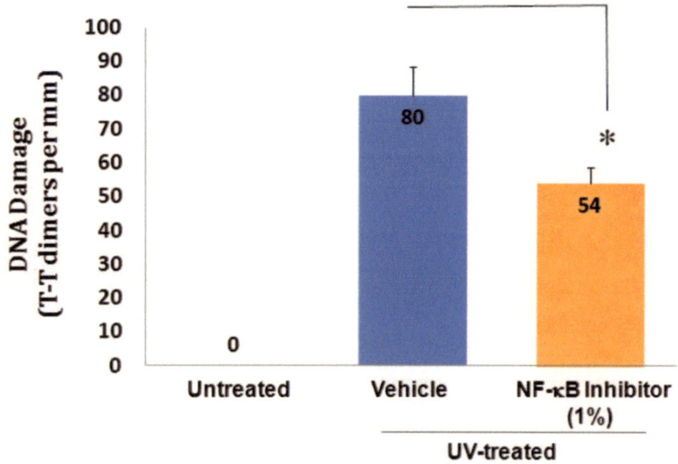

(a)

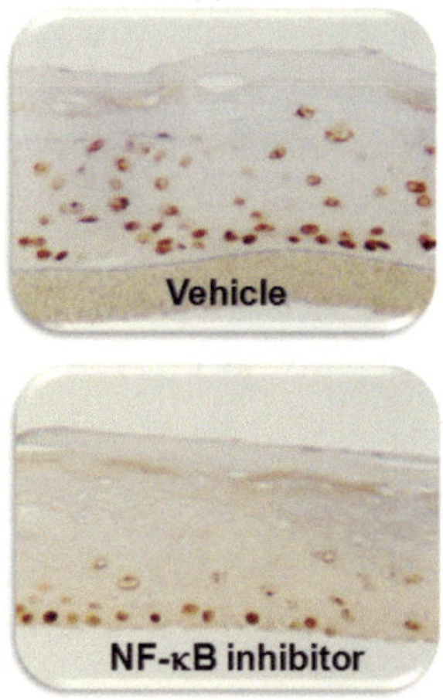

(b)

Figure 1. Topical pretreatment of skin equivalents with an NF-κB inhibitor reduces UV-induced DNA damage Human epidermal skin equivalents were pre-treated with vehicle or NF-κB inhibitor (4-hexyl-1,3-phenylenediol) for 2 hr prior to UV exposure, and DNA damage assessed by Thymine (T-T) dimer staining followed by blinded quantification. *P<0.05 using Student's t-test.

Among the various types of DNA damage, repairing double strand breaks can be particularly challenging to cells [41, 42], and may contribute to genomic instability associated with most cancers [42-45]. Wiesmuller et al., have shown that NF-κB is involved in double strand removal and repair via a stimulatory action on homologous repair, involving the targets

ATM and the tumor suppressor gene BRCA2 [46]. NF-κB is known to bind to the BRCA2 promoter and activate BRCA2 gene expression [47]. The role of NF-κB in ATM function and DNA repair was demonstrated by Siervi et al., in T-cells where levels of ATM mRNA and protein were significantly reduced by NF-κB blockade [48]. Activation of NF-κB by ATM results in an anti-apoptotic signal in the cells. Wiesmuller et al. have also described that NF-κB utilizes multiple mechanisms to enhance homologous recombination, including stimulation of the activity of CtIP–BRCA1 complexes to trigger DNA end processing, and upregulation of ATM and BRCA2 for strand transfer [46].

The nuclear factor p53 controls several physiological processes including DNA repair and cell cycle arrest. Cross-talk between NF-κB and p53 has been established by multiple groups ([49, 50]; see review by [51]), including results that suggest NF-κB may have both anti- and pro-apoptotic roles. Only a limited number of studies have investigated the role of NF-κB in DNA damage and repair in skin cells (including: [38, 39, 52-55]). Evaluation of the p53-NFκB cross-talk by Puszynski et al. in HaCat keratinocytes cells showed that inactivation of NF-κB improved p53-mediated DNA repair and prevented arsenite-induced malignant transformation of HaCaT cells [54]. Marwaha et al. have shown that in primary skin cells, such as dermal fibroblasts and keratinocytes, treatment with T-oligos led to the up-regulation and activation of p53, coinciding with decreased NF-κB DNA binding activity and inhibition of transcription from NF-κB-driven promoter constructs [53]. Thyss et al. have demonstrated that the sequential activation of NF-κB, Egr-1 and Gadd45 cascade induces UVB-mediated cell death in epidermal cells [55], a process that was crucial in order to eradicate the cells that bear the risk of becoming tumorigenic. In HaCat keratinocytes, hydroxytyrosol (main component of olive oil described as an inhibitor of NF-κB), has been shown to significantly reduce the DNA strand breaks caused by UVB, and also attenuate the expression of p53 and NF-κB in a concentration-dependent manner [52]. And finally, pharmacological inhibition of NF-κB increased the DNA repair capacity of primary human keratinocytes suggesting a potential inhibitory role of the NF-κB pathway on NER /BER in skin cells (Figure 2).

6. NF-κB and the decrease in DNA repair capacity of dermal fibroblasts: A role in accelerating the skin aging process?

Aging of the dermal compartment of skin is generally associated with fibroblast aging. Indeed in skin biopsies of aged donors, a general decrease in collagen synthesis activity is observed as well as an accumulation of senescent cells that display a catabolic phenotype [56, 57]. We have recently shown that there is a general decrease in DNA repair capacity in aging dermal fibroblasts. Indeed, using two different types of DNA repair measurement that directly measure the activity on human dermal fibroblasts nuclear extracts on plasmid [58] and oligonucleotides [59, 60] bearing specific damages, we showed that the level of NER and BER are dramatically reduced in dermal fibroblasts from a group of female volunteers with age comprised between 40 and 50 years old compared to a results obtained in a younger group 20-30 years old for both chronically UV-exposed skin or non-exposed skin site [61, 62]. Sauvaigo et al. also demonstrated that SSB repair decreased with aging in dermal fibroblasts [60]. This suggests that the depression in the repair capacity of skin cells may contribute significantly to a lower resistance of aged tissue to DNA damage and thus accelerate the aging process of the skin tissue. The decreased DNA repair may also increase the occurrence of senescent cells as we have seen that on average subjects with the low DNA repair activity display more severe signs of skin aging such as wrinkle, overall photo-damage and firmness (Unpublished results).

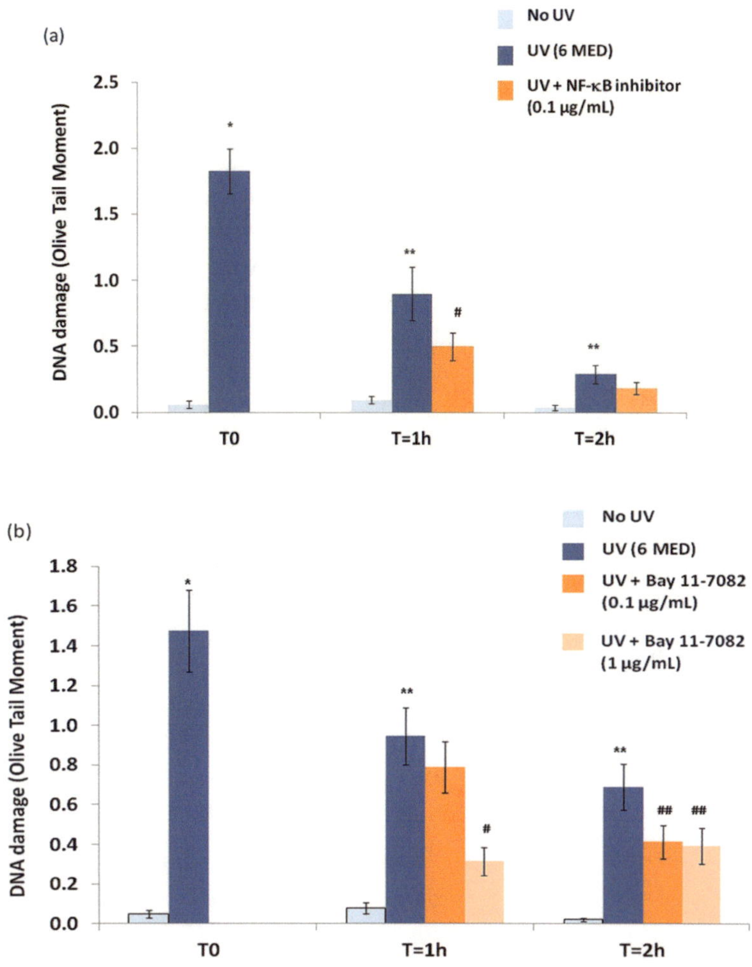

Figure 2. Treatment of primary human keratinocytes with NF-κB inhibitors increased repair of UV-induced DNA damage. Primary human keratinocytes were exposed to UV, followed by immediate treatment with the NF-κB inhibitors 4-hexyl-1,3-phenylenediol (Figure 2A) or BAY11-7082 (Figure 2B). DNA damage was assessed by Comet assay at T= 0, 1 and 2 hours after treatment with NF-κB inhibitors

While the mechanisms contributing to the decreased DNA repair in aged skin are not known, in parallel we have observed that in aging dermal fibroblasts there was an increased activation of the NF-κB pathways which directly induced a transcriptional repression of the collagen gene expression [63]. Taken together, it could be hypothesized that the elevation of NF-κB transcriptional activity may contribute to the decrease in DNA repair capacity of skin cells and thereby lead to accelerated skin aging. Since NF-κB is activated by DNA damage, there is a potential for a vicious circle to take place as more NF-κB may decrease the capacity of the cell to repair damages and lead to a longer persistence of the DNA damages.

7. NF-κB and the development of resistance to alkylating agent-based chemotherapy

In addition to the putative role of NF-κB and the decreased DNA repair capacity of skin cells leading to skin aging, NF-κB regulation of DNA repair may also contribute to chemoresistance. Studies of chemotherapeutic resistance have shown a significant correlation exists between NF-κB activation and the decreased effectiveness of some chemotherapeutic agents. Agents such as taxol and irradiation treatments upregulate the transcription factor NF-κB which leads to promoting survival and chemoresistance in solid tumor cancers [64]. The mechanism for this chemoresistance is through the activation NF-κB which can subsequently mediate cell survival, proliferation, invasion, and metastasis [65].

Sphingosine kinase may be of therapeutic interest in the context of inflammatory disease and drug resistant cancers. Sphingolipid metabolism has been shown to be aberrant in breast cancer tumor samples, resulting from an increase of sphingosine kinase expression [66]. The sphingosine kinase cascade pathway was first linked to the NF-κB pathway in 1998 via demonstration that TNF induced adhesion was mediated through sphingosine kinase signaling, which links to downstream NF-κB activation [67]. Using a novel selective Sphk2 inhibitor, ABC294640, Antoon et al. demonstrated inhibition of NF-κB activation via inhibition of Sphk2 [68]. In vivo testing in a well-established immunocompromised xenograft model for tumor growth, demonstrated that this inhibitor showed lower proliferation of cancerous cells, and no tumor growth when compared to control. This establishes the underlying pathways including the inhibition of NF-κB activation, as viable target for otherwise chemoresistant tumors [68]

Curcumin, a natural phenol that is present in turmeric has been shown to sensitize tumor cells to several anti-cancer drugs via modulation of NF-κB and histone deacetylase. Curcumin suppresses activation of NF-κB through IkB kinase (IKK) activity inhibition [69]. In a xenograft model, curcumin plus paclitaxel significantly suppressed the incidence of breast cancer metastasis in lung tissue, and also demonstrated in these lung tissues was the reduction of the p65 subunit of NF-κB [70]. By combining compounds which can either directly or indirectly inhibit the NF-KB signaling pathway concomitant with chemotherapy, the resulting synergistic treatment may allow lower doses of the toxic chemotherapeutic agents to be used, improving patient responses [71]. These data help to demonstrate that down regulation of the NF-κB pathway could lead to the tumor cells

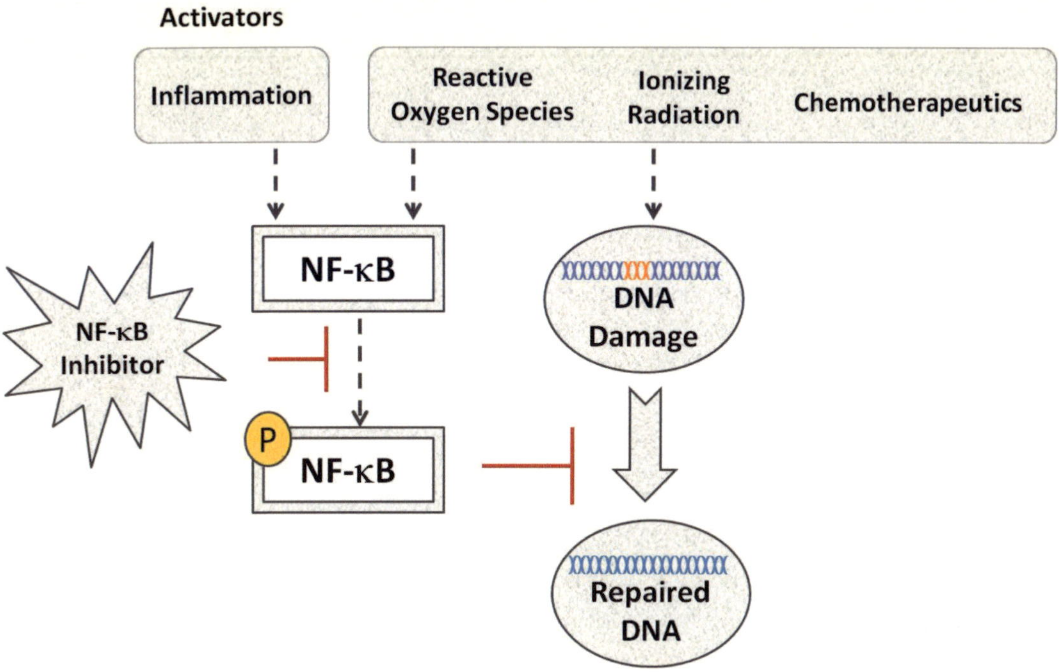

Figure 3. Model showing the effects of NF-κB on DNA damage and repair

becoming more susceptible to current chemotherapies, and allow for lower doses of these therapies, leading to better patient outcomes.

8. Summary: The regulation of DNA damage and DNA repair by NF-κB

Skin is under continuous assault from a variety of damaging environmental factors including ultraviolet irradiation and atmospheric pollutants. Extrinsic factors, particularly sunlight, have been demonstrated to accelerate the intrinsic aging process by increasing free radical production and decreasing antioxidant protections which can result in DNA damage and can affect the repair of damaged DNA. The age-related accumulation of somatic damage is worsened by sun exposure, leading to an increased incidence of skin disorders, skin cancer and potentially skin aging. New findings on the molecular mechanisms involved in the regulation of DNA damage and the subsequent repair of damaged DNA in the skin can help identify new targets to modulate DNA repair activity and thereby have a significant effect on skin physiology. The NF-κB pathway is a key regulator of inflammatory mediators in skin cells and has been reported to be the final common pathway for the conversion of environmental insults into inflammation in the skin. Through the ability to regulate processes that result in increased DNA damage and decrease the repair of damaged DNA, the NF-κB pathway may be a primary pathway linking inflammation and DNA damage.

Pharmacological inhibition of NF-κB therefore may provide protection to skin from the numerous external aggressions encountered daily and reduce the DNA damage to oxidatively challenged and aging skin by increasing endogenous DNA repair processes.

Acknowledgements

The authors would like to thank Dr. Paul Khavari (Department of Dermatology, Stanford University) and Hélène Wong (Johnson and Johnson) for discussions on NF-κB regulation and DNA Damage

Author details

Simarna Kaur[1], Thierry Oddos[2], Samantha Tucker-Samaras[1] and Michael D. Southall[1]

1 Johnson & Johnson Skin Research Center, CPPW, a Division of Johnson & Johnson Consumer Companies, Inc. Skillman, New Jersey, USA

2 Johnson & Johnson Skin Research Center, CPPW, a Division of Johnson & Johnson Consumer Companies, Inc. Skillman, New Jersey, France

References

[1] Patrick, M.H., Studies on thymine-derived UV photoproducts in DNA--I. Formation and biological role of pyrimidine adducts in DNA. Photochem Photobiol, 1977. 25(4): p. 357-72.

[2] Johnson & Johnson Santé Beauté France. Campus de Maigrement 27100 Val de Reul. France

[3] Berquist, B.R. and D.M. Wilson, 3rd, Pathways for repairing and tolerating the spectrum of oxidative DNA lesions. Cancer Lett.

[4] Hanawalt, P.C., Subpathways of nucleotide excision repair and their regulation. Oncogene, 2002. 21(58): p. 8949-56.

[5] Dogliotti, E., et al., The mechanism of switching among multiple BER pathways. Prog Nucleic Acid Res Mol Biol, 2001. 68: p. 3-27.

[6] Mitra, S., et al., Complexities of the DNA base excision repair pathway for repair of oxidative DNA damage. Environ Mol Mutagen, 2001. 38(2-3): p. 180-90.

[7] Li, X. and W.D. Heyer, Homologous recombination in DNA repair and DNA damage tolerance. Cell Res, 2008. 18(1): p. 99-113.

[8] Kleijer, W.J., et al., Incidence of DNA repair deficiency disorders in western Europe: Xeroderma pigmentosum, Cockayne syndrome and trichothiodystrophy. DNA Repair (Amst), 2008. 7(5): p. 744-50.

[9] Robbins, J.H., et al., Xeroderma pigmentosum. An inherited diseases with sun sensitivity, multiple cutaneous neoplasms, and abnormal DNA repair. Ann Intern Med, 1974. 80(2): p. 221-48.

[10] Lehmann, A.R., D. McGibbon, and M. Stefanini, Xeroderma pigmentosum. Orphanet J Rare Dis. 6: p. 70.

[11] Bender, K., et al., Sequential DNA damage-independent and -dependent activation of NF-kappaB by UV. EMBO J, 1998. 17(17): p. 5170-81.

[12] Mabb, A.M., S.M. Wuerzberger-Davis, and S. Miyamoto, PIASy mediates NEMO sumoylation and NF-kappaB activation in response to genotoxic stress. Nat Cell Biol, 2006. 8(9): p. 986-93.

[13] McCool, K.W. and S. Miyamoto, DNA damage-dependent NF-kappaB activation: NEMO turns nuclear signaling inside out. Immunol Rev. 246(1): p. 311-26.

[14] Piret, B., S. Schoonbroodt, and J. Piette, The ATM protein is required for sustained activation of NF-kappaB following DNA damage. Oncogene, 1999. 18(13): p. 2261-71.

[15] Kripke, M.L., et al., Pyrimidine dimers in DNA initiate systemic immunosuppression in UV-irradiated mice. Proc Natl Acad Sci U S A, 1992. 89(16): p. 7516-20.

[16] Niedernhofer, L.J., Tissue-specific accelerated aging in nucleotide excision repair deficiency. Mech Ageing Dev, 2008. 129(7-8): p. 408-15.

[17] Nouspikel, T., DNA repair in mammalian cells : Nucleotide excision repair: variations on versatility. Cell Mol Life Sci, 2009. 66(6): p. 994-1009.

[18] Abdel-Malek, Z.A., et al., alpha-MSH tripeptide analogs activate the melanocortin 1 receptor and reduce UV-induced DNA damage in human melanocytes. Pigment Cell Melanoma Res, 2009. 22(5): p. 635-44.

[19] Dong, L., et al., Melanocyte-stimulating hormone directly enhances UV-Induced DNA repair in keratinocytes by a xeroderma pigmentosum group A-dependent mechanism. Cancer Res. 70(9): p. 3547-56.

[20] Chen, L., et al., Eradication of murine bladder carcinoma by intratumor injection of a bicistronic adenoviral vector carrying cDNAs for the IL-12 heterodimer and its inhibition by the IL-12 p40 subunit homodimer. J Immunol, 1997. 159(1): p. 351-9.

[21] Meeran, S.M., et al., Interleukin-12-deficient mice are at greater risk of UV radiation-induced skin tumors and malignant transformation of papillomas to carcinomas. Mol Cancer Ther, 2006. 5(4): p. 825-32.

[22] Nastala, C.L., et al., Recombinant IL-12 administration induces tumor regression in association with IFN-gamma production. J Immunol, 1994. 153(4): p. 1697-706.

[23] Siders, W.M., et al., T cell- and NK cell-independent inhibition of hepatic metastases by systemic administration of an IL-12-expressing recombinant adenovirus. J Immunol, 1998. 160(11): p. 5465-74.

[24] Piao, M.J., et al., Silver nanoparticles down-regulate Nrf2-mediated 8-oxoguanine DNA glycosylase 1 through inactivation of extracellular regulated kinase and protein kinase B in human Chang liver cells. Toxicol Lett. 207(2): p. 143-8.

[25] Huang, T.T. and A.D. D'Andrea, Regulation of DNA repair by ubiquitylation. Nat Rev Mol Cell Biol, 2006. 7(5): p. 323-34.

[26] Sen, R. and D. Baltimore, Inducibility of kappa immunoglobulin enhancer-binding protein Nf-kappa B by a posttranslational mechanism. Cell, 1986. 47(6): p. 921-8.

[27] Karin, M., Nuclear factor-kappaB in cancer development and progression. Nature, 2006. 441(7092): p. 431-6.

[28] Baeuerle, P.A. and D. Baltimore, NF-kappa B: ten years after. Cell, 1996. 87(1): p. 13-20.

[29] Karin, M. and Y. Ben-Neriah, Phosphorylation meets ubiquitination: the control of NF-[kappa]B activity. Annu Rev Immunol, 2000. 18: p. 621-63.

[30] Baeuerle, P.A. and V.R. Baichwal, NF-kappa B as a frequent target for immunosuppressive and anti-inflammatory molecules. Adv Immunol, 1997. 65: p. 111-37.

[31] Bowie, A. and L.A. O'Neill, The interleukin-1 receptor/Toll-like receptor superfamily: signal generators for pro-inflammatory interleukins and microbial products. J Leukoc Biol, 2000. 67(4): p. 508-14.

[32] Lu, Y., et al., Role of nuclear factor-kappaB in interleukin-1-induced collagen degradation by corneal fibroblasts. Exp Eye Res, 2006. 83(3): p. 560-8.

[33] Okamoto, T., et al., Regulation of NF-kappa B and disease control: identification of a novel serine kinase and thioredoxin as effectors for signal transduction pathway for NF-kappa B activation. Curr Top Cell Regul, 1997. 35: p. 149-61.

[34] Pahl, H.L., Activators and target genes of Rel/NF-kappaB transcription factors. Oncogene, 1999. 18(49): p. 6853-66.

[35] Baumann, L., Cosmetic dermatology : principles and practice. 2002, New York: McGraw-Hill. xii, 226 p.

[36] Habraken, Y. and J. Piette, NF-kappaB activation by double-strand breaks. Biochem Pharmacol, 2006. 72(9): p. 1132-41.

[37] Brach, M.A., et al., Ionizing radiation induces expression and binding activity of the nuclear factor kappa B. J Clin Invest, 1991. 88(2): p. 691-5.

[38] Wang, J., et al., RelA/p65 functions to maintain cellular senescence by regulating genomic stability and DNA repair. EMBO Rep, 2009. 10(11): p. 1272-8.

[39] Seitz, C.S., et al., Alterations in NF-kappaB function in transgenic epithelial tissue demonstrate a growth inhibitory role for NF-kappaB. Proc Natl Acad Sci U S A, 1998. 95(5): p. 2307-12.

[40] Zhang, J.Y., et al., CDK4 regulation by TNFR1 and JNK is required for NF-kappaB-mediated epidermal growth control. J Cell Biol, 2005. 168(4): p. 561-6.

[41] Brzoska, K. and I. Szumiel, Signalling loops and linear pathways: NF-kappaB activation in response to genotoxic stress. Mutagenesis, 2009. 24(1): p. 1-8.

[42] Halazonetis, T.D., V.G. Gorgoulis, and J. Bartek, An oncogene-induced DNA damage model for cancer development. Science, 2008. 319(5868): p. 1352-5.

[43] Li, Y., et al., The repressive effect of NF-kappaB on p53 by mot-2 is involved in human keratinocyte transformation induced by low levels of arsenite. Toxicol Sci. 116(1): p. 174-82.

[44] Guha Mazumder, D.N., et al., Arsenic levels in drinking water and the prevalence of skin lesions in West Bengal, India. Int J Epidemiol, 1998. 27(5): p. 871-7.

[45] Hartwig, A., et al., Modulation of DNA repair processes by arsenic and selenium compounds. Toxicology, 2003. 193(1-2): p. 161-9.

[46] Matsui, M., et al., The role of oxidative DNA damage in human arsenic carcinogenesis: detection of 8-hydroxy-2'-deoxyguanosine in arsenic-related Bowen's disease. J Invest Dermatol, 1999. 113(1): p. 26-31.

[47] Volcic, M., et al., NF-kappaB regulates DNA double-strand break repair in conjunction with BRCA1-CtIP complexes. Nucleic Acids Res. 40(1): p. 181-95.

[48] Wu, K., et al., Induction of the BRCA2 promoter by nuclear factor-kappa B. J Biol Chem, 2000. 275(45): p. 35548-56.

[49] De Siervi, A., et al., Identification of new Rel/NFkappaB regulatory networks by focused genome location analysis. Cell Cycle, 2009. 8(13): p. 2093-100.

[50] Mayo, M.W., et al., Requirement of NF-kappaB activation to suppress p53-independent apoptosis induced by oncogenic Ras. Science, 1997. 278(5344): p. 1812-5.

[51] Wu, H. and G. Lozano, NF-kappa B activation of p53. A potential mechanism for suppressing cell growth in response to stress. J Biol Chem, 1994. 269(31): p. 20067-74.

[52] Schneider, G. and O.H. Kramer, NFkappaB/p53 crosstalk-a promising new therapeutic target. Biochim Biophys Acta. 1815(1): p. 90-103.

[53] Guo, W., et al., The protective effects of hydroxytyrosol against UVB-induced DNA damage in HaCaT cells. Phytother Res. 24(3): p. 352-9.

[54] Marwaha, V., et al., T-oligo treatment decreases constitutive and UVB-induced COX-2 levels through p53- and NFkappaB-dependent repression of the COX-2 promoter. J Biol Chem, 2005. 280(37): p. 32379-88.

[55] Puszynski, K., R. Bertolusso, and T. Lipniacki, Crosstalk between p53 and nuclear factor-B systems: pro- and anti-apoptotic functions of NF-B. IET Syst Biol, 2009. 3(5): p. 356-67.

[56] Thyss, R., et al., NF-kappaB/Egr-1/Gadd45 are sequentially activated upon UVB irradiation to mediate epidermal cell death. EMBO J, 2005. 24(1): p. 128-37.

[57] Dekker, P., et al., Stress-induced responses of human skin fibroblasts in vitro reflect human longevity. Aging Cell, 2009. 8(5): p. 595-603.

[58] Dumas, M., et al., In vitro biosynthesis of type I and III collagens by human dermal fibroblasts from donors of increasing age. Mech Ageing Dev, 1994. 73(3): p. 179-87.

[59] Millau, J.F., et al., A microarray to measure repair of damaged plasmids by cell lysates. Lab Chip, 2008. 8(10): p. 1713-22.

[60] Guerniou, V., et al., Repair of oxidative damage of thymine by HeLa whole-cell extracts: simultaneous analysis using a microsupport and comparison with traditional PAGE analysis. Biochimie, 2005. 87(2): p. 151-9.

[61] Sauvaigo, S., et al., DNA repair capacities of cutaneous fibroblasts: effect of sun exposure, age and smoking on response to an acute oxidative stress. Br J Dermatol, 2007. 157(1): p. 26-32.

[62] Pons, B., et al., Age-associated modifications of Base Excision Repair activities in human skin fibroblast extracts. Mech Ageing Dev. 131(11-12): p. 661-5.

[63] Sauvaigo, S., et al., Effect of aging on DNA excision/synthesis repair capacities of human skin fibroblasts. J Invest Dermatol. 130(6): p. 1739-41.

[64] Bigot, N., et al., NF-kappaB Accumulation Associated with COL1A1 Transactivators Defects during Chronological Aging Represses Type I Collagen Expression through a -112/-61-bp Region of the COL1A1 Promoter in Human Skin Fibroblasts. J Invest Dermatol.

[65] Murray, S., et al., Taxane resistance in breast cancer: Mechanisms, predictive biomarkers and circumvention strategies. Cancer Treat Rev.

[66] Wang, C.Y., et al., Control of inducible chemoresistance: enhanced anti-tumor therapy through increased apoptosis by inhibition of NF-kappaB. Nat Med, 1999. 5(4): p. 412-7.

[67] Ruckhaberle, E., et al., Microarray analysis of altered sphingolipid metabolism reveals prognostic significance of sphingosine kinase 1 in breast cancer. Breast Cancer Res Treat, 2008. 112(1): p. 41-52.

[68] Xia, P., et al., Tumor necrosis factor-alpha induces adhesion molecule expression through the sphingosine kinase pathway. Proc Natl Acad Sci U S A, 1998. 95(24): p. 14196-201.

[69] Antoon, J.W., et al., Targeting NFkB mediated breast cancer chemoresistance through selective inhibition of sphingosine kinase-2. Cancer Biol Ther. 11(7): p. 678-89.

[70] Jobin, C., et al., Curcumin blocks cytokine-mediated NF-kappa B activation and proinflammatory gene expression by inhibiting inhibitory factor I-kappa B kinase activity. J Immunol, 1999. 163(6): p. 3474-83.

[71] Aggarwal, B.B., et al., Curcumin suppresses the paclitaxel-induced nuclear factor-kappaB pathway in breast cancer cells and inhibits lung metastasis of human breast cancer in nude mice. Clin Cancer Res, 2005. 11(20): p. 7490-8.

[72] Royt, M., et al., Curcumin sensitizes chemotherapeutic drugs via modulation of PKC, telomerase, NF-kappaB and HDAC in breast cancer. Ther Deliv. 2(10): p. 1275-93.

Section 2

Interface with Replication, Transcription, Telomeres, and Cell Cycle Regulation

Chapter 9

Relation of the Types of DNA Damage to Replication Stress and the Induction of Premature Chromosome Condensation

Dorota Rybaczek and
Magdalena Kowalewicz-Kulbat

Additional information is available at the end of the chapter

http://dx.doi.org/10.5772/54020

1. Introduction

Any integrated view of the diversity of biochemical reactions involved in the faithful replication of eukaryotic chromosomes and their accurate mitotic segregation is not possible without careful consideration of the molecular mechanisms that are responsible for repairing damaged DNA. In order to arrange and order the sequence of events, in which the various levels of organization are only stages of the same molecular pathway, there is a need for both a timely switching on of numerous genes and the precise cooperation of large numbers of proteins. An important clue concerning the nature of the competitive interaction between these different elements comes from looking at the response to DNA damage.

The present chapter is a review of the types of DNA damage generated under stressful conditions and experimental approaches to the relation of these types of DNA damage to hydroxyurea treatment and caffeine-induced premature chromosome condensation (PCC). In this chapter, an attempt is also made to explain the molecular base of DNA damage and to present experimental procedures allowing the illustration of DNA damages at the cell level, especially with the use of histochemical and immunocytochemical methods. It will be experimentally shown, among others, that replication stress mainly leads to the generation of double-strand breaks in DNA (DSBs), while the breakage of restrictive interactions of checkpoints during PCC induction results in the accumulation of single-strand breaks (SSBs).

2. The types and molecular base of DNA damage

DNA can be damaged by the action of endogenous (intrinsic) or exogenous (extrinsic) stress factors. The endogenous factors include, among others, errors generated during replication and reactive oxygen species (ROS). The exogenous (environmental) factors are divided into (i) physical factors, e.g. UV and ionizing radiation (X, γ); (ii) chemical factors, i.e. mutagenic polycyclic aromatic hydrocarbons (PAH), nitrosamines, dioxins, analogues of bases and alkylating agents; and (iii) biological factors, such as viruses.

Stress-induced damage includes spontaneous depurination and deamination, oxidation, formation of DNA adducts induced by alkylating agents, formation of cyclobutane dimers, single- and double-strand damage, as well as errors made during replication, repair, reverse transcription and recombination. DNA is also subject to covalent modifications that may affect nitrogen bases and lead to changes in base pairing between DNA strands, or even entirely preventing base pairing. Genomic instability may also be associated with chromosomal rearrangements which result from changes that occur in the *trans* position (including replication, DNA repair and S phase checkpoint pathways) or from changes that act in the *cis* position, i.e. in the regions of chromosomal instability, known as hotspots, for example breaks or fragile sites and highly transcribed DNA sequences (Aguilera & Gómez-González, 2008).

Plants, due to their 'settled' lifestyles are exposed to many environmental factors that cause disturbances in the cell cycle. They are often threatened by excessive salinity, drought, extreme low or high temperatures, as well as fungal or bacterial infections (Vashisht & Tuteja, 2006). Each of these burdens leads to the mobilization of defense responses: (1) activation of cell cycle checkpoints and DNA repair factors, (2) inhibition of cell growth, or (3) initiation of the apoptosis pathway (Deckert et al., 2009 and references therein).

Recognition of double-stranded breaks depends on the MRN complex (Mre11-Rad50-Nbs1), necessary for binding chromatin-remodeling factors (Schiller et al., 2012). MRN complex acts as a stabilizing platform for broken endings of DNA molecules. It binds to the sites of damage and ATM kinase, and promotes phosphorylation of histone H2A (H2AX-Ser139) and the processing of DNA. Processing of ends can either rely on their alignment, necessary to continue the connection through the induction of non-homologous end joining, or long single-stranded fragments for homologous recombination. Eukaryotic organisms use many types of DNA repair: (i) 3'-5' exonuclease activity of DNA polymerase; (ii) reversion repair (RR); (iii) mismatch repair (MMR); (iv) base excision repair (BER); (v) nucleotide excision repair (NER), (vi) non-homologous end joining (NHEJ); (vii) homologous recombination (HR); (viii) translesion synthesis (TLS). The methods also include: photoreactivation; methylguanine methyltransferase (MGMT), catalyzing the reaction of demethylation of methylated guanine bases; double strand break repair (DSBR); synthesis-dependent strand annealing (SDSA) and break-induced replication (BIR).

3. Replication stress and activation of checkpoint signaling pathways

Under the conditions of replication stress, the rate of DNA synthesis is slowed down and the possibility of entry into mitosis is blocked until the expression of specific genes and activation of repair factors. The control over DNA synthesis then involves a system of intra-S phase checkpoint, activated after the detection of DNA damage - in particular double strand breaks (DSBs) or single-strand breaks (SSBs) [Figure 1; (Bartek et al., 2004; Osborn et al., 2002; comp. Rybaczek & Kowalewicz-Kulbat, 2011)].

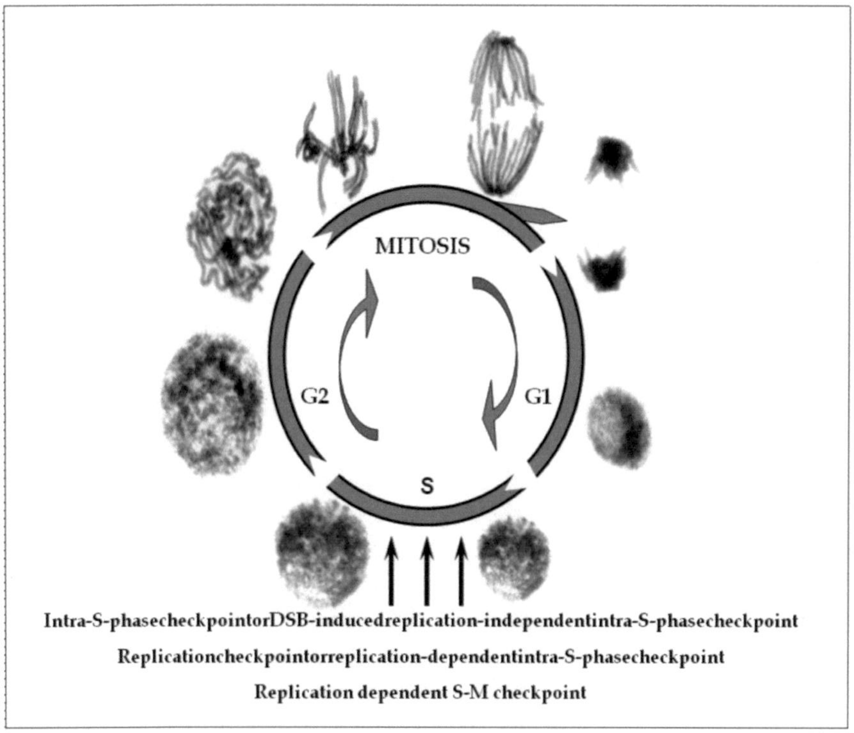

Figure 1. The three major S-phase checkpoints within the cell cycle

Further stages of the cell cycle are blocked until the repair of detected damage (Adamsen et al., 2011; Herrick & Bensimon, 2008). It has also been shown that any disruption of structural nature (e.g. DSB or SSB) induces a slowdown in the replication fork movement and further DNA damage, e.g. through the influence of replication inhibitors, may result in total inhibition of the cycle in the intra-S phase checkpoint (Blow & Hodgson, 2002; Elledge, 1996). Then checkpoint sensory factors trigger a signal transduction cascade, delivering a signal of DNA damage to effector proteins via transmitters (Mordes & Cortez, 2008; Nojima, 2006).

Thus, the detection of DSBs activates an ATM-dependent pathway (*Ataxia Telangiectasia Mutated*) and a slightly more slowly activated parallel ATR-dependent pathway (*Ataxia Telan-*

giectasia mutated – Rad3-related). The target substrate for both these sensory kinases is Cdc25 phosphatase (Cortez, 2003). The function of ATR kinase is not limited solely to the transmission of signals in response to DNA double breaks in the S phase checkpoint. This enzyme is activated during each S phase and plays an active role in regulating the initiation of DNA replication under physiological conditions. In addition, it is involved in the recognition of single-stranded DNA molecules (ssDNA; Shechter et al., 2004). ATR occurs in a durable complex with ATR-interacting protein (ATRIP), focusing in the area of the nucleus in regions corresponding to the sites of DNA damage (Myers et al., 2007). Research carried out on cytoplasmic extracts of *Xenopus* oocytes revealed that ATR associates with chromatin during DNA replication, and dissociates after its completion (Freire et al., 2006; Harper & Elledge, 2007; reviewed by Marheineke & Hyrien, 2004). The association of ATR and DNA breaks is also a result of the elimination of the replication factor A (RPA), while its appearance is independent of the presence of α-type DNA polymerase. Therefore it seems that the "recruitment" of ATR occurs after a partial generation of replication forks in the *origin* region, but before Polα association (Luciani et al., 2004; Namiki & Zaou, 2006; Zou & Elledge, 2003). Although ATR-ATRIP complexes can bind to certain DNA structures, their participation in the activation of cell responses to replication stress is not possible without the participation of two other factors: replication factor C (RFC) and proliferating-cell-nuclear-antigen-like proteins (PCNA-like). During replication, RFC recognizes the binding sites between primers/starters of RNA and DNA matrix and assembles PCNA, a toroidal homotrimer protein encircling DNA – also known as a "sliding clamp" which determines the processivity of the related DNA polymerases (Majka & Burgers, 2004; Tan et al., 2012). In the cells of *S. pombe*, Rad17 (RFC1 factor and four small subunits RFC2-5) and Rad9/Hus1/Rad1 (PCNA-like 9-1-1 complex), participate not only in the functional organization of the intra-S phase checkpoint, but also other cell cycle checkpoints whose function is to monitor the structural DNA damage [e.g. G2 (Majka et al., 2006, reviewed by Lin & Dutta, 2007)]. Recruitment of PCNA-like complexes to the sites of DNA damage in a molecule is, perhaps, independent of the activation of ATR and Chk1 (Niimi et al., 2008; Scorah et al., 2008), but is an important element of the mechanism signaling the appearance of structural disorders. In the cells of *S. pombe* and in mammals, Rad17 and Hus1 are factors determining the possibility of phosphorylation of Chk1 kinase by ATR. Rad17 is also a substrate of ATR. Although both these proteins bind to chromatin in intact cells, phosphorylation of Rad17 by ATR significantly increases with the increasing volume of PCNA-like complexes, following the occurrence of DNA conformational disorders. It therefore appears that the first stage of the then triggered signaling pathway is the independent localization of Rad17 and ATR-ATRIP complexes in the regions of damage; the next stage is a Rad17-dependent assembly of PCNA-like complexes around the DNA. PCNA-like complexes enable the activation of ATR molecules and - consequently - the phosphorylation of ATR substrates located within chromatin, such as Rad17 and Rad9 (Majka et al., 2006; Niida & Nakanishi, 2006). In addition to ATM and ATR kinases in humans, and their homologues in yeast cells, the PIKK family of signaling proteins includes also DNA-dependent protein kinase (DNA-PK). This enzyme consists of a DNA-PK catalytic subunit (DNA-PKCS,) and a heterodimeric subunit Ku70-Ku80. DNA-PKCS is a DNA-dependent serine-threonine kinase, showing a relatively weak ability to bind to DNA free ends; however, this affinity is enhanced and stabilizes under the influence of heterodimer Ku70-Ku80. It is believed that DNA-PK participates primarily in the repair of double-strand breaks (DSBs) by non-homologous end-joining [NHEJ (Müller et al., 2007; Pawelczak & Turchi, 2008; Shimura et al., 2007)].

Replication protein A (RPA) binds to all single-strand DNAs in the nucleus, including the parts of ssDNA formed during DNA replication and repair (Costanzo et al., 2003). The association of RPA and ssDNA (RPA-ssDNA) is an important component of signaling and the place to which the ATR molecule binds (this mechanism occurs both in human cells and in *S. cerevisiae*; Zou & Elledge, 2003). However, recognition of RPA-ssDNA structures and recruitment of other proteins to these complexes occur through the activity of ATRIP which occurs in conjunction with the ATR kinase. Biochemical studies indicate that ATRIP binds to the N-terminal part of the large subunit of RPA via its conserved acidic alpha-helix domain (Ball et al., 2007). The RPA-ssDNA complex is not a sufficient stimulus for binding the ATR-ATRIP complex and does not activate ATR. The induction and transmission of the signal "down" depends on ATR-ATRIP interaction with another protein complex, i.e. 9-1-1, which recognizes the DNA end adjacent to the RPA-coated ssDNA. The 9-1-1 complex is also responsible for recruiting TopBP1 protein, the main activator of ATR-ATRIP complex in the cells of vertebrates (Kumagai et al., 2006). In addition, the RPA-ssDNA platform recruits RAD17 and claspin, proteins strongly interacting with ATR, leading to the phosphorylation of ATR substrates, including Chk1 kinase (Bartek et al., 2004). Thus the presence of RPA is crucial for the specific recruitment of signaling factors to the 5' end of the damaged DNA (Ellison & Stillman, 2003). In this case, it is single-strand DNA fragments that are responsible for the activation of the checkpoint. Structures of this type are generated as a result of impaired DNA polymerase activity during replication, during the formation of double strand DNA breaks, at the ends of telomeres, and even during DNA repair via nucleotide excision. All of these factors activate the ATR kinase to recruit repair proteins (Byun et al., 2005; Cimprich & Cortez, 2008; Nedelcheva et al., 2005). Recent studies have shown that for the effective recruitment and signaling in response to DNA damage, ATR kinase requires continuous cooperation with its sister sensory ATM kinase, showing some similarity in structure and function (Cimprich & Cortez, 2008). These kinases also share phosphorylation substrates, e.g. H2AX histones (Burma et al., 2001; Ward & Chen, 2001).

4. Premature chromosome condensation and overriding of cell cycle checkpoint

The initiation of mitotic chromosome condensation in normal cells is preceded by the completion of all processes related to DNA replication and repair of abnormal DNA structures generated during the S phase. The main task of the checkpoint in G2 phase is to block cell entry into mitosis in the event of an anomaly in the genetic material. The common elements of the biochemical pathway that control the G2/M transition and of the S-phase checkpoint, are ATM and ATR kinases, and their role is to maintain the MPF complex, i.e. M-phase promoting factor (CDK1 kinase with cyclin B) in an inactive state

(Raleigh & Connell, 2000). Both in animal cells and in yeast, the activation of the CDK2-cyclin B complex, induced by phosphatase Cdc25, is a necessary condition for the initiation of mitotic chromosome condensation. The activation of ATM and ATR kinases during the G2 phase causes a cascade of phosphorylation. Similar to DNA replication, the substrates of these sensory kinases are the kinases Chk2 (for ATM) and Chk1 (for ATR). Chk1 kinase (active form) phosphorylates Cdc25 phosphatase by blocking its enzymatic activity (Cdc25 is then not able to carry out the activating dephosphorylation of CDK1 kinase; De Veylder et al., 2003). Phosphorylation of the phosphatase Cdc25 can lead to its degradation through ubiquitin-dependent proteolysis, or to association with 14-3-3 protein and consequently to its removal from the nucleus (Boutros et al., 2006). At the same time, ATM and ATR kinases induce gene expression of Wee1 kinase (responsible for blocking cell cycle progression in G2 phase), thus gaining the time required to repair defective DNA structures. Probably, the activation of Wee1 kinase also involves the activity of kinases Chk1 and Chk2 (De Schutter et al., 2007). In animal cells, ATM kinase also activates the p53 pathway. This factor is involved, among others, in the regulation of responses to replication stress, altered DNA structure, oxidative stress and osmotic shock, and disturbances in the integrity of cell membranes. Because of its multiple functions in cell cycle regulation, p53 has been termed 'the guardian of the genome' (Han et al., 2008).

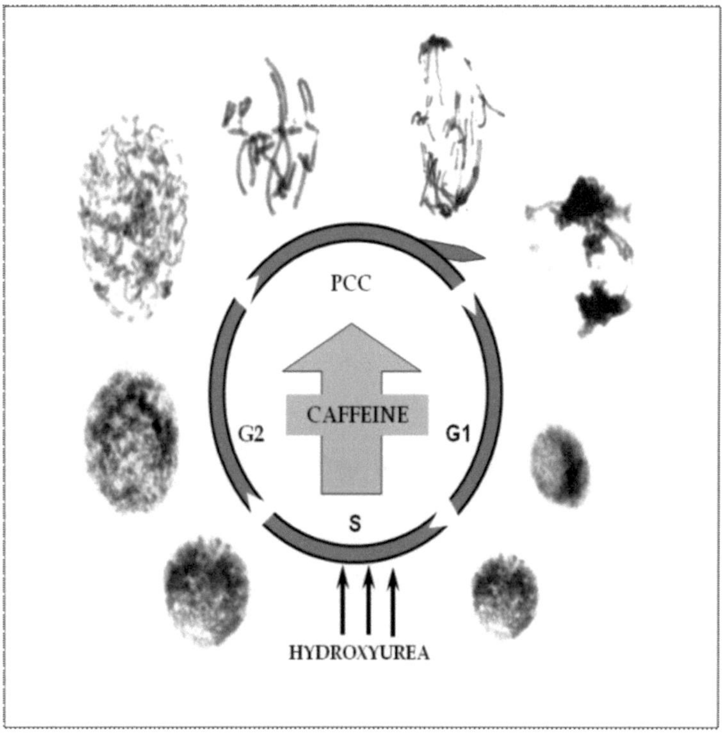

Figure 2. Overview of the induction of premature chromosome condensation (PCC)

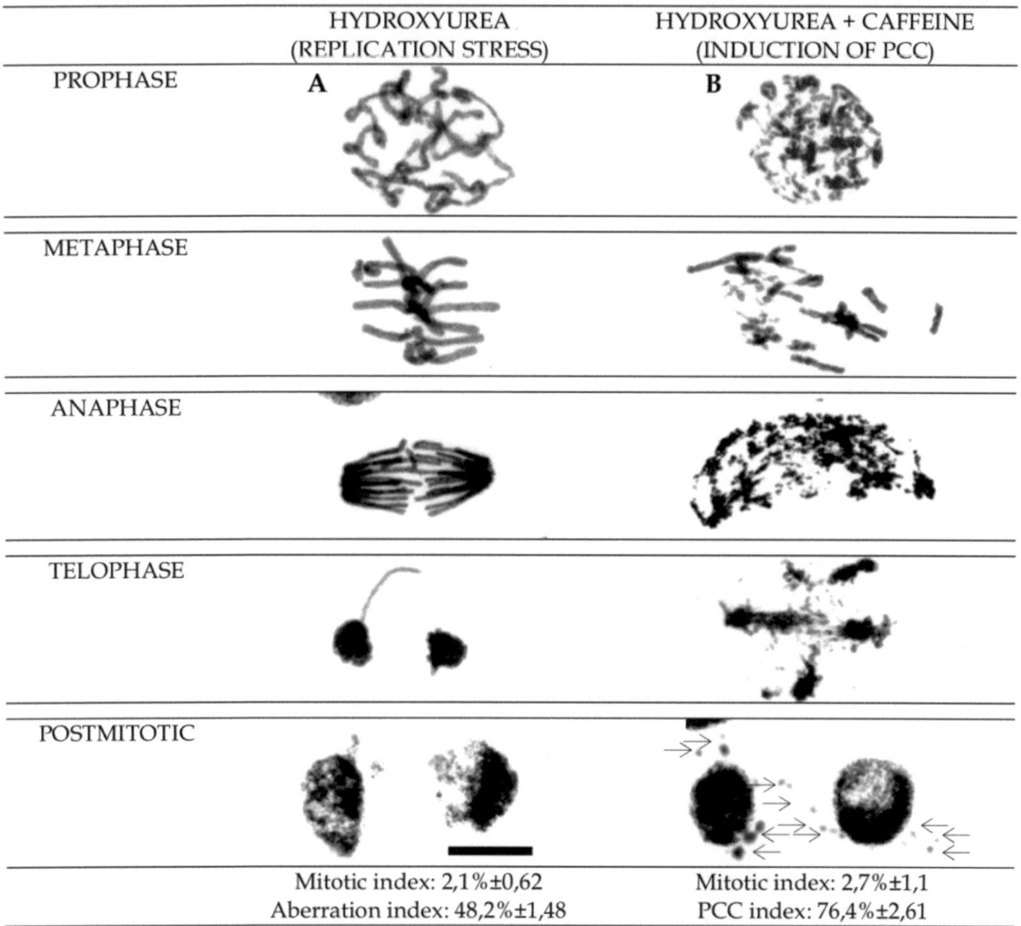

Figure 3. Feulgen-stained root meristem cells of *Vicia faba*: (A) hydroxyurea-treated (2.5 mM, 24 h); (B) caffeine-induced PCC (2.5 mM HU for 24 h $\rightarrow$ the mixture of 2.5 mM HU and 5 mM CF for 8 h). The array of aberrations in serie 'A' included a relatively small number of breakpoints per cell nucleus ($\leq$ 5). The full array of aberrations ($\geq$ 25 per cell nucleus) in serie 'B' included chromosomal breaks, irregular condensation/decondensation of chromatin, lost and lagging chromatids and chromosomes as well as segregation defects. Micronucleus formation (arrows), were found significantly increased in comparison either with the control or HU treatment (comp. Rybaczek & Kowalewicz-Kulbat, 2011; Rybaczek et al., 2008). The mitotic index was calculated as the percent ratio between the number of dividing cells and the entire meristematic cell population. Index of aberrations was calculated as the percent ratio between the number of cells showing chromosome aberrations and all mitotic cells. PCC index was calculated as the percent ratio between the number of cells showing chromosome aberrations typical of premature mitosis and all mitotic cells. Experimental procedure of Feulgen staining: root tips were fixed in cold absolute ethanol and glacial acetic acid (3:1, v/v) for 1 h, washed several times with ethanol, rehydrated, hydrolysed in 4 M HCl (1.5 h), and stained with Schiff's reagent (pararosaniline; Sigma-Aldrich) according to standard methods. After rinsing in SO_2-water (3 times) and distilled water, 1.5 mm long apical segments were cut off, placed in a drop of 45% acetic acid, and squashed onto microscope slides. Following freezing with dry ice, coverslips were removed and the dehydrated dry slides were embedded in Canada Baume. Slides were analysed under the light microscope to count mitotic cells that had characteristic features of either normal mitosis or PCC. *Bar* 20 µm

In a cell there are also mechanisms responsible for DNA damage tolerance (DDT), which allow the completion of the replication of genetic material despite the damage to DNA that blocks replicase complex. In addition, disruption of the efficiency of the intra-S phase checkpoint, following the action of chemical agents, leads to the induction of premature chromosome condensation (PCC; Figure 2), specifically via overriding of the control over the stability of the genome, even despite the uncompleted S phase and not implemented post-replication repair processes in G2 phase (Figure 3A). The successive phases of prematurely initiated mitosis follow an aberration course because the unreplicated regions of the genome are manifested in the form of losses or breaks in chromosomes [(Figure 3B) comp. Rybaczek et al., 2008; Rybaczek, 2011]. Caffeine (CF) is a particularly effective PCC inducer. It blocks the activity of kinases ATM/ATR (Cortez, 2003), by which they can not phosphorylate their downstream kinases (i.e. Chk1 and Chk2; Rybaczek & Kowalewicz-Kulbat, 2011; Rybaczek et al., 2007) and, consequently, catalytic activity of Cdc25 phosphatases is maintained - phosphatases which serve as inducers of complexes CDK1-cyclin B (MPF; M-phase Promoting Factor) and trigger mitotic phosphorylations (Gotoh & Durante, 2006; Rybaczek & Kowalewicz-Kulbat, 2011).

The overriding of the checkpoint function induced by the action of caffeine leads to the selective sensibilization of pro-oncogenic cells deprived of p53 protein and tumorous cells to the action of antineoplastic factors and the effect of ionizing radiation (Yao et al. 1996). The test results obtained by Wang and co-workers (1999) show that the effectiveness disturbance of the S-M control system induced by caffeine in *S. pombe* cells is connected with the activation of Cdc2 kinase (due to the removal of phosphate group from Tyr15 within the ATP-binding pocket) and with the septation process that during a normal course of cell cycle of *S. pombe* results from the transfer through mitosis.

5. Labeling of DNA damages following hydroxyurea-induced stress and caffeine-induced premature chromosome condensation

One of the basic protective mechanisms of the replicative apparatus are foci concentrating molecules of phosphorylated histones H2AX (Rybaczek & Maszewski, 2007a; Rybaczek & Maszewski, 2007b). The generation of γ-H2AX molecules as a result of exposure to stressors is a rapid process. Half of the γ-H2AX histones appear as early as after 1 min of irradiation and a maximum level is reached with 3 to 10 minutes of exposure; then, in terms of 1 Gy radiation, γ-phosphorylation concerns approximately 1% of histone H2AX molecules, which is equivalent to about $2x10^6$ base pairs of DNA in the region of the double-strand break (DSB). It is assumed that each grouping of these molecules determines a single DSB region (Paull et al., 2000; Rogakou et al., 1998). Phosphorylated histone H2AX binds cohesin and chromatin-modifying complex NuA4. The acetylation of histones follows, which allows connection of the INO80 complex, which removes histones in the area of the damaged DNA, thereby creating single-strand regions. This greatly simplifies the recruitment of proteins of the pathway of response to DNA damage and repair proteins. Then TIP60 complex is connected, followed by the removal of dimers H2AX/H2B and insertion of non-phosphorylated histone H2A, and thus switching off the signal of the DNA structure checkpoint and - after the completion of repair - restoration of the correct chromatin structure. The results of testing using antibodies recognizing phosphorylated histone H2AX (α-H2AX^{S139}) - microscopic images of immunofluorescence in meristematic root cells of *Allium porum, Vicia faba, Raphanus sativum,* and HeLa cells, and strong signals obtained using a Western blot – provide, above all, the next example of homology of organization of cellular systems in animals and plants - the similarities in their structural elements, systems, and hence, similarities of biochemical regulatory mechanisms (Rybaczek & Kowalewicz-Kulbat, 2011; Rybaczek & Maszewski, 2007a). Our studies have shown that a significant level of Ser139 phosphorylation in histone H2AX appears after hydroxyurea treatment, as it was the case with phosphorylations of Chk1 serines 317 and 345. Correlation of immunolabeling using anti-Chk1 (Ser317) and anti-H2AX (Ser139) antibodies, especially evident at the boundaries of nucleolar and perinucleolar regions of chromatin, seems to indicate that both regions overlap with the areas of an increased activity of Chk1 kinase (Rybaczek & Maszewski, 2007b). It was also concluded that as opposed to *V. faba* and *A.porrum* (both representing a 'reticulate' type of DNA package) the diffuse chromatin in chromocentric cell nuclei of *R. sativus* may be more vulnerable both to generate DSBs and to recruit repair factors (Rybaczek & Maszewski, 2007a). The formation of histone H2AX foci phosphorylated at Ser139 is therefore a sensitive test showing the presence of structural damage to the genome (Figure 4A, B). An equally sensitive test detecting single-strand DNA damage is labeling nuclei by antibodies recognizing single-stranded DNA (anti-single-stranded DNA, Figure 4A, B) or antibodies recognizing *PARP2* gene product, i.e. Poly(ADP-Ribose) Polymerase-2 (PARP-2;Figure 5A, B).

Comparisons of means were made using nonparametric Mann-Whitney U tests, due to the fact that some series had a skewed distribution (Figure 4A). The following has been indicated: (i) a significant increase in the DSB series compared to SSB in the control series ($U = 6.23$; $P \leq 0.001$), (ii) a significant increase in the DSB series compared to SSB after a 24-hour activity of 2.5 mM hydroxyurea ($U = 8.61$; $P \leq 0.001$), and (iii) a significant increase in SSB compared to DSB in the series in which PCC induction was performed under the influence of 5 mM caffeine (under constant sustained hydroxyurea stress; $U = 8.61$; $P \leq 0.001$).

Additionally, the presence of double-stranded breaks (DSBs) in the nuclei of cells undergoing PCC suggests also that premature entry into mitosis occurs before the completion of DNA repair (Rybaczek et al. 2007; Rybaczek et al. 2008). The key target of S-M checkpoint is the activity of the cyclin B/Cdk1 complexes (MPF), but similar effects can result from the change in the activity balance of protein kinases and phosphatases brought about, e.g. by the hyperexpression of *cdc25* genes (Forbes et al. 1998).

PARP activation is an immediate cellular response to chemical or radiation-induced DNA SSB damage. PARP-2 is a nuclear protein whose main role is to detect and signal SSB to the enzymatic machinery involved in the SSB repair. Once PARP detects a SSB, it binds to the DNA, and, after a structural change, begins the synthesis of a Poly(ADP-Ribose) chain (PAR) as a signal for other DNA-repairing enzymes such as DNA ligase III (LigIII), DNA polymerase beta (polβ), and scaffolding proteins such as X-ray cross-complementing gene 1 (XRCC1). After repairing, the PAR chains are degraded via PAR glycohydrolase [(PARG) Isabelle et al., 2010].

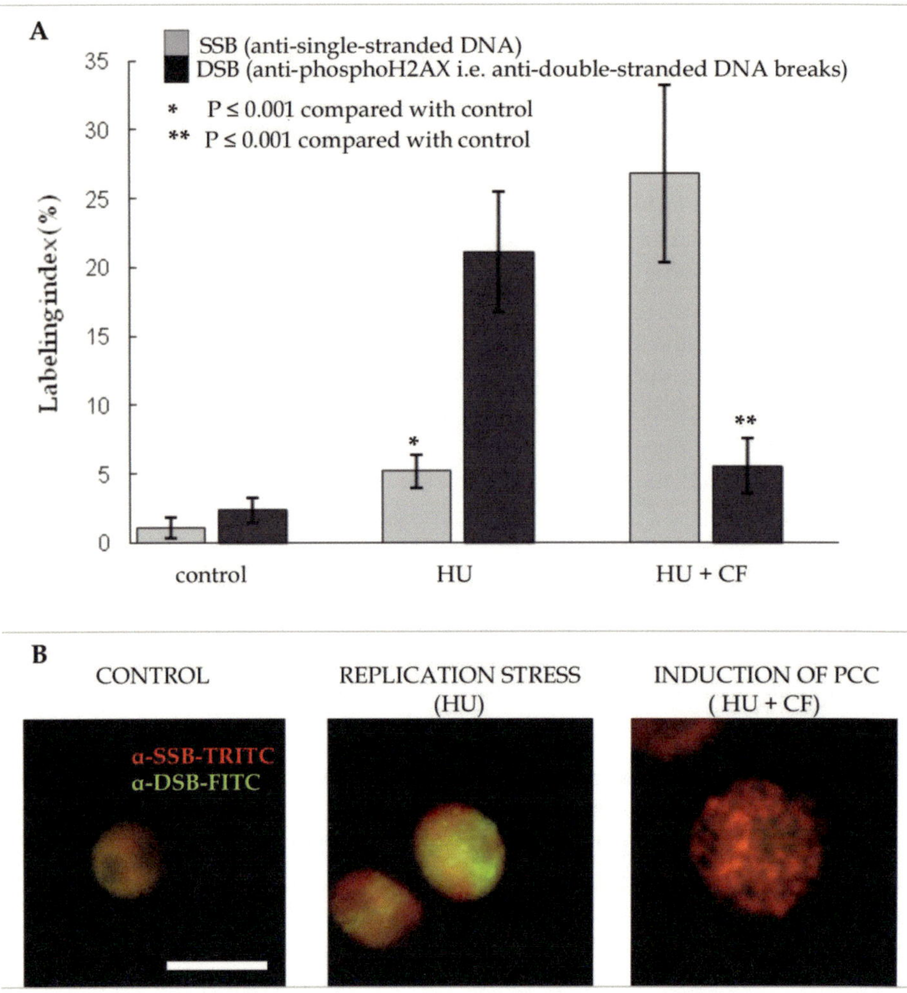

Figure 4. Immunolabeling indices (%) estimated for *Vicia faba* stained with anti-ssDNA [red, TRITC-labeled] and anti-H2AX(Ser139) [green, FITC-labeled] antibodies. *Columns*, mean from five independent experiments; *bars*, SD. For immunocytochemical detection of single-standed DNA and phospho-H2AX histone cells were fixed for 45 min in 4% formaldehyde buffered with PBS. Excised apical parts of roots were then placed in a citric acid-buffered digestion solution (pH 5.0; 37°C for 45 min) containing 2.5% pectinase (Fluka), 2.5% cellulase (Onozuka R-10; Serva) and 2.5% pectoliase (ICN). The cells were pre-treated in a blocking buffer (10% horse serum, 1% bovine serum albumin; BSA, 0.02% NaN_3, 1 x PBS) for 1 h at room temperature to minimize the non-specific adsorption of the antibodies to the coverslip, and were incubated overnight in a humidified atmosphere (4°C) with primary antibody. Mouse monoclonal antibody to single-stranded DNA was used at 1:200 (MILLIPORE), rabbit polyclonal antibody to phospho-H2AX (Ser139) was used at 1:750 (CELL SIGNALING). Secondary antibodies, including FITC-conjugated goat anti-rabbit (for H2AX), and TRITC-conjugated goat anti-mouse antibodies (for ssDNA), were used at 1:1000 for 1 h at room temperature in the dark. Secondary antibodies were from Sigma-Aldrich. The labeling index was calculated as the ratio of immunofluorescence-labeled cells to all cells in a meristematic population. *Bar* 20 μm

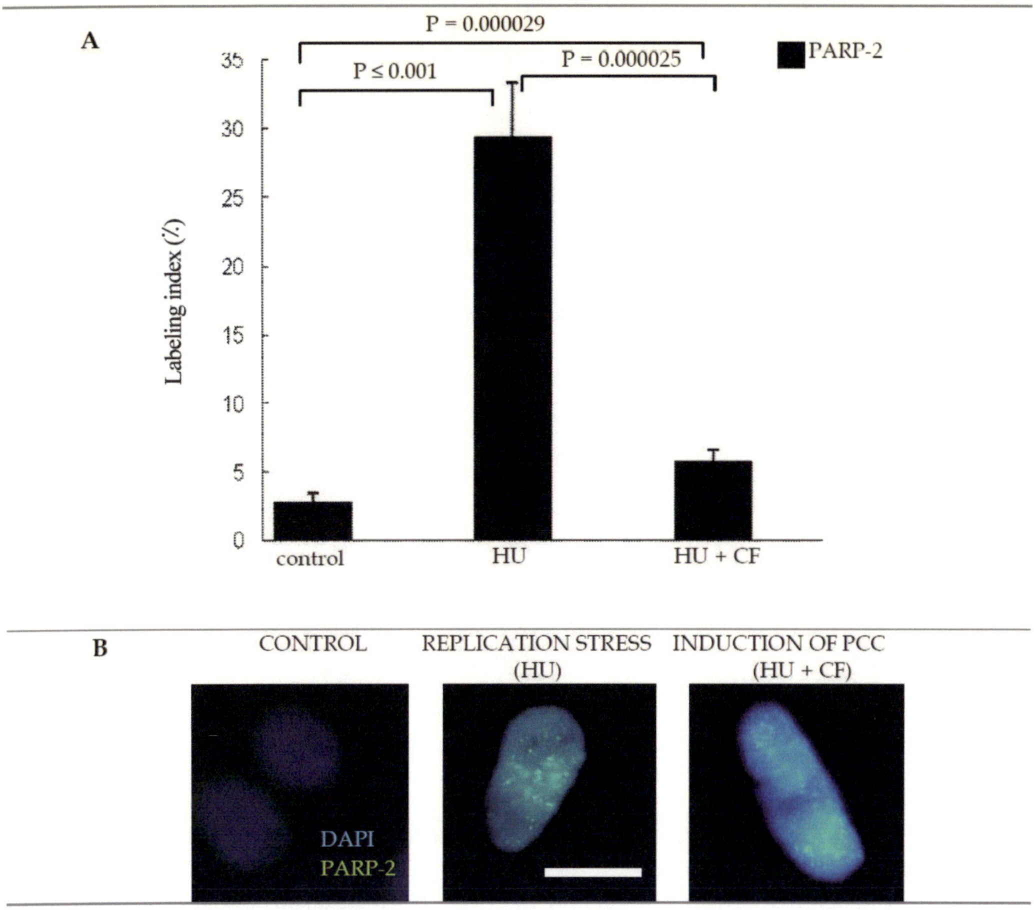

Figure 5. Fig. 5. Immunolabeling indices (%) estimated for *Vicia faba* stained with anti-PARP-2 antibody [green, DyLight®488] and DAPI [blue]. *Columns*, mean from five independent experiments; *bars*, SD. For immunocytochemical PARP-2 (Poly[ADP-Ribose] Polymerase-2) cells were fixed for 45 min in 4% formaldehyde buffered with PBS. Excised apical parts of roots were then placed in a citric acid-buffered digestion solution (pH 5.0; 37°C for 45 min) containing 2.5% pectinase (Fluka), 2.5% cellulase (Onozuka R-10; Serva) and 2.5% pectoliase (ICN). The cells were pre-treated in a blocking buffer (10% horse serum, 1% bovine serum albumin; BSA, 0.02% NaN_3, 1 x PBS) for 1 h at room temperature to minimize the non-specific adsorption of the antibodies to the coverslip, and were incubated overnight in a humidified atmosphere (4°C) with primary antibody. Rabbit polyclonal antibodies specific to PARP-2 were purchased from AGRISERA (at a dilution of 1:50). Bound primary antibodies were detected with secondary goat anti-rabbit IgG DyLight®488 antibody (AGRISERA; at a dilution of 1:1000, for 1 h at 18°C). Nuclear DNA was stained with 4′,6-diamidino-2-phenyl-indole (DAPI, 0.4 μg/ml; Sigma-Aldrich). The labeling index was calculated as the ratio of immunofluorescence-labeled cells to all cells in a meristematic population. *Bar* 20 μm

Nonparametric Kruskal-Wallis tests were used for analysis of variance ($H = 78.9$; $P \leq 0.001$; Figure 5A). Comparisons between groups were made using post hoc tests (Figure 5A). A statistically significant increase in the fluorescence labeling index of the anti-PARP2 in series HU and PCC was observed relative to the control, as well as a significantly higher labeling index for HU compared to the PCC series (Figure 5A).

In summary, this chapter aims to review how the nature of the damage to nucleobases influences DNA repair with regards to DSB and SSB generation (Figures 4, 5). Reports, literature and our own research results show histone H2AX phosphorylated at Ser139 is the marker of double-strand breaks (Figure 4A, C). It was shown that rapid and sensitive detection of single-strand damage is possible thanks to immunocytochemical reaction performed using commercially available antibodies recognizing ssDNA (anti-ssDNA, MILLIPORE, Figure 4B, C), or another similarly useful SSBs marker, Poly(ADP-Ribose) Polymerase-2 (AGRISERA, Figure 5A, B). We demonstrate that replication stress leads mainly to the generation of double-strand breaks in DNA (DSBs), while the breakage of restrictive interactions of checkpoints during PCC induction results in the accumulation of single-strand breaks (SSBs).

6. Future perspectives and the key questions that remain unanswered

The formation of DNA damage is a continuous process. Out of necessity, it must be perceived in terms of temporal and spatial chromatin dynamics, and as coupled with the activation of checkpoints (Zhou & Elledge, 2000; Liu et al., 2006). The consequence of this activation is possibly the most efficient (i.e. fast and effective) initiation of the repair processes. Maintaining the efficiency is important, as any decrease in DNA repair efficiency, for example resulting from mutations in genes encoding repair proteins, may lead to neoplasia.

Most recent studies on DNA repair have been aimed at achieving various strategic objectives, most often concerned with strengthening the effects of widely understood radio and chemotherapy (Legerski, 2010). Thoms and Bristow (2010) describe the achievement of the "therapeutic ratio" as the primary aim of their investigations. Other researchers emphasize the benefits of mathematical methods in either future experimental studies of DNA repair or clinical studies of drug resistance (Lavi et al., 2012).

DNA repair processes have been studied using (i) different experimental systems, e.g. *in vitro* model (Garner & Costanzo, 2009), (ii) different cell types, e.g. human stem cells (Rocha et al., 2013) or even neurons (McMurray, 2005); (iii) model organisms, e.g. *Arabidopsis thaliana* cells, *Xenopus laevis* egg cell free extract (Garner & Costanzo, 2009); (iv) different proteins e.g. cyclin-dependent kinases (CDKs; Yata & Esashi, 2009), histone variants (Shi & Oberdoerffer, 2012) or cell cycle checkpoints connected proteins (Liu et al., 2006); as well as (v) the context of chromatin condensation (Shi & Oberdoerffer, 2012).

Most (although not all) molecular mechanisms involved in DNA repair appear to be evolutionarily conservative. However, many important questions still remain unanswered. This is particularly evident in studies on chromatin adopting different conformations and damaged - with varying intensity - by various factors and various states of condensation. This variety makes it difficult to draw definite conclusions with regard to the processes of DNA repair in chromatin fibres. In addition, the common features of almost all types of repair (concerning

http://dx.doi.org/10.5772/54020

either SSBs or DSBs) is that they involve large protein complexes, and that the repaired DNA is subject to many structural changes not only initially but also during repair itself (e.g. unwinding or nucleolytic processing). Finally, control systems of higher plant cell cycles involve regulatory factors related to the "permanently embryonic" nature of meristematic zones, autotrophic metabolism, spatial stabilization, the presence of cellulose wall and the resulting specific intertissue dependencies (Jacobs, 1992). Hopefully, cutting-edge research techniques will soon make it possible to reveal many of the still unknown mechanisms of DNA repair and to formulate really definite conclusions.

7. Conclusion

The instability of the genome, visible in chromosome mutations and rearrangements, is usually associated with a pathological disorders, but is also of key importance for evolution. Processes that make up the cell cycle (replication, chromatin condensation, anaphase-telophase chromosome segregation and cytokinesis) occur in a sequential manner and are subject to precise control. However, the cell cycle includes several functionally different cycles that are inherently related to the cell cycle but independent of each other, for example, nuclear DNA cycle, nuclear membrane cycle, nucleolus cycle, microtubular cycle, a cycle of biosynthesis and segregation of cell organelles, and the use of sucrose like highly-energetic substances. Despite the enormous diversity of processes occurring in the cell cycle, the mechanisms responsible for the integrity of the genome exhibit a remarkable homology and coherence of action in reducing the effects of DNA damage. This results in the evolutionary development of organisms and an increase in their productivity in the expansion to new and more demanding environments.

Acknowledgement

The work was funded by "POMOST" fellowship from the Foundation for Polish Science (the contract no. POMOST/2011-4/8).

Author details

Dorota Rybaczek[1] and Magdalena Kowalewicz-Kulbat[2]

1 Department of Cytophysiology, Faculty of Biology and Environmental Protection, University of Łódź, Łódź, Poland

2 Department of Immunology and Infectious Biology, University of Łódź, Łódź, Poland

References

[1] Adamsen, B.L., Kravik, K.L. & De Angelis, P.M. (2011) DNA damage signaling in response to 5-fluorouracil in three colorectal cancer cell lines with different mismatch repair and TP53 status. *Int J Oncol* 39, 673-682.

[2] Aguilera, A. & Gómez-González, B. (2008) Genome instability: a mechanistic view of its causes and consequences. *Nat Rev Genet* 9, 204-217.

[3] Ball, H.L., Ehrhardt, M.R., Mordes, D.A., Glick, G.G., Chazin, W.K. & Cortez, D. (2007) Function of a conserved checkpoint recruitment domain in ATRIP proteins. *Mol Cell Biol* 27, 3367-3377.

[4] Bartek, J., Lukas, C. & Lukas, J. (2004) Checking on DNA damage in S phase. *Nat Rev Mol Cell Biol* 5, 792-804.

[5] Blow, J.J. & Hodgson, B. (2002) Replication licensing – defining the proliferative state? *Trends Cell Biol* 12, 72-78.

[6] Boutros, R., Dozier, C. & Ducommun, B. (2006) The when and where of CDC25 phosphatases. *Curr Opin Cell Biol* 18, 185-191.

[7] Burma, S., Chen, B.P., Murphy, M., Kurimasa, A. & Chen, D.J. (2001) ATM phosphorylates histone H2AX in response to DNA double-strand breaks. *J Biol Chem* 276, 42462-42467.

[8] Byun, T.S., Pacek, M., Yee, M.C., Walter, J.C. & Cimprich, K.K. (2005) Functional uncoupling of MCM helicase and DNA polymerase activities activates the ATR-dependent checkpoint. Genes Dev 19, 1040-1052.

[9] Cimprich, K.A. & Cortez, D. (2008) ATR: An essential regulator of genome integrity. *Nat Rev Mol Cell Biol* 9, 616-627.

[10] Cortez, D. (2003). Caffeine inhibits checkpoint responses without inhibiting the ataxia-telangiectasia-mutated (ATM) and ATM- and Rad3-related (ATR) protein kinases. *J Biol Chem* 278, 37139-37145.

[11] Costanzo, V., Shechter, D., Lupardus, P.J., Cimprich, K.A., Gottesman,m M. & Gautier, J. (2003) An ATR- and Cdc7-dependent DNA damage checkpoint that inhibits initiation of DNA replication. *Mol Cell* 11, 203-213.

[12] De Schutter, K., Joubes, J., Cools, T., Verekest, A., Corellou, F., Babiychuk, E., Van Der Schueren, E., Beeckman, T., Kushnir, S., Inzé, D. & De Veylder, L. (2007) *Arabidopsis* WEE1 kinase controls cell cycle arrest in response to activation of the DNA integrity checkpoint. *Plant Cell* 19, 211-225.

[13] De Veylder, L., Joubès, J. & Inzé, D. (2003) Plant cell cycle transitions. *Curr Opin Plant Biol* 6, 536-543.

[14] Deckert, J., Pawlak, S. & Rybaczek, D. (2009) The nucleus as a 'headquarters' and target in plant cell stress reactions, In: *Compartmentation of Responses to Stresses in Higher*

Plants, True or False, Waldemar Maksymiec, pp.61-90, Transworld Research Network, ISBN: 978-81-7895-422-6, Kerala, India.

[15] Elledge, S.J. (1996) Cell cycle checkpoint: preventing an identity crisis. *Science* 274, 1664-1672.

[16] Ellison, V. & Stillman, B. (2003) Biochemical characterization of DNA damage checkpoint complexes: clamp loader and clamp complexes with specificity for 5′ recessed DNA. *PLoS Biol* 1, 231-243.

[17] Freire, R., van Vugt, M.A.T.M., Mamely, I. & Medema, R.H. (2006) Claspin. Timing the cell cycle arrest when the genome is damaged. *Cell Cycle* 5, 2831-2834.

[18] Forbes, K.C., Humphrey, T. & Enoch, T. (1998) Supressors of Cdc25p overexpression identify two pathways that influence the G2/M checkpoint in fission yeast. *Genet Soc Amer* 150, 1361-1375.

[19] Garner, E. & Costanzo, V. (2009) Studying the DNA damage response using *in vitro* model systems. *DNA Repair* 8, 1025-1037.

[20] Gotoh, E. & Durante, M. (2006) Chromosome condensation outside of mitosis: mechanisms and new tools. *J Cell Physiol* 209, 297-304.

[21] Han, E.S., Muller, F., Pérez, V.I., Qi, W., Liang, H., Xi, L., Fu, C., Doyle, E., Hickey, M., Cornell, J., Epstein, C.J., Roberts, L.J., Van Remmen, H. & Richardson, A. (2008) The *in vivo* gene expression signature of oxidative stress. *Physiol Genomics* 34, 112-126.

[22] Harper, J.W. & Elledge, S.J. (2007) The DNA damage response: ten years after. Mol *Cell* 28, 739-745.

[23] Herrick, J. & Bensimon, A. (2008) Global regulation of genome duplication in eukaryotes: an over-view from the epifluorescence microscope. *Chromosoma* 117, 243-260.

[24] Isabelle, M., Moreel, X., Gagné, J-P., Rouleau, M., Ethier, C., Gagné, P., Hendzel, M.J. & Poirier, G.G. (2010) Investigation of PARP-1, PARP-2, and PARG interactomes by affinity-purification mass spectrometry. Proteome Science 8, 22 doi: 10.1186/1477-5956-8-22.

[25] Jacobs, T. (1992) Why do plant cells divide? *Plant Cell* 9, 1021-1029.

[26] Kumagai, A., Lee, J., Yoo, H.Y. & Dunphy, W.G. (2006) TopBP1 activates ATR-ATRIP complex. *Cell* 124, 943-955.

[27] Lavi, O., Gottesman, M.M. & Levy, D. (2013) The dynamics of drug resistance: a mathematical perspective. *Drug Resist Updat* 15, 90-97.

[28] Legerski, R.J. (2010) Repair of DNA interstrand cross-links during S phase of the mammalian cell cycle. *Environ Mol Mutagen* 51, 540-551.

[29] Lin, J.J. & Dutta, A. (2007) ATR pathway is the primary pathway for activating G_2/M checkpoint induction after re-replication. *J Biol Chem* 282, 30357-30362.

[30] Liu, W-F., Yu, S-S., Chen, G-J. & Li, Y-Z. (2006) DNA damage checkpoint, damage repair, and genome stability. *Acta Genetica Sinica* 33, 381-390

[31] Luciani, M.G., Oehlmann, M. & Blow, J.J. (2004) Characterization of a novel ATR-dependent, Chk1-idependent, intra-S-phase checkpoint that suppresses initiation of replication in *Xenopus*. *J Cell Sci* 117, 6019-6030.

[32] Majka, J. & Burgers, P.M. (2004) The PCNA-RFC families of DNA clamps and clamp loaders. *Prog Nucleic Acid Res Mol Biol* 78, 227-260.

[33] Majka, J., Niedziela-Majka, A. & Burgers, P.M.J. (2006) The checkpoint clamp activates Mec1 kinase during initiation of the DNA damage checkpoint. *Mol Cell* 24, 891-901.

[34] Marheineke, K. & Hyrien, O. (2004) Control of replication origin density and firing time in *Xenopus* egg extracts: role of a caffeine-sensitive, ATR-dependent checkpoint. *J Biol Chem* 279, 28071-28081.

[35] McMurray, C.T. (2005) To die or not to die: DNA repair in neurons. Mutat Res 577, 260-274.

[36] Mordes, D.A. & Cortez, D. (2008) Activation of ATR and related PIKKs. *Cell Cycle* 7, 2809-2812.

[37] Müller, B., Blackburn, J., Feijoo, C., Zhao, X. & Smythe, C. (2007) DNA-activated protein kinase functions in a newly observed S phase checkpoint that links histone mRNA abundance with DNA replication. *J Cell Biol* 179, 1385-1398 [Erratum in: *J Cell Biol* (2008) 180, 843].

[38] Myers, J.S., Zhao, R., Xu, X., Ham, A-J.L. & Cortez, D. (2007) Cyclin-dependent kinase 2-dependent phosphorylation of ATRIP regulates the G_2-M checkpoint response to DNA damage. *Cancer Res* 67, 6685-6690.

[39] Namiki, Y. & Zou, L. (2006) ATRIP associates with replication protein A-coated ssDNA through multiple interactions. *Proc Natl Acad Sci USA* 103, 580-585.

[40] Nedelcheva, M.N., Roguev, A., Dolapchiev, L.B., Shevchenko, A., Taskov, H.B., Shevchenko, A., Stewart, A.F. & Stoynov, S.S. (2005) Uncoupling of unwinding from DNA synthesis implies regulation of MCM helicase by Tof1/Mrc1/Csm3 checkpoint complex. *J Mol Biol* 347, 509-521.

[41] Niida, H. & Nakanishi, M. (2006) DNA damage checkpoints in mammals. *Mutagenesis* 21, 3-9.

[42] Niimi, A., Brown, S., Sabbioneda, S., Kannouche, P.L., Scott, A., Yasui, A., Green, C.M. & Lehmann, A.R. (2008) Regulation of proliferating cell nuclear antigen ubiquitination in mammalian cells. *Proc Natl Acad Sci USA* 105, 16125-16130.

[43] Nojima, H. (2006) Protein kinases that regulate chromosome stability and their downstream targets. *Genome Dyn* 1, 131-148.

[44] Osborn, A.J., Elledge, S.J. & Zou, L. (2002) Checking on the fork: the DNA-replication stress-response pathway. *Trends Cell Biol* 12, 509-516.

[45] Paull, T.T., Rogakou, E.P., Yamazaki, V., Kirchgessner, C.U., Gellert, M. & Bonner, W.M (2000) A critical role for histone H2AX in recruitment of repair factors to nuclear foci after DNA damage. *Curr Biol* 10, 886-895.

[46] Pawelczak, K.S. & Turchi, J.J. (2008) A mechanism for DNA-PK activation requiring unique contributions from each strand of a DNA terminus and implications for micrphomology-mediated nonhomologous DNA end joining. *Nucleic Acids Res* 36, 4022-4031.

[47] Raleigh, J.M. & O'Connell, M.J. (2000) The G2 DNA damage checkpoint targets both Weel and Cdc25. *J Cell Sci* 113, 1727-1736.

[48] Rocha, C.R.R., Lerner, L.K., Okamoto, O.K., Marchetto, M.C. & Menck, C.F.M. (2012) The role of DNA repair in the pluripotency and differentiation of human stem cells. *Mutat Res* 752, 25-35.

[49] Rogakou, E.P., Pilch, D.R., Orr, A.H., Ivanova, V.S. & Bonner, W.M. (1998) DNA double-stranded breaks induce histone H2AX phosphorylation on serine 139. *J Biol Chem* 273, 5858-5868.

[50] Rybaczek, D. (2011) Eidetic analysis of the premature chromosome condensation process, In: *DNA Repair*, Inna Kruman, pp.185-204, InTech, ISBN: 978-953-307-697-3, Rijeka, Croatia.

[51] Rybaczek, D. & Kowalewicz-Kulbat, M. (2011) Premature chromosome condensation induced by caffeine, 2-aminopurine, staurosporine and sodium metavanadate in S-phase arrested HeLa cells is associated with a decrease in Chk1 phosphorylation, formation of phospho-H2AX and minor cytoskeletal rearrangements. *Histochem Cell Biol* 135, 263-280.

[52] Rybaczek. D., Bodys, A. & Maszewski, J. (2007) H2AX foci in late S/G2- and M-phase cells after hydroxyurea- and aphidicolin-induced DNA replication stress in *Vicia*. *Histochem Cell Biol* 128, 227-241.

[53] Rybaczek, D. & Maszewski, J. (2007a) Phosphorylation of H2AX histones in response to double-strand breaks and induction of premature chromatin condensation in hydroxyurea-treated root meristem cells of *Raphanus sativus*, *Vicia faba*, and *Allium porrum*. *Protoplasma* 230, 31-39.

[54] Rybaczek, D. & Maszewski, J. (2007b) Induction of foci of phosphorylated H2AX histones and premature chromosome condensation after DNA damage in *Vicia faba* root meristem. *Biol Plantarum* 51, 443-450.

[55] Rybaczek, D., Żabka, A., Pastucha, A. & Maszewski, J. (2008) Various chemical agents can induce premature chromosome condensation in *Vicia faba*. *Acta Physiol Plant* 30, 663-672.

[56] Schiller, C.B., Lammens, K., Guerini, I., Coordes, B., Feldmann, H., Schlauderer, F., Möckel, C., Schele, A., Strässer, K., Jackson, S.P. & Hopfner, K.P. (2012) Structure of Mre11-Nbs1 complex yields insights into ataxia-telangiectasia-like disease mutations and DNA damage signaling. *Nat Struct Mol Biol* 19, 693-700.

[57] Scorah, J., Dong, M-Q., Yates, III jr, Scott, M., Gillespie, D. & McGowan, Ch. (2008) A conserved PCNA-interacting protein sequence in Chk1 is required for checkpoint function. *J Biol Chem* 283: 1725-17259.

[58] Shechter, D., Costanzo, V. & Gautier, J. (2004) Regulation of DNA replication by ATR: signaling in response to DNA intermediates. *DNA Repair* 3, 901-908.

[59] Shi, L. & Oberdoertter, P. (2012) Chromatin dynamics in DNA double strand breaks repair. *Biochim Biophys Acta* 1819, 811-819.

[60] Shimura, T., Martin, M.M., Torres, M.J., Gu, C., Pluth, J.M., DiBernardi, M.A., McDonald, J.S. & Aladjem, M.J. (2007) DNA-PK is involved in repairing a transient surge of DNA breaks induced by deceleration of DNA replication. *J Mol Biol* 367, 665-680.

[61] Tan, Z., Wortman, M., Dillehay, K.L., Seibel, W.L., Evelyn, C.R., Smith, S.J., Malkas, L.H., Zheng, Y., Lu, S. & Dong, Z. (2012) Small-molecule targeting of proliferating cell nuclear antigen chromatin association inhibits tumor cell growth. *Mol Pharmacol* 81, 811-819.

[62] Thoms, J. & Bristow, R.G. (2010) DNA repair targeting and radiotherapy: a focus on the therapeutic ratio. *Semin Radiat Oncol* 20, 217-222.

[63] Vashisht, A.A. & Tuteja, N. (2006) Stress responsive DEAD-box helicases: a new pathway to engineer plant stress tolerance. *J Photochem Photobiol B.* 84, 150-160.

[64] Wang, S.-W., Norbury, C., Harris, A.L. &Toda, T. (1999) Caffeine can override the S-M checkpoint in fission yeast. *J Cell Sci* 112, 927-937.

[65] Ward, I.M. & Chen, J. (2001) Histone H2AX is phosphorylated in an ATR-dependent manner in response to replicational stress. *J Biol Chem* 276, 47759-47762.

[66] Yao, T., Utsunomiya, T., Nagai, E., Oya, M. & Tsuneyoshi, M. (1996) p53 expression patterns in colorectal adenomas and early carcinomas: a special reference to depressed adenoma and non-polyploid carcinoma. *Phatol Int* 46, 962-967.

[67] Yata, K. & Esashi, F. (2009) Dual role of CDKs in DNA repair: To be, or not to be. *DNA Repair* 8, 6-18.

[68] Zhou, B.B. & Elledge, S.J. (2000) The DNA damage response: putting checkpoints in perspective. *Nature* 408, 433-439.

[69] Zou, L. & Elledge, S.J. (2003) Sensing DNA damage through ATRIP recognition of RPA-ssDNA complexes. *Science* 300, 1542-1548.

Chapter 10

p21^{CDKN1A} and DNA Repair Systems: Recent Findings and Future Perspectives

Micol Tillhon, Ornella Cazzalini, Ilaria Dutto,
Lucia A. Stivala and Ennio Prosperi

Additional information is available at the end of the chapter

http://dx.doi.org/10.5772/54173

1. Introduction

After exposure to genotoxic agents, cells activate DNA damage response pathways consisting of a signaling cascade (cell cycle checkpoints), and of DNA repair processes able to recognize and remove a great number of DNA lesions [1].

DNA repair is characterized by an impressive high number of different proteins necessary to perform specialized biochemical reactions, which are different according to the type of lesion to be repaired [2]. Thus, the nucleotide excision repair (NER) mechanism will repair bulky lesions, such as the cyclobutane pyrimidine dimers (CPDs) produced by UV-C irradiation, or other types of adducts produced by the interaction of chemicals with DNA. Base excision repair (BER) is instead involved in the removal of bases damaged by alkylating, or oxidative agents, while the repair of single and double strand breaks is performed through the pathway of homologous recombination, or via the non homologous end-joning (NHEJ) repair. In addition, cells repair errors introduced during DNA replication with the mechanism of mismatch repair (MMR).

Among the many factors involved in these defense processes against DNA damage, p21^{CDKN1A} protein – known also as p21$^{(WAF1/CIP1/SDI1)}$ – plays a key role in several fundamental biological processes, such as cell cycle control, DNA replication/repair, gene transcription, apoptosis, and cell motility [3-6]. This protein is a cyclin-dependent kinase (CDK) inhibitor belonging to the Cip/Kip family; it was first described as a potent inhibitor of cell proliferation and DNA replication, both in physiological conditions and after DNA damage [7,8]. Homologs are found in several organisms, including *Xenopus* (Xic1), *Drosophila* (Dacapo), as well as *C. Elegans* (CKI-1). In mammals, p21 was previously known as CDK-interacting protein 1 (CIP1), wild type p53-activated fragment (WAF1), senescent cell-derived inhibitor 1 (SDI1), and melanoma differentiation-associated protein 6 (MDA-6); all these names have been substituted by a new terminology including all CDK inhibitors, and p21 is now named CDKN1A.

Due to the lack of a defined tertiary structure, p21 protein may adopt an extended conformation [9], which may explain its ability to interact with a number of proteins involved in several important biological processes [3-6] (Figure 1).

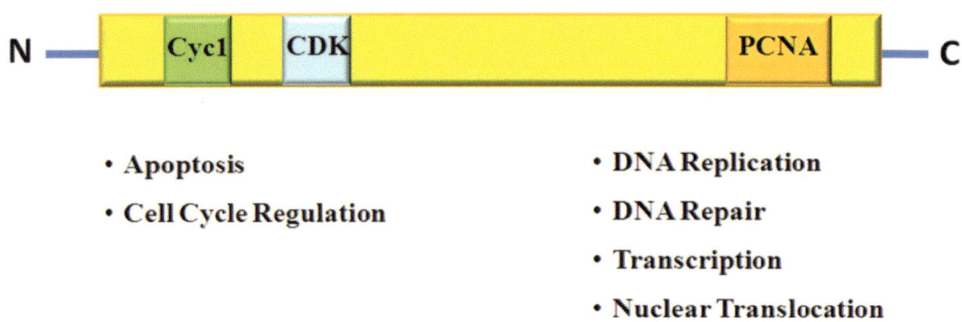

Figure 1. Schematic structure of p21 protein showing the regions responsible for binding to Cyclins, CDK and PCNA. Below the N- and C-terminal regions are indicated the processes in which they are involved, respectively.

2. p21 biology and functions

The main role of p21 is cell-cycle regulation, performed by inhibiting the activity of cyclin-CDK complexes thanks to direct interaction through specific sequences (termed CDK and Cy motifs) in the N-terminal domain of the protein [10-13]. Cell cycle progression may be also regulated, independently of cyclins and CDKs, thanks to the strong affinity binding to proliferating cell nuclear antigen (PCNA) [14-17], a protein playing a central role in DNA replication and repair, as well as in other processes of DNA metabolism [18,19]. This association may interfere with PCNA-dependent enzyme activities involved in DNA synthesis [18,19]. In contrast with the negative cell-cycle regulation, p21 may also serve as an assembly factor for cyclin D-CDK4/6 complexes, thus promoting cyclin D-dependent events, and downstream activation of cyclin E-CDK2 [7,8].

CDKN1A gene inactivation studies performed with experimental models, and in particular with knock-out mice, have confirmed the tumor suppressor functions of this protein [20,21]. The p21-null mice showed a normal development and did not show any spontaneous tumor formation until 7-month of age [20]. However, embryonic fibroblasts derived from these animals were deficient in G1 checkpoint arrest following DNA damage [20]. Subsequent studies in this model were extended to a longer time frame and the observations reported that p21-deficient mice developed spontaneous tumors at a median age of 16 months. The most common malignancies occurring in these animals were hemopoietic (B-cell lymphoma), endothelial, and epithelial tumors [21]. In addition, accelerated tumor formation and an increased capacity of tumor metastasis, respectively induced by urethane or by gamma radiation, were found in $p21^{-/-}$ mice [22,23]. Accelerated tumorigenesis, and promotion of lung metastasis was also found in correlation with cytoplasmic p21 in the mammary epitelium of mice expressing the MMTV/*neu* oncogene [24]. Tumor suppression functions of p21 were also confirmed by studies in the skin and in the colon of p21-deficient mice [25,26]. Furthermore, spontaneous tumor formation in p21-null mice was also found to occur in combination with other knock-out genetic backgrounds, such as $Muc2^{-/-}$ (mice lacking mucin 2), and $Apc^{1638+/-}$ (mutant allele of the adenomatosis polyposis gene) mice [27,28].

In addition to enhanced tumor formation, further investigations showed that loss of p21 caused exhaustion of blood stem cells [29], and induced development of Systemic Lupus Erythematosus in female animals [30]. Thus, the results obtained from transgenic mice, clearly indicated the tumor suppressor role of p21, although other studies have provided contrasting results [6,31]. As an example, p21-null mice crossed with knock-in PML-RAR mice, showed an oncogenic role of p21 in maintaining self-renewal of leukemic stem cells [32]. The dual behaviour of p21 most probably occurs because of its participation in several cellular processes, and it is dependent on different factors [6,31].

An important aspect for determining the target of p21 activity is the intracellular localization. Early studies indicated that lack of p21 expression, or cytoplasmic localization of the protein, promoted anchorage-independent growth, and drug resistance [5,6,31]. Human p21 protein is located predominantly in the nucleus; however, it is also present in the nucleolus and in the cytoplasm. In the nucleus, in addition to inhibit CDK2 and binding to PCNA, p21 may also associate with transcriptional regulators [4]. In the nucleolus, p21 was found to colocalize with cyclin E [33], and to accumulate after DNA damage, as a consequence of inhibition of nuclear export [34]. Interestingly, growing body of evidence indicates that the cytoplasmic localization of p21 is linked to drug resistance [6,31], thus suggesting that in this compartment the protein may have a tumor-promoting function [35]. Cellular localization of p21 is regulated mainly by post-translation modifications. In fact, nuclear translocation appears to be counteracted by different kinases phosphorylating Thr145 and Ser146 residues located near the NLS region of p21 [36-38]. These modifications are responsible for cytoplasmic localization of p21, as well as for the loss of interaction with PCNA [39]. An important role in p21 phosphorylation is played by AKT1/PKB, which also mediates stability of the protein [36,37]. Another relevant modification of p21 (i.e ubiquitination) regulating its degradation, has been shown to occur predominantly in the nucleus, because p21 mutant in the NLS region exhibited enhanced stability [40].

A summary of the most important functions performed by p21 protein is reported in the following paragraphs.

Cell-cycle regulation

As the principal mediator of cell cycle arrest in response to DNA damage, p21 not only acts by inactivating G_1-phase cyclins/CDKs complexes, but also by inhibiting cell cycle progression through other mechanisms. These possibly include direct interaction with PCNA to inhibit DNA replication, and indirect effects mediated by interaction with other cell cycle regulators. In addition, p21 has been shown to play a role in the maintenance of G_2-phase arrest, through multiple mechanisms [3,5,6].

The demonstration that p21 is involved in cell response to DNA damage, mediated through transcriptional activation by p53, was first obtained in mammalian cells [41,42]. The main role of p21 in the G_1 checkpoint resides in its ability to inhibit the activity of cyclin E, and cyclin A/CDK2 complexes required for the G_1/S phase transition, thereby contributing to G_1-phase arrest [43]. Accordingly, mouse embryonic fibroblasts (MEFs) obtained from p21-null mice fail to arrest in G_1 phase, in response to DNA damage [20,44]. Recently, it has been demonstrated that CDK2$^{-/-}$ MEFs, as well as regenerating liver cells in CDK2$^{-/-}$ mice, are able to arrest at the G_1/S checkpoint in response to γ-irradiation. This response has been found to depend on the ability of CDK1 to substitute for CDK2, and on p21, which may associate with, and inhibit nuclear CDK1 at the G_1/S transition [45].

p21 potentially participates in the G_1/S checkpoint also by blocking directly DNA synthesis, thanks to its ability to bind the central region (interdomain connecting loop) of PCNA [46,47]. *In vitro* studies showed that the C-terminal domain of p21 is sufficient to displace DNA replication enzymes from PCNA, thereby blocking processive DNA synthesis [47,48]. *In vivo* expression of C- vs N-terminal truncated forms of p21, as well as of CDK- or PCNA-binding deficient p21 mutants, indicated that p21 interaction with PCNA could indeed arrest cell cycle [49–51]. In particular, interaction with PCNA localized at DNA replication sites could prevent loading of DNA polymerase δ, but occurrence of this mechanism was observed in a limited number of cells [52], and never proved with endogenous p21, whose levels are significantly reduced in S phase [53,54]. Other mechanisms of p21-mediated G_1/S checkpoint activation after DNA damage have been reported. A direct interaction between p21 and the p50 non-catalytic subunit of human DNA polymerase δ was found both *in vitro* and *in vivo* [55]. It was concluded that p21 might be recruited to the DNA replication complex via direct interaction with p50, thereby facilitating the binding to PCNA. However, this interpretation does not take into account p21 degradation in S phase [53,54]. Another suggested explanation for p50–p21 interaction was the inhibition of cyclinA/CDK2 complex associated with DNA polymerase δ [55]. An additional mechanism of p21-mediated arrest at the G_1/S transition was described in HCT116 cells treated with adriamycin. ICBP90 (Inverted CCAAT box binding protein) is a 90 kDa nuclear protein that binds to the promoter of topoisomerase IIα gene, and that was suggested to be important in the G_1/S transition, due to partial colocalization with PCNA [56]. Expression of p21 directly down-regulated the levels of ICBP90 protein, both through the reduction of E2F-mediated transcription and the promotion of ubiquitin-dependent proteolytic degradation [56]. Thus, downregulation of ICBP90 by p21 might constitute another level of checkpoint control of S-phase entry.

It has been shown that p21 is also essential to sustain the G_2 phase checkpoint after DNA damage in human cells, as well as in preventing G_2-arrested cells from undergoing additional S-phase [57-59].

Cyclin B-CDK1 complex has a relatively low affinity for p21 when compared with the other cyclin-CDK complexes [60], and a low amount of cyclin B/CDK1 was found to be associated with p21 after activation of the G_2 checkpoint [61]. However, p21 has been demonstrated to contribute to CDK1 inactivation by inhibiting the CDK-activating kinase (CAK) and, consequently, the CDK1-activating Thr161 phosphorylation. Thus, p21/CAK pathway appears to be essential in sustaining the G_2 arrest in response to DNA damage [61]. Other likely targets of p21 in G_2 phase are cyclin A-CDK1/2 complexes [62,63]. As an additional mechanism of G_2 arrest, p21 was also suggested to mediate nuclear retention of cyclin B1-CDK1 complex in response to genotoxic stress, thus preventing its activation by Cdc25 and CAK [64]. Recently, it has been also proposed that p21 contributes to G_2 arrest by mediating cyclin B degradation in response to DNA damage [65]. Furthermore, a new p21-dependent mechanism to maintain G_2 arrest after DNA damage has been shown to involve Emi1 protein, an inhibitor of the Anaphase Promoting Complex (APC) whose destruction controls progression through mitosis to G_1 phase [66]. It has been reported that p21 down-regulates Emi1 in cells arrested in G_2 by DNA damage, thereby contributing to APC activation and degradation of key substrates, including cyclins A2 and B1. Thus, p21 controls positively this checkpoint preventing G_2-arrested cells from entering mitosis [66].

Another important function of p21 is related to the control of basal proliferation in specific cell types. In particular, the stem cell self-renewal of keratinocytes [67], of the haematopoietic system [29], and of the mouse forebrain and hyppocampus [68,69], have been shown to depend on p21 protein. In fact, studies in CDKN1A knock-out mice showed that p21 restricts the self-renewal potential of stem cell population, and promotes their irreversible commitment to differentiation [67]. In the absence of p21, an increase in stem cell proliferation with a consequent exhaustion of the population was observed in different cell types [67-70]. Interestingly, p21 is also able to maintain the self-renewal potential of leukemic stem cells, and to protect them from DNA damage accumulation, thereby demonstrating an oncogenic activity of the protein [32].

Cell quiescence and senescence are other processes in which p21 plays a fundamental role by keeping cells arrested in G_0, or G_0-like state, in order to prevent untimely DNA replication [71,72]. Accordingly, loss of p21 has been shown to facilitate cell cycle entry from a quiescence state, at the expense of replication stress [73]. Interestingly, lack of p21 expression has been found to link cell cycle control with appendage regeneration in mice, since $p21^{-/-}$ animals showed a phenotype similar to that of regenerating mouse strains [74].

p21 also plays a complex role in cell differentiation. In fact, its expression is induced in differentiating cells of the skin and of the intestinal epithelium, as well as in cultured epidermal cells, while down-regulation has been observed at late stages of differentiation [75,76]. However, p21 appears to play a positive role in promoting differentiation of human promyelocytic leukaemia cells [77], mouse skeletal muscle and cartilage cells [78,79], and oligodendrocytes [80]. The whole body of evidence indicates that p21 plays either positive or negative roles in differentiation, independently of cell cycle control, but depending on cell type and specific stage of differentiation. This regulatory function may involve specific interactions of p21 with critical regulators of differentiation [3,6].

In contrast with the CDK inhibitory function, a cell growth promoting effect has also been demonstrated [81]. In fact, p21 may serve as an assembly factor for cyclin D/CDK4 complex, thereby promoting its nuclear translocation, kinase activation, and cell proliferation [81]. This function has been suggested to potentially confer an oncogenic activity to p21 [6,31,35].

Transcriptional regulation

In addition to the role of CDK inhibitor, p21 functions as a transcriptional cofactor that may regulate transcription, either positively or negatively [3-5,82]. This activity of p21 may occur through three different mechanisms: i) by inhibition of cyclin/CDK complexes; ii) by direct binding to several transcription factors, such as NF-kB, Myc, E2F, STAT3, and estrogen receptors [2-5]; iii) by regulating the activity of transcriptional co-activators, such as p300/CBP [5,82]. According to the first mechanism, CDK inhibition will prevent the phosphorylation of Rb-family proteins, thereby inactivating E2F-dependent transcription [4,5]. In the second mechanism, p21 acts as a co-factor that physically interacts with, and represses the activity of transcription factors. As an example, interaction of p21 with STAT3 proteins inhibits their transcriptional activity; overexpression of p21 was shown to reduce the transcriptional activity of STAT3 proteins, without modifying their DNA binding activity [83]. In addition, it was shown that p21 may specifically repress E2F-dependent transcription [84], not only through inhibition of cyclin/CDK activity and substrate association, but also through a direct interaction with E2F factor [85], which could function as an anchor for p21 [3]. Another important example is the binding of p21 to the N-terminus of c-Myc, resulting in the interference of c-Myc-Max association, and in the suppression c-Myc-dependent transcription. At the same time, the interaction between c-Myc and p21 may directly counteract p21-dependent inhibition of DNA synthesis, as c-Myc binds p21 in competition with PCNA [86]. A general correlation has been observed between p21 inhibitory effects and specific DNA sequences in the promoter of some genes showing a cell cycle-dependent transcriptional regulation by p21 [87]. For example, it has been shown that p21 functions as transcriptional repressor of the myc and cdc25A genes upon DNA damage, being recruited to the promoter of these genes. This was associated with inhibition of p300 recruitment, and down-regulation of histone H4 acetylation [88]. p21 may also bind to other transcription factors and modulate positively their function. An example is given by the estrogen receptor (ERα)-dependent transcription which may be enhanced by p21 through CDK-dependent and independent mechanisms [89,90]. The third mechanism occurs by modulation of a repression domain in p300, which occurs independently of the CDK inhibitor effect on the phosphorylation of p300 [91,92]. This protein is an essential co-activator that stimulate gene expression through its acetyl transferase activity, or through its ability to interact with components of the transcriptional machinery [93]. It has been shown that p21 prevents the recruitment of p300, causing histone hypoacetylation and transcriptional repression [94].

After UV-induced DNA damage, p21 has been shown to directly interact and to regulate the histone acetyl transferase activity (HAT) activity of p300 [95], which provides accessibility of NER machinery to DNA damage sites through histone acetylation [96]. For this activity, full-length p21 protein is required and its binding to p300 is not dependent on interaction with PCNA [95]. It is known that both p21 and PCNA may bind p300 at basal levels, and that

PCNA inhibits the transcriptional activity of p300 [97]. After DNA damage, p21 may restore p300-HAT activity by disrupting the inhibitory interaction with PCNA, thereby allowing p300 to participate in NER [5].

Finally, p21 also up-regulates multiple genes that have been associated with senescence or implicated in age-related diseases, in which a DNA damage response seems to occur [98].

Apoptosis

p21 is a major inhibitor of p53-dependent as well as p53-independent apoptosis [2-6,31]. In fact, reduction in p21 expression was shown to lead to apoptosis in DNA-damaged human cancer cells [99-101]. The cleavage and inactivation of p21 is mediated by caspase-3 in human normal cells, and in cancer cell lines [99,100]. However, the inhibitory function is not absolute since, under some circumstances (e.g. enforced overexpression), p21 may promote the signaling apoptotic pathway that ultimately determines cell death [99,100]. Initial work provided the evidence that in the absence of p21, DNA-damaged cells underwent cell cycle arrest followed by typical apoptotic cell death [59,102]. These findings suggested that p21 could exert an anti-apoptotic function in response to DNA damage. The mechanism by which p21 negatively regulates DNA damage-induced death machinery relies on its ability to bind key regulatory proteins involved in the apoptotic process (e.g. protease precursors and specific kinases) [100]. Indeed, p21 physically interacts, through its first N-terminal 33 aminoacids, with pro-caspase 3, i.e. the inactive precursor of the apoptotic executioner caspase 3 [103,104]; when bound to p21, the inactive pro-caspase cannot be converted into the active protease and apoptosis is inhibited [104]. Caspase 2, which acts upstream caspase 3, is also kept in a repressed status by p21 [105]. The strict relationship between p21 and caspases is also supported by the observation that p21 itself is cleaved by caspases early during DNA damage induced apoptosis; proteolysis involves the p21 NLS region, and impairs p21 translocation into the nucleus [106-108].

The p53-independent expression of p21 in several human cell lines, induce not only cell cycle inhibition, but also suppression of apoptosis [99,100]. Two mechanisms of action are responsible for this phenomenon: *i*) the interaction with pro-apoptotic regulatory proteins, such as pro-caspase-3, caspase-8 or apoptosis signal-regulating kinase-1 (ASK-1), with their consequent inhibition [103,104,109]. *ii*) the inhibition of apoptotic events, such as chromatin condensation, cell shrinkage and loss of adhesion, by targeting caspase-dependent activation of CDKs [110].

In the first case, p21 forms a complex with ASK-1 within the cytoplasm [111]. In the second one, p21 seems to have an anti-apoptotic activity through the inhibition of CDK activity required for activation of the caspase cascade downstream of mitochondria [112,113].

An important consequence of the inhibitory activity of apoptosis in a variety of systems is that p21 could dramatically impair the effectiveness of chemotherapeutic agents acting by damaging DNA. In this respect, an innovative strategy to kill cancer cells is based on the direct or indirect attenuation of p21 (obtained by different approaches) before chemotherapy [114-116].

In contrast with the anti-apoptotic role, p21 appears to possess pro-apoptotic functions under certain conditions, and in specific systems [5,6,31]. In fact, p21 overexpression in thymocytes induced hypersensitivity to p53-dependent cell death in response to X-rays and UV radiation [117]. Overexpression of p21 was shown to enhance the apoptotic response induced by a variety of stimuli and in different cell systems [5,6,31]. Other studies reported the pro-apoptotic role of p21 after targeted overexpression of the protein [118,119] or by showing a decrease in apoptosis after p21 gene disruption [99,100]. A pro-apoptotic effect of p21 was also observed in breast cancer cells treated with sodium butyrate, which is an inducer of p21 expression; interestingly, in these cells the pro-apoptotic effect required the interaction of p21 with PCNA [120]. However, the mechanism(s) by which p21 may promote apoptosis are still to be clarified.

Finally, p21 may also play an important role in regulating another type of cell death, i.e. autophagy, a process in which cell organelles are enclosed and destroyed in vesicles [121]. This mechanism appears to be regulated by p21 by maintaining autophagic proteins in an inactive state [122].

Cell motility

One of the most recently described functions of p21 is the regulation of actin-based cell motility. Cytoplasmic p21 has been shown to influence cell motility and neuronal neurite outgrowth by interfering with substrate adhesion through the inhibition of Rho kinase [123]. Degradation of cytoplasmic p21 favors a nonmotile cell behavior. In tumor cells, high levels of p21 localized in the cytoplasm will favor Rho inhibition with consequent enhanced cell movement [124]. This effect has been shown to contribute to tumor metastasis and invasion, thus suggesting another mechanism by which p21 may play an oncogenic role [5,31].

DNA repair

The role of p21 in DNA repair, has been debated for a long period, since both negative or absent effects, in contrast with studies supporting a positive role of p21, have been reported. Recent lines of evidence obtained using different experimental models (with and without overexpression systems), and particularly those performed with untransformed cells, support a positive role for p21 in DNA repair. As already stated, the idea that p21 could play a role in DNA repair was first suggested by the evidence showing that p21 interacts with PCNA [10-17]. Since this binding results in competition and displacement of PCNA-interacting proteins thereby inhibiting DNA synthesis [14-16,125], it was proposed that p21 could inhibit DNA repair, in a similar way as it affects DNA replication in vitro. However, a number of direct interactions between p21 and specific factors participating in different processes of DNA repair have indicated that p21 may mediate the DNA damage response also at this level.

As described in the introductory section, there are different mechanisms of DNA repair which are essentially able to remove specific lesions, thereby restoring the correct genetic information. Given their peculiarity, the lines of evidence suggesting the participation of p21 in each process will be described individually.

3. p21 and Nucleotide Excision Repair (NER)

The first biochemical studies showed that high p21 levels could inhibit the NER process in a reconstituted *in vitro* system [126,127]. A similar effect was observed when purified p21 protein was introduced into cells by electroporation [128]. Other studies performed on p21-null murine fibroblasts, or on p21$^{-/-}$ HCT116 tumor cell line, reported that the NER process was not significantly affected in the absence of the protein, thus implying that p21 was not involved in NER [129-132].

In contrast with these findings, a careful *in vitro* analysis showed that a reconstitued NER reaction was insensitive to p21, given the non-processive DNA synthesis of NER [133,134]. In addition, early studies using ectopic expression of the protein showed that p21 did not inhibit NER [135,136]. In particular, cells expressing a p21 mutant form unable to bind PCNA were deficient in NER, but when the wild type protein was expressed, cells became proficient for repair [135]. A positive role for p21 in NER, was also suggested by the co-localization and interaction of p21 with PCNA in actively repairing normal fibroblasts [137,138], and by increased DNA repair in cells treated with DNA-damaging drugs, after p21 overexpression [139]. Accordingly, deletion of p21 gene in primary human fibroblasts resulted in increased sensitivity to UV radiation, together with reduced DNA repair efficiency, namely in the global genome excision repair sub-pathway [140]. Overall, the discrepancy of these results may be attributed to the different experimental conditions in biochemical assays (e.g. low vs high concentrations of p21 in *in vitro* reactions), and to the different cell model systems utilized (e.g. tumor vs normal cells, murine vs human cells), that could have introduced biasing factors, such as reduced NER efficiency in tumor cells, and the reduced global genome repair pathway in rodent cells [141].

Results obtained more recently with *in vivo* systems, i.e. by investigating the behavior of a p21 protein tagged with Green Fluorescent Protein (GFP) in living cells challenged with DNA damaging radiation, have shed more light on the role of p21 in DNA repair. In fact, spatio-temporal analysis of p21-GFP autofluorescence by time-lapse microscopy showed that p21 protein was rapidly recruited to nuclear regions where a local DNA damage was induced with the micropore irradiation technique, or with a laser beam [142] Interestingly, in experimental settings in which p21-GFP was co-expressed with PCNA tagged with Red Fluorescent Protein (RFP-PCNA), the dynamics of the process of p21-GFP recruitment was temporally similar to that of RFP-PCNA. In fact, the kinetics of p21-GFP accumulation at DNA damage sites was very rapid, and closely followed (though with a little delay) that of PCNA, suggesting that p21 was required at a later step after PCNA recruitment. Interestingly, the protein accumulation at DNA damage sites was found to be dependent on the previous recruitment of PCNA since a p21 mutant protein unable to interact with PCNA (p21^{PCNA-}) did not accumulate at sites of DNA damage [142]. In addition, the involvement of p21 was clearly related to the DNA repair process, since p21 recruitment did not occur in NER-deficient XPA fibroblasts [142]. Another important feature of p21 is that both endogenous p21 in normal fibroblasts, as well as ectopic p21 protein expressed in HeLa cells, were found to co-localize with NER factors interacting with PCNA (e.g. XPG, DNA polymerase δ, and CAF-1), and to be present in complexes containing these NER factors. Finally, conditions inducing an increase in endogenous p21 protein, or its ectopic expression, did not result in inhibition of NER [142].

An independent confirmation that p21 does not affect NER, and that the protein co-localizes with NER factors, like XPB, has been recently obtained with a similar approach of micropore irradiation in U2OS cells expressing myc-tagged p21 protein [143]. Another study showed that the p21 recruitment after UV damage in human melanoma SK-MEL-1 and SK-MEL-2 cell lines occurred via translocation to the nucleus and interaction with PCNA, which was found to save p21 from degradation, and to enhance DNA repair [144].

A further step in clarifying what could be the role of p21 in DNA repair has been recently obtained by investigating common interactors of p21 and PCNA. One such protein was found to be p300, a transcriptional co-activator endowed with HAT activity [95]. This protein was suggested to have a role in DNA repair synthesis [145], probably acting as a p53-dependent regulator of chromatin accessibility to NER machinery [96]. p21 has been found to regulate HAT activity required during DNA repair, by dissociating the p300-PCNA interaction [95]. Since it was previously shown that PCNA inhibits both the HAT and transcriptional activity of p300 [97], it has been suggested that a function played by p21 in NER could be the removal of the inhibitory effect of PCNA on HAT activity [95]. Since p300 has been shown to acetylate a number of proteins involved in BER [5,95], our group has recently investigated whether also NER proteins are acetylated. The results have shown that XPG, the PCNA-interacting endonuclease involved in the incision step of NER, is indeed acetylated by p300, and that p21 regulates the interaction between XPG and p300 in a PCNA-dependent manner [146]. Interestingly, *in vitro* experiments have also shown that PCNA is able to inhibit the acetylation of XPG. Therefore, these results suggest that p21 may help in removing the inhibitory effect of PCNA on the acetylation of XPG. This function may serve to facilitate NER completion, since lack of XPG acetylation induced by knocking-down p300 expression and activity in human fibroblasts, has been found to result in the accumulation of the endonuclease at DNA damage sites [146]. Concomitantly, knock-down of p300/CBP expression, has been shown to significantly impair NER efficiency, suggesting that in addition to acetylate histone for chromatin accessibility, p300/CBP may also acetylate NER factors to facilitate DNA repair.

Taken together, these lines of evidence indicate that p21 accumulates at sites of DNA damage similarly to DNA repair factors [147], and suggest a regulatory role in NER based on p21 ability to control, perhaps both spatially and temporally, the interaction of repair factors with PCNA (Figure 2).

4. p21 and Base Excision Repair (BER)

Further pieces of evidence suggesting that p21 is involved in other DNA repair pathways by regulating PCNA interacting proteins, were obtained by investigating the effect of p21 in the BER process. *In vitro* experiments showed that p21 inhibited PCNA-directed stimulation of

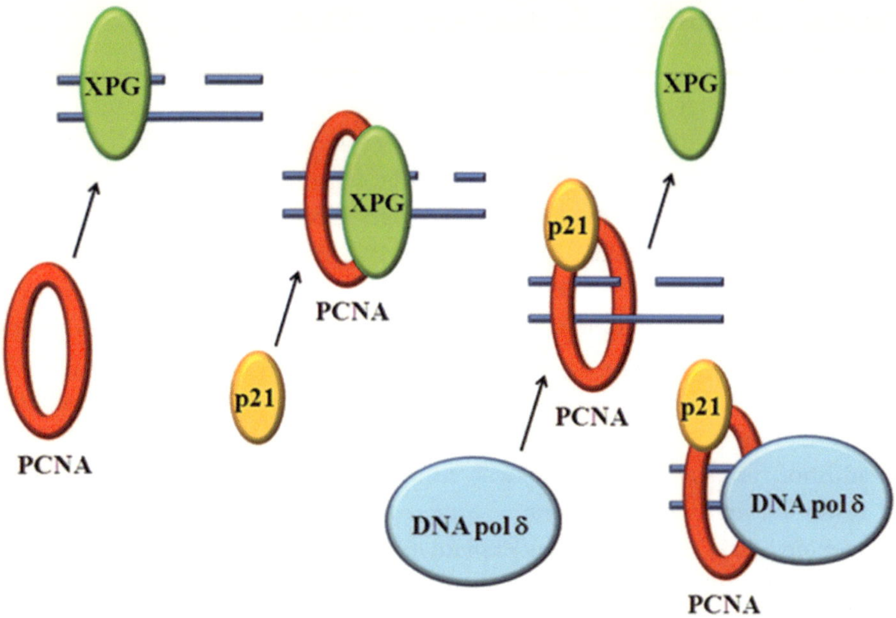

Figure 2. Schematic representation of interplay between PCNA, p21 and PCNA-interacting proteins, during NER. In this example, XPG endonuclease is shown. From left to right, are depicted the steps of the binding of PCNA to XPG, followed by the arrival of p21, which then displaces XPG from PCNA, to leave space for binding of the next partner, i.e. DNA polymerase δ.

DNA polymerase δ long-patch BER, but not in the presence of AP endonuclease 1, indicating a regulatory role of p21 in BER [148]. The requirement of p21 in BER is further supported by several findings: first, a direct physical association between p21 and poly(ADP-ribose) polymerase 1 (PARP-1), another important player in BER, was described. In particular, p21 was shown to compete with PARP-1 for binding to PCNA *in vitro*, and an association between p21 and PARP-1 was also found in normal fibroblasts treated with alkylating agents [149]. In addition, both PCNA and p21 were found to inhibit the ADP-ribosylating activity of PARP-1 [149]. We recently observed that p21-null human fibroblasts were more sensitive to DNA damage, and deficient in DNA repair induced by alkylating agents [150]. These results prompted us to investigate whether p21 might regulate the interaction of BER factors with PARP-1. The recruitment of PARP-1 and PCNA to damaged DNA was found to occur to a greater extent in $p21^{-/-}$ fibroblasts than in $p21^{+/+}$ parental cells. The PARP-1 accumulation in $p21^{-/-}$ cells was also accompanied by a higher activity of PARP-1, concomitantly with a persistent interaction of PARP-1 with BER factors, such as XRCC1 and DNA polymerase β [150]. Since an excess of PARP-1 antagonizes the activity of DNA polymerase β, these results suggest that prolonged association of PARP-1 with BER factors reduced the DNA repair efficiency observed in $p21^{-/-}$ fibroblasts [150]. These results indicate that p21 regulates the interaction between PARP-1 and BER factors, to promote efficient DNA repair.

5. p21 and Double-Strand Breaks Repair (DSBR)

Most of the evidence that p21 is rapidly accumulated at sites of DNA damage, have been obtained with UV-C irradiation, a typical means that primarily activates the NER pathway. However, p21 has been shown to behave in a similar way also in cells which have sustained other types of DNA lesions that are removed through different DNA repair pathways. Interestingly, the irradiation of normal human fibroblasts with heavy-ions inducing single (SSB) and double DNA strand breaks (DSB), stimulated the recruitment of p21 to sites of energy deposition [151]. Co-localization of p21 with proteins involved in double-strand break repair (i.e. Mre11, Rad50 and PCNA) was observed in these cells [151], thus lending further support to the accumulation of p21 at sites of DNA damage. This process has been shown to occur independently of p53 and core NHEJ factors (such as Ku70, Ku80, and DNA PKcs) [152]. In addition, after exposure to X-rays, recruitment of p21 was found to occur at foci spatially distinct from those containing histone γ-H2AX and 53BP1, suggesting no relation with DSB repair [153]. This result was explained by the production of differenty types of DNA lesions, according to the energy source employed. However, p21 recruitment occurred depending on its ability to bind PCNA [153]. Since results have shown that PCNA is required for initiation of recombination-associated DNA synthesis [154], it is thus likely that the role of p21 is related to this step of DSB repair.

6. p21 and Translesion DNA Synthesis (TLS)

The translesion DNA synthesis (TLS) is a process taking place at arrested replication forks in a PCNA-dependent manner, and that allows the bypass of the lesion by a mechanism of DNA polymerase switch. In this process, which actually it is not a repair reaction, the high fidelity replicative DNA polymerase is replaced by a low-fidelity enzyme able to synthetize DNA past a lesion [155,156]. Independent researches investigating the mechanisms controlling this reaction obtained results indicating the participation of p21 also in this process. In particular, it was suggested that p21 was required to limit the level of mutations arising from the error-prone lesion bypass; interestingly, the interaction with PCNA was shown to be important for the regulatory role of p21 in TLS [157]. This function of p21 has been suggested to control the loading of DNA polymerase η on PCNA, thereby contributing to limit TLS activity and the associated mutagenesis effect [143,158]. In addition, p21 was shown to modulate the level of PCNA ubiquitination occurring during TLS. Impaired PCNA ubiquitination was observed when p21 was knocked-down by RNA interference [157], but also when a nondegradable form of p21 was expressed [159]. These apparently opposite results may be explained by the different experimental approach and model system, yet they indicate that p21 protein must be finely regulated in order to fulfill its functions in the DNA damage response.

7. Proteasomal degradation of p21 protein

The most important post-translational modification of p21, i.e. ubiquitination, induces its proteasomal degradation [160]. However, both ubiquitin-dependent and -independent mechanisms have been reported [53,161,162]. The ubiquitin-dependent mechanisms have been described to occur via different E3 ubiquitin ligases, namely SCF^{Skp2}, APC/C^{Cdc20} and CRL^{Cdt2}, both in basal conditions (e.g. in S phase) [53,163,164], and after DNA damage induced by UV or ionizing radiation [165-167]. An ubiquitin-independent degradation of p21 has been shown to be mediated by direct association with the C8α-subunit of the proteasome complex [168], or with MDM2, yet independently of its E3 ligase activity [169,170]. Degradation via the C8α-subunit was protected by the interaction with PCNA [168,171]. In contrast, $CRL4^{Cdt2}$-mediated (ubiquitin-dependent) degradation of p21 required the interaction with PCNA [165,166]. The relative role of these different mechanisms is not fully understood, especially in S phase [172]. To complicate these findings, p21 degradation may be dependent on the different cell model systems investigated (p21 degradation was more pronounced in transformed cell lines) [167], as well as on the overexpression system that may result in reduced degradation [167,171,173].

It was suggested that p21 destruction was required for efficient DNA repair, implying an adverse effect, in particular on the NER process [174]. However, as previously discussed, other studies have shown that p21 does not inhibit NER [142,143,173], and that p21 is required for efficient NER in normal untransformed cells [95,140]. More recently, it has been shown that degradation of p21 after DNA damage is triggered by the extent of DNA damage rather than the type of lesion, and is not required for DNA repair, in normal human fibroblasts [173]. In fact, it has been shown that by inhibiting p21 degradation with caffeine (obtained through inhibition of ATM activity [174]), the NER efficiency was not significantly reduced [174]. In agreement with these findings, a recent report showed that inhibition of p21 degradation by deletion of CUL4A (a component of the CRL4 ubiquitin ligase complex with DDB1 and DDB2), resulted in NER stimulation [175]. These lines of evidence, while indicating that p21 degradation occurs after DNA damage, still do not clarify the actual role of the process in the context of DNA repair. In fact, p21 degradation appears to be a phenomenon independent of DNA repair, since it occurs also in NER-deficient fibroblasts [176].

8. p21 degradation, DDB2 and DNA repair

Although there is no doubt that p21 is degraded after DNA damage, several aspects of this process suggest that it is not a pre-requisite for DNA repair, but it may be related to a more general response to DNA damage. A particular consideration to be made is that another important protein involved in NER, i.e. the UV-induced DNA damage binding protein 2 (DDB2) has been indicated as an important mediator of the cell fate following DNA damage [177]. DDB2 protein is mutated in Xeroderma pigmentosum group E patients, and cells derived from these individuals show a partial deficiency in NER [178]. DDB2 protein exhibits a high affinity for damaged DNA and mediates binding of the CUL4A-DDB1 complex to target histone H2A ubiquitination in chromatin [179]. In addition, DDB2-DDB1-CUL4A complex ubiquitinates p21 for proteasomal degradation [165,166]. Deletion of DDB2 in mice (*DDB2*$^{-/-}$ cells), similarly to that of CUL4A, results in accumulation of p21 protein; however, it was also suggested that NER was restored when deleting concomitantly CDKN1A gene (*DDB2*$^{-/-}$ *p21*$^{-/-}$) [180]. This result was again taken as the indication that p21 must be degraded for optimal DNA repair. However, it must be noted that absence of p21 resulted in an increased cell entry into S-phase [175], thus confounding the type of DNA synthesis (i.e. replicative vs repair) observed [180]. It is also worth noting that in most studies investigating p21 degradation, cells were exposed to irradiation conditions inducing extensive DNA damage [165,166,170,174]. In contrast, cell exposure to sub-lethal DNA damaging conditions, does not lead to evident p21 degradation [142,173,181]. Since p21 is also involved in the regulation of the apoptotic process, it appears evident that p21 accumulation may inhibit apoptosis. Thus, p21 degradation after extensive DNA damage may be more considered a pro-apoptotic response rather than a pre-requisite for DNA repair [5]. In fact, DDB2-deficient cells have been shown to be apoptosis-resistant [177], and to be significantly impaired in undergoing premature senescence [182]. Accordingly, p21 degradation, as stimulated after DNA damage by E3 ligases associated with MKRN1 or DDB2, has been shown to facilitate the apoptotic cell death pathway, as opposed to the cell cycle arrest and senescence [176,183,184]. Overall, these lines of evidence seem to suggest that p21 degradation is indeed induced to avoid inhibition of the apototic process when cells have accumulated an irrepairable extent of DNA damage. In contrast, when the amount of DNA lesions are low enough to be worth attempting to repair them, p21 is not degraded and may help in DNA repair [5].

9. Future directions

The involvement of p21 in DNA repair processes is linked to its ability to bind PCNA which is a central hub for the majority of the factors participating in these processes. Due to its peculiar ability to displace PCNA-interacting proteins, it is likely that p21 may play a regulatory role in orchestrating the PCNA interactions. A clear example of this function is the p21 regulation of the interaction between p300 and PCNA, which has been shown to inhibit the acetyl transferase activity. The influence of p21 is useful for histone acetylation, and for chromatin remodeling function of p300 in DNA repair [95,185]. However, since also DNA repair factors are acetylated by p300/CBP [5,186], the role of p21 in this context could be to remove the inhibition exerted by PCNA. This function is important for DNA repair regulation, and the inability to perform this job is likely to impair DNA repair. In fact, in p21-null human fibroblasts the NER factor XPG (the endonuclease involved in lesion incision) accumulates at the sites of DNA damage, in a manner similar to that observed after knock-down of p300/CBP activity [146]. These results support a regulatory role by which p21 may influence XPG acetylation and consequently its retention on chromatin. Studies are under way to establish the link between XPG acetylation and NER efficiency; however, it is clear that in the absence of p21, as well as after silencing of p300/CBP, DNA repair is inefficient [140,146].

If p21 plays a regulatory role in DNA repair, how this function may be related/coupled to p21 degradation? One possibility is that p21 could be degraded after execution of its function, in order to avoid the persistence of the PCNA/p21 complex onto DNA. Prolonging the DNA residence time of this complex may be detrimental to the genome, since additional unwanted reactions might occur under these circumstances. This hypothesis is supported by findings showing that p21 has been found to co-localize with, and participate in protein complexes containing factors such as XPG, DNA polymerase δ and CAF-1 [142], all of which are known to interact with PCNA. Therefore, coupling DNA repair with protein degradation could fulfil this function. This speculation needs a formal proof, since some DNA repair factors are ubiquitinated, while others are not. Thus, this hypothesis requires appropriated future experimentation on the effects of p21 ubiquitination on DNA repair synthesis.

Acknowledgements

The Authors wish to thank the collaborators (I.A. Scovassi, T. Nardo, D. Necchi) that have participated in the investigations described in this chapter. Research in the Author laboratory has been funded in the past by MIUR grant, and currently by The Italian Association for Cancer Research (AIRC), grants no. IG 5126 and 11747 (to E. P.). M.T. is a PhD student from "Dottorato in Scienze Genetiche e Biomolecolari" (University of Pavia), supported by AIRC.

Author details

Micol Tillhon[1], Ornella Cazzalini[2], Ilaria Dutto[1], Lucia A. Stivala[2] and Ennio Prosperi[1*]

*Address all correspondence to: prosperi@igm.cnr.it

1 CNR Institute of Molecular Genetics (IGM-CNR), Pavia, Italy

2 Dept. of Molecular Medicine, lab Pathology, University of Pavia, Pavia, Italy

References

[1] Bartek J, Lukas J. DNA damage checkpoints: from initiation to recovery or adaptation. Current Opinion in Cell Biology 2007;19(2) 238-245.

[2] Hoeijmakers JH. Genome maintenance mechanism for preventing cancer. Nature 2001;411(6835) 366-374.

[3] Dotto GP. p21(WAF1/Cip1): more than a break to the cell cycle? Biochimica Biophysica Acta 2000;1471(1) M43-56.

[4] Coqueret O. New roles for p21 and p27 cell-cycle inhibitors: a function for each cell compartment? Trends in Cell Biology 2003;13(2) 65-70.

[5] Cazzalini O, Scovassi AI, Savio M, Stivala LA, Prosperi E. Multiple roles of the cell cycle inhibitor p21^{CDKN1A} in the DNA damage response. Mutation Research/Reviews in Mutation Research 2010;704(1-3) 12-20.

[6] Stivala LA, Cazzalini O, Prosperi E. The Cyclin-Dependent Kinase Inhibitor p21CDKN1A as a target of anti-cancer drugs. Current Cancer Drug Targets 2012;12(2) 85-96.

[7] Sherr CJ, Roberts JM. CDK inhibitors: positive and negative regulators of G1 phase progression. Genes & Development 1999;13(12) 1501-1512.

[8] Besson A, Dowdy SF, Roberts JM. CDK inhibitors: cell cycle regulators and beyond. Developmental Cell 2008;14(2) 159-169.

[9] Kriwacki, R.W.; Hengst, L.; Tennat, L.; Reed, S.I.; Whight, P.E. Structural studies of p21$^{waf1/cip1/Sdi1}$ in the free and Cdk2-bound state: conformational disorder mediates binding diversity. Proceedings of the National Academy of Sciences of USA 1996;93(21), 11504-11509.

[10] Chen J, Jackson PK, Kirschner MW, Dutta A. Separate domains of p21 involved in the inhibition of Cdk kinase and PCNA. Nature 1995;374(6520) 386-388.

[11] Goubin F, Ducommun B. Identification of binding domains on the p21Cip1 cyclin-dependent kinase inhibitor. Oncogene 1995;10(12) 2281-2287.

[12] Chen J, Saha P, Kornbluth S, Dynlacht BD, Dutta A. Cyclin-binding motifs are essential for the function of p21Cip1. Molecular and Cellular Biology 1996;16(9) 4673-4682.

[13] Fotedar R, Fitzgerald P, Rousselle T, Cannella D, Dore M, Messier H, Fotedar A. p21 contains independent binding sites for cyclin and cdk2: both sites are required to inhibit cdk2 kinase activity. Oncogene 1996;12(10) 2155-2164.

[14] Flores-Rozas H., Kelman Z, Dean FB, Pan ZQ, Harper JW, Elledge SJ, O'Donnell M, Hurwitz J. Cdk-interacting protein 1 directly binds with proliferating cell nuclear antigen and inhibits DNA replication catalyzed by the DNA polymerase delta holoenzyme. Proceedings of the National Academy of Sciences of USA 1994;91(18) 8655-8659.

[15] Waga S, Hannon GJ, Beach D, Stillman B. The p21 inhibitor of cyclin-dependent kinases controls DNA replication by interaction with PCNA. Nature 1994;369(6481) 574-578.

[16] Luo Y, Hurwitz J, Massagué J. Cell-cycle inhibition by independent CDK and PCNA binding domains in p21. Nature 1995;375(6527) 159-161.

[17] Chen L., Akamatsu M, Smith ML, Lung FDT, Duba D, Roller PP, Fornace AJ, O'Connor PM. Characterization of p21Cip1/Waf1 peptide domains required for cyclin E/cdk2 and PCNA interactions. Oncogene 1996;12(3) 595-607.

[18] Prosperi E. The fellowship of the rings: distinct pools of proliferating cell nuclear antigen (PCNA) trimer at work. FASEB Journal 2006;20(7) 833-837.

[19] Moldovan GL, Pfander B, Jentsch S. PCNA, the maestro of replication fork. Cell 2007;129(4) 665-679.

[20] Deng G, Zhang P, Harper JW, Elledge SJ, Leder P. Mice lacking p21CIP1/WAF1 undergo normal development, but are defective in G1 checkpoint control. Cell 1995;82(4) 675-684.

[21] Martin-Caballero J, Flores JM, Garcìa-Palencia P, Serrano M. Tumour susceptibility of p21waf1/cip1-deficient mice. Cancer Research 2001;61(16) 6234-6238.

[22] Jackson RJ, Adnane J, Coppola D, Cantor A, Sebti SM, Pledger WJ. Loss of the cell cycle inhibitors p21(Cip1) and p27(Kip1) enhances tumorigenesis in knockout mouse models. Oncogene 2002;21(55) 8486-8497.

[23] Jackson RJ, Engelman RW, Coppola D, Cantor AB, Wharton W, Pledger WJ. p21Cip1 nullizygosity increases tumor formation in irradiated mice. Cancer Research 2003;63(12) 3021-3025.

[24] Chen K, Xia W, Yang JY, Hsu JL, Chou CK, Sun HL, Wyszomierski LS, Mills GB, Muller WJ, Yu D, Hung MC. Activation of p21(CIP1/WAF1) in mammary epithelium accelerates mammary tumorigenesis and promotes lung metastasis. Biochemical Biophysical Reserach Communications 2010;403(1) 103-107.

[25] Weinberg WC, Fernandez-Sala E, Morgan DL, Shalizi A, Mirosh E, Stanulis E, Deng C, Hennings H, Yuspa SH. Genetic deletion of p21WAF1 enhances papilloma formation but not malignant conversion in experimental mouse skin carcinogenesis. Cancer Research 1999;59(9) 2050-2054.

[26] Poole AJ, Heap D, Carroll RE, Tyner AL. Tumor suppressor functions for the Cdk inhibitor p21 in the mouse colon. Oncogene 2004;23(49) 8128-8134.

[27] Yang W, Velcich A, Lozonschi I, Liang J, Nicholas C, Zhuang M, Bancroft L, Augenlicht LH. Inactivation of p21WAF1/cip1 enhances intestinal tumor formation in Muc2-/- mice. American Journal of Pathology 2005;166(4) 1239-1246.

[28] Yang WC, Mathew J, Velcich A, Edelmann W, Kucherlapati R, Lipkin M, Yang K, Augenlicht LH. Targeted inactivation of the p21WAF1/cip1 gene enhance Apc-initiated tumor formation and the tumor-promoting activity of a Western-style high-risk diet by altering cell maturation in the intestinal mucosal. Cancer Research 2001;61(2) 565-569.

[29] Cheng T, Rodriguez N, Shen H, Yang Y, Bombkowski D, Sykes M, Scadden DT. Hematopoietic stem cell quiescence maintained by p21cip1/waf1. Science 2000;287(5459) 1804-1808.

[30] Balomenos D, Martìn-Caballero J, Garcìa MI, Prieto I, Flores JM, Serrano M, Martinez-AC. The cell cycle inhibitor p21 controls T-cell proliferation and sex-linked lupus development. Nature Medicine 2000;6(2) 171-176.

[31] Abbas T, Dutta A. p21 in cancer: intricate networks and multiple activities. Nature Reviews of Cancer 2009;9(6) 400-414.

[32] Viale A, De Franco F, Orleth A, Cambiaghi V, Giuliani V, Bossi D, Ronchini C, Ronzoni S, Muradore I, Monestiroli S, Gobbi A, Alcalay M, Minucci S, Pelicci PG. Cell-cycle restriction limits DNA damage and maintains self-renewal of leukaemia stem cells. Nature 2009;45(7225) 751-756.

[33] Cazzalini O, Perucca P, Valsecchi F, Stivala LA, Bianchi L, Vannini, V, Prosperi, E. Intracellular localization of the cyclin-dependent kinase inhibitor $p21^{CDKN1A}$-GFP fusion protein during cell cycle arrest. Histochemistry and Cell Biology 2004;121(5) 377-381.

[34] Abella N, Brun S, Calvo M, Tapia O, Weber JD, Berciano MT, Lafarga M, Bachs O, Agell N. Nucleolar disruption ensures nuclear accumulation of p21 upon DNA damage. Traffic 2010;11(6) 743-755.

[35] Abukhdeir AM, Park BH. p21 and p27, roles in carcinogenesis and drug resistance. Expert Reviews in Molecular Medicine 2008;10 e19.

[36] Zhou BP, Liao Y, Xia W, Spohn, B, Lee, MH, Hung, M.C. Cytoplasmic localization of p21Cip1/WAF1 by Akt-induced phosphorylation in HER-2/neu-overexpressing cells. Nature Cell Biology 2001;3(3) 245-252.

[37] Li Y, Dowbenko D, Lasky LA. AKT/PKB phosphorylation of p21Cip/WAF1 enhances protein stability of p21Cip/WAF1 and promotes cell survival. The Journal of Biological Chemistry 2002;277(13) 11352-11361.

[38] Zhang Y, Wang Z, Magnuson NS. Pim-1 kinase-dependent phosphorylation of p21Cip1/WAF1 regulates its stability and cellular localization in H1299 cells. Molecular Cancer Research 2007;5(9) 909-922.

[39] Scott MT, Morrice N, Ball KL. Reversible phosphorylation at the C-terminal regulatory domain of p21(Waf1/Cip1) modulates proliferating cell nuclear antigen binding. The Journal of Biological Chemistry 2000; 275(15) 11529-11537.

[40] Rodríguez-Vilarrupla A, Díaz C, Canela N, Rahn HP, Bachs O, Agell N. Identification of the nuclear localization signal of p21(cip1) and consequences of its mutation on cell proliferation. FEBS Letters 2002;531(2) 319-323.

[41] El-Deiry W, Tokino T, Velculescu VE, Levy DB, Parsons R, Trent JM, Lin D, Mercer WE, Kinzier KW, Volgestein B. WAF1, a potential mediator of p53 tumor suppressor. Cell 1993;75(4) 817-825.

[42] Waldman T, Kinzler KW, Vogelstein B. p21 is necessary for the p53-mediated G1 arrest in human cancer cells. Cancer Research 1995;55(22) 5187-5190.

[43] Brugarolas J, Moberg K, Boyd SD, Taya Y, Jacks T, Lees JA. Inhibition of cyclindependent kinase 2 by p21 is necessary for retinoblastoma protein-mediated G1 arrest after gamma-irradiation. Proceedings of the National Academy of Sciences USA 1999;96(3) 1002-1007.

[44] Brugarolas J, Chandrasekaran C, Gordon JI, Beach D, Jacks I, Hannon GJ. Radiation-induced cell cycle arrest compromised by p21 deficiency. Nature 1995;377(6549) 552-557.

[45] Satyanarayana A, Hilton MB, Kaldis P. p21 inhibits CDK1 in the absence of Cdk2 to maintain the G1/S phase DNA damage checkpoint. Molecular Biology of the Cell 2008;19(1) 65-77.

[46] Gulbis JM, Kelman Z, Hurtwitz J, O'Donnel M, Kuriyan J. Structure of the C terminal region of p21waf1/cip1 complexed with human PCNA. Cell 1996;87(2) 297-306.

[47] Warbrick E, Lane DP, Glover DM, Cox LS. A small peptide inhibitor of DNA replication defines the site of interaction between the cyclin-dependent kinase inhibitor p21WAF1 and proliferating cell nuclear antigen. Current Biology 1995;5(3) 275-282.

[48] Chen J, Peters R, Saha P, Lee P, Theodoras A, Pagano M, Wagner G, Dutta A. A 39 amino acid fragment of the cell cycle regulator p21 is sufficient to bind PCNA and partially inhibit DNA replication in vivo. Nucleic Acids Research 1996;24(9) 1727-1733.

[49] Cayrol C, Knibiehler M, Ducommun B. p21 binding to PCNA causes G1 and G2 cell cycle arrest in p53-deficient cells. Oncogene 1998;16(3) 311-320.

[50] Rousseau D, Cannella D, Boulaire J, Fitzgerald P, Fotedar A, Fotedar R. Growth inhibition by CDK-cyclin and PCNA binding domains of p21 occurs by distinct mechanisms and is regulated by ubiquitin-proteasome pathway. Oncogene 1999;18(30) 4313-4325.

[51] Mattock H, Lane DP, Warbrick E. Inhibition of cell proliferation by the PCNA-binding protein region of p21 expressed as a GFP miniprotein. Experimental Cell Research 2001;265(2) 234-241.

[52] Cazzalini O, Perucca P, Riva F, Stivala LA, Bianchi L, Vannini V, Ducommun B, Prosperi E. p21CDKN1A does not interfere with loading of PCNA at DNA replication sites, but inhibits subsequent binding of DNA polymerase d at the G1/S phase transition. Cell Cycle 2003;2(6) 596-603.

[53] Bornstein G, Bloom J, Sitry-Ahevah D, Nakayama K, Pagano M, Hershko A. Role of the SCFSkp2 ubiquitin ligase in the degradation of p21Cip1 in S phase. The Journal of Biological Chemistry 2003;278(28) 25752-25757.

[54] Gottifredi V, McKinney K, Poyurovsky MV, Prives C. Decreased p21 levels are required for efficient restart of DNA synthesis after S phase block. The Journal of Biological Chemistry 2004;279(7) 5802-5810.

[55] Li H, Xie B, Rahmeh A, ZhouY, Lee MYWT. Direct interaction of p21 with p50, the small subunit of human DNA polymerase delta. Cell Cycle 2006;5(4) 428-436.

[56] Arima Y, Hirota T, Bronner C, Mousli M, Fujiwara T, Niwa S, Ishikawa H, Saya H. Down-regulation of nuclear protein ICBP90 by p53/p21cip1/waf1-dependent DNA-damage checkpoint signals contributes to cell cycle arrest at G1/S transition. Genes Cells 2004;9(2) 131-142.

[57] Bunz F, Dutriaux A, Lengauer C, Waldman T, Zhou S, Brown JP, Sedivy JM, Kinzler KW, Vogelstein B. Requirement for p53 and p21 to sustain G2 arrest after DNA damage. Science 1998;282(5393) 1497-1501.

[58] Niculescu AR, Chen X, Smeets M, Hengst L, Prives C, Reed SI. Effects of p21Cip1/Waf1 at both the G2/S and the G1/M cell cycle transitions: pRb is a critical determinant in blocking DNA replication and in preventing endoreduplication. Molecular and Cellular Biology 1998;18(1) 629-643.

[59] Waldman T, Lengauer C, Kinzler KW, Vogelstein B. Uncoupling of S phase and mitosis induced by anticancer agents in cells lacking p21. Nature 1996;381(6584) 713-716.

[60] Harper JW, Elledge SJ, Keyomarsi K, Dynlacht B, Tsai LH, Zhang P, Dobrowolski S, Bai C, Connell-Crowley L, Swindell E, Fox MP, Wei N. Inhibition of cyclin-dependent kinases by p21. Molecular Biology of the Cell 1995;6(4) 387-400.

[61] Smits VA, Klompmaker R, Vallenius T, Rijksen G, Makela TP, Medema RH. p21 inhibits Thr161 phosphorylation of Cdc2 to enforce the G2 DNA damage checkpoint. The Journal of Biological Chemistry 2000;275(39) 30638-30643.

[62] Dulic' V, Stein GH, Far DF, Reed SI. Nuclear accumulation of p21Cip1 at the onset of mitosis: a role at the G2/M-phase transition. Molecular and Cellular Biology 1998;18(1) 546-557.

[63] Baus F, Gire V, Fisher D, Piette J, Dulic V. Permanent cell cycle exit in G2 phase after DNA damage in normal human fibroblasts. The EMBO Journal 2003;22(15) 3992-4002.

[64] Charrier-Savournin FB, Château MT, Gire V, Sedivy J, Piette J, Dulic V. p21-Mediated nuclear retention of cyclin B1-Cdk1 in response to genotoxic stress. Molecular Biology of the Cell 2004;15(9) 3965–3976.

[65] Gillis LD, Leidal AM, Hill R, Lee PWK. p21waf1/cip1 mediates cyclin B1 degradation in response to DNA damage. Cell Cycle 2009;8(2) 253-256.

[66] Lee J, Kim AK, Barbier V, Fotedar A, Fotedar R. DNA damage triggers p21WAF1-dependent Emi1 down-regulation that maintains G2 arrest. Molecular Biology of the Cell 2009;20(7) 1891-1902.

[67] Topley GI, Okuyama R, Gonzales JG, Conti C, Dotto GP. p21WAF1/Cip1 functions as a suppressor of malignant skin tumor formation and a determinant of keratinocyte stem-cell potential. Proceedings of the National Academy of Sciences of U.S.A. 1999;96(16) 9089-9094.

[68] Kippin TE, Martens DJ, van der Kooy D. p21 loss compromises the relative quiescence of forebrain stem cell proliferation leading to exhaustion of their proliferation capacity. Genes & Development 2005;19(6) 756-767.

[69] Pechnick RN, Zonis S, Wawrowsky K, Pourmorady J, Chesnokova V. p21Cip1 restricts neuronal proliferation in the subgranular zone of the dentate gyrus of the hyppocampus. Proceedings of the National Academy of Sciences of U.S.A. 2008;105(4) 1358-1363.

[70] Choudhury AR, Ju Z, Djojosubroto MW, Schienke A, Lechel A, Schaetzlein S, Jiang H, Stepczynska A, Wang C, Buer J, Lee HW, von Zglinicki T, Ganser A, Schirmacher P, Nakauchi H, Rudolph KL. Cdkn1a deletion improves stem cell function and lifespan of mice with dysfunctional telomeres without accelerating cancer formation. Nature Genetics 2007;39(1) 99- 105.

[71] Roninson IB. Oncogenic functions of tumour suppressor p21(Waf1/Cip1/Sdi1), association with cell senescence and tumour-promoting activities of stromal fibroblasts. Cancer Letters 2002;179(1) 1-14.

[72] Herbig U, Sedivy JM. Regulation of growth arrest in senescence: telomere damage is not the end of the story. Mechanisms of Ageing and Development 2006;127(1) 16-24.

[73] Perucca P, Cazzalini O, Madine M, Savio M, Laskey RA, Vannini V, Prosperi E, Stivala LA. Loss of p21CDKN1A impairs entry to quiescence and activates a DNA damage response in normal fibroblasts induced to quiescence. Cell Cycle 2009;8(1) 105-114.

[74] Bedelbaeva K, Snyder A, Gourevitch D, Clark L, Zhang XM, Leferovich J, Cheverud JM, Lieberman P, Heber-Katz E. Lack of p21 expression links cell cycle control and appendage regeneration in mice. Proceedings of the National Academy of Sciences of U.S.A. 2010;107(13) 5845-5850.

[75] Di Cunto F, Topley G, Calautti E, Hsiao J, Ong L, Seth PK, Dotto GP. Inhibitory function of p21Cip1/WAF1 in differentiation of primary mouse keratinocytes independent of cell cycle control. Science 1998;280(5366) 1069-1072.

[76] Gartel AL, Serfas MS, Gartel M, Goufman E, Wu GS, el-Deiry WS, Tyner AL. p21(WAF1/CIP1) expression is induced in newly nondividing cells in diverse epithe-

lia and during differentiation of the Caco-2 intestinal cell line. Experimental Cell Research 1996;227(2) 171-181.

[77] Casini T, Pelicci PG. A function of p21 during promyelocytic leukemia cell differentiation independent of CDK inhibition and cell cycle arrest. Oncogene 1999;18(21) 3235-3243.

[78] Zhang P, Wong C, Liu D, Finegold M, Harper JW, Elledge SJ. p21(CIP1) and p57(KIP2) control muscle differentiation at the myogenin step. Genes & Development 1999;13(2) 213-224.

[79] Negishi Y, Ui N, Nakajima M, Kawashima K, Maruyama K, Takizawa T, Endo H. p21Cip-1/SDI-1/WAF-1 gene is involved in chondrogenic differentiation of ATDC5 cells in vitro. The Journalof Biological Chemistry 2001;276(35) 33249-33256.

[80] Zezula J, Casaccia-Bonnefil P, Ezhevsky SA, Osterhout DJ, Levine JM, Dowdy SF, Chao MV, Koff A. p21cip1 is required for the differentiation of oligodendrocytes independently of cell cycle withdrawal. EMBO Reports 2001;2(1) 27-34.

[81] LaBaer J, Garrett MD, Stevenson LF, Slingerland JM, Sandhu C, Chou HS, Fattaey A, Harlow E. New functional activities for the p21 family of CDK inhibitors. Genes & Development 1997;11(7) 847-862.

[82] Perkins ND. Not just a CDK inhibitor: regulation of transcription by p21(WAF1/CIP1/SDI1). Cell Cycle 2002;1(1) 39-41.

[83] Coqueret O, Gascan H. Functional interaction of STAT3 transcription factor with the cell inhibitor p21WAF1/CIP1/SDI1. The Journal of Biological Chemistry 2000;275(25) 18794-18800.

[84] Shiyanov P, Bagchi S, Adami G, Kokontis J, Hay N, Arroyo M, Morozov A, Raychaudhuri P. p21 disrupts the interaction between cdk2 and the E2F-p130 complex. Molecular and Cellular Biology 1996;16(3) 737-744.

[85] Delavaine L, La Thangue NB. Control of E2F activity by p21Waf1/Cip1. Oncogene 1999;18(39) 5381-5392.

[86] Kitaura H, Shinshi M, Uchikoshi Y, Ono T, Iguchi-Ariga SM, Ariga H. Reciprocal regulation via protein–protein interaction between c-Myc and p21(cip1/waf1/ sdi1) in DNA replication and transcription. The Journal of Biological Chemistry 2000;275(14) 10477-10483.

[87] Zhu H, Chang BD, Uchiumi T, Roninson IB. Identification of promoter elements responsible for transcriptional inhibition of polo-like kinase 1 and topoisomerase II alpha genes by p21(WAF1/CIP1/SDI1). Cell Cycle 2002;1(1) 59-66.

[88] Vigneron A, Cherier J, Barre` B, Gamelin E, Coqueret O. The cell cycle inhibitor p21waf1 binds to the myc and cdc25A promoters upon DNA damage and induces

transcriptional repression. The Journal of Biological Chemistry 2006;281(46) 34742-34750.

[89] Perkins ND, Felzien LK, Betts JC, Leung K, Beach DH, Nabel GJ. Regulation of NF-kappaB by cyclin-dependent kinases associated with the p300 coactivator. Science 1997;275(5299) 523-527.

[90] Redeuilh G, Attia A, Mester J, Sabbah M. Transcriptional activation by the estrogen receptor alpha is modulated through inhibition of cyclin-dependent kinases. Oncogene 2002;21(37) 5773-5782.

[91] Snowden AW, Anderson LA, Webster GA, Perkins ND. A novel transcriptional repression domain mediates p21WAF1/CIP1 induction of transactivation. Molecular and Cellular Biology 2000;20(8) 2676-2686.

[92] Gregory DJ, Garcia-Wilson E, Poole JC, Snowden AW, Roninson IB, Perkins ND. Induction of transcription through the CRD1 motif by p21WAF1/CIP1 is core promoter specific and cyclin dependent kinase independent. Cell Cycle 2002;1(5) 343-350.

[93] Martinez-Balba´s MA, Bannister AJ, Martin K, Haus-Seuffert P, Meisterernst M, Kouzarides T. The acetyltransferase activity of CBP stimulates transcription. The EMBO Journal 1998;17(10) 2886-2893.

[94] Devgan V, Mammucari C, Millar SE, Brisken C, Dotto GP. p21WAF1/Cip1 is a negative transcriptional regulator of Wnt4 expression downstream of Notch1 activation. Genes & Development 2005;19(12) 1485-1495.

[95] Cazzalini O, Perucca P, Savio M, Necchi D, Bianchi L, Stivala LA, Ducommun B, Scovassi AI, Prosperi E. Interaction of p21(CDKN1A) with PCNA regulates the histone acetyltransferase activity of p300 in nucleotide excision repair. Nucleic Acids Research 2008;36(5) 1713-1722.

[96] Rubbi CP, Milner J. p53 is a chromatin accessibility factor for nucleotide excision repair of DNA damage. The EMBO Journal 2003;22(4) 975-986.

[97] Hong R, Chakravarti D. The human proliferating cell nuclear antigen regulates transcriptional coactivator p300 activity and promotes transcriptional repression. The Journal of Biological Chemistry 2003;278(45) 44505-44513.

[98] Chang BD, Watanabe K, Broude EV, Fang J, Poole JC, Kalinichenko TV, Roninson IB. Effects of p21Waf1/Cip1/Sdi1 on cellular gene expression: implications for carcinogenesis, senescence, and age-related diseases. Proceedings of the National Academy of Sciences of U.S.A. 2000;97(8) 4291-4296.

[99] Gartel AL, Tyner AL. The role of the cyclin-dependent kinase inhibitor p21 in apoptosis. Molecular Cancer Therapeutics 2002;1(8) 639-649.

[100] Liu S, Bishop WR, Liu M. Differential effects of cell cycle regulatory protein p21(WAF1/Cip1) on apoptosis and sensitivity to cancer chemotherapy. Drug Resistance Updates 2003;6(4) 183-195.

[101] Garner E, Raj K. Protective mechanisms of p53–p21–pRb proteins against DNA damage-induced cell death. Cell Cycle 2008;7(3) 277–282.

[102] Waldman T, Zhang Y, Dillehay L, Yu J, Kinzler K, Vogelstein B, Williams J. Cell cycle arrest versus cell death in cancer therapy. Nature Medicine 1997;3(9) 1034-1036.

[103] Suzuki A, Tsutomi Y, Akahane K, Araki T, Miura M. Resistance to Fas-mediated apoptosis: activation of caspase 3 is regulated by cell cycle regulator p21WAF1 and IAP gene family ILP. Oncogene 1998;17(8) 931-939.

[104] Suzuki A, Tsutomi Y, Miura M, Akahane K. Caspase 3 inactivation to suppress Fas-mediated apoptosis: identification of binding domain with p21 and ILP and inactivation machinery by p21. Oncogene 1999; 18(5) 1239–1244.

[105] Baptiste-Okoh N,Barsotti AM, Prives C. Caspase 2 is both required for p53- mediated apoptosis and downregulated by p53 in a p21-dependent manner. Cell Cycle 2008;7(9) 1133-1138.

[106] Gervais JL, Seth P, Zhang H. Cleavage of CDK inhibitor p21(Cip1/Waf1) by caspases is an early event during DNA damage-induced apoptosis. The Journal of Biological Chemistry 1998;273(30) 19207-19212.

[107] Levkau B, Koyama H, Raines EW, Clurman BE, Herren B, Orth K, Roberts JM, Ross R. Cleavage of p21Cip1/Waf1 and p27Kip1 mediates apoptosis in endothelial cells through activation of Cdk2: role of a caspase cascade. Molecular Cell 1998;1(4) 553-563.

[108] Jin YH, Yoo KJ, Lee YH, Lee SK. Caspase 3-mediated cleavage of p21WAF1/CIP1 associated with the cyclin A-cyclin-dependent kinase 2 complex is a prerequisite for apoptosis in SK-HEP-1 cells. The Journal of Biological Chemistry 2000;275(39) 30256–30263.

[109] Xu SQ, El-Deiry WS. p21(WAF1/CIP1) inhibits initiator caspase cleavage by TRAIL death receptor DR4. Biochemical and Biophysical Research Communications 2000;269(1) 179-190.

[110] Harvey KJ, Lukovic D, Ucker DS. Caspase-dependent Cdk activity is a requisite effector of apoptotic death events. The Journal of Cell Biology 2000;148(1) 59-72.

[111] Asada M, Yamada T, Ichijo H, Delia D, Miyazono K, Fukumuro K,Mizutani S. Apoptosis inhibitory activity of cytoplasmic p21(Cip1/WAF1) in monocytic differentiation, The EMBO Journal 1999;18(5) 1223-1234.

[112] Le HV, Minn AJ, Massague J. Cyclin-dependent kinase inhibitors uncouple cell cycle progression from mitochondrial apoptotic functions in DNA-damaged cancer cells. The Journal of Biological Chemistry 2005;280(36) 32018-32025.

[113] Sohn D, Essmann F, Schulze-Osthoff K, Janicke RU. p21 blocks irradiation induced apoptosis downstream of mitochondria by inhibition of cyclin-dependent kinase-mediated caspase-9 activation. Cancer Research 2006;66(23) 11254-11262.

[114] Seoane J, Le HV, Massaguè J. Myc suppression of the p21(Cip1) Cdk inhibitor influences the outcome of the p53 response to DNA damage. Nature 2002;419(6908) 729-734.

[115] Weiss RH. p21Waf1/Cip1 as a therapeutic target in breast and other cancers. Cancer Cell 2003;4(6) 425-429.

[116] Janicke RU, Essmann F, Schulze-Osthoff K. The multiple battles fought by antiapoptotic p21. Cell Cycle 2007;6(4) 407-413.

[117] Fotedar R, Brickner H, Saadatmandi N, Rousselle T, Diederich L, Munshi A, Jung B, Reed JC, Fotedar A. Effect of p21waf1/cip1 transgene on radiation induced apoptosis in T cells. Oncogene 1999;18(24) 3652-3658.

[118] Hingorani R, Bi B, Dao T, Bae Y, Matsuzawa A, Crispe IN. CD95/Fas signaling in T lymphocytes induces the cell cycle control protein p21cip-1/WAF-1, which promotes apoptosis. Journal of Immunology 2000;164(8) 4032-4036.

[119] Chinery R, Brockman JA, Peeler MO, Shyr Y, Beauchamp RD, Coffey RJ. Antioxidants enhance the cytotoxicity of chemotherapeutic agents in colorectal cancer, a p53-independent induction of p21WAF1/CIP1 via C/EBPbeta. Nature Medicine 1997;3(11) 1233-1241.

[120] Chopin V, Toillon RA, Jouy N, Le Bourhis X. P21(WAF1/CIP1) is dispensable for G1 arrest, but indispensable for apoptosis induced by sodium butyrate in MCF-7 breast cancer cells. Oncogene 2004;23(1) 21-29.

[121] Giansanti V, Torriglia A, Scovassi AI. Conversation between apoptosis and autophagy, "Is it your turn or mine?" Apoptosis 2011;16(4) 321-333.

[122] Fujiwara K, Daido S, Yamamoto A, Kobayashi R, Yokoyama T, Aoki H, Iwado E, Shinojima N, Kondo Y, Kondo S. Pivotal role of the cyclin-dependent kinase inhibitor p21WAF1/CIP1 in apoptosis and autophagy. The Journal of Biological Chemistry 2008;283(1) 388-397.

[123] Lee S, Helfman DM. Cytoplasmic p21Cip1 is involved in Ras-induced inhibition of the ROCK/LIMK/Cofilin pathway. The Journal of Biological Chemistry 2004;279(3) 1885-1891.

[124] Starostina NG, Simpliciano JM, McGuirk MA, Kipreos ET. CRL2^{LRR-1} targets a CDK inhibitor for cell cycle control in C. elegans and actin-based motility regulation in human cells. Developmental Cell 2010;19(5) 753-764.

[125] Oku T, Ikeda S, Sasaki H, Fukuda K, Morioka H, Ohtsuka E, Yoshikawa H, Tsurimoto T. Functional sites of human PCNA which interact with p21 (Cip1/Waf1), DNA polymerase delta and replication factor C. Gene Cells 1998;3(6) 357-369.

[126] Pan ZQ, Reardon JT, Li L, Flores-Rozas H, Legerski R, Sancar A, Hurwitz J. Inhibition of nucleotide excsion repair by cyclin-dependent kinase inhibitor p21. The Journal of Biological Chemistry 1995;270(37) 22008-22016.

[127] Podust VN, Podust L, Goubin F, Ducommun B, Hübscher H. Mechanism of inhibition of proliferating cell nuclear antigen-dependent DNA synthesis by the cyclin-dependent kinase inhibitor p21. Biochemistry 1995;34(27) 8869-8875.

[128] Cooper MP, Balajee AS, Bohr VA. The C-terminal domain of p21 inhibits nucleotide excision repair in vitro and in vivo. Molecular and Cellular Biology 1999;10(7) 2119-2129.

[129] Smith L, Ford JM, Hollander MC, Bortnick RA, Amounson SA, Seo YR, Deng C, Hanawalt PC, Fornace AJ. p53-mediated DNA repair responses to UV radiation: studies of mouse cells lacking p53, p21, and/or gadd45 genes. Molecular and Cellular Biology 2000;20(10) 3705-3714.

[130] Adimoolam S, Lin CX, Ford JM. The p53 regulated Cyclin-dependent kinase inhibitor, p21 (cip1,waf1,sdi1), is not required for global genomic and transcriptional coupled nucleotide excision repair of UV-induced DNA photoproducts. The Journal of Biological Chemistry 2001;276(28) 25813-25822.

[131] Therrien JP, Loignon M, Drouin R, Drobetsky EA. Ablation of p21waf1cip1 expression enhances the capacity of p53-deficient human tumor cells to repair UVB-induced DNA damage. Cancer Research 2001;61(9) 3781-3786.

[132] Wani MA, Wani G, Yao J, Zhu Q, Wani A. Human cells deficient in p53 regulated p21waf/cip1 expression exhibit normal nucleotide excision repair of UV-induced DNA damage. Carcinogenesis 2002;23(3) 403-410.

[133] Shivji MKK, Grey SJ, Strausfeld UP, Wood RD, Blow JJ. Cip1 inhibits DNA replication but not PCNA-dependent nucleotide excision repair. Current Biology 1994;4(12) 1062-1068.

[134] Shivji MKK, Ferrari E, Ball K, Hübscher U, Wood RD. Resistance of human nucleotide excision repair synthesis in vitro to p21CDKN1. Oncogene 1998;17(22) 2827-2838.

[135] McDonald ER, Wu GS, Waldman T, El-Deiry WS. Repair defect of p21waf1/cip1$^{-/-}$ human cancer cells. Cancer Research 1996;56(10) 2250-2255.

[136] Sheikh MS, Chen YQ, Smith ML, Fornace AJ. Role of p21waf/cip1/sdi1 in cell death and DNA repair as studied using a tetracycline-inducible system in p53-deficient cells. Oncogene 1997;14(15) 1875-1882.

[137] Li R, Hannon GJ, Beach D, Stillman B. Subcellular distribution of p21 and PCNA in normal and repair-deficient cells following DNA damage. Current Biology 1996;6(2) 189-199.

[138] Savio M, Stivala LA, Scovassi AI, Bianchi L, Prosperi E. p21waf1/cip1 protein associates with the detergent-insoluble form of PCNA concomitantly with disassembly of PCNA at nucleotide excision repair sites. Oncogene 1996;13(8) 1591-1598.

[139] Ruan S, Okcu MF, Ren JP, Chiao P, Andreeff M, Levin V, Zhang W. Overexpressed WAF1/Cip1 renders glioblastoma cells resistant to chemotherapy agents 1,3-bis(2-chloroethyl)-1-nitrosourea and cisplatin. Cancer Research 1998;58(7) 1538-1543.

[140] Stivala LA, Riva F, Cazzalini O, Savio M, Prosperi E. p21waf1/cip1-null human fibroblasts are deficient in nucleotide excision repair downstream the recruitment of PCNA to DNA repair sites. Oncogene 2001;20(5) 563–570.

[141] Hanawalt PC. Revisiting the rodent repairadox. Environmental and Molecular Mutagenesis 2001;38(2-3) 89-96.

[142] Perucca P, Cazzalini O, Mortusewicz O, Necchi D, Savio M, Nardo T, Stivala LA, Leonhardt H, Cardoso MC, Prosperi E. Spatiotemporal dynamics of p21CDKN1A protein recruitment to DNA-damage sites and interaction with proliferating cell nuclear antigen. Journal of Cell Science 2006;119(8) 1517-1527.

[143] Soria G, Speroni J, Podhajcer OL, Prives C, Gottifredi V. p21 differentially regulates DNA replication and DNA-repair-associated processes after UV irradiation. Journal of Cell Science 2008;121(19) 3271-3282.

[144] Lee JY, Kim HK, Kim JY, Sohn J. Nuclear translocation of p21WAF1/CIP1 protein prior to its cytosolic degradation by UV enhances DNA repair and survival. Biochemical and Biophysical Research Communications 2009;390(4) 1361-1366.

[145] Hasan S, Hassa PO, Imhof R, Hottiger MO. Transcription coactivator p300 binds PCNA and may have a role in DNA repair synthesis. Nature 2001;410(6826) 387-391.

[146] Tillhon M, Cazzalini M, Nardo T, Necchi D, Sommatis S, Stivala LA, Scvassi AI, Prosperi E. p300/CBP acetyl transferases interact with and acetylate the nucleotide excision repair factor XPG. DNA Repair 2012;11(10) 844-852.

[147] Mocquet V, Lainé JP, Riedl T, Yajin Z, Lee MY, Egly JM. Sequential recruitment of the repair factors during NER: the role of XPG in initiating the resynthesis step. The EMBO Journal 2007;27(1) 155-167.

[148] Tom S, Ranalli TA, Podust VN, Bambara RA. Regulatory roles of p21 and apurinic/apyrimidinic endonuclease 1 in base excision repair. The Journal of Biological Chemistry 2001;276(52) 48781-48789.

[149] Frouin I, Maga G, Denegri M, Riva F, Savio M, Spadari S, Prosperi E, Scovassi AI. Human proliferating cell nuclear antigen, Poly(ADP-ribose) polymerase 1, and p21waf1/cip1. A dynamic exchange of partners. The Journal of Biological Chemistry 2003;278(41) 39265-39268.

[150] Cazzalini O, Donà F, Savio M, Tillhon M, Maccario C, Perucca P, Stivala LA, Scovassi AI, Prosperi E. p21CDKN1A participates in base excision repair by regulating the activity of poly(ADP-ribose) polymerase 1. DNA Repair 2010;9(6) 627-35.

[151] Jakob B, Scholz M, Taucher-Scholz G. Characterization of CDKN1A (p21) binding to sites of heavy-ion-induced damage: colocalization with proteins involved in DNA repair. International Journal of Radiation Biology 2002;78(2) 75-88.

[152] Koike M, Yutoku Y, Koike A. Accumulation of p21 proteins at DNA damage sites independent of p53 and core NHEJ factors following irradiation. Biochemical and Biophysical Research Communications 2011;412(1) 39-43.

[153] Wiese C, Rudolph JK, Jakob B, Fink D, Tobias F, Blattner C, Taucher-Scholz G. PCNA-dependent accumulation of CDKN1A into nuclear foci after ionizing irradiation. DNA Repair 2012;11(5) 511-521.

[154] Li X, Stith CM, Burgers P, Heyer WD. PCNA is required for initiation of recombination-associated DNA synthesis by DNA polymerase δ. Molecular Cell 2009;36(4) 704-713.

[155] Sale JE, Lehmann AR, Woodgate R. Y-family DNA polymerases and their role in tolerance of cellular DNA damage. Nature Reviews Molecular Cell Biology 2012;13(3): 141-152.

[156] Lehmann AR, Niimi A, Ogi T, Brown S, Sabbioneda S, Wing JF, Kannouche PL, Green CM. Translesion synthesis: Y-family polymerases and the polymerase switch. DNA Repair 2007;6(7) 891-899.

[157] Avkin S, Sevilya Z, Toube L, Geacintov N, Chaney SG, Oren M, Livneh Z. p53 and p21 regulate error-prone DNA repair to yield a lower mutation load. Molecular Cell 2006;22(3) 407–413.

[158] Prives C, Gottifredi V. The p21 and PCNA partnership. A new twist for an old plot. Cell Cycle 2008;7(24) 3840–3846.

[159] Soria G, Podhajcer O, Prives C, Gottifredi V. p21Cip1/WAF1 downregulation is required for efficient PCNA ubiquitination after UV irradiation. Oncogene 2006;25(20) 2829–2838.

[160] Blagosklonny MV, Wu GS, Omura S, el-Deiry WS. Proteasome-dependent degradation of p21 $^{WAF1/CIP1}$ expression, Biochemical and Biophysical Research Communications 1996;227(2) 564-569.

[161] Sheaff RJ, Singer JD, Swanger J, Smitherman M, Roberts JM, Clurman BE. Proteasomal turnover of p21Cip1 dose not require p21 Cip1 ubiquitination. Molecular Cell 2000;5(2) 403-410.

[162] Bloom J, Amador V, Bartolini F, DeMartino G, Pagano M. Proteasome-mediated degradation of p21 via N-terminal ubiquitinylation. Cell 2003;115(1) 71-82.

[163] Amador V, Ge S, Santamaria PG, Guardavaccaro D, M. Pagano APC/C ^{Cdc20} controls the ubiquitin-mediated degradation of p21 in prometaphase, Molecular Cell 2007;27(3) 462-473.

[164] Kim Y, Starostina NG, Kipreos ET. The CRL4 ^{Ctdt2} ubiquitin ligase targets the degradation of p21 ^{Cip1} to control replication licensing. Genes & Development 2008;22(18) 2507-2519.

[165] Abbas T, Sivaprasad U, Terai K, Amador V, Pagano M, DuttaA. PCNA-dependent regulation of p21 ubiquitylation and degradation via the CRL4 ^{Cdt2} ubiquitin ligase complex. Genes & Development 2008;22(18) 2496-2506.

[166] Nishitani H, Shiomi Y, Iida H, Michishita M, Takami T, TsurimotoT. CDK inhibitor p21 is degraded by a PCNA coupled Cul4-DDB1 ^{Cdt2} pathway during S phase and after UV irradiation. The Journal of Biological Chemistry 2008;283(43) 29045-29052.

[167] Stuart SA, Wang JYJ. Ionizing radiation induces ATM-independent degradation of p21 ^{Cip1} in transformed cells. The Journal of Biological Chemistry 2009;284(22) 15061-15070.

[168] Touitou R, Richardson J, Bose S, Nakanishi M, Rivett J, Allday MJ. A degradation signal located in the C-terminus of p21 $^{WAF1/CIP1}$ is a binding site for the C8 α-subunit of the 20S proteasome. The EMBO Journal 2001;20(10) 2367-2375.

[169] Zhang Z, Wang H, Li M, Agrawal S, Chen X, Zhang R. MDM2 is a negative regulator of p21WAF1/CIP1, independent of p53. The Journal of Biological Chemistry 2004;279(16) 16000-16006.

[170] Lee H, Zeng SX, Lu H. UV induces p21 rapid turnover independently of ubiquitin and Skp2. The Journal of Biological Chemistry 2006;281(37) 26876-26883.

[171] Cayrol C, Ducommun B. Interaction with cyclin-dependent kinases and PCNA modulates proteasome-dependent degradation of p21. Oncogene 1998;17(19) 2437-2444.

[172] Havens CG, Walter JC. Mechanism of CRL4(Cdt2), a PCNA-dependent E3 ubiquitin ligase. Genes & Development 2011;25(15) 1568-1582.

[173] Savio M, Coppa T, Cazzalini O, Perucca P, Necchi D, Nardo T, Stivala LA, Prosperi E. Degradation of p21CDKN1A after DNA damage is independent of type of lesion, and is not required for DNA repair. DNA Repair 2009;8(7) 778-785.

[174] Bendjennat M, Boulaire J, Jascur T, Brickner H, Barbier V, Sarasin A, Fotedar A, Fotedar R. UV irradiation triggers ubiquitin-dependent degradation of $p21^{WAF1}$ to promote DNA repair. Cell 2003;114(5) 599-610.

[175] Liu L, Lee S, Zhang J, Peters SB, Hannah J, Zhang Y, Yin Y, Koff A, Ma L, Zhou P. Cul4A abrogation augments DNA damage response and protection against skin carcinogenesis. Molecular Cell 2009;34(4) 451-460.

[176] McKay BC, Ljungman M, Rainbow AJ. Persistent DNA damage induced by ultraviolet light inhibits $p21^{waf1}$ and bax expression: implications for DNA repair, UV sensitivity and the induction of apoptosis. Oncogene 1998;17(5) 545-555.

[177] Stoyanova T, Roy N, Kopanja D, Bagchi S, Raychaudhuri P. DDB2 decides cell fate following DNA damage. Proceedings of the National Academy of Sciences USA 2009;106(26) 10690-10695.

[178] Sugasawa K. Regulation of damage recognition in mammalian global nucleotide excision repair. Mutation Research 2010;685(1-2) 29-37.

[179] Kapetanaki MG, Guerrero-Santoro J, Bisi DC, Hsieh CL, Rapić-Otrin V, Levine AS. The DDB1-CUL4ADDB2 ubiquitin ligase is deficient in xeroderma pigmentosum group E and targets histone H2A at UV-damaged DNA sites. Proceedings of the National Academy of Sciences USA 2006;103(8) 2588-2593.

[180] Stoyanova T, Yoon T, Kopanja D, Mokyr MB, Raychaudhuri P. The xeroderma pigmentosum group E gene product DDB2 activates nucleotide excision repair by regulating the level of p21Waf1/Cip1. Molecular and Cellular Biology 2008;28(1) 177-187.

[181] Itoh T, Linn S. The fate of $p21^{CDKN1A}$ in cells surviving UV-irradiation. DNA Repair 2005;4(12) 1457-1462.

[182] Roy N, Stoyanova T, Dominguez-Brauer C, Park HJ, Bagchi S, Raychaudhuri P. DDB2, an essential mediator of premature senescence. Molecular and Cellular Biology 2010;30(11) 2681-2692.

[183] Lee EW, Lee MS, Camus S, Ghim J, Yang MR, Oh W, Ha NC, Lane DP, Song J. Differential regulation of p53 and p21 by MKRN1 E3 ligase controls cell cycle arrest and apoptosis. The EMBO Journal 2009;28(14) 2100-2113.

[184] Stoyanova T, Roy N, Bhattacharjee S, Kopanja D, Valli T, Bagchi S, Raychaudhuri P. p21 cooperates with DDB2 protein in suppression of ultraviolet ray-induced skin malignancies. The Journal of Biological Chemistry 2012;287(5) 3019-3028.

[185] Das C, Lucia MS, Hansen KC, Tyler JK. CBP/p300-mediated acetylation of histone H3 on lysine 56. Nature 2009;459(7243) 113-117.

[186] Arif M., Senapati P, Shandilya J, Kundu TK. Protein lysine acetylation in cellular function and its role in cancer manifestation. Biochimica Biophysica Acta 2010;1799(10-12), 702-716.

Chapter 11

The Role of P53 Exonuclease in Accuracy of DNA Synthesis and Sensitivity to Nucleoside Analogs in Various Compartments of Cells

Galia Rahav and Mary Bakhanashvili

Additional information is available at the end of the chapter

http://dx.doi.org/10.5772/54220

1. Introduction

Genomic DNA is susceptible to a variety of mutagenic processes. The maintenance of the stability of genetic material, which is an important and essential feature of every living organism, depends on an accurate DNA replication [1]. Organisms across all kingdoms have developed diverse and highly efficient repair mechanisms to safeguard the genome from deleterious consequences of various kinds of stresses that might tend to destabilize the integrity of the genome. DNA is constantly being damaged. A low fidelity of DNA synthesis in various compartments of the cells by main replicative DNA polymerases leads to genomic instability (mutator phenotype) [2]. The errors produced during DNA synthesis could result from three fidelity determining processes: a)nucleotide misinsertion into the nascent DNA, b)lack of exonucleolytic proofreading activity, i.e the mechanism to identify and excise incorrect nucleotide incorporated during DNA synthesis, and c)extension of mismatched 3′-termini of DNA [3]. Failure to repair DNA can lead to mutations, genomic instability, chromosomal abnormalities, progression of cancer and premature aging.

Mutator phenotypes (with the potential for cancer progression) have been reported for cells that lack a proofreading 3′→5′ exonuclease activity associated with the DNA polymerase [4]. Certain organisms with a deficiency of exonucleolytic proofreading, have an increased susceptibility to cancer, especially under conditions of stress. Since cancer cells typically have many mutations compared to a non-cancer cell, it was proposed that one of the earliest changes in the development of a cancer cell is a mutation that increases the spontaneous mutation rate [5]. Inactivation of 3′→ 5′ exonuclease activity in the mouse DNA pol δ in nucleus appears to produce replication errors that can drive evolution of a cancer. Mitochondrial DNA (mtDNA) alterations have been associated with various human diseases with impaired mitochondrial function [6]. Mitochondrial DNA polymerase γ (pol γ) is responsible for replication of mtDNA and is implicated in all repair processes [7]. Mitochondrial DNA is prone to mutations, since it is localized near the inner mitochondrial membrane in which reactive oxygene species are generated. Additionally, mtDNA lacks histone protection and the highly efficient DNA repair mechanisms [8]. The mutation rate of mtDNA is estimated to be about 20-100-fold higher than that of nuclear DNA [9]. The mutagenic mechanisms were shown to be replication errors caused by misinsertion (as a result of a dNTP excess), or decreased proofreading efficiency [10,11]. The biological importance of the 3′→5′ exonuclease activity of pol γ to mtDNA integrity is illustrated by the fact that mice encoding an exonuclease-deficient form of pol γ have strongly elevated rates of base substitutions in mtDNA and undergo accelerated aging [12].

Virulence, pathogenesis and the ability to develop effective antiretroviral drugs and vaccines are largely dependent on genetic diversity in viruses [13]. Retroviruses are RNA viruses that replicate through a DNA intermediate in a process catalyzed by the viral reverse transcriptase (RT) in cytoplasm [14]. Human immunodeficiency virus type 1 (HIV-1), the etiological agent of AIDS, exhibits exceptionally high mutation frequencies [15]. The accepted explanations for the inaccuracy of HIV-1 RT are the relatively low fidelity of the enzyme during DNA synthesis and the deficiency of intrinsic 3′→5′ exonuclease activity [16-18]. A strong mutator phenotype is also observed for herpes viral DNA polymerase mutants with reduced intrinsic 3′→5′ exonuclease activity [19].

Thus, in various compartments of the cell increased DNA replication accuracy provided by DNA polymerase proofreading activity is an essential activity for the maintenance of genomic integrity for many organisms.

2. Exonucleases in protecting genome stability

The effect of misinsertion of a wrong nucleotide on the polymerase reaction can be either inhibitory, leading to nascent chain termination and primer dissociation or non-inhibitory, leading to mispair extension (resulting in the fixation of either transition or transversion mutations) (Fig 1). Exonucleolytic proofreading of polymerization errors is one of the major determinants of genome stability [20]. The physiological role for the exonucleolytic proofreading has been proposed to be to increase the fidelity of DNA synthesis by excising incorrectly polymerized nucleotides. Following the incorporation of a non-complementary nucleotide at the 3′ end of the primer, exonucleolytic correction can occur by intrinsic exonuclease through intramolecular shuttling of the DNA substrate from the polymerase to the 3′→5′ exonucleolysis active site of the enzyme (*e.g.* pol γ, pol δ and pol ε) [1,4]. However, there are DNA polymerases that do not possess an intrinsic proofreading function, *e.g.* cellular DNA polymerases α and β, retroviral RTs [17,21,22]. Hence, during *in vitro* DNA synthesis by an inaccurate DNA polymerases, following the polymerase dissociation at a mispair, misincorporated nucleotides could be removed by two kinds of an "external" proofreading carried out by the 3′→ 5′ exonuclease activity of other DNA polymerase [23] and/or by separate protein serving as a proofreading exonuclease [24,25]. The lack of intrinsic proofreading, combined with delayed chain elongation of mispaired 3'-ends could provide the opportunity for a separate exonuclease to bind to the nascent DNA ends and excise the mispaired nucleotides. Enzymes that contain 3′–5′ exonuclease activities are involved in maintaining genome stability. Proofreading in trans is a very efficient process, which has a potential to allow exonuclease-proficient enzyme/protein to proofread for 3′→ 5′ exonuclease-deficient DNA polymerases. Proteins with intrinsic proofreading activity may be important for both, 3′→5′ exonuclease-deficient and exonuclease-proficient DNA polymerases. The p53 protein is a member of external proteins that by intrinsic 3′→5′ exonuclease activity may serve as proofreader and could be actively involved in DNA repair thereby significantly expanding the role of p53 as a guardian of the genome [26].

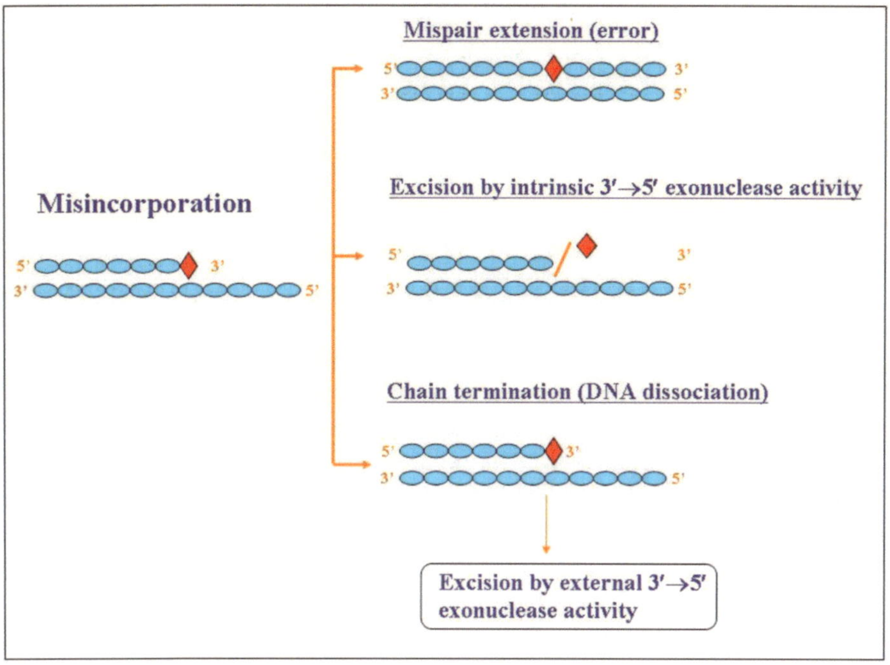

Figure 1. The outcomes of the misincorporation. DNA polymerases following a misincorporation of the wrong nucleotide, can either continue chain elongation beyond the mismatch or remove the mispaired terminus (if a proofreading exonuclease is associated with DNA replication machinery) or block the DNA synthesis by dissociating from the template-primer.

3. p53 and DNA repair

The tumor suppressor protein p53 represents a central factor for the maintenance of genome stability and for the suppression of cancer [27,28]. Under normal conditions within the cell p53 is present at low levels, but after exposure to various stress signals, the protein is stabilized and functionally activated by a series of post-translational modifications, resulting in p53 accumulation at nuclear and extranuclear sites [29,30]. The cellular level of p53 and the nature of DNA damage can dictate the response of the cell. As p53 is a pleiotropic regulator, it affects many processes. The biological outcomes of p53 functions as a sequence-specific transcription factor include cell cycle arrest, apoptosis or DNA repair [31]. Apparently, cell cycle arrest mediated by p53 in response to DNA damage allows time for the cells to repair DNA. If the cells are unable to repair DNA damage, apoptosis is triggered by a p53-dependent pathway to eliminate the cells that contained damaged DNA. These processes together ensure the integrity of the genome. p53 can affect DNA repair processes through its ability to transactivate genes involved in these processes [28]. Mutations in p53 are the most frequent molecular alterations detected in human cancers. The loss of the functional p53 may be responsible for genetic instability and the development of cancer [32].

Appropriate subcellular localization is critical for regulating function of p53. p53 is actively transported between the nucleus and cytoplasm. Furthermore, p53 translocates to mitochondria. The sub-cellular localization of p53 and the interaction with other cellular or viral proteins plays a central role in the regulation of its various biological activities [26]. p53 may modulate DNA repair through processes, which are independent of its transactivation function. p53 can directly interact with DNA repair related cellular factors including DNA polymerase β, AP endonuclease, Rad 51, and mammalian homologs of the RecQ helicase family and Wrn proteins [33-36]. In addition, full range of various intrinsic biochemical features of the p53 protein support its possible roles in DNA repair. After DNA damage: (a) p53 is able to recognize and bind sites of DNA damage, such as single-stranded (ss) DNA and double-stranded (ds) DNA ends [37,38], (b) p53 catalyzes DNA and RNA strand transfer and promotes the annealing of complementary DNA and RNA single-strands [39,40], (c) p53 binds insertion/deletion mismatches and bulges [41] and (d) it can bind DNA in a non-sequence-specific manner [42]. Evidence suggesting a direct role in DNA repair is supported by observations that (1) p53 increases transcription-coupled nucleotide excision repair [43]; (2) p53, like classical mismatch repair factors, checks the fidelity of homologous recombination processes by specific mismatch recognition [44]; (3) p53 can markedly stimulate base excision repair [33,45]; (4) p53 exhibits 3'→ 5' exonuclease activity and wild-type p53, but not mutant p53, enhanced the replication fidelity of various DNA polymerases in an *in vitro* replication assay, strongly supporting the idea that p53 can act as an exogenous proofreader for the replicases [46,47].

4. Characterization of p53 exonuclease activity

Highly purified p53 protein from different sources displays 3′→ 5′ exonuclease activity. p53 has no associated polymerase activity and catalyzes the excision of nucleotides from DNA exclusively in the 3 ′to 5′direction [46]. This activity is dependent on the presence of Mg^{2+} and is intrinsic to the wtp53, since no exonuclease activity was detected with mutant p53 protein, *e.g.* 273His and 175His mutant p53s. Importantly, the exonuclease activity could be

http://dx.doi.org/10.5772/54220

reconstituted from SDS gel-purified and urea-renatured p53 protein. While p53 exhibits optimal transactivation as tetramer, it displays exonuclease activity as monomer [48]. Notably, the oligomarization status of p53 may be important in determining whether protein may act as transcription activator (tetramer) or as exonuclease (monomer).

p53 removes 3′-terminal nucleotides from various nucleic acids substrates: ssDNA, dsDNA RNA/DNA template-primer, ssRNA and dsRNA [46-52]. A unique property of p53 is its ability to excise nucleotides non-processively (on DNA <17 nucleotides) and processively (on DNA >17 nucleotides) [48]. The purified wtp53 exhibits all hallmarks of a genuine proofreading activity [49]. First, the protein shows a preference for degradation of ssDNA over dsDNA substrate. Second, on partial duplex structures, the p53 exonuclease activity displays a marked preference for excision of a mismatched versus a correctly paired 3′ terminus, which enables the protein to act as a proofreader. The intrinsic ability of p53 exonuclease to sequentially remove incorrect 3′ terminal nucleotides from DNA strands before primer extension is important for subsequent elongation of primers during error correction and renders the p53 protein essential in DNA replication, repair, and recombination. Third, p53 acts coordinately with the DNA polymerase to enhance the fidelity of DNA synthesis by excision of mismatched nucleotides from the nascent DNA strand.

The proofreading capacity of p53 was observed during ongoing DNA synthesis *in vitro;* p53 exonuclease has a marked impact on the extent of mispair formation and on the extension from specific mispaired termini by DNA polymerase [49]. Recombinant, as well as endogenous wtp53 can proofread for exonuclease-deficient cellular or viral DNA polymerases (*e.g.* DNA polymerase α, DNA polymerase α-primase, HIV-1 RT) and exonuclease-proficient DNA polymerase (*e.g.* pol γ), thus enhancing the accuracy of DNA synthesis by excising incorrectly polymerized nucleotides [53-57]. Apparently, the exonuclease activity of p53, by removal of a mismatched nucleotide incorporated by a DNA polymerase, might provide a biochemical basis for its direct involvement in the correction of replication errors. Notably, the exonuclease activity of p53 must not be restricted to its non-induced state, but might also be exerted by a subclass of p53 after DNA damage when the protein is able to display its full range of possible biochemical activities [26]. Remarkably, p53 exonuclease excises nucleotides from RNA/DNA template-primers, a property which distinguishes it from the large majority of the known exonucleases [50]. The fact that p53 is reactive with both DNA/DNA and RNA/DNA suggests that it may functionally interact with substrates participating in the reverse transcription process during the replication of retroviruses.

p53 is capable of excising 3'-terminal mispaired nucleotides in direct exonuclease assay independent of DNA polymerase; p53 is very active when first binding to a 3′-terminus [49,50].. Some template-primers with terminal mispairs remain unextended by the polymerase. Interestingly, unextended free template-primers (already dissociated from the enzyme following the misinsertion) may be further recognized by other DNA polymerase (*e.g.* HIV-1 RT) molecules and undergo a rebinding process with a subsequent 3'-mismatch extension [58]. The fact that p53 excises terminal nucleotides independent of DNA polymerase [49,55] suggests that the dissociated unextended 3'-mismatch containing template-primer may be recognized and utilized by p53 to remove terminal mispairs generating the correctly base-paired 3'-termini necessary for continued DNA synthesis [49]. The recognition and binding to 3′ mismatched ends is a prerequisite for the excision of mismatched or damaged nucleotides [42]. Endogenous p53 displays intrinsic 3'-terminal mispaired DNA binding activity. Since p53 binds directly to various 3'-terminal purine:pyrimidine and purine:purine mispairs to an equal extent, it can be considered a general 3'-mismatched DNA binding protein. Intrinsic 3'-terminal mismatched DNA binding capacity of p53 extends the spectrum of DNA damage sites that p53 can recognize and bind. Through the binding p53 participates in damage recognition, which serves as a signal for DNA repair. Thus, the role of p53 in proofreading is two fold — to excise terminal mismatches, but also to prevent extension of mismatched primer ends by DNA polymerase.

p53 intrinsic exonuclease activity, like sequence-specific DNA binding, was mapped to the central conserved core domain of protein, which is the target for most of the missense mutations inactivating the tumor suppressor function of p53 [59]. It is noteworthy that bacterially expressed, i.e., nonphosphorylated, p53 is virtually devoid of sequence-specific DNA binding activity but exerts exonuclease activity [46], pointing to the possibility that the p53 exonuclease activity might be exerted by hypo- or even nonphosphorylated p53. Treatments activating sequence-specific DNA binding of full-length p53 strongly inhibited its exonuclease activity, indicating that p53 exonuclease and sequence-specific DNA binding are distinct features of the p53 core domain, regulated in opposite manners. Apparently, p53 exerts two complementary functions in maintaining the integrity of the genome. After damage different functional subclasses of p53 will exist within the same cell, then the increase of p53 protein levels not only will activate the potential of p53 to transcribe p53 target genes, leading to growth arrest, but will also increase the amount of p53 with a 3'→5' proofreading exonuclease activity. As its basal function in maintaining genetic stability, p53 participates actively in repair processes of endogenous DNA damage and the prevention of mutational events resulting from such damage, through activities not related to sequence-specific DNA binding, specifically through its exonuclease activity [26]. Such p53 then could enhance the accuracy of DNA repair synthesis performed by the error-prone DNA polymerases, e.g. pol α and β. At another level of control, cellular stress activates the functions of p53 generally associated with growth arrest and apoptosis.

Mutant H115N p53, showed markedly reduced exonuclease activity [60]. Surprisingly, purified H115N p53 protein was found to be significantly more potent than wild-type p53 in binding to DNA. Interestingly as well, non-specific DNA binding by the core domain of H115N p53 is superior to that of wild-type p53. Unexpectedly, in contrast to wtp53, H115N p53 was markedly impaired in causing apoptosis when cells were subjected to DNA damage facilitating apoptosis, further supporting the idea that the exonuclease activity and transcriptional activation functions of p53 can be separated. The impact of deficiency of exonuclease activity in p53 is not known. This might be partly due to the observation that tumor derived hot-spot mutants not only fail to function as transcriptional activators but also were reported to be deficient in exonuclease activity. p53 hot spot mutants were categorized into two classes; structural and functional mutants [61]. Since representative members of both classes were defective in exonuclease activity, it is likely that both, structural integrity of the protein and DNA binding activity are essential for each of these two biochemical functions.

5. p53 exonuclease provides proofreading during DNA synthesis in various compartments of cells

p53 activities are extended to normal and cancer cells and they efficiently contribute to genome stability even in the absence of stresses. p53 is expressed constitutively in the cell and is distributed in the nucleus, cytoplasm and mitochondria of unstressed and stressed cells.

5.1. p53 exonuclease activity in nucleus

The observation that p53 protein is co-located with the DNA replication machinery and may preferentially remove mismatched nucleotides from DNA, suggests a link between p53 and DNA replication fidelity [62]. The localization of p53 in nucleus is essential for its normal function in growth inhibition or induction of apoptosis. The low accuracy of DNA polymerases and imbalance of intracellular dNTP pools are major factors in causing replication errors [3]. The proofreading for such replication errors by the 3′→ 5′ exonuclease activity associated with the DNA replication machinery is extremely important in reduction the occurrence of mutations. DNA polymerase α is lack of proofreading activity and is prone to making replication errors [63]. p53 specifically interacts with DNA polymerase α and has been shown to preferentially excise mismatched nucleotides from DNA and enhance the DNA replication fidelity of DNA polymerase α *in vitro* [47]. The fact that p53 is able to enhance the replication fidelity of pol α *in vitro* suggests that p53 may serve a proofreading function during DNA replication in intact cells.

It is conceivable that cells lacking p53 exonuclease activity can demonstrate high mutation frequency under stress conditions and the mutations should be reduced by introduction of wild type p53 into the cells. Hydroxyurea (HU), an inhibitor of ribonucleotide reductase involved in the *de novo* synthesis of deoxynucleotides, was used to induce dNTP pool imbalance and to cause mutations in the cells due to misincorporation of unpaired deoxynucleotides into DNA [54]. Cells with different states of p53 expression, either endogenously or ectopically, were exposed to HU. The analysis of the rates of HU-induced mutations in H1299 (p53-null) and H460 (wtp53) cells revealed substantially increased mutation rates in H1299 cells. Furthermore, the HU-induced mutation frequency was significantly reduced by introduction of wild type p53 expression vector into the p53-null H1299 cells. Thus, wild type p53 expression was associated with a reduction of mutations caused by replication errors under the stress of dNTP pool imbalance [54]. p53, presumably, may play an important role in reduction mutations caused by misincorporation of unpaired nucleotides. This biological function of p53 in whole cells is consistent with its biochemical activity in preferential removal of mismatched nucleotides from DNA by 3′→ 5′ exonuclease activity and enhancing replication fidelity of DNA polymerase α in vitro. The reported association of replication error phenotype with p53 mutations in mucosa-associated lymphoid tissue lymphomas is consistent with the proofreading function of p53 [64].

It was shown that in the early steps of cellular transformation process high incidences of mutations occur, which may be due to misinsertion and proofreading deficiency of DNA polymerases [65]. The existence of complex pol-prim- p53 *in vivo,* identified by immonoprecipitation experiments, suggests that p53 might cooperate with DNA polymerase to maintain the genetic information in cells [53]. The functional interaction of DNA polymerase and exonuclease activity was observed with p53/pol-prim complex. p53-containing DNA pol-prim complex excised preferentially a 3′-mispaired primer end over a paired one and replaced it with a correctly paired nucleotide. In contrast, a pol-prim complex containing the hot spot mutant p53R248H did not display exonuclease activity and did not elongate a mispaired 3′-end, indicating that the p53 exonuclease from the p53/pol-prim complex was mandatory for the subsequent elongation of the primer by DNA polymerase. These findings support the view that p53 might fulfill a proofreading function for pol-prim and suggest that the defect in proofreading function of p53 may contribute to genetic instability associated with cancer development and progression.

Notably, the non-genotoxic stress may include a long-lasting, moderate accumulation of p53 in nucleus. In contrast, acute genotoxic stress may induce rapid and transient accumulation of very high levels of p53 with preferential activation of target genes involved in apoptosis. The *in vivo* experiments showed that while expression of low levels of p53 facilitate BER activity, higher levels reduced it and instead induced apoptosis, suggesting that p53 mediating various activities are correlated with the levels of the p53 protein in the cells [66]. In this regard, it is possible that the accumulation of p53 in nucleus allows the protein to function in several ways: as a regulator of transcription, as a facilitator of BER and as an exonucleolytic proofreader. Moreover, there is a possibility that both transcription-independent pathways act in synergy thereby amplifying the potency of involvement of p53 in DNA repair. The presence of p53 was demonstrated in different nuclear compartments and suggested that the p53 population not engaged in transcriptional regulation could exert functions other than induction of growth arrest or apoptosis and directly participate in processes of repair via its various biochemical activities [26].

5.2. p53 exonuclease activity in cytoplasm

p53 is retained in the cytoplasm during part of the normal cell cycle. Wild-type p53 occurs in cytoplasm in a subset of human tumor cells such as breast cancers, colon cancers and neuroblastoma [67-69]. Notably, cytoplasmic sequestration of p53 in tumor cells (that do not have mutated p53), besides structural mutation and the functional inactivation of wtp53, was suggested to be an important mechanism in abolishing p53 function and in tumorigenesis [67,70]. Shuttling between nucleus and cytoplasm not only regulates protein localization, but also often impacts on protein function. Analyses of various cell lines (MCF-7 human breast cancer cells – expressing high levels of wtp53 in nucleus, LCC2-subclone derived from MCF-7 cells-expressing high levels of wtp53 in cytoplasm, MDA cells-expressing high levels of mutant p53 or H1299-p53-null cells), demonstrated that the cytoplasmic extracts of non-stressed LCC2 cells, exert high level of 3′→ 5′ exonuclease activity [55,56]. Interestingly, the 3′→ 5′ exonuclease in the cytoplasmic fraction from LCC2 cells displays identical biochemical functions characteristic for recombinant wtp53 [56]: 1)it removes 3′-terminal nucleotides from various nucleic acid substrates: ssDNA, dsDNA, and RNA/DNA template-primers, 2)it hydrolyzes ssDNA in preference to dsDNA and RNA/DNA template-primers, 3)it shows a marked preference for excision of a mismatched vs correctly paired 3′ terminus with RNA/DNA and DNA/DNA substrates, 4)it exerts the preferential excision of purine-purine (transversion) mispairs over purine-pyrimidine (transition) mispairs, 5)it excises nucleotides from various nucleic acid substrates independently from DNA polymerase, 6) it fulfils the requirements for proofreading function; acts coordinately with the exonuclease-deficient viral (*e.g.* MLV RT, HIV-1 RT) and cellular DNA polymerases – (*e.g.* pol α and β) (unpublished results) to enhance the fidelity of DNA synthesis by excision of mismatched nucleotides from the nascent DNA strand [55,56]. It is noteworthy, that in non-stressed cells p53 is constitutively expressed and exists in transcriptional inert state. Thus, the protein exerts exonuclease activity independently of p53 functions in transcription.

Interestingly, p53 protein in cytoplasmic extracts of MCF-7 cells displays a relatively high level of 3′→ 5′ exonuclease activity in comparison to nuclear lysates of LCC2 cells [55]. The biochemical difference between the p53 in nuclear and cytoplasmic compartments raises questions whether nuclear p53 loses exonuclease function of cytoplasmic p53 or acquires an additional functions (*e.g.* efficient sequence-specific DNA binding and transactivation). The disparity in expression of p53 exonuclease activity may be attributable to the different post-transcriptional events: a)post-translational modifications (*e.g.* phosphorylation, acetylation) may regulate the ability of p53 to serve as an exonuclease in the nucleus and in the cytoplasm; b) The alteration of p53 protein conformation from mutant (in cytoplasm) to wild-type (in nucleus) may be responsible for low level of exonuclease activity in nucleus [71]. c) the interaction of p53 with other proteins and/or DNA polymerases may affect on expression its various biochemical activities.

5.3. p53 exonuclease activity in mitochondria

Mitochondrial DNA mutations can arise from different sources, including errors made by pol γ, the enzyme that replicates the mitochondrial genome. The mitochondrial pol γ belongs to a family A DNA polymerase, and as observed for other family A DNA polymerases, this enzyme excises the terminal nucleotide at a much slower rate than observed for the potent 3′→5′ exonuclease-proficient T4 DNA polymerase [72]. The mutagenic mechanisms were shown to be replication errors caused by incorporation of wrong nucleotide (as a result of a dNTP excess), or decreased proofreading efficiency. Furthermore, a potentially important source of replication infidelity is damage due to reactive oxygen species. Among several known oxidized dNTPs, one that is particularly common and potentially highly mutagenic is 8-oxo-7,8-dihydro-2'-deoxyguanosine (8-oxodG) [73]. Incorrect 8-oxo-dGTP-A base pairing can lead to A-T to C-G transversions if the incorporated 8-oxo-dGMP escapes proofreading and any subsequent repair. pol γ, was demonstrated to stably misincorporate 8-oxo-dGTP opposite template adenine in a complete DNA synthesis reaction *in vitro* [74]. Low-fidelity DNA synthesis in mitochondria was observed despite the presence of the intact proofreading exonuclease, thus indicating that the 8-oxo-GMP-A mismatch was not efficiently proofread.

A certain fraction of p53 translocates to mitochondria. Mitochondrial localization of p53 was observed in both stressed and non-stressed cells [75,76], where p53 was shown to physically and functionally interact with both, the mtDNA and pol γ in response to mtDNA damage induced by exogenous and endogenous insults [77]. p53 is localized in mitochondria to the inside face of the inner membrane i.e, in matrix, the compartment in which mtDNA is located [57,77]. The functional cooperation of p53 and pol γ during DNA replication was studied using the mitochondrial fraction of p53-null H1299 cells, as the source of pol γ [57]. p53 affected the accuracy of DNA replication by promoting excision of misincorporated nucleotides which increased in the presence of either added recombinant wild-type p53, or endogenous p53 provided by the cytosolic extracts from H1299 cells over-expressing wild-type p53, but not from cells expressing the exonuclease-deficient mutant p53–R175H. Endogenous p53 in mitochondrial extracts of HCT116 (p53+/+) cells had increased exonuclease activity compared with that from HCT116(p53-/-) cells and adding exogenous p53 complemented the HCT116(p53-/-) mitochondrial extract mediated mispair excision. Furthermore, nucleotide misincorporation was reduced in the mitochondrial extracts of HCT116 (p53+/+) cells compared with that of HCT116(p53-/-) cells. Irradiation-induced mitochondrial translocation of endogenous p53 in HCT116(p53+/+) cells correlated with the enhancement of error-correction activities. This evidence strongly supports a direct role of p53 in mitochondria providing exonuclease activity for DNA repair required for error-repair pathway [57]. Therefore, p53 not only serves as guardian of the nuclear genome but also of the mitochondrial genome.

p53 interacts physically with mtDNA and pol γ in response to mtDNA damage induced by endogenous insults including oxidative stress. The intrinsic exonuclease activity of pol γ does not efficiently proofread 8-oxodG misinserted opposite adenine [78]. Once 8-oxo-dGMP is incorporated opposite adenine by pol γ it is preferentially extended rather than excised, which increases its mutagenic potential. Interestingly, human mitochondrial single-stranded DNA binding protein (HmtSSB) was identified as a novel protein-binding partner of p53 in mitochondria. HmtSSB enhances intrinsic 3'→5' exonuclease activity of p53, particularly in hydrolysing 8-oxodG present at 3'-end of DNA, suggesting that p53 is directly involved in DNA repair within mitochondria during oxidative stress.

5.4. p53 exonucleolytic proofreading may affect the mutation spectra of DNA polymerase

The accuracy of DNA synthesis reflects complex interactions between the parameters of the catalytic "triad" involved in DNA polymerization: DNA polymerase, the nature of the mispair and proofreading exonucleases (fidelity–enhancing accessory component) [1,22]. DNA polymerase catalyzed both, misinsertion and mismatch extension reactions and the extent of proofreading depend on the type of the mispair, and the influence of surrounding sequences of the template. Various cellular and viral DNA polymerases share common pattern of mispair formation and extension: namely, purine-pyrimidine mispair (*e.g.* A:C mispair) is easily inserted and more efficiently extended than the purine-purine (*e.g.* A:A or A:G mispair) or pyrimidine-pyrimidine mispair (e.g. C:C or C:T) [79,80]. Thus, the general trend of mispair extension is A:C>A:A>A:G. Interestingly, p53 displays variation in excision of mismatched base pairs; the protein exhibits preferential excision of purine-purine transversion mispairs (*e.g.* A:A, A:G) over purine-pyrimidine transition mispairs (*e.g.* A:C, G:T) [49]. Apparently, the variances in the extension and excision spectrum generated are different for these two reactions. The mispair excision pattern (A:G>A:A>A:C) detected with p53 is an interesting observation with respect to the contribution of proofreading to fidelity; it is compatible with the mispair extension specificity obtained with this particular sequence studied.

The importance of the mispair extension efficiency as a fidelity parameter was illustrated by the fact that an increased forward polymerization capacity for transition A:C mispair, as compared to transversion A:G mispair, overcomes the ability of p53 exonuclease activity in cytoplasm to excise nucleotide mispairs under the similar exonuclease to polymerase ratios [56]. Indeed, the purine-pyrimidine mispair A:C (the most easily formed and extended) is less efficiently excised and the purine-purine A:A and A:G mispairs (less efficiently formed and extended), are rather efficiently excised. Therefore, it is conceivable that the structural feature that make the mismatched terminus a poor substrate for elongation (polymerization) is a good substrate for degradation (exonucleolysis) [81].

Remarkably, p53 exonuclease displays the same pattern of mispair excision specificity with RNA/DNA substrate observed with DNA/DNA template-primer [50]. The mispair excision pattern obtained with identical RNA and DNA sequences indicates that the p53 exonuclease activity for different mismatches is dependent upon the nature of the mispair. The same relative order obtained during replication in extracts and in reconstituted reaction, demonstrates the reproducibility of the observations, thus indicating that this specificity reflects the proofreading potential of human replication apparatus.

Among the base substitution mutations, 80% are transitions and 20% are transversions [13]. An interesting observation is that external proofreading activity in the replication apparatus may preferentially correct some of the misincorporated beses to reduce the rates of transversions. p53 may affect the mutation spectra of DNA polymerase (*e.g.* HIV-1 RT) by acting as an external proofreader [56]. Indeed, HIV-1 RT gains significant benefit from proofreading with A:G mispair (about 15-fold decrease in A:G mispair extension) as compared with A:C mipair (about 2.8-fold decrease), since the enzyme has difficulty extending from this particular mispair. Furthermore, the low mispair extension capacity implies that DNA polymerase has a substantially higher probability of dissociation from the transversion mispairs. Dissociation would prevent mutation fixation, because the mispairs would be subject to removal by the external p53 proofreading activity. Thus, base substitutions that produce transversions may be decreased in the presence of p53, indicating that the mutation spectra might be generated through the actions of RT (DNA polymerase) and cytoplasmic p53 (exonuclease).

The mutational spectra and error rates during DNA synthesis probably depends on the composition and position of mispair, since each position provides a new set of protein-DNA contacts. There is the possibility that neighboring nucleotide sequence may influence recognition of the altered geometry of the mismatch by the enzyme/protein responsible for the proofreading or/and proofreading efficiency. The fact that p53 binds mismatch in the two different sequence contexts tested, indicates that the recognition and binding of 3'-terminally mismatched DNA substrates by p53 might be independent of the sequence context. Since formation of exonuclease complexes requires "melting" of the terminal three base pairs at the primer end, the nature of mismatch at the primer end and the A+T- or G+C-richness of the primer terminus affect the rate for formation of exonuclease complexes. It has been proposed that high A-T content of the primer terminus compared with high G-C content increases excision rates by assisting the strand separation process. Hence, a comprehensive study of various DNA substrates are needed to determine the effect of local sequence context on the substrate specificity of the p53 exonuclease and whether p53 could take advantage of A+T richness to prepare duplex DNA for the hydrolysis reaction.

6. Intermolecular pathway of proofreading by p53 exonuclease

Following the incorporation of wrong nucleotide the DNA polymerase stalling and the kinetic delay allows error correction by intramolecular or/and intermolecular pathway [3]. The intramolecular pathway entails "movement" of the primer end from the polymerase to the intrinsic exonuclease active site (without dissociating from the DNA). In this way, DNA polymerase functions as a "self-correcting" enzyme that removes its own polymerization errors as it moves along the DNA. The intermolecular proofreading may occur when misinsertion is followed by polymerase dissociation from the mismatched template-primer, leaving the 3′ terminal mispair accessible to the external exonuclease for binding and error correction. In both cases, the efficiency of editing misinserted nucleotides by a 3′→ 5′ exonuclease would be directly dependent on the DNA polymerase capacity to extend from a misincorporated nucleotide.

Polymerase dissociation at a mispair is an important consideration for proofreading for both exonuclease-deficient and exonuclease-proficient polymerases, thus allowing error correction by a separate 3′→ 5′ exonuclease. The formation of exonuclease complex with the primer end of the mismatched DNA participates in error correction during DNA synthesis [42]. A functional interaction between the p53 exonuclease and DNA polymerase activities was observed. The 3'-terminal mismatched DNA binding and exonuclease activities of p53 are implicated in the recognition and excision step of mismatch repair. It is conceivable that the binding of p53 to mismatched DNA and preferential excision of mismatched nucleotides may be a relevant event in the biological function of the protein in DNA repair. The experiments in which DNA polymerases, either exonuclease-deficient (*e.g.* HIV-1 RT) or exonuclease-proficient (*e.g.* pol γ) were tested for the extension of preformed 3′- terminally mispaired substrates in the presence of p53 (conditions that mimic a situation of intermolecular editing), points to a mechanism of mismatch correction prior to polymerization [56,57]. Under DNA replication conditions the un-extended 3'-terminal mismatched DNA produced following misincorporation, dissociated from the DNA polymerase and was recognized by p53 (Fig.2). Upon excision of the mispair, p53 exonuclease dissociates and the corrected primer could be transferred to the polymerase and undergo a rebinding process by the DNA polymerase with a subsequent DNA polymerization.

It is important to note, that DNA polymerase could gain enormous benefit from proofreading even from a relatively weak exonuclease, if the polymerase has difficulty extending from a particular mispair [20]. Exonuclease has a dramatic impact on the accuracy of polymerase by preventing the occurrence of base substitutions during continues DNA replication. All that is required is discrimination against extension from a mispair within the polymerase active site.

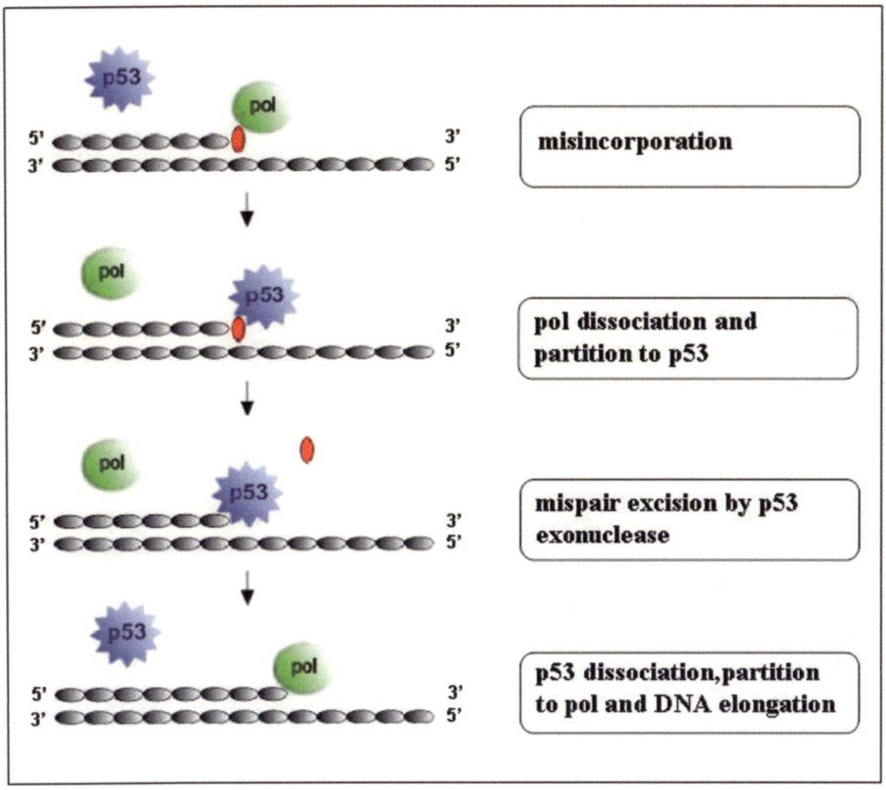

Figure 2. Model for error-correction by p53. The incorporation of wrong nucleotide ( ) into DNA results in DNA polymerase (pol) dissociation from the template-primer, leaving the 3'-terminal mispair accessible to the p53. Upon excision of the mispair, the p53 dissociates thus allowing the DNA polymerase to re-associate with the correct 3'-terminus and resume DNA synthesis.

7. Hallmarks of proofreading and p53 exonuclease activity

Two variables might affect the efficiency of excision from the mispair [1]. First, one hallmark of proofreading is the "next-nucleotide effect". Increased proofreading at the expense of

DNA replication is observed at low concentrations of dNTPs, a condition which prevents error production during replication *in vivo* by antimutator DNA polymerases. The enhancement of the extent of polymerizing activity at the expense of proofreading activity can be achieved by the presence of high concentrations of dNTPs and dNTP pool imbalances; both conditions are mutagenic. Increasing the concentration of the next correct nucleotide to be incorporated following the mispair enhances the probability of mismatch extension, thereby decreasing proofreading efficiency. Increased polymerizing activity reduces proofreading even in the presence of a fully functional exonuclease activity. Since a decrease in accuracy of DNA synthesis with increasing next correct dNTP concentration is a well-established phenomena of proofreading, the observed dependence of fidelity of DNA synthesis by exonuclease-deficient DNA polymerase *e.g.* HIV-1 RT on next nucleotide concentration, implies that the 3′→ 5′ exonuclease of p53 in cytoplasm might be effective in eliminating polymerase-catalyzed base-substitution errors [56]. This effect supports a coordinated action of the p53-exonuclease in cytoplasm with HIV-1 RT during DNA synthesis.

Second, the polymerase/exonuclease ratio serves as an important enzymatic "marker' of polymerase fidelity [1]. Exonucleolytic proofreading is a major determinant of replication fidelity. The balance between the DNA polymerizing and 3′→ 5′ exonuclease reactions usually affects the overall accuracy of DNA synthesis to ensure optimal DNA replication efficiency and to prevent excessive DNA degradation of correctly synthesized DNA. The high ratio of exonuclease to polymerase at the constant dNTP concentrations may increase the fidelity of DNA synthesis.

Cellular responses to DNA damage include repair processes that act coordinately prior to, during and after DNA replication, to maintain genomic stability. The accuracy of DNA synthesis might respond to alterations in composition of replication complex. p53 function may be regulated by controlling where the protein is in the cell. Various stress conditions may trigger distinct signaling pathways in controlling p53 nucleo–cytoplasmic-mitochondrial translocation, thus contributing to heterogeneity of p53-dependent responses. The identification of the p53 protein in cytoplasm or in mitochondria that may enhance the fidelity of DNA polymerase suggests that the accuracy of DNA synthesis by the enzyme may respond to alterations in composition of replication complex. Most probably, p53 in nucleus or cytoplasm or mitochondria might have a transient interaction with replication complex. Therefore, the DNA synthesis in each compartment may be dynamic process with p53 component binding and dissociating the DNA polymerization complex during dsDNA synthesis, thus affecting the polymerase/exonuclease (p53) ratio. The change in the ratio of DNA polymerase vs exonuclease (p53) could be achieved through a reduction in polymerization efficiency of DNA polymerase due to mutations, or from over-expression of p53, or through p53 gene induction (increase in p53 concentration) or p53 targeting (increase in local nuclear or cytoplasmic or mitochondrial concentration). p53 is able to excise 3'-terminal nucleotides during the ongoing DNA synthesis *i.e.* coupled with DNA polymerization and following direct binding to template-primer *i.e.* independent of DNA polymerase, thus increasing the potency of involvement of the protein during the DNA replication by acting as an external proofreader in each cellular compartment. Consequently, the presence of p53 in nucleus/

cytoplasm/mitochondria, by carrying these properties, may be relevant to the accuracy of DNA synthesis by various DNA polymerases.

8. Excision of nucleoside analogs from DNA by p53 protein

Many nucleoside analogs (NAs), potent anti-cancer and antiviral drug compounds, include a variety of purine and pyrimidine nucleoside derivatives which may compete with physiological nucleosides. Nucleoside analogs, clinically active in cancer chemotherapy (*e.g.* Ara-C, in the treatment of hematological malignancies, or gemcitabine-dFdC, against a variety of solid tumors) and in treatment of virus infections (*e.g.* 3′-azido-2,3,-deoxythymidine-AZT, 2,3-dideoxycitidine-ddC, inhibitors of HIV-1 RT), are incorporated into DNA and cause cell death or inhibition of viral replication [82,83]. These drugs are intracellularly converted to the active analog trophosphates, which are then incorporated into replicating DNA. The incorporated NA, structurally mimicing a mismatched nucleotide at the 3'-terminus, blocks further extension of the nascent strand (chain termination) and causes stalling of replication forks with higher probability to the dissociation of the enzyme from template-primer. The high toxicity of dideoxynucleotide compounds may be caused by high rates of incorporation of the NA into mtDNA and the persistence of these analogs in mtDNA due to inefficient excision. Analysis of the processes involved in the removal of NAs and repair of stalled forks is important to better understand the mechanisms that spare toxicity to these drugs.

Proofreading exonuclease activity is capable of removing wrong nucleotides from DNA, providing a mechanism that potentially causes drug resistance. In general, the amount of NAs presented at the DNA termini depends on the efficiency of the incorporation of the compounds by DNA polymerases and on the rate of excision by 3′→5′ exonucleases [83]. The excision of the incorporated NA from the 3′-end of DNA by exonucleases may decrease their potential for chain termination and may be viewed as a potential cellular mechanism of resistance to anti-viral drugs or anti-cancer NAs. The role of p53 exonuclease in maintaining genomic stability in mammalian cells is particularly relevant with respect to the development of anticancer and antiviral therapies.

Many anticancer agents induce cellular cytotoxicity by causing DNA damage. Cells developed several repair mechanisms to facilitate the excision of incorporated NAs. The cytotoxic activity of gemcitabine (2'2'-difluorodeoxycitidine, dFdC) was strongly correlated with the amount of dFdCMP incorporated into cellular DNA. Interestingly, dFdCTP incorporation by human DNA polymerase α results in "masked termination" of DNA synthesis, where following a single dFdCTP incorporation into DNA, the primer is extended by only one additional dNTP before polymerization is inhibited [84]. The p53 protein recognizes dFdCMP-DNA in whole cells, as evidenced by the fact that p53 protein rapidly accumulated in the nuclei of the gemcitabine treated ML-1 cells [85]. Although, the excision of the dFdCMP at the penultimate position from the 3′-end of the DNA was slower than the excision of matched or mismatched nucleotides in whole cells with wtp53 (ML-1) and not detectable in CEM cells harboring mutant p53. ML-1 cells were more sensitive to the cytotoxic effect of the drugs compared to the p53-null or mutant cells. Transfection of p53-null cells with wild-type p53 expression vector enhanced the sensitivity of the cells to gemcitabine. Taken together, these authors concluded that recognition of the incorporated NAs in DNA by wild-type p53 did not confer resistance to gemcitabine, but may have facilitated the apoptotic cell death process. It was reported that treatment with gemcitabine resulted in an increased production of DNA-dependent protein kinase (DNA-PK) and p53 complex in nucleus, that interacts with the gemcitabine-containing DNA [86]. DNA-PK and p53 sensor complex may serve as a mechanism to activate the pro-apoptosis function of p53. Apparently, the prolonged existence of the NA-stalled DNA end induced the kinase activity, which subsequently phosphorylated p53 and activated the downstream pathways leading to apoptosis.

Remarkably, p53 present in complex with DNA-PK exhibited 3′→5′ exonuclease activity with mismatched DNA, however the active p53 was unable of excising efficiently the incorporated drug from NA-DNA construct containing gemcitabine at the penultimate site and a matched pair at the 3′-end [86]. It should be noted, that the specific effects of gemcitabine exposure appeared to vary depending on the duration of treatment and upon the cell line. The drug-induced apoptosis were further compared in two lines derived from the MCF-7 cells: MN-1 cells with wild-type p53 and MDD2 cells containing mutant p53 [87]. The MDD2 cells were significantly more resistant to gemcitabine induced cytotoxicity than the MN-1 cells. Unexpectedly, MDD2 cells accumulated more gemcitabine than MN-1 cells, with higher incorporation into nucleic acids. The activation of gemcitabine to its phosphorylated form was similar in both cell lines and it was suggested that the absence of 3′→5′ exonuclease activity in the mutant p53 cell line accounted for the enhanced incorporation into nucleic acids. The presence of a dysfunctional p53, presumably, allows the cells that accumulate DNA damage to continue proliferating. It should be pointed out, that wild-type p53 in ML-1 cells removed the purine nucleoside analog fludarabine (F-ara-A) more efficiently than gemcitabine [85]. Further studies are needed to assess the role of p53 in cellular response to various anti-cancer purine and pyrimidine NA-induced DNA damage.

HIV-1 RT readily utilizes many NAs and the incorporation of nucleoside RT inhibitors (NRTIs) into the 3′-end of viral DNA leads to chain termination of viral DNA synthesis in cytoplasm [88]. The ability of p53 exonuclease activity to excise NA from DNA was studied. A decrease in incorporation of the NA (*e.g.* ddTTP or ddATP) into DNA by HIV-1 RT was shown during both RNA-dependent and DNA-dependent DNA polymerization reactions in the presence of either purified recombinant p53 or endogenous protein provided by cytoplasmic fraction of LCC2 cells [89]. Furthermore, p53 in the cytoplasm was able to excise the incorporated 3′-terminal NAs, although less efficiently than the matched or mismatched nucleotides; longer incubation times were required for excision of the terminally incorporated analogs. In control experiments, no reduction in incorporation of either ddTTP or ddATP was observed in the presence of cytoplasmic fraction of H1299 (p53-null) cells. These data suggest that p53 in cytoplasm may act as an external proofreader for NA incorporation and confer cellular resistance mechanism to the anti-viral compounds.

http://dx.doi.org/10.5772/54220

Acquired mitochondrial toxicity occurs as a consequence of incorporation of anti-cancer or anti-viral NA into mtDNA and/or inhibition of mtDNA replication [90,91]. NRTIs, in addition to the target viral polymerase in cytoplasm (antiviral activity), can be incorporated into a mtDNA by pol γ, leading to termination of mtDNA synthesis and mitochondrial dysfunction (host toxicity). Mitochondrial toxicity may be caused by termination of the growing nascent DNA strand after incorporation of the NRTIs into mtDNA or by inhibition of pol γ exonucleolytic proofreading [90,91]. DNA synthesis/repair proceeding in nucleus-free mitochondria, relies upon a preassembled DNA replication machinery of pol γ and multiple proteins to maintain mtDNA integrity. p53 in mitochondria may functionally interact with pol γ, thus providing a proofreading function during mtDNA replication for excision of NAs [92]. Indeed, increased excision of the incorporated NAs from DNA was detected with H1299mit in the presence of recombinant or endogenous wild-type p53 but not exonuclease-deficient mutant p53-R175H: Mitochondrion-localized elevation of p53 following the IR-stress stimuli correlates with the low incorporation of NA. The fact that p53 localizes to the mitochondria and interacts with mtDNA and pol γ, taken together with observations that the presence of p53 (provided by recombinant or endogenous p53) reduces the amount of incorporation of NA in H1299mit, suggests that p53 may potentially participate in NA excision. p53 in mitochondria probably have a transient interaction with replication complex; the DNA synthesis may be dynamic process with p53 component binding and dissociating the polymerization complex during DNA synthesis, thus affecting the polymerase (pol γ)/exonuclease(p53) ratio. Consequently, the decrease in the ratio of pol γ/p53 due to the increase in local p53 concentration in mitochondria, may enhance the proofreading efficiency and excision of NA by external p53. Knowledge of the mechanism of inhibition of pol γ may be utilized to obtain selectivity for HIV-1 RT over pol γ. The removal of the incorporated NRTI by p53 exonuclease, indicates that the presence of the cellular component-p53 in mitochondria may be important in defining the cytotoxicity of NRTIs toward mitochondrial replication, thus affecting risk-benefit approach (NRTI toxicity versus viral inhibition).

Although dFdC is not a chain terminator, the extension of a dFdCMP-terminated primer is 25-fold slower than the extension of a canonical DNA primer in mitochondria. Moreover, the primer 3′-dFdCMP was excised with a 50-fold slower rate than the matched 3′-dCMP. Given that mtDNA repair is limited and inefficient [93], persistence of dFdCMP within mtDNA is predicted to be likely. The toxicological profile of gemcitabine resembles that of many other anti-viral nucleoside analogs and frequently mimics the symptoms of heritable mitochondrial defects. The mitochondria may be able to remove chain-terminating nucleoside analogs and resume normal mtDNA replication, but nucleoside analogs that do not chain terminate, and therefore can become part of the mitochondrial genome, may exert long term toxicity [85]. pol γ was able to extend a DNA primer containing 3′-dFdCMP although with decreased nucleotide incorporation efficiency at the first two downstream positions. p53 is able to remove the incorporated anti-cancer drug arabinosylcytosine (Ara-C) (pyrimidine analog) from DNA incorporated by pol γ in mitochondrial fraction of p53-null cells [92]. The binding and removal of chemically active anti-cancer and anti-viral NAs from DNA by p53 may lead to either drug resistance or activation of p53 pro-apoptotic functions (Fig.3).

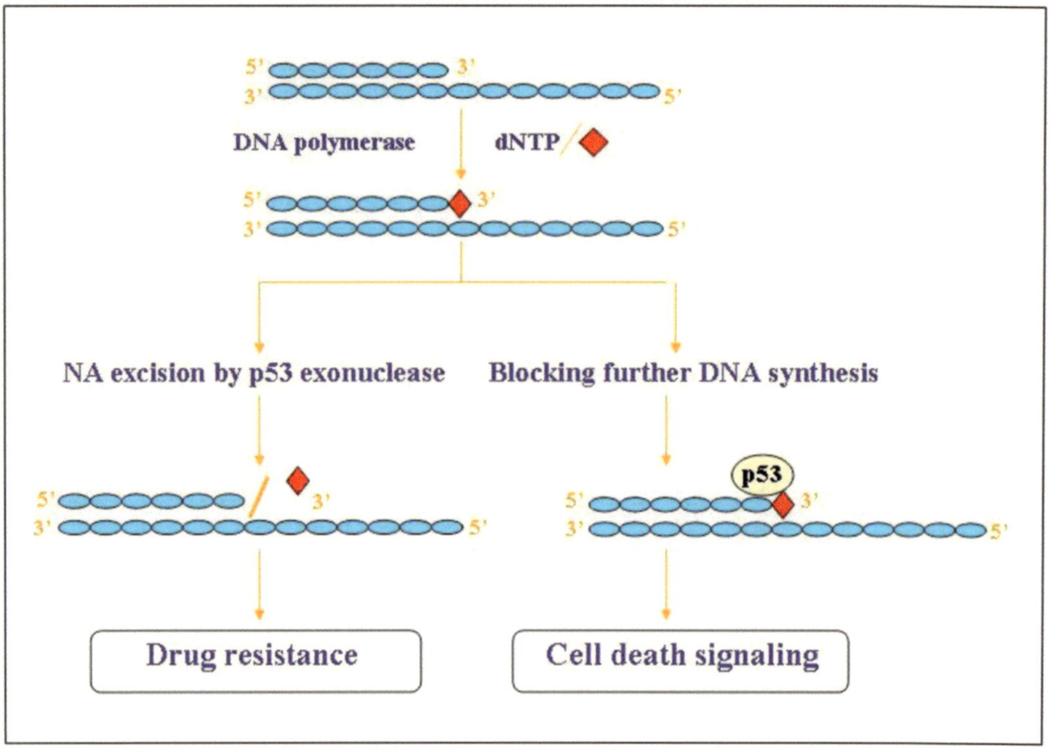

Figure 3. The potential functions of p53 in response to nucleoside analog-induced DNA damage. The p53 protein, following the recognition and preferential binding to the drug-containing DNA could display two different functions: the removal of the incorporated NA from DNA, thus conferring the resistance to the drugs, or may serve as a mechanism to activate the pro-apoptosis function of p53 and trigger the cell death program.

p53 is a multifunctional protein with positive and negative effects. In general, drug resistance that occurs in cancer chemotherapy and antiviral therapy is a negative event that will decrease the efficacy of the treatment. The behavior of p53 exonuclease probably depends on the sub-cellular localization of the p53, local concentration, nature of NA (purine, pyrimidine), position of the NA (3'-terminal NA, analog residue at the penultimate position and nature of the subsequent correct nucleotide) and on the local DNA sequence composition. The recognition and removal of NA from drug-containing DNAs by p53 exonuclease activity in various compartments of the cell may play a role in decreasing drug activity, leading to various biological outcomes: 1)the excision of the incorporated NA from DNA in nucleus may confer resistance to the drugs (negative effect) [85]; 2)the removal of the NA by p53 from DNA incorporated by HIV-1 RT in cytoplasm may confer resistance to the drugs by non-viral mechanism (negative effect) [89] and 3)the excision of NAs from mitochondrial DNA may decrease the potential for chain termination and host toxicity (positive effect) [92]. Apparently, the presence of p53 in mitochondria may be important, since the excision of the mispair and NA by p53 is favorite event for mitochondrial function.

9. Conclusions and perspectives

Nature has devised multiple strategies to safeguard the genetic information and developed intricate repair mechanisms and pathways to reverse an array of different DNA lesions, including mismatches. An accessory proofreading exonuclease would be critical for the removal of the mispairs and therefore, for the maintenance of genomic integrity. The high incidence of mutations may be due to misinsertion and proofreading deficiency of DNA polymerases [65]. Mammalian cells have evolved several repair mechanisms for the maintenance of genomic integrity to prevent the fixation of genetic damage induced by endogenous and exogenous mutagens [3]. Cells may have several 3′→5′ exonucleases to preserve genomic integrity during DNA synthesis. Under conditions where the activity of one exonuclease is inactivated, the function of another exonuclease might be important for correcting errors produced during DNA replication. p53 was shown to be an example of accessory protein that may enhance the fidelity of DNA synthesis by exonuclease-deficient DNA polymerase, *e.g.* HIV-1 RT [56] and exonuclease-proficient DNA polymerase, *e.g.* pol γ [57] in various compartments of the cell: nucleus, cytoplasm and mitochondria. The preferential excision of mismatched nucleotides from the replicating DNA strand by p53, implies that this cellular error-correction pathway may compensate for a lack of effective proofreading of DNA polymerase induced replication errors. In addition, the proofreading activity of p53 may limit the tranversion mutations, indicating that p53 may affect the mutation spectra of DNA polymerase by acting as an external proofreader. The mutagenic capacity of a low fidelity DNA polymerase will be decreased through increase in exonuclease concentration or exonuclease targeting (increase in local p53 concentration).

p53 plays a pivotal role in the regulation of cell fate determination in response to a variety of cellular stresses. p53 may exert the functional heterogeneity in its non-induced and in its activated state. Furthermore, p53 is able to elicit a spectrum of different biological effective pathways in nucleus, cytoplasm and mitochondria. The increase of p53 protein levels will increases the amount of p53 with a 3′→5′ exonuclease activity. Hence, it is of interest to elucidate 3′→ 5′ exonuclease activity nucleus, cytoplasm and mitochondria of the cells with activated p53 induced by drug treatments (in the absence of DNA damage) or following UV irradiation (in the presence of DNA damage).

The role of p53 is particularly relevant with respect to the development of anticancer and antiviral therapies. The potency of NAs is dependent upon their incorporation at the 3′ ends of replicating DNA. However, clinical drug resistance limits the efficacy of these compounds. Cells have evolved several repair mechanisms to facilitate the excision of misincorporated nucleotides or nucleoside analogs. Uncovering the mechanisms, which are responsible for DNA repair of NA-induced DNA damage will have therapeutic value. The stress induced activation of p53 that occurs during cancer chemotherapy has negative and positive effects. The p53 protein is able to remove incorporated NA. Therapeutic strategies based on p53 are particularly interesting because they exploit the cancer cell's intrinsic genome instability and predisposition to cell death-apoptosis. p53 may remove incorporated therapeutic NAs from DNA or trigger apoptosis. The knowledge regarding functions of p53 in genome integrity and cancer evolution may facilitate drug screening and better design of therapeutic approaches.

10. Future directions

The functional interaction between p53 and DNA polymerase may have important consequences for the maintenance of genomic integrity and pose significant challenges to the development of p53-targeting cancer therapies. Mutant p53 can be classified as a loss-of-function or gain-of-function protein depending on the type of mutation [27,28]. Characterization of exonuclease-deficient H115N mutant p53 revealed that although exonuclease-mutant H115N p53 can induce cell cycle arrest more efficiently than wild-type p53, its ability to produce apoptosis in DNA damaged cells is markedly impaired [60]. Does exonuclease-mutant p53 promote mismatch genetic instabilities? What is the ultimate phenotypic result of this genomic instability? Is it truly contributing to the increased proliferation, seen in tumors of mutp53 mice, and can these results be extended to human tumors? In order to answer these questions, more studies must be conducted on the biology of various mutant p53's and their interaction with the factors involved in DNA repair and apoptosis. Characterizing the instability phenotype of cells after perturbing these interactions will lead to a better understanding of the main causes of mutant p53-mediated genomic instabilities, which might also be point mutant-specific. p53 have a dual role in response to therapy, as exonuclease that by excision of incorporated anti-cancer drugs may confer resistance to drugs or as mediator of cell death induced by chemotherapy [85]. These features could serve as a template for the development of p53-targeting cancer therapies.

A major focus in the future would be to characterize the cellular and biological functions of p53 in mitochondria in response to various stresses. There are many missing points about the biological roles of p53 in mitochondria that still remain to be identified. How p53 can be imported into mitochondria? Whether p53 determines the percent of mutated mtDNA (heteroplasmy in a cell)? Uncovering the mechanisms by which pol γ-mediated mtDNA mutations and depletion are manifested in tissues in the absence and presence of p53 is the next step in understanding causes for mtDNA –related diseases. Understanding how p53 can be imported into mitochondria, will be important and could contribute towards the design of new therapies for cancer and other diseases.

The control of the viral mutation rate could be a viable anti-retroviral strategy. Still more work needs to be done in order to understand the molecular mechanisms involved in controlling fidelity not only at a molecular level (*i.e.*, intrinsic RT fidelity), but also related to the cytoplasmic p53 protein that can modulate the viral mutation rate and affect the incorporation of NRTIs into viral DNA. New understandings of the sub-cellular localization of p53, its role in the fidelity of proviral DNA synthesis in cytoplasm and drug resistance, therefore, may have broad implications for cellular and molecular biology as well as medicine. It may form the basis for new strategies in targeted antiviral therapy that focus on the sub-cellular context of p53 in cells.

Depletion and mutation of mitochondrial DNA during chronic NRTI therapy may lead to cellular respiratory dysfunction and release of reactive oxidative species, resulting in cellular damage [91]. Future NRTIs should provide higher specificity for HIV-RT and lower incorporation by pol γ to minimize mitochondrial toxicity. Whether the effective targeting of p53 in mitochondria may result in decrease of mitochondrial toxicity in response to conventional anti-viral therapies? Further studies are needed to elucidate if p53, by error-correction functions in mitochondria, can decrease mitochondrial toxicity.

Acknowledgements

This research was supported by grant from Israel Cancer Research Fund (ICRF) and by grant from Israel Cancer Association.

Author details

Galia Rahav and Mary Bakhanashvili*

*Address all correspondence to: bakhanus@yahoo.com

Infectious Diseases Unit, Sheba Medical Center, Tel Hashomer Israel; The Mina and Everard Goodman Faculty of Life Sciences, Bar-Ilan University, Ramat-Gan, Israel

References

[1] Echols H, Goodman MF. (1991) Fidelity mechanisms in DNA replication. Ann. Rev. Biochem. 60: 477-511.

[2] Reha-Krantz. (2010) DNA polymerase proofreading: Multiple roles maintain genome stability. BBA 1804: 1049-1063.

[3] McElhinny SAN, Pavlov Y, Kunkek T. (2006) Evidence for extrinsic exonucleolytic proofreading. Cell Cycle 5: 958-962.

[4] Shevelev IV, Hubscher U. (2002) The 3′→5′ exonucleases. Nat.Rev. 3: 1-12.

[5] Jackson AL, Loeb LA. (1998) The mutation rate and cancer. Genetics 148: 1483-1490.

[6] Copeland WC, Ponamarev MV, Nguyen D, Kunkel TA, Longley MJ. (2003)Mutations in DNA polymerase gamma cause error-prone DNA synthesis in human disorders. Acta Biochim Pol. 50:155-167.

[7] Kaguni LS. (2004) DNA polymerase γ, the mitochondrial replicase. Ann. Rev. Biochem. 73: 293-320.

[8] Singh KK. (2004) Mitochondria damage checkpoint in apoptosis and genome stability. FEMS Yeast Res.5: 127-132.

[9] Pesole G, Gissi C, De Chirico A, Saccone C. (1999) Nucleotide substitution rate of mammalian mitochondrial genomes. J Mol Evol 48: 427-434.

[10] Johnson A, Johnson K. (2001a) Fidelity of nucleotide incorporation by human mitochondrial DNA polymerase. J Biol. Chem. 276: 38090-38106.

[11] Johnson A, Johnson K. (2001b) Exonuclease proofreading by human mitochondrial DNA polymerase. J Biol. Chem. 276: 38097-38107.

[12] Trifunovic A, Wredenberg A, Falkrnberg M, Spelbrink JN, Rovio AT, Bruder CE, et al. (2004) Somatic mtDNA mutations cause aging phenotypes without affecting reactive oxygen species production. Nature 429: 417-423.

[13] Svarovskaya ES, Cheslock SR, Zhang W, Hu W, Pathak VK (2003) Retrovira mutation rates and reverse transcriptase fidelity. Front. Biosci.8: d117-d134.

[14] Katz R, Skalka AM. (1990) Generation of diversity in retroviruses. Ann. Rev. Genet. 24: 409-445.

[15] Menéndez-Arias L. (2009) Mutation rates and intrinsic fidelity of retroviral reverse transcriptases. Viruses. 1: 1137–1165.

[16] Perrino FW, Preston BD, Sandell LL, Loeb LA. (1989) Extension of mismatched 3′ termini of DNA is a major determinant of the infidelity of human immunodeficiency virus type 1 reverse transcriptase. Proc. Natl. Acad. Sci. USA 86: 8343-8347.

[17] Bakhanashvili M, Hizi A (1992) Fidelity of the reverse transcriptase of human immunodeficiency virus type. FEBS Lett. 306: 151-156.

[18] Bakhanashvili M, Hizi A. (1993) Fidelity of DNA synthesis exhibited in vitro by the reverse transcriptase of the lentivirus equine infectious anemia virus. Biochemistry 32: 7559-7567.

[19] Tian W, Hwang YT, Hwang CBC. (2008) The enhanced DNA replication fidelity of a mutant herpes simplex virus type 1 DNA polymerase is mediated by an improved nucleotide selectivity and reduced mismatch extension ability. J Virology 82: 8937-8941.

[20] Kunkel T. (1988) Exonucleolytic proofreading. Cell 53: 837-840.

[21] Brutlag D, Kornberg A. (1972) Enzymatic synthesis of deoxyribonucleic acid 36. A proofreading function for the 3′ leads to 5′ exonuclease activity in deoxyribonucleic acid polymerases. J. Biol. Chem. 247: 241-248.

[22] Hubscher U, Maga G, Spadari S. (2002) Eukaryotic DNA polymerases. Ann. Rev. Biochem. 71: 133-163.

[23] Joyce C.M. (1989) How DNA travels between the separate polymerase and 3′→5′ exonuclease sites of DNA polymerase I (Klenow fragment). J. Biol. Chem. 264: 858-866.

[24] Perrino FW, Loeb LA. (1990) Hydrolysis of 3′ -terminal mispairs in vitro by the 3′→5′exonuclease of DNA polymerase δ permits subsequent extension by DNA polymerase α. Biochemistry 29: 5226-5231.

[25] Maki H, Kornberg A. (1987) Proofreading by DNA polymerase III of Escherichia coli depends on cooperative interaction of the polymerase and exonuclease subunits. Proc. Natl. Acad. Sci. USA 84: 4389-4392.

[26] Albrechtsen N, Dornreiter L, Grosse F, Kim E, Wiesmuller L, Deppert W (1999) Maintenance of genomic integrity by p53: complementary roles for activated and non-activated p53. Oncogene 18: 7706-7717.

[27] Oren M (1999) Regulation of the p53 tumor suppressor protein. J Biol. Chem. 274: 36031-36034.

[28] Vousden KH, Prives C (2009) Blinded by the Light: The Growing Complexity of p53. Cell 137: 413-431.

[29] Soussi T (1995) The p53 tumor suppressor gene: from molecular biology to clinical investigation. In Molecular genetics of cancer (Cowell, J.K., ed.), p135-178, Bios. Scientific, Oxford, UK.

[30] Taira N, Yoshoda K. (2012) Post-translational modifications of p53 tumor suppressor: determinants of its functional targets. Histol Histopathol. 27: 437-443.

[31] Levine AJ. (1997) P53, the cellular gatekeeper for growth and division. Cell 88: 323-331.

[32] Freed-Pastor WA, Prives C. (2012) Mutant p53: one name, many proteins. Genes. Dev. 26: 1268-1286.

[33] Zhou J, Ahn J, Wilson SH, Prives C. (2001) A role for p53 in base excision repair. EMBO J. 20: 914–923.

[34] Gaiddon C, Moorthy NC, Prives C. (1999)Ref-1 regulates the transactivation and pro-apoptotic functions of p53 in vivo. EMBO J. 18: 5609–5621.

[35] Linke SP, Sengupta S, Khabie N, Jeffries BA, Buchhop S, Miska S, et al. (2003) p53 interacts with hRAD51 and hRAD54, and directly modulates homologous recombination. Cancer Res. 63: 2596–2605.

[36] Yang Q, Zhang R, Wang XW, Spillare EA, Linke SP, Subramanian D, et al. (2002) The processing of Holliday junctions by BLM and WRN helicases is regulated by p53. J Biol. Chem. 277: 31980–31987.

[37] Kern SE, Kinzler KW, Baker SJ, Nigro JM, Rotter V, Levine AJ, Friedman P, Prives C. Vogelstein B. (1991) Mutant p53 binds DNA abnormally. Oncogene 6: 131-136.

[38] Steinmeyer K, Deppert W. (1988) DNA binding properties of murine p53. Oncogene 3: 501-507.

[39] Bakalkin G, Yakovleva T, Selivanova G, Magnusson KP, Szekely L, Kiseleva E, Klein G, Terenius L, Wiman KG. (1994) p53 binds single-stranded DNA endsand catalyzes DNA renaturation and strand transfer. Proc. Natl. Acad. Sci. USA 91: 413-417.

[40] Oberosler P, Hloch P, Rammsperger U, Stahl H. (1993) p53-catalyzed annealing of complementary single-stranded nucleic acids. EMBO J 12: 2389-2396.

[41] Lee S, Elenbaas B, Levine A, Griffith J (1995) p53 and its 14kDa C-terminal domain recognize primary DNA damage in the form of insertion/deletion mismatches. Cell 81: 1013-1020.

[42] Bakhanashvili M, Hizi A, Rahav G. (2010) The interaction of p53 with 3'-terminal mismatched DNA. Cell Cycle 9, 1380-1389.

[43] Hwang BJ, Ford J.M, Hanawalt PC, Chu G. (1999) Expression of the p48 xeroderma pigmentosum gene is p53-dependent and is involved in global genomic repair. Proc. Natl. Acad. Sci. USA, 96: 424-428.

[44] Dudenhoffer C, Rohaly G, Will K, Deppert W, Wiesmullar L. (1998) Specific mismatch recognition in heteroduplex intermediates by p53 suggests a role in fidelity control of homologous recombination. Mol.Cell.Biol. 18: 5332-5342.

[45] Offer H, Wolkowicz R, Matas D, Blumenstein S, Livneh Z, Rotter V. (1999) Direct involvement of p53 in the base excision repair pathway of the DNA repair machinery. FEBS Lett. 450: 197-204.

[46] Mummenbrauer T, Janus F, Muller B, Wiesmuller L, Deppert W, Gross F. (1996) p53 protein exhibits 3′→5′ exonuclease activity. Cell 85: 1089-1099.

[47] Huang P. (1998) Excision of mismatched nucleotides from DNA: a potential mechanism for enhancing DNA replication fidelity by the wild-type p53 protein. Oncogene 17: 261-270.

[48] Skalski V, Lin Z, Choi BY, Brown KR. (2000) Substrate specificity of the p53-associated 3′→5′ exonuclease. Oncogene 19: 3321-3329.

[49] Bakhanashvili M. (2001) Exonucleolytic proofreading by p53 protein. Eur.J Biochem. 268: 2047-2054.

[50] Bakhanashvili M. (2001) p53 enhances the fidelity of DNA synthesis by human immunodeficiency virus type 1 reverse transcriptase. Oncogene 20: 7635-7644.

[51] Bakhanashvili M, Gedelovich R, Grinberg S, Rahav G. (2008) Exonucleolytic degradation of RNA by the tumor suppression protein p53 in cytoplasm. J Molec. Medicine 86: 75-88.

[52] Grinberg S, Teiblum G, Rahav G, Bakhanashvili M. (2010) p53 in cytoplasm exerts 3′→5′ exonuclease activity with dsRNA. Cell cycle 9: 2442-2455.

[53] Melle C, Nasheuer H. (2002) Physical and functional interactions of the tumor suppressor protein p53 and DNA polymerase α-primase. Nucleic Acids Res. 30: 1493-1499.

[54] Ballal K, Zhang W, Mukhopadyay T, Huang P.(2002) Suppression of mismatched mutation by p53: a mechanism guarding genomic integrity. J. Mol. Med. 80: 25-32.

[55] Lilling G, Novitsky E, Sidi Y, Bakhanashvili M. (2003) p53-associated 3′→5′ exonuclease activity in nuclear and cytoplasmic compartments of the cells. Oncogene 22, 233-245.

[56] Bakhanashvili M, Novitsky E, Lilling G, Rahav G. (2004) p53 in cytoplasm may enhance the accuracy of DNA synthesis by human immunodeficiency virus type 1 reverse transcriptase. Oncogene 23: 6890-6899.

[57] Bakhanashvili M. Grinberg S, Bonda E, Simon AJ, Moshitch-Moshkovitz S, Rahav G. (2008) p53 in mitochondria enhances the accuracy of DNA synthesis. Cell Death Diff. 15: 1865-1874.

[58] Bakhanashvili M, Hizi A. (1996) The interaction of the reverse transcriptase of humanimmunodeficiency virus type 1 with 3′-terminally mispaired DNA. Arch. Bioch. Bioph. 334: 89-96.

[59] Janus F, Albrechtsen N, Knippschild U, Wiesmuller L, Grosse F, Deppert W. (1999) Different regulation of the p53 core domain activities 3′ to 5′ exonuclease and sequence-specific DNA binding. Mol. Cell. Biol. 19: 2155-2168.

[60] Ahn J, Poyurovsky MV, Baptiste N, Beckerman R, Cain C, Mattia M, et al. (2009) Dissection of the sequence-specific DNA binding and exonuclease activities reveals a superactive yet apoptotically impaired mutant p53 protein. Cell Cycle 8: 1603-1615.

[61] Cho Y, Gorina S, Jeffrey PD, Pavletich NP. (1994) Crystal structure of a p53 tumor suppressor-DNA complex: understanding tumorigenic mutations. Science 265: 346–355.

[62] Cox LS, Hupp T, Midgley CA, Lane DP (1995) A direct effect of activated human p53 on DNA replication. EMBO J 14: 2099-2105.

[63] Syvaoja J, Suomensaari S, Nishida C, Goldsmith JS, Chui GS, Jain S, Linn S. (1990) DNA polymerases alpha, delta, and epsilon: three distinct enzymes from Hela cells. Proc. Natl Acad. Sci. USA 87: 6664-6668.

[64] Peng H, Chen G, Du M, Singh N,Isaacson PG, Pan L. (1996) Replication error phenotype and p53 gene mutation in lymphoma of mucosa associated lymphoid tissue. Am.J Pathol. 148: 643-648.

[65] Stoler DL, Chen N, Basik M, Kahlenberg M, Rodriguez-Bigas MS, Petrelli NJ, Anderson GR. (1999) The onset and extent of genomic instability in sporadic colorectal tumor progression. Proc. Natl. Acad. Sci. USA. 96: 15121-15126.

[66] Offer H, Milyavsky M, Erez N, Matus D, Zurer I, Harris CC, Rotter V. (2001) Structural and functional involvement of p53 in BER in vitro and in vivo. Oncogene 20: 581-589.

[67] Stenmark-Askmalm M, Stal O, Sullivan S, Ferraud L, Sun XF, Carstensen J, Nordenskjold B. (1994) Cellular accumulation of p53 protein: an independent prognostic factor in stage II breast cancer. Eur. J Cancer 30A: 175-180.

[68] Moll UM, LaOuglia M, Benard, Riou G. (1995) Wild-type p53 protein undergoes cytoplasmic sequestration in undifferentiated neuroblastomas but not in differentiated tumors. Proc. Natl. Acad. Sci. US, 92: 4407-4411.

[69] Bosari S, Viale G, Roncalli M, Graziani D, Borsani G, Lee AK, Coggi G. (1995) p53 gene mutations, p53 protein accumulation and compartmentalization in colorectal adenocarcinoma. Am. J Pathol. 147: 790-798.

[70] Sun XF, Cartensen J.M, Zhang H, Stal O, Wingren S, Hatschek T, Nordenskjold B. (1992) Prognostic significance of cytoplasmic p53 oncoprotein in colorectal adenocarcinoma. Lancet 340: 1369-1373.

[71] Gaitonde SV, Riley JR, Qiao D, Martinez JD. (2000) Conformational phenotype of p53 is linked to nuclear translocation. Oncogene 19: 4042-4049.

[72] Braithwaite DK, Ito J (1993) Compilation, alighnment and phylogenetic relationships of DNA Polymerases. Nucleic Acids Res. 21: 787-802.

[73] Loft S, Poulsen HE. (1999) Markers of oxidative damage to DNA: antioxidants and molecular damage. Methods Enzymol. 300: 166-184.

[74] Katafuchi A, Nohmi T. (2010) DNA polymerases involved in the incorporation of oxidized nucleotides into DNA: their efficiency and template base preference. Mutat Res. 703: 24-31.

[75] Marchenko ND, Zaika A, Moll UM. (2000) Death signal-induced localization of p53 protein to mitochondria. A potential role in apoptotic signaling. J. Biol. Chem. 275: 16202-16212.

[76] Mahyar-Roemer M, Fritzsche C, Wagner S, Laue M, Roemer K. (2004) Mitochondrial p53 levels parallel total p53 levels independent of stress response in human colorectal carcinoma and glioblastoma cells. Oncogene 23: 6226-6236.

[77] Achanta G, Sasaki R, Feng L, Carew JS, Lu W, Pelicano H, et al. (2005) Novel role of p53 in maintaining mitochondrial genetic stability through interaction with DNA pol γ. EMBO J 24: 3482-3492.

[78] Wong TS, Rajagopalan S, Townsley FM, Freund SM, Petrovich M, Loakes D, Fersht AR. (2009) Physical and functional interactions between human mitochondrial single-stranded DNA binding protein and tumor suppressor p53. Nucleic Acids Res. 37: 568-581.

[79] Mendelman LV, Petruska JS, Goodman MF. (2009) Base mispair extension kinetics. Comparison of DNA polymerase alpha and reverse transcriptase. J. Biol. Chem. 265:2338- 2346.

[80] Perrino FW, Loeb LA. (1989) Proofreading by the ε subunit of Escherichia coli DNA polymerase III increases the fidelity of calf thymus DNA polymerase α. Proc. Natl. Acad. Sci. USA 86: 3085-3088.

[81] Sloane DL, Goodman MF, Echols H. (1988) The fidelity of base selection by the polymerase subunit of DNA polymerase III holoenzyme. Nucleic Acid Res. 16: 6465-6475.

[82] Keating MJ. (1997) In: Nucleoside Analogs in Cancer Therapy. Cheson BD. Keating, Plunkett W. (eds). Marcel Dekker, Inc., New York, pp201-226.

[83] Sluis-Cremer N, Arion D, Parniak MA. (2000) Molecular mechanisms of HIV-1 resistance to nucleoside reverse transcriptase inhibitors (NRTIs). Cell. Mol. Life Sci. 57: 1408-1422.

[84] Zhou Y, Achanta G, Pelicano H, Gadhi V, Plunkett W, Huang P. (2002) Action of (E)-2′-Deoxy-2′-(fluoromethylene) cytidine on DNA metabolism: incorporation, excision and cellular response. Mol. Pharmacology 61: 222-229.

[85] Feng L, Achanta G, Pelicano H, Zhang W, Plunkett W, Huang P. (2000) Role of p53 in cellular response to anticancer nucleoside analog-induced DNA damage. Int. J Molec Medicine 5: 597-604.

[86] Achanta G, Pelicano H, Feng L, Plunkett W, Huang P.(2001) Interaction of p53 and DNA-PK in response to nucleoside analogues: potential role as a sensor complex for DNA damage. Cancer Res 61: 8723-8729.

[87] Galmarini CM, Clarke ML, Falette N, Puisieux A, Mackey JR, Dumontet C. (2002) Expression of a non-functional p53 affects the sensitivity of cancer cells to gemcitabine. Int. J Cancer. 97: 439-445.

[88] Sluis-Cremer N, Arion D, Parniak MA. (2000) Molecular mechanisms of HIV-1 resistance to nucleoside reverse transcriptase inhibitors (NRTIs). Cell. Mol. Life Sci. 57: 1408-1422.

[89] Bakhanashvili M, Novitsky E, Rubinstein E, Levy I, Rahav G. (2005) Excision of nucleoside analogs from DNA by p53 protein, a potential cellular mechanism of resistance to inhibitors of human immunodeficiency virus type 1 reverse transcriptase. Antimic. Agents and Chem. 49:1576-1579.

[90] Fowler JD, Brown JA, Johnson KA, Suo Z. (2008) Kinetic investigation of the inhibitory effect of gemcitabine on DNA polymerization catalyzed by human mitochondrial DNA polymerase. J Biol. Chem. 283: 15339-15348.

[91] Lewis W, Day BJ, Copeland WC. (2003) Mitochondrial toxicity of NRTI antiviral drugs: an integrated cellular perspectives. Nature Reviews 2: 812-822.

[92] Bakhanashvili M, Grinberg S, Bonda E, Rahav G. (2009) Excision of nucleoside analogs in mitochondria by p53 protein. AIDS 23: 779-788.

[93] Ewald B, Sampath D, Plunkett W. (2008) Nucleoside amalogs: molecular mechanisms signaling cell death, Oncogene 27: 6522-6537.

Chapter 12

Biological Systems that Control Transcription of DNA Repair and Telomere Maintenance-Associated Genes

Fumiaki Uchiumi, Steven Larsen and
Sei-ichi Tanuma

Additional information is available at the end of the chapter

http://dx.doi.org/10.5772/53905

1. Introduction

A variety of transcription factor binding sequences instead of the authentic TATA- or TATA-like elements are present in large numbers of 5′-flanking or regulatory regions of the human genes [1]. Our previous research showed that several human gene promoter regions of the DNA repair-associated genes, including *PARP*, *PARG*, *ATR*, and *RB1*, contain duplicated GGAA-motifs or ETS binding sequences, although they have no obvious TATA-like elements [2]. On the other hand, surveillance of a human genomic DNA database revealed that 5′-flanking regions of the human genes encoding telomerase and telomere maintenance factors, which are called as shelterins, are TATA-less but most of them carry GC-boxes and/or Sp1-binding sequences [3]. These observations suggest that the expression of the DNA repair and telomere maintenance factor-encoding genes is likely to be regulated by a TATA-independent mechanism.

The molecular mechanisms of effect induced by caloric restriction (CR) mimetic drugs, including Resveratrol (Rsv), have been well studied [4]. It was suggested that the CR mimetic compounds activate NAD^+ dependent deacetylase sirtuins, or inhibits cAMP phosphodiesterases to improve mitochondrial functions [5]. Thus, it is supposed that Rsv affects cellular senescence to elongate lifespan of various organisms [4]. It should be noted that mitochondrial functions cross-talk with telomeres in which telomere-shortening causes chromosomal instability and leads to cellular senescence [6]. We have reported that caloric restriction (CR) mimetics, 2-deoxy-D-glucose (2DG) and Rsv up-regulate promoter activities of the 5′-flanking regions of genes encoding telomere-maintenance factors including shelterin complex proteins [3]. Moreover, we observed that telomerase activity in HeLa S3 cells was moderately induced by the 2DG and Rsv [7,8]. Additionally, it has been reported that tumor suppressor p53, which is encoded by the *TP53* gene, is phosphorylated and then it induces ERK1/2 activation in response to Rsv treatment [9]. Interestingly, the *TP53* promoter contains GGAA (TTCC)-duplication adjacent to the transcription start site (Table 1). Taken together, these observations suggest that the anti-aging effect of CR mimetic compounds stems from up-regulation of *TP53* expression *via* duplicated GGAA (TTCC) elements, in accordance with the moderate induction of expression of genes encoding telomere maintenance factors possibly through GC-box or Sp1-binding elements.

In this review article, we will discuss the contribution of *cis*-elements, namely duplicated GGAA and GC-boxes, in regulation of DNA-repair- and telomere maintenance-associated gene expression that is thought to control cellular senescence and aging of organisms.

2. Transcription of eukaryotic cells

2.1. General transcription factors and TATA-dependent and independent transcription mechanisms

Transcription or synthesis of RNAs is known to be regulated at several steps, including chromosomal modification, transcription initiation, elongation, and termination [10]. Eukaryotic transcription of mRNAs is catalyzed by RNA polymerase II (Pol II) and the molecular mechanisms are well studied [11]. Initiation of transcription is executed by transcription machinery complex consisting of Pol II and general transcription factors (GTFs), such as TFIIA, TFIIB, TFIID, TFIIE, TFIIF, and THIIH. Transcription is thought to start from the formation of pre-initiation complex (PIC), which contains GTFs and Pol II, at the transcription start site (TSS) [11]. The most studied eukaryotic promoter regions contain TATA- or TATA-like sequences that are recognized by TATA binding protein (TBP). Binding of TBP to the TATA-box results in recruitment of TFIID and TAFs [12], then it provokes the formation of the PIC, precisely determining the TSS. Although TATA-dependent transcription initiating mechanisms have been extensively characterized by a variety of experiments, 76% of the TSSs in human genomes have no obvious TATA or TATA-like elements [1]. This fact clearly indicates that eukaryotic transcription is initiated by either TATA-dependent or independent mechanisms.

2.2. TATA-less promoters-genome wide analyses by ChIP experiment

Recent study of PICs in *Saccharomyces* by genome wide ChIP analysis revealed that they are positioned at TATA-boxes or TATA-like elements in TATA-less promoters [13]. In contrast, from the analysis of human DNA sequence data base, it was shown that only 2.6% of human promoters contain the TATA-consensus 7-mer TATAAA around their TSSs [14]. Moreover, surveillance of the human genome database revealed that a total of 174 different DNA sequence motifs are found in promoter regions, and that no obvious TATA-like elements are listed in the top 50 most common of these motifs [15]. These observations imply that appropriate cooperation between transcription factor (TF) binding sites would determine TSSs and tissue specific transcription in mammalian cells as TATA-element determines. In other words, TATA-box might be one of the *cis*-elements that specify where TSSs should be located in the human gene promoter regions. The concept that multiple *cis*-elements and their combinations determine the location of TSS and tissue specificity is consistent with the transcription model that is driven by enhanceosome in several gene promoters including *IFNB* promoter [16].

3. Promoter regions of the human DNA-repair associated genes

We have been studying the regulatory mechanism of the human *PARG* gene expression, and isolated its promoter region [17]. Deletion and mutagenesis analyses narrowed the core promoter region, and indicated an important role for duplicated GGAA motifs in the TATA-less *PARG* promoter function. The *PARG* gene encodes a poly(ADP-ribose) glycohydrolase (PARG) that degrade the poly(ADP-ribose) (PAR) which is synthesized by enzyme reaction catalyzed by poly(ADP-ribose) polymerase, PARP protein [18]. Interestingly, no obvious TATA-box but a duplicated GGAA-motif is found around the TSS of the human *PARP1* gene [19].

Poly(ADP-ribosyl)ation is thought to be involved in the process of DNA-repair, which is dependent on both poly(ADP-ribose) synthesis and degradation [18]. Given that the *PARP1* and *PARG* genes encode proteins that work cooperatively in the PAR-dependent DNA-repair system, their expression would be similar in response to the same DNA-damaging signal. Therefore, it is natural that the 5′-upstream regions of the two genes resemble each other containing duplicated GGAA (TTCC) element but TATA-box. We thus speculate that other promoters of PAR-dependent DNA-repair system associated genes might contain GGAA-duplication instead of the TATA-box.

3.1. Surveillance of 5′-upstream regions of the PARP and PAR-associated protein encoding genes

At first, we understood that the duplicated GGAA is a sequence that should be associated with macrophage-like differentiation of HL-60 cells induced by 12-*O*-tetradecanoylphorbol-13-acetate (TPA) [17]. The expression of several genes are up-regulated during the TPA-induced differentiation of HL-60 cells, as shown by DNA-microarray experiments [20]. Interestingly, *RB1* gene, which encodes a tumor suppressor and cell cycle regulator protein Rb1, is included in the late response genes [20]. The Rb1 protein is also suggested to control cell fate by inducing differentiation and inhibiting apoptosis [21]. Thus, we examined the 5′-flanking region of the *RB1* gene, and found that a duplication of the GGAA-motif is essential for the promoter activity [2]. We have also reported that duplicated GGAA-motifs are contained in the promoter regions of the human *XPB* and *ATR* genes that are involved in DNA-repair synthesis and DNA-damage response signal, respectively [2]. These genes are known to be involved in the DNA repair synthesis.

PARP modifies itself and various target proteins by addition of a PAR using NAD^+ as the substrate [18]. This modification is important for the recruitment of base excision repair (BER) associating factors, including XRCC1 [22]. Therefore, expression of the genes encoding PARP target proteins or PAR-associating proteins might be similarly regulated as in *PARP1* and *PARG* genes. In this context, it should be emphasized that PAR binds to p53 altering its associatiation with DNA [23].

Genes	Sequence (5′ to 3′)
ADPRHL2 (ADH3)	GATGGGGAACACTATTCCTCCGA, CGGACGGAAGTAGGGAAACTGT
APEX1 (APE1)	CAGCTTTCCGGAGCGCAGAGGAAGCTGG, CACTGGGAAAGACACCGCGGAACTCCC, CCGTTTTCCTATCTCTTTCCCGTGG
ATM	CAGCAGGAACCACAATAAGGAACAAGA, CCTTCGGAACTGTCGTCACTTCCGTCCT
ATR	CGGTGGGAACGTGAGGAACTTTT, ACGGCTTCCCGGCTTCCCCCGG
BRCA1	ATGCTGGAAATAATTATTTCCCTCCA, AATTCTTCCTCTTCCGTCTCTTTCCTTTTA, TTGGTTTCCGTGGCAACGGAAAAGCGCGGGAATTACA
BRCA2	GACAAGGAATTTCCTTTCG
CHEK1	TTTTTTTCCTACGGAATCATG, TCGCCTTCCCAAAGTGCTGGAATTACA, CTTATTTCCATTTTTCCTATTT
DCLRE1C (Artemis)	TAAACGGAAGAGGGAATTAATAGTTCCTGAAT, AAGCAGGAAGCGGAACGAAG, TCGATTTCCCTTCCCGCGA, GCGGCTTCCCGGAAGTGGC
E2F4	TGGCAGGAAGTGAGGGATAGGAATAGAT, AAAATGGAAAAGGAACAGGT, GGCAAGGAAAGTTCCGATGG, CCACGTTCCCTGGAAGGCGC, GGGACGGAAGCGGAAGCAGT, GGCCAGGAACGGAAGCGGAAGTGGC
E2F6	CCCTGTTCCCTTCCTCTGGAATTCGG, ACCTCTTCCTTTTCCTTTGC
FANCD2	CGGCCTTCCACTTCCGGCGCGGAAGTTGG
NBN (NBS1)	CAGGTGGAAGTGGAAAGGAAGGGTA, CTAGATTCCAAAGGAATACCT, TGCTGTTCCTTTTCCAACCA
PARG	GCCGCTTCCCCCGCCTCCTTCCATGGT, TGACCTTCCGGGCGCCGGTTCCCGTTA, GCCCCGGAAGCTGGAAGCGCC, CAGCTTTCCGGTGGTGGGAAAGTGA
PARP1	GCGGGTTCCGTGGGCGTTCCCGCGG
POLB	CCCGTTTCCCCTTCTAGGGAAAGGATTCCAGATA, AGGTCTTCCCATAGGAAGGCCC
PRKDC (DNA-PK_{CS})	ATCGAGGAACAAACTTGGAACTCTT, CGTTTTTCCTTAGGTTTCCATGTT, CCCCGGGAAAGTTCCTGCCG
RB1	CAGGTTTCCCAGTTTAATTCCTCATG, CGGGCGGAAGTGACGTTTTCCCGCGG
TERT	TCCCCTTCCTTTCCGCGGC
RTEL1 (RTEL)	GCGGGGGAACAGTTTCCGCCGG, GGACCGGAAGTGGGGGGCGGAAGTGCA
TDP1	TCTCCGGAAGGGGAAGGGGC
TP53	ATTACGGAAAGCCTTCCTAAAA, CTTTCTTCCTTCCACCCT, TCCATTTCCTTTGCTTCCTCCGG
WRN	AGGTGGGAAGATGGGAATGAGG
XRCC1	GCTAAGGAACGCAGCGCTCTTCCCGCTC
XRCC5 (Ku80)	CAGAGTTCCGGGGCACGGTTTCCCCGCC
ZC3HAV1	GCTCTTTCCGGGAATGGGT

Table 1. Duplicated GGAA motifs in the 5′-upstream regions of human DNA-repair associated genes

PARP1 has been reported to regulate G1 arrest in response to DNA damage *via* poly(ADP-ribosyl)ation of the p53 [24]. Furthermore, XRCC1 and ATM (Ataxia telangiectasia mutated) proteins, which play roles in the DNA-damage response signaling system, are also known to interact with PAR [25]. Moreover, cooperation of PARP and DNA-dependent protein kinase (DNA-PK) during DNA strand break repair has been also demonstrated [26]. Not surprisingly, duplicated GGAA-motifs are found in the 5'-upstream regions of the *ATM, PRKDC* (*DNA-PK*$_{CS}$), *TP53* and *XRCC1* genes encoding the PARP/PAR associating proteins (Table 1). Although degradation of PAR in nuclei is thought to be mainly catalyzed by the PARG, it should be noted that ARH3 catalyzes the degradation of PAR on the mitochondrial matrix [27]. As GGAA duplication is contained in the 5'-flanking region of the *ADPRHL2* (*ARH3*) gene (Table 1), we predict that it functions in response to DNA-damage signals.

3.2. Surveillance of the DNA repair associated gene promoter regions

XRCC1, which is a 70-kDa X-ray cross-complementing group 1 protein, is thought to act as a scaffold protein for BER and DNA single strand break repair (SSBR) [28]. Various proteins are involved in the XRCC1-associated DNA-repair processes, including APEX1 (APE1), TDP1, PCNA, RFC, POLB (DNA-pol β), WRN, ERCC6 (CSB), and E2F family proteins [28]. We previously reported that the *WRN* promoter region contains GGAA duplications [7], and after analyses of several other DNA-repair related genes found that *APEX1, TDP1, POLB* and *E2F4* gene promoters also harbor duplicated GGAA-motifs (Table. 1).

Additionally, GGAA-duplications around the TSSs of the human *ATM* and *ATR* genes were discovered (Table 1). Both ATM and ATR are check point kinases with critical roles in DNA repair *via* homologous recombination repair (HRR) at the sites of double-strand breaks (DSBs) [29]. Cancer and genetic studies highlighted the roles for the FANC proteins, Rad51, BRCA1, BRCA2, CHEK1 (CHK1), CHEK2 (CHK2), NBN (NBS1), RecQL4, WRN, XRCC5 (Ku80), and XRCC6 (Ku70) in HRR [29]. Therefore, we examined the sequences of each 5'-upstream region of these HRR/DSB associated genes and revealed that the duplicated GGAA-motifs are contained in the 5'-flanking region of the *BRCA1, BRCA2, CHEK1, DCLRE1C (Artemis), FANCD2, NBN* and *XRCC5 (Ku80)* genes (Table 1). Although the *CHEK2, LIG4* and *XRCC4* genes are not listed in Table 1, duplicated GGAA (TTCC) motifs, which are distant within thirteen nucleotides, are located near their TSSs.

3.3. Possible roles of the duplicated GGAA motif in the 5'-upstream regions of DNA-repair genes as a bidirectional initiation element

It has been shown that the human *PARG* gene is head-head linked with the *TIM23* gene, which encodes a mitochondrial inner membrane translocase 23 [17,30]. Moreover, we reported that a duplicated GGAA motif is located in the region of a head-head junction of the human *IGHMBP2* and *MRPL21* promoters [31]. Furthermore, many cancer or DNA repair associated genes are regulated by bidirectional promoters, for example tandem repeat binding sites for ETS family proteins were identified in the bidirectional promoter regions of *PERLD1/ERBB2* and *CIDEC/FANCD2* genes in breast and ovarian cancers [32]. We also identified several head-head oriented genes whose promoter regions contain duplicated GGAA-motifs [33]. Several examples of bidirectional partners of the DNA repair-associated genes those are oriented in a head-head manner are summarized in Table 2. Given that specific TFs are linked to the regulation of bidirectional promoters [34], the TF-binding elements in these promoter regions may determine whether they function as bidirectional or unidirectional promoters dependent on the prevailing TF-expression of the cell. Although it has not been shown yet, functions of transcribed RNAs or translated proteins from these bidirectional partners might be associated with cellular responses that are required against DNA damaging agent.

DNA repair genes (GENE ID)	Partner genes (GENE ID)
ADPRHL2 (ADH3) (54936)	*TEKT2* (27285)
APEX1 (APE1) (328)	*OSGEP* (55644)
ATM (472)	*NPAT* (4863)
BRCA1 (672)	*NBR2* (10230)
CHEK2 (11200)	*HSCB* (150274)
FANCD2 (2177)	*CIDECP* (152302)
LIG4 (3981)	*ABHD13* (84945)
PARG (8505)	*TIM23B* (653252)
PCNA (5111)	*CDS2* (8760)
PRKDC (DNA-PK$_{CS}$) (5591)	*MCM4* (4173)
TP53 (7157)	*WRAP53* (55135)
XRCC6 (Ku70) (2547)	*DESI1* (27351)

Table 2. Bidirectional promoter partner genes with the human DNA-repair associated genes

3.4. Multiplicity of GGAA motifs may play a role in the formation of specific chromosomal structures

It is well known that various repetitive sequences are providing special features at specific regions of eukaryotic chromosomes. Telomeres are composed of TTAGGG repeats and they are maintained by specific structures that are known as T- and D-loops [35]. Other example is that the centromeres, in which the (CENP) B box is located, have specific structures that function to segregate chromosomes accurately [36]. Interestingly, the 17-bp sequence of (CENP) B box, which is recognized by CENP-B protein, contains GGAA motif, and this (CENP) B box appear every other α-satellite repeat (171-bp sequence) in human chromosomes [37,38]. Thus, repetitive sequences play roles in the formation of specific chromosomal structures and they are generally referred as microsatellites.

It is noteworthy that repetitive GGAA motifs or GGAA-microsatellites are targets of the oncogenic fusion protein EWS/FLI, whose mRNA is transcribed from the result of aberrant chromosomal translocation, t(11;22)(q24;q12) [39,40]. The GGAA-microsatellites are located in the promoter regions of several genes, including *DAX1/NR0B1, FCGRT, CAV1, CACNB2,*

http://dx.doi.org/10.5772/53905

FEZF1, *KIAA1797*, and *GSTM4* [41-43]. The EWS/FLI binds to these promoter regions activating their transcription [44]. Although, the function of GGAA-microsatellites in the formation of specific structures of human chromosomes has not been clearly shown, DNA damage is reported to be introduced non-randomly or heterogeniously [45], suggesting that sensitivities to oxidative damages are partly dependent on DNA sequences or the structures. Oxidative damages to DNA, which might cause microsatellite instability, inhibition of methylation, and telomere shortening, do not only generate 8-OH-Gua, but also modulate transcription by altering redox status in cells [45]. Furthermore, given that telomere repeat sequence TTAGGG changes DNA conformation to form G-quadruplex structure [46], the repetitive GGAA motifs might also play a part in maintaining specific structures of chromosomes. Thus it could be hypothesized that the duplicated GGAA motifs in the 5′-upstream regions of the DNA-repair genes affect chromosomal structures, which might be altered by DNA-damage causing agents. Alternatively, affinities of GGAA-binding TFs with the duplicated GGAA motifs may be altered by oxidative damages. Yet these possibilities are to be elucidated by further experimental analyses.

4. Promoter regions of the human telomere maintenance factor-encoding genes

Human telomeres are unique structures of chromosomal ends where telomere binding proteins and telomere maintenance factors are associated to control chromosomal integrity, and their shortening is thought to cause instability of chromosomes leading to cellular senescence [35,47]. It has been shown that telomeres form a T-loop configuration [47,48], which are protected by shelterin proteins, including TRF1, TRF2, Rap1, TIN2, TPP1 and POT1 [49,50]. Recently, conditional knock down experiments demonstrated that shelterin proteins function as repressors or inhibitors of ATM/ATR signaling, non-homologous end joining (NHEJ), alt-NHEJ, HRR and resection [51]. Given that shelterin proteins have similar functions in protecting telomeres from DNA-damage, shelterin genes might be regulated in a similar manner to each other. In addition, their gene expression needs to be regulated by a unique system that is different from those of ATM/ATR signaling, NHEJ, alt-NHEJ, HRR and resection.

4.1. GC-box or Sp1 binding element is a common TF binding motif within the 5′-upstreams of the telomere maintenance factor-encoding genes

Previously, we have isolated 300 to 500-bp 5′-upstream regions of the human *TERT*, *TERC*, *DKC1*, *POT1*, *RAP1*, *TANK1*, *TANK2*, *TIN2*, *TPP1*, *TRF1*, and *TRF2* genes [3,7]. Sequence analyses of the PCR-amplified DNA fragments showed that they have no apparent TATA-box or TATA-like element except for the *TERC* gene promoter [3]. Similar to the 5′-upstream region of the human *WRN* gene, GC-boxes or Sp1-binding elements are found adjacent to the TSSs of the *TERT*, *TERC*, *DKC1*, *RAP1*, *TANK1*, *TIN2*, *TPP1*, *TRF1* and *TRF2* genes but not in the *POT1* and *TANK1* promoter regions [3]. Instead, OCT-binding elements are located in the 5′-flanking regions of both these genes. We have also isolated the 5′-upstream region of the human *RTEL1* gene [2], which encodes a DNA helicase motif containing protein with telomere D-loop dissociation and telomere G-quadruplex contracting activity [52,53]. Therefore, the mechanism for maintenance of telomere integrity by RTEL1 would be different from that of the shelterin proteins. It is noteworthy that duplicated GGAA motifs are located near the TSS of the *RTEL1* gene (Table 1) and one of them functions as an essential *cis*-element for transcription [2], suggesting that GC-box binding TFs are not the main regulators of *RTEL1* gene expression, rather the contribution by GGAA motif-binding TFs are of greater importance, in a similar manner as the DNA-repair associated genes, *ATM*/*ATR* and *Rb1*.

4.2. TATA-independent regulatory mechanisms of DNA-repair associated genes and telomere maintenance factor-encoding genes

Clustering analysis of TF-binding sites in human promoters revealed that a TATA-box is totally absent in promoters containing an ETS binding motif [14]. The most frequently found sequence co-localized with ETS binding motifs in human promoters is the Sp1 element with 28.4% occurrence [14], next is the ETS binding motif itself (18.7%). In addition, occurrences of Sp1 motif with the other Sp1 motifs in human promoters was estimated at 61.2%. These lines of evidences suggest that Sp1 family and ETS family proteins synergistically control promoters containing both elements.

However, comparison of common TF-binding motifs in the 5'-flanking regions of the DNA-repair and telomere associated genes suggest that they are individually regulated by GGAA-binding factors and GC-box-binding factors, respectively. In addition, most of these promoters do not have an authentic TATA or TATA-like element. We can speculate that through the evolution of organisms, GGAA-duplicated motifs have become selectively utilized for regulation of gene expression of the DNA-repair factor encoding genes, while GC-box might have developed to be a regulator for telomere maintenance factor-encoding genes (Fig. 1). TATA-dependent transcription may have been disadvantageous in control of DNA damage inducible genes with a distinct ability to sustain or maintain integrity of genomes, including chromosomes and telomeres.

5. Caloric restriction induced signals that affect transcription of the telomere associated genes

It is well established that loss of function mutations on the *WRN* gene that encodes telomere regulating RecQ helicase can lead to cancer or premature aging syndrome [54,55]. On the other hand, caloric restriction (CR) can extend life spans of various organisms [56], and thus CR mimetic drugs are expected to have an anti-aging effect. We therefore hypothesized that CR or CR mimetic drugs might induce signals acting on transcription of telomere-associated genes. We previously reported that the relative promoter activities of the human shelterin encoding genes compared with that of the *PIF1* gene are up-regulated by 2-deoxy-D-glucose (2DG) or Resveratrol (Rsv) in HeLa S3 cells [3].

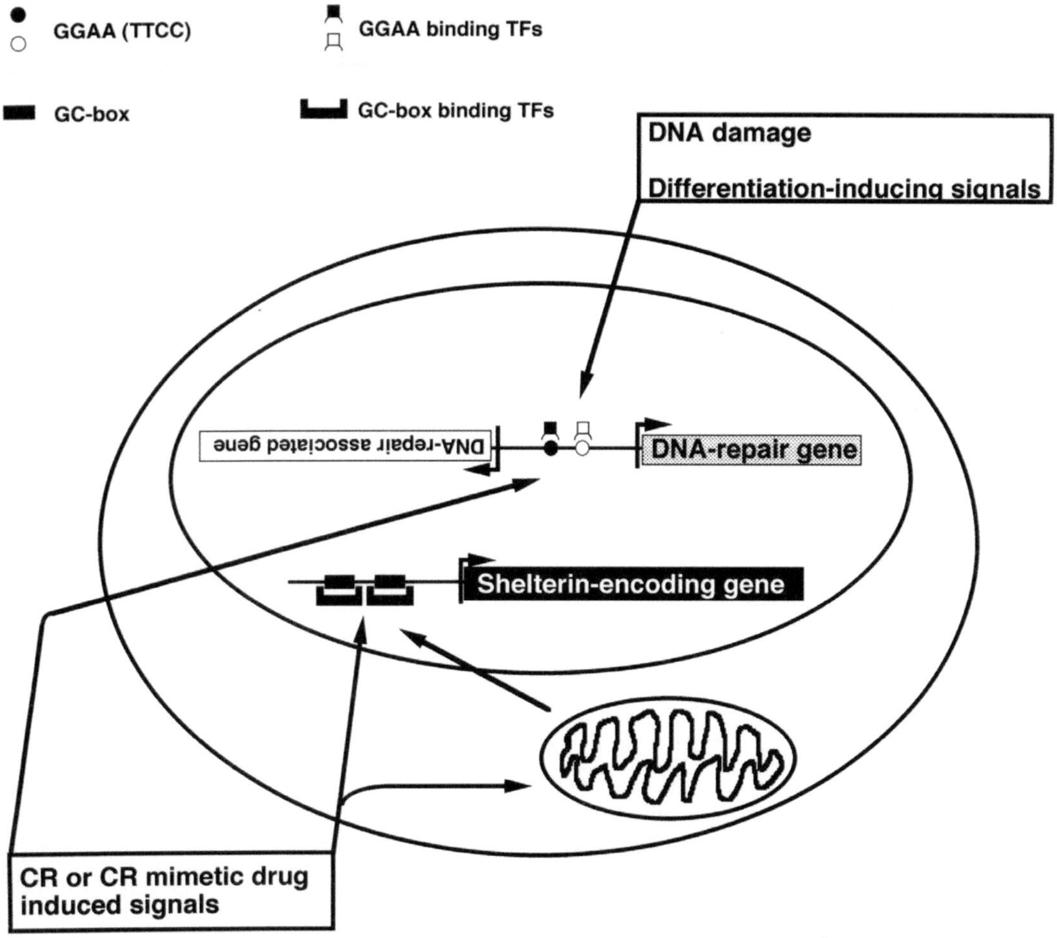

Figure 1. Hypothetical model of transcription of DNA-repair and telomere maintenance associated genes in response to biological stress signals. Duplicated GGAA motifs in the 5'-upstream regions of DNA-repair genes could respond to DNA damaging or differentiation-inducing signals. In the case that the duplicated GGAA elements are located in the commomn gene regulatory region of two head-head oriented genes, bidirectional transcription would be evoked by various GGAA motif binding TFs. On the other hand, GC-boxes that are contained in the human shelterin-encoding gene promoters could respond to CR-induced signals. In turn, the CR-induced signals may affect mitochondria to provoke modulation of GC-box-mediated transcription. The 5'-flanking regions of the human *WRN*, *SIRT1*, and *TERT* genes contain duplicated GGAA motifs with GC-boxes, implying that they are required for circumstances in which DNA damage or shortening of telomeres occurs.

5.1. Effect of CR mimetic drugs on telomere associated protein-encoding gene promoters

2DG and Rsv, which are known as a potent inhibitors of glucose metabolism [56], and an activator of sirtuin-mediated deacetylation [4], respectively, are referred as CR mimetic drugs. It has been shown that telomerase activity in HeLa S3 cells was moderately activated by 2DG and by Rsv [7,8]. These observations suggest that CR mimetic drugs have protective effects on telomeres by inducing telomerase activity along with up-regulating expression of the telomere maintenance factor-encoding genes. Up to present, human *TERT* (h*TERT*) promoter region has been well characterized with c-Ets, GC-box, E-box and other TF-binding elements that are located in its 5′-flanking region [57,58]. GC-boxes and Sp1-binding sites are not the only commonly found elements in the human *TERT* and *WRN* promoter regions [59], but also duplicated GGAA elements which are found adjacent to both TSSs (Table 1).

Interestingly, both duplicated GGAA-motif and GC-boxes are contained within 500-bp upstream of the TSS of the human *SIRT1* gene [60]. It is suggested that human *SIRT1* gene expression is regulated by PPARβ/γ through Sp1 binding elements [61]. SIRT1, which belongs to sirtuin protein family, is proposed to regulate aging and the healthspan of organisms [62]. The biologically important function of the SIRT1 is its NAD^+ dependent deacetylating activity targeting various proteins including histones, PGC-1α, FOXO1, p53 and HIF1α [62]. These findings imply that the signals provoked by CR or CR mimetic drugs might induce Sp1 or GC-box binding TFs, thus simultaneously up-regulating expression of *TERT*, *WRN*, *SIRT1*, and the shelterin-encoding genes. Given that the CR causes stress response for cells due to the lack of nutrients or energy to survive, cells need to stop growing but need to keep the integrity of chromosomes and telomeres without replication of their genome. Therefore, agents with ability to induce telomere maintenance factor encoding genes might be lead compounds to design anti-aging drugs.

5.2. Mechanisms that regulate aging or lifespan *via* mitochondria and metabolic stress

Genetic studies of *C. elegans* implied that the insulin/IGF-1 signaling pathway regulates the lifespan of animals [63]. Insulin/IGF-1 signaling and glucose metabolism are thought to be associated with several diabetes/obesity controlling factors, including AKT, FOXO, mTOR and AMPK [64]. The mTOR is a component of mTORC1 and mTORC2 that play key roles in signal transduction in response to changes in energy balance [64]. Recently, it was reported that mTORC1 in the Paneth cell niche plays a role in calorie intake by modulating cADPR release from cells [65]. AMPK is known to be a sensor for energy stress and DNA damage, which acts by phosphorylating various TFs, such as FOXO, PGC-1α, CREB and HDAC5 [64,66]. Moreover, AMPK regulates SIRT1 activity by modulating NAD^+ metabolism [66].

It has been shown that mitochondrial functions can control lifespan [67]. Furthermore, it was suggested that a cross talk system between telomeres and mitochondria functions in the regulation of aging [68]. This concept was implied from a *Tert* knock down experiment that indicate telomere dysfunction causes suppression of PGC-1α in a p53-mediated manner [6]. The tumor suppressor p53 has been suggested to affect aging of organisms as a pro-aging factor [69]. Moreover, it is noteworthy that p53 regulates mitochondrial functions including respiration and glycolysis [70,71]. Taken together, these lines of evidences strongly suggest that p53-mediated signaling is transferred to telomeres and mitochondria in order to affect cellular senescence. Although canonical GC-box motif is not found near the TSS, duplicated GGAA-motifs are located in the human *TP53* promoter (Table 1). Therefore, transcription of genes that need to respond to the energy stress might be classified into two types, namely duplicated GGAA-motif- and GC-box-controlled system, which activates p53/DNA repair/mitochondria and telomere maintenance, respectively.

http://dx.doi.org/10.5772/53905

6. Conclusions

Here we discussed the TF-binding elements in the 5′-upstream regions of DNA-repair factor- and telomere maintenance factor-encoding genes, and proposed that duplicated GGAA in conjugation with the GC-box/Sp1-regulatory motifs are common sequences required for their gene regulation (Table 1). Moreover, duplicated GGAA-motifs are frequently found in the bidirectional promoter regions of head-dead oriented DNA-repair genes (Table 2). GGAA containing sequences are known as a target for ETS family proteins, and the GC-box can be recognized by multiple proteins, including Sp1 family. Therefore, multiple TFs may access and bind to the duplicated GGAA or GC-box when cells were exposed to DNA damage or energy stress (Fig. 1). Therefore, we hypothesize that these genes are required to respond promptly and accurately when cells encounter stress signals, such as DNA damage or lack of energy source. This might in part explain why they have common *cis*-elements in the gene regulatory regions. However, detailed molecular mechanism(s) how expression of these DNA-repair genes and telomere maintenance genes is regulated are yet to be elucidated. Thus, revealing the regulatory mechanisms behind expression of these genes should contribute to the development of novel drugs for cancer, obesity, diabetes and an anti-aging treatment in the future.

Acknowledgements

The authors are grateful to Takahiro Oyama and Midori Konno for discussion and outstanding technical assistance. This work was supported in part by a Research Fellowship from the Research Center for RNA Science, RIST, Tokyo University of Science.

Author details

Fumiaki Uchiumi[1,2], Steven Larsen[2] and Sei-ichi Tanuma[2,3,4]

1 Department of Gene Regulation, Faculty of Pharmaceutical Sciences, Tokyo University of Science, Yamazaki, Noda, Chiba, Japan

2 Research Center for RNA Science, RIST, Tokyo University of Science, Yamazaki, Noda, Chiba, Japan

3 Department of Biochemistry, Faculty of Pharmaceutical Sciences, Tokyo University of Science, Yamazaki, Noda, Chiba, Japan

4 Genome and Drug Research Center, Tokyo University of Science, Yamazaki, Noda, Chiba, Japan

References

[1] Yang, C., Bolotin, E., Jiang, T., Sladek, F.M. & Martinez, E. (2007). Prevalence of the initiator over the TATA box in human and yeast genes and identification of DNA motifs enriched in human TATA-less core promoters, *Gene* 389. (1): 52-65.

[2] Uchiumi, F., Watanabe, T. & Tanuma, S. (2010). Characterization of various promoter regions of the human DNA helicase-encoding genes and identification of duplicated *ets* (GGAA) motifs as an essential transcription regulatory element, *Exp. Cell Res.* 316. (9): 1523-1534.

[3] Uchiumi, F., Oyama, T., Ozaki, K. & Tanuma, S. (2011). Chapter 29, Characterization of 5′-flanking regions of various human telomere maintenance factor-encoding genes, in Kruman, I. (ed.), *DNA repair*, InTech, Rijeka, Croatia, pp. 585-596.

[4] Stefani, M., Markus, M.A., Lin, R.C., Pinese, M., Dawes, I.W. & Morris, B.J. (2007). The effect of resveratrol on a cell model of human aging. *Ann. NY Acad. Sci.* 1114. (10): 407-418.

[5] Park, S.J., Ahmad, F., Philp, A., Baar, K., Williams, T., Luo, H., Ke, H., Rehmann, H., Taussig, R., Brown, A.L., Kim, M.K., Beaven, M.A., Burgin, A.B., Manganiello, V. & Chung, J.H. (2012). Resveratrol ameliorates aging-related metabolic phenotypes by inhibiting cAMP phosphodiesterases, *Cell* 148. (3): 421-433.

[6] Sahin, E., Colla, S., Liesa, M., Moslehi, J., Müller, F.L., Guo, M., Cooper, M., Kotton, D., Fabian, A.J., Walkey, C., Maser, R.S., Tonon, G., Foerster, F., Xiong, R., Wang, Y.A., Shukla, S.A., Jaskelioff, M., Martin, E.S., Heffernan, T.P., Protopopov, A., Ivanova, E., Mahoney, J.E., Kost-Alimova, M., Perry, S.R., Bronson, R., Liao, R., Mulligan, R., Shirihai, O.S., Chin, L. & DePinho, R.A. (2011). Telomere dysfunction induces metabolic and mitochondrial compromise, *Nature* 470. (7334): 359–365.

[7] Zhou, B., Ikejima, T., Watanabe, T., Iwakoshi, K., Idei, Y., Tanuma, S. & Uchiumi, F. (2009). The effect of 2-deoxy-D-glucose on Werner syndrome RecQ helicase gene, *FEBS Lett.* 583. (8): 1331-1336.

[8] Uchiumi, F., Watanabe, T., Hasegawa, S., Hoshi, T., Higami, Y. & Tanuma, S. (2011). The effect of resveratrol on the werner syndrome RecQ helicase gene and telomerase activity, *Curr. Aging Sci.* 4. (1): 1–7.

[9] Lin, H.Y., Tang, H.Y., Davis, F.B. & Davis, P.J., Resveratrol and apoptosis, *Ann. NY Acad. Sci.* 1215. (1): 79-88.

[10] Turner, B.M. (2001). Transcription in eukaryotes: The problems of complexity. In *Chromatin and Gene Regulation: Mechanisms in Epigenetics*. Blackwell Science Ltd. pp. 25-43.

[11] Carey, M.F., Peterson, C.L. & Smale, S.T. (2009). Chapter 1, A primer on transcriptional regulation in mammalian cells. In *Transcriptional Regulation in Eukaryotes*. 2nd ed. Cold Spring Harbor Laboratory Press, New York, pp. 1-45.

[12] Albright S.R. & Tjian, R. (2000). TAFs revisited: More data reveal new twists and confirm old ideas, *Gene* 242. (1-2): 1-13.

[13] Rhee, H.S. & Pugh, B.F. (2012). Genome-wide structure and organization of eukaryotic pre-initiation complexes, *Nature* 483. (7389): 295-301.

[14] FitzGerald, P.C., Shlyakhtenko, A., Mir, A.A. & Vinson, C. (2004). Clustering of DNA sequences in human promoters, *Genome Res.* 14. (8): 1562-1574.

[15] Xie, X., Lu, J., Kulbokas, E.J., Golub, T.R., Mootha, V., Lindblad-Toh, K., Lander, E.S. & Kellis, M. (2005). Systematic discovery of regulatory motifs in human promoters and 3′ UTRs by comparison of several mammals, *Nature* 434. (7031): 338-345.

[16] Merika, M. & Thanos, D. (2001). Enhanceosomes. *Curr. Opin. Genet. Dev.* 11. (2): 205-208.

[17] Uchiumi, F., Sakakibara, G., Sato, J. & Tanuma, S. (2008). Characterization of the promoter region of the human *PARG* gene and its response to PU.1 during differentiation of HL-60 cells, *Genes to Cells* 13. (12): 1229-1248.

[18] Gibson, B.A. & Kraus, W.L. (2012). New insights into the molecular and cellular functions of poly(ADP-ribose) and PARPs, *Nat. Rev. Mol. Cell Biol.* 13. (7):411-424.

[19] Soldatenkov, V.A., Albor, A., Patel, B.K., Dreszer, R., Dritschilo, A. & Notario, V. (1999). Regulation of the human poly(ADP-ribose) polymerase promoter by the ETS transcription factor, *Oncogene* 18. (27): 3954-3962.

[20] Zheng, X., Ravatn, R., Lin, Y., Shih, W.C., Rabson, A., Strair, R., Huberman, E., Conney, A. & Chin, K.V. (2002). Gene expression of TPA induced differentiation in HL-60 cells by DNA microarray analysis, *Nucleic Acids Res.* 30. (20): 4489-4499.

[21] Goodrich, D.W. (2006). The retinoblastoma tumor-suppressor gene, the exception that proves the rule. *Oncogene* 25. (38): 5233-5243.

[22] Curtin, N.J., Mukhopadhyay, A., Drew, Y., Plummer, R. (2012). Chapter 4, The role of PARP in DNA repair and its therapeutic exploitation. In Kelley, M.R. (ed.) *DNA Repair in Cancer Therapy*, Academic Press, London, UK, pp. 55-73.

[23] Malanga, M., Pleschke, J.M., Kleczkowska, H.E. & Althouse F.R. (1998). Poly(ADP-ribose) binds to specific domains of p53 and alters its DNA binding functions, *J. Biol. Chem.* 273. (19): 11839-11843.

[24] Wieler, S., Gagné, J.P., Vaziri, H., Poirier, G.G. & Benchimol, S. (2003). Poly(ADP-ribose) polymerase-1 is a positive regulator of the p53-mediated G_1 arrest response following ionizing radiation, *J. Biol. Chem.* 278. (21): 18914-18921.

[25] Masson, M., Niedergang, C., Schreiber, V., Muller, S., Mennissier-de Murcia, J. & de Murcia, G. (1998). XRCC1 specifically associated with poly(ADP-ribose) polymerase and negatively regulates its activity following DNA damage, *Mol. Cell Biol.* 18. (6): 3563-3571.

[26] Morrison, C., Smith, G.C., Stingl, L., Jackson, S.P., Wagner, E.F. & Wang, Z.Q. (1997). Genetic interaction between PARP and DNA-PK in V(D)J recombination and tumorigenesis, *Nat. Genet.* 17. (4): 479-482.

[27] Niere, M., Mashimo, M., Agledal L, Dölle, C., Kasamatsu, A., Kato, J., Moss, J. & Ziegler, M. (2012). ADP-ribosylhydrolase 3 (ARH3), not poly(ADP-ribose) glycohydrolase (PARG) isoforms, is responsible for degradation of mitochondrial matrix-associated poly(ADP-ribose), *J. Biol. Chem.* 287. (20): 16088-16102.

[28] Zhang, Y & Chen. D. (2011). Chapter 8, The involvement of E2F1 in the regulation of XRCC1-dependent base excision DNA repair, in Kruman, I. (ed.), *DNA repair*, InTech, Rijeka, Croatia, pp. 125-142.

[29] Willers, H., Pfäffle, H.N. & Zou, L. (2012). Chapter 7, Targeting homologous recombination repair in cancer. In Kelley, M.R. (ed.) *DNA Repair in Cancer Therapy*, Academic Press, London, UK, pp. 119-160.

[30] Meyer, R.G., Meyer-Ficca, M.L., Jacobson, E.L. & Jacobson, M.K. (2003). Human poly(ADP-ribose) glycohydrolase (PARG) gene and the common promoter sequence it shares with inner mitochondrial membrane translocase 23 (TIM23), *Gene* 314. : 181-190.

[31] Uchiumi, F., Enokida, K., Shiraishi, T., Masumi, A. & Tanuma, S. (2010). Characterization of the promoter region of the human *IGHMBP2* (*Sμbp-2*) gene and its response to TPA in HL-60 cells, *Gene* 463. (1-2): 8-17.

[32] Yang, M.Q., Koehly, L.M. & Elinitski, L.L. (2007). Comprehensive annotation of bidirectional promoters identifies co-regulation among breast and ovarian cancer genes, *PLoS Computat. Biol.* 3. (4): e72.

[33] Uchiumi, F., Miyazaki, S. & Tanuma, S. (2011). The possible functions of duplicated ets (GGAA) motifs located near transcription start sites of various genes, *Cell. Mol. Life Sci.* 68. : 2039-2051.

[34] Welch, L.R., Koehly, L.M. & Elnitski L. (2011). Chapter 5, Shared regulatory motifs in promoters of human DNA repair genes, in Kruman, I. (ed.), *DNA repair*, InTech, Rijeka, Croatia, pp. 67-84.

[35] Blackburn, E.H. (2000). The end of the (DNA) line, *Nat. Struct. Biol.* 7. (10): 847-850.

[36] Warburton, P.E. (2001). Epigenetic analysis of kinetochore assembly on variant human centromeres, *Trends Genet.* 17. (5): 243-247.

[37] Sugimoto, K., Shibata, A. & Himeno, M. (1998). Nucleotide specificity at the boundary and size requirement of the target sites recognized by human centromere protein (CENP-B) *in vitro*, *Chromosome Res.* 6. (2): 133-140.

[38] Ohzeki, J., Nakano, M., Okada, T. & Masumoto, H. (2002). CENP-B box is required for de novo centromere chromatin assembly on human alphoid DNA, *J. Cell Biol.* 159. (5): 765-775.

[39] Delattre, O., Zucman, J., Plougastel, B., Desmaze, C., Melot, T., Peter, M., Kovar, H., Joubert, I., de Jong, P., Rouleau, G., Aurias, A. & Thomas, G. (1992). Gene function with an ETS DNA-binding domain caused by chromosome translocation in human tumors, *Nature* 359. (6391): 162-165.

[40] Gangwal, K., Sankar, S., Hollenhorst, P.C., Kinsey, M., Haroldsen, S.C., Shah, A.A., Boucher, K.M., Watkins, W.S., Jorde, L.B., Graves, B.J. & Lessnick, L. (2008). Microsatellites as EWS/FLI response elements in Ewing's sarcoma, *Proc. Natl. Acad. Sci. USA* 105. (29): 10149-10154.

[41] Guillon, N., Tirode, F., Boeva, V., Zynovyev, A., Barillot, E. & Delattre, O. (2009). The oncogenic EWS-FLI1 protein binds *in vivo* GGAA microsatellite sequences with potential transcriptional activation function, *PLoS One* 4. (3): e4932.

[42] Luo, W., Gangwal, K., Sankar, S., Boucher, K.M., Thomas, D. & Lessnick, S.L. (2009). *GSTM4* is a microsatellite-containing EWS/FLI target involved in Ewing's sarcoma oncogenesis and therapeutic resistance, *Oncogene* 28. (46): 4126-4132.

[43] Garcia-Aragoncillo, E., Carrillo, J., Lalli, E., Agra, N., Gomez-Lopez, G., Pestana, A. & Alonso, J. (2008). DAX1, a direct target of EWS/FLI1 oncoprotein, is a principal regulator of cell-cycle progression in Ewing's tumor cells, *Oncogene* 27. (46): 6034-6043.

[44] Gangwal, K., Close, D., Enriquez, C.A., Hill, C.P. & Lessnick, S.L. (2010). Emergent properties of EWS/FLI regulation via GGAA microsatellites in Ewing's sarcoma, *Genes Cancer* 1. (2): 177-187.

[45] Evans, M.D. & Cooke, M.S. (2004). Factors contributing to the outcome of oxidative damage to nucleic acids, *BioEssays* 26. (5): 533-542.

[46] Rhodes, D. (2006). Chapter 11, The structural biology of telomeres, in de Lange, T., Lundblad, V. & Blackburn, E. (ed.), *Telomeres (second ed.)*, Cold Spring Harbor Laboratory Press, New York, pp. 317-343.

[47] de Lange, T. (2006). Mammalian telomeres, in de Lange, T., Lundblad, V. & Blackburn, E. (ed.), *Telomeres (second ed.)*, Cold Spring Harbor Laboratory Press, New York, pp. 387-431.

[48] Griffith, J.D., Comeau, L., Rosenfield, S., Stansel, R.M., Bianchi, A., Moss, H. & de Lange, T. (1999). Mammalian telomeres end in a large duplex loop, *Cell* 97. (4): 503-514.

[49] Gilson, E. & Geli, V. (2007). How telomeres are replicated, *Nat. Rev. Mol. Cell. Biol.* 8. (10): 825-838.

[50] O'Sullivan, R.J. & Karlseder, J. (2010). Telomeres: protecting chromosomes against genome instability, *Nat. Rev. Mol. Cell. Biol.* 11. (3): 171-181.

[51] Sfeir, A. & de Lange, T. (2012). Removal of shelterin reveals the telomere end-protection problem, *Science* 336. (6081): 593-597.

[52] Ding, H., Schertzer, M., Wu, X., Gertsenstein, M., Selig, S., Kammori, M., Pourvali, R., Poon, S., Vulto, I., Chavez, E., Tam, P.P.L., Nagy, A. & Lansdorp, P.M. (2004). Regulation of murine telomere length by *Rtel*: an essential gene encoding a helicase-like protein, *Cell* 117. (7): 873-886.

[53] Vannier, J.B., Pavicic-Kaltenbrunner, V., Petalcorin, M.I.R., Ding, H. & Boulton, S.J. (2012). RTEL1 dismantles t loops and counteracts telomeric G4-DNA to maintain telomere integrity, *Cell* 149. (4): 795-806.

[54] Yu, C., Oshima, J., Fu, Y.H., Wijsman, E.M., Hisama, F., Alisch, R., Matthews, S., Nakura, J., Miki, T., Ouais, S., Martin, G.M., Mulligan, J. & Schellenberg, G.D. (1996). Positional cloning of the Werner's syndrome gene, *Science* 272. (5259): 258–262.

[55] Crabbe, L., Verdun, R.E., Haggblom, C.I. & Karlseder, J. (2004). Defective telomere lagging strand synthesis in cells lacking WRN helicase activity, *Science* 306. (5703): 1951-1953.

[56] Roth, G.S., Ingram, D.K. & Lane, M.A. (2001). Caloric restriction in primates and relevance to humans, *Ann. NY Acad. Sci.* 928. (4): 305-315.

[57] Dwyer, J., Li, H., Xu, D. & Liu, J.P. (2007). Transcriptional regulation of telomerase activity, *Ann. NY Acad. Sci.* 1114. (10): 36-47.

[58] Nicholls, C., Li, H., Wang, J.Q. & Liu, J.P. (2011). Molecular regulation of telomerase activity in aging, *Protein Cell* 2. (9): 726-738.

[59] Uchiumi, F., Higami, Y. & Tanuma, S. (2010). Regulations of telomerase activity and *WRN* gene expression, *in* Gagnon, A.N. (ed.), *Telomerase: Composition, Functions and Clinical Implications*, Nova Science Publishers, Inc., Hauppauge, NY, pp. 95–103.

[60] Uchiumi, F., Tachibana, H., Larsen, S. & Tanuma, S. (2012). Effect of lignin glycosides extracted from pine cones on the human *SIRT1* promoter, *Pharm. Anal. Acta.* S8. : 001.

[61] Okazaki, M., Iwasaki, Y., Nishiyama, M., Taguchi, T., Tsugita, M., Nakayama, S., Kambayashi, M., Hashimoto, K. & Terada, Y. (2010). PPARβ/γ regulates the human SIRT1 gene transcription via Sp1, *Endoc. J.* 57. (5): 403-413.

[62] Houtkooper, R.H., Pirinen, E & Auwerx, J. (2012). Sirtuins as regulators of metabolism and healthspan, *Nat. Rev. Mol. Cell Biol.* 13. (4): 225-238.

[63] Kenyon CJ. (2010). The genetics of aging, *Nature* 464. (7288): 504–512.

[64] Zoncu, R., Efeyan, A., & Sabatini, D.M. (2011). mTOR: from growth signal integration to cancer, diabetes and aging, *Nat. Rev. Mol. Cell Biol.* 12. (1): 21–35.

[65] Yilmaz, Ö.H., Katajisto, P., Lamming, D.W., Gültekin, Y., Bauer-Rowe, K.E., Sengupta, S., Birsoy, K., Dursun, A., Yilmaz, V.O., Selig, M., Nielsen, G.P., Mino-Kenudson, M., Zukerberg, L.R., Bhan, AK., Deshpande, V. & Sabatini, D.M. mTORC1 in the Paneth cell niche couples intestinal stem-cell function to calorie intake, *Nature* 486. (7404): 490-495.

[66] Cantó, C., Auwerx, J. (2010). AMP-activated protein kinase and its downstream transcriptional pathways, *Cell. Mol. Life Sci.* 67. (20): 3407–3423.

[67] Robb, E.L., Page, M.M. & Stuart, J.A. (2009). Mitochondria, cellular stress resistance, somatic cell depletion and lifespan, *Curr. Aging Sci.* 2. (1): 12-27.

[68] Sahin, E. & DePinho, R.A. (2012). Axis of aging: telomerase, p53 and mitochondria, *Nat. Rev. Mol. Cell. Biol.* 13. (6): 397-404.

[69] Vijg, J. (2007). Genome instability and accelerated aging, *in* Vijg, J. (ed.), *Aging of the Genome*, Oxford University Press, Oxford, pp. 151–180.

[70] Bensaad, K., Tsuruta, A., Selak, M.A., Vidal, M.N.C., Nakano, K., Bartrons, R., Gottlieb, E. & Vousden, K.H. (2006). TIGAR, a p53-inducible regulator of glycolysis and apoptosis, *Cell* 126. (1): 107-120.

[71] Matoba, S., Kang, J.G., Patino, W.D., Wragg, A., Boehm, M., Gavrilova, O., Hurley, P.J., Bunz, F. & Hwang, P.M. (2006). p53 regulates mitochondrial respiration, *Science* 312. (5780): 1650-1653.

Chapter 13

The Endothelin Axis in DNA Damage and Repair: The Cancer Paradigm

Panagiotis J. Vlachostergios and
Christos N. Papandreou

Additional information is available at the end of the chapter

http://dx.doi.org/10.5772/53977

1. Introduction

Maintenance of genomic stability is central to cellular homeostasis and self defense from environmental or intracellular inducers of DNA damage. Depending on the type of DNA lesion, several DNA repair mechanisms exist. Each major DNA repair process involves the detection of DNA damage, the accumulation of DNA repair factors at the site of damage and finally the physical repair of the lesion [1, 2].

The simplest, single enzyme DNA repair pathway is direct reversal or repair (DR) which is effected by O6-methylguanine-methyltransferase (MGMT), which is an enzyme that directly reverses DNA alkylation damage at the O6 position of guanine residues [2].

The mismatch repair (MMR) pathway is responsible for repair of 'insertion and deletion' loops that form during DNA replication [3]. These errors cause base 'mismatches' in the DNA sequence that distort the helical structure of DNA. Key MMR proteins MSH2 and MLH1 are involved in detection of this distortion and excision of the mismatch site which is then followed by new DNA synthesis.

DR is closely associated with MMR as a reduction in MGMT expression resulting from gene promoter methylation in some tumors, such as gliomas, results in recognition of resultant DNA mismatches by MMR and ultimate stimulation of pro-apoptotic signals after treatment with the alkylating agent temozolomide [4].

Repair of DNA alkylation products, oxidative lesions and single strand breaks (SSBs) is orchestrated by the base excision repair (BER) pathway. BER comprises a first step of removal of the damaged base from the double DNA helix which is followed by excision of the "damaged" area and replacement with newly synthesized DNA [5]. The enzymes poly (ADP-ribose) polymerase 1 and 2 (PARP1 and PARP2) play a key role in this process, acting as sensors of DNA damage and signal transducers for subsequent repair. Bulky SSBs, including those caused by ultraviolet radiation are repaired by the nucleotide excision repair (NER) pathway [6]. NER is divided into two sub-pathways, transcription-coupled repair (TCR) and global-genome repair (GGR). TCR is involved in repair of lesions that block the elongating RNA polymerase during transcription, whereas GGR repairs lesions that disrupt base pairing and distort the DNA helix. The actual mechanism through which NER is effected involves surrounding of the lesion, excision by the protein Excision repair cross-complementing protein 1 (ERCC1) and replacement with the use of the normal DNA replication machinery [6].

As opposed to SSBs, repair of double strand breaks (DSBs) depends on homologous recombination (HR) and non-homologous end joining (NHEJ) repair pathways. Homologous recombination involves the resection of DNA sequence around the lesion using the homologous sister chromatid as a template for new DNA synthesis. Most important HR repair factors include BRCA1, BRCA2, RAD51 and PALB2 [7]. With regard to NHEJ, DNA repair involves direct ligation of the ends between DSBs in an error-prone manner. As such, deletion or mutation of DNA sequences at or around the DSB site may occur [8].

Translesion synthesis and template switching are another two DNA repair pathways which allow DNA to continue to replicate in the presence of DNA lesions that would otherwise halt the process. In translesion synthesis, low-fidelity 'translesion' DNA polymerases are recruited to the DNA damage site in order to enable DNA synthesis during DNA replication. When the replication fork passes the DNA damage site, the low-fidelity DNA polymerases are replaced with the usual high-fidelity enzyme to allow normal DNA synthesis. Template switching involves bypass of the DNA damage at the replication fork by leaving a gap in DNA synthesis opposite the lesion. When the replication fork passes the DNA damage site, the single-strand gap is repaired using template DNA on a sister chromatid, as in HR repair [2].

The concept of targeting DNA repair pathways is supported by an increasing amount of evidence as a potent contributor to the effectiveness of conventional chemotherapy or radiotherapy and even as a promising monotherapy in tumors with known DNA repair deficiencies. Thus, sensitization of cancer cells to DNA damaging agents with DNA repair inhibitors is an evolving field of cancer research [9]. Further to clinical development of newly synthesized agents, the exploitation of already existing targeted agents inhibiting growth signaling pathways would seem a reasonable strategy, given that in most cases of genotoxic stress, anti-apoptotic and prosurvival signals are activated, rendering the DNA repair machinery a vital cellular tool for survival and proliferation.

The endothelin (ET) axis is such a drugable target and comprises three 21-amino acid peptides, endothelin-1 (ET-1), ET-2 and ET-3, two G-protein coupled receptor (GPCR) subtypes, endothelin A (ETRA) and endothelin B (ETRB) and the endothelin-converting enzyme (ECE), which catalyzes the generation of active ET [10]. The ET axis has been previously implicated in the response of endothelial cells to ionizing radiation and it could be used as a biomarker for irradiation of endothelial tissues, based on evidence of transient increase of ET-1 mRNA accumulation in human vein endothelial cells (HUVECs), followed by a net increase of ET-1 and big ET-1 peptides in the cytoplasm after irradiation [11]. In addition, ETRA downregulation was recently identified as part of the transcriptional response of endothelial lymphatic cells exhibiting a chronic oxidative stress signature in radiation-induced post-radiotherapy breast angiosarcomas [12]. In general, the ET axis is a key regulator of oncogenic processes, as it was shown to be expressed and active in various cancer and stromal cells leading to autocrine and paracrine feedback signaling loops promoting tumor growth and cell proliferation, escape from apoptosis, angiogenesis, invasion and metastatic dissemination, aberrant osteogenesis and modification of nociceptive stimuli [13]. ET-1 is the most prevalent and well-studied ET family member. ET-1 downstream signaling is mediated by ETRA and ETRB whereas ET-1 clearance uses two pathways: a) ETB-mediated uptake and subsequent lysosomal degradation [14] b) ET-1 cleavage by the extracellular membrane enzyme neutral endopeptidase 24.11 (NEP, neprilysin, CD10) [15].

Aberration of the ET axis, particularly in terms of ET-1 overexpression or/and pertubation of ETRA to ETRB expression ratio have been consistently associated with malignant transformation and progression in colorectal and prostate tissues. ET-1 plasma levels were found to be increased in patients with colorectal cancer as well as in a rat model of colorectal cancer in which inhibition of ETAR with a selective antagonist (BQ123) significantly reduced tumour weight of metastatic lesions to the liver. Further, ETBR gene promoter hypermethylation is a frequent event leading to reduced or absent receptor expression [16-18]. Increased ETAR expression was observed with advancing tumour stage and grade in patients with local and metastatic prostate cancer [19]. In addition, reduced ET-1 clearance due to attenuated levels of ETBR and NEP expression further promote increased local ET-1 levels [19, 20]. ET-1 and ETRA are greatly involved in ovarian carcinogenesis and progression and were both found to be overexpressed in primary and metastatic ovarian tumours [21-23].

With regard to ET-2, emerging data have demonstrated an association between upregulation of ET-2 transcript levels in human breast cancer cell lines [24] as well as in basal cell carcinoma as a result of increased Hedgehog signaling [25]. Investigation of the role of ET-3 in cancer has recently revealed a significant reduction in both ET-3 transcript and protein levels in breast cancer tissues compared with normal tissue, due to hypermethylation of the ET-3 promoter and subsequent gene silencing [26]. Thus, ET-3 might be considered a signaling factor with tumor suppressor properties, as opposed to ET-1 and ET-2 [27].

2. DNA damage and the Endothelin Axis

The best example of the involvement of the ET axis in the cellular response after exposure to DNA damage is the tanning response. After UV irradiation of keratinocytes, upregulation of a plethora of growth and survival factors occurs, including ET-1, bFGF, NGF, MSH, ACTH, P-LPH and P-endorphin. The essential roles of the tanning response are prevention of further DNA damage or/and apoptosis of stressed cells and induction of melanogenesis [28-30]. A better understanding of the signaling events following UV-mediated stimulation of melanogenesis might enable selective manipulation of these signaling events with the aim of reducing or/and preventing the damaging effects of UV skin irradiation.

ET-1 has emerged as an excellent inducer of melanogenesis and melanocyte growth, promoting increased tyrosinase activity after binding to a high-affinity surface receptor [31]. ET-1 was also shown to enhance melanocyte dendricity and to act synergistically with other factors in UV-irradiated keratinocyte-conditioned medium, whereas this effect was abolished by addition of anti - ET-1 antibodies [30]. Thus, ET-1 is the major additional dendricity factor produced by UV- irradiated keratinocytes, although it is not a major factor in the absence of ultraviolet irradiation. Further, incubation of human melanocytes with the same medium resulted in substantial increase in melanin synthesis which was abrograted by anti - ET-1 antibodies [30]. Treatment of cultured melanocytes alone with ET-1 rapidly increased tyrosinase activity and melanogenesis and was responsible for transcriptional upregulation of tyrosinase and tyrosine-related protein -1 (TRP-1) [32]. Exposure of human epidermis to a moderate dose of UV radiation led to a significant upregulation of ET-1, interleukin (IL)-1 and tyrosinase gene transcripts. Given that UV irradiation induces IL-1 in keratinocytes, and IL-1 promotes ET-1 expression in an autocrine manner in the same cells, it is most likely that subsequent ET-1 release to neighboring melanocytes leads to increased tyrosinase mRNA, protein and activity, as well as to an increase in melanocyte population. This sequence of events, in which ET-1 seems to play a key role, has been suggested as a proposed model of the tanning response *in vivo* [32, 33].

A key transcriptional factor responsible for skin homeostasis after UV exposure is retinoid X receptor a (RXRa). Retinoids have been shown to regulate skin development, differentiation, and homeostasis, which are mediated by nuclear receptors such as retinoid acid receptors and retinoid X receptors (RXRs) [34, 35]. RXRa is the most abundant RXR isoform in skin and is implicated in the regulation of oxidative DNA damage and skin apoptosis and proliferation mechanisms of epidermal and dermal melanocytes following UV irradiation. This is mostly effected through regulation of secreted paracrine factors involved in the crosstalk between keratinocytes and melanocytes. Increased secretion of mitogenic paracrine factors, including ET-1, from mutated keratinocytes lacking RXR led to a significant increase in melanocytes after culture with conditioned keratinocyte medium following UV irradiation. Given that ET-1 was previously shown to regulate melanocyte proliferation and melanogenesis [36, 37] and that p53 upregulates ET-1 in UV irradiated keratinocytes [38, 39], it was suggested that p53 might be the link between RXRa and ET-1. However no recruitment of RXRa was found on the p53 promoter [40]. It is therefore possible that RXRa may directly or indirectly modulate expression of ET-1 and other paracrine survival factors to regulate melanocyte homeostasis [41].

ETRB was found to be expressed in human glioma cells [42, 43]. Based on this finding, treatment with ETRB inhibitors led to induction of cell cycle arrest and apoptosis. This was at least partially explained by DNA damage-mediated induction of genes encoding Growth Arrest and DNA Damage-inducible (GADD)153, GADD45A, GADD34, sestrin 2 and death receptor 5 (DR5). Up-regulation of the same genes was also observed in human melanoma

http://dx.doi.org/10.5772/53977

cell lines under the same conditions [44]. This evidence suggests that ETRB inhibition causes induction of DNA damage response mediators.

The central role of ET axis signaling in glioblastoma (GBM) was further evidenced by the emergence of ET-3 overexpression in GBM stem cells (GSC). Serum-induced proliferation and subsequent differentiation was associated with reduced ET-3 secretion and down-regulation of genes related with stemness, while upregulation of ET-1 and YKL-40 gene products. This was also evidenced in tissues from patients with GBM which were found to have low ET3 but high ET-1 and YKL-40 transcript levels. When the ET3/ETRB cascade was blocked either with the use of an ETRB antagonist or ET-3 RNA interference (siRNA), a plethora of genes were found to be downregulated, most of which were involved in cytoskeleton organization, pause of growth and differentiation, and DNA repair. With regard to the latter, most important DNA damage control and repair genes involved were found to be NIPBL (Nipped-B homolog), DHX9 [DEAH (Asp-Glu-Ala-His) box polypeptide 9], GTSE1 (G-2 and S-phase expressed 1), and RIF1 (RAP1 interacting factor homolog). These data support the existence of an intimate relation between ET-3/ETB signaling and maintenance of GSC phenotype in terms of migration, undifferentiation, and survival [45]. A simplified schema of the role of ET axis in DNA damage control and repair in GBM cells is depicted in Figure 1.

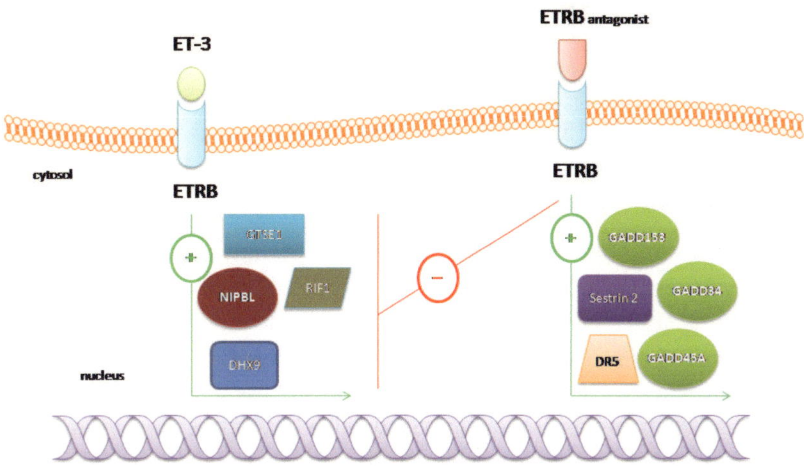

Figure 1. Simplified schema of the DNA damage control and repair transcriptional regulation by the ET axis in GBM cells.

An intriguing part of the association between ETRB and response to DNA damage in both glioma and melanoma cells is that cellular death was not found to be dependent on ETRB signaling. First, treatment with ETRB antagonists was able to reduce cell viability at higher doses compared to the ones required to inhibit the ET-1–ETRB ligation. Second, ETRB antagonism in glioma cells with undetectable ETRB was able to induce cell death. Third, experimental reduction of ETRB expression in other cell lines by >90% had no effect on cell viability of glioma or melanoma cells [44]. It might be hypothesized that melanoma and glioma cells follow a distinct pattern of response to treatment with ETRB antagonists that should be further elucidated.

3. DNA repair and the Endothelin axis

A significant amount of data supports a pro-survival effect of ET-1 after UV irradiation on human melanocytes. The anti-apoptotic role of ET-1 was shown to be a receptor-mediated effect, unrelated to ET-1-mediated mitogenic or melanogenic events, as it was replicated on melanocytes with no significant increase of cell proliferation as well as in melanocytes that lacked the ability to synthesize melanin. ET-1 treatment rescued melanocytes from UV-induced apoptosis as evidenced by reduced Annexin V staining and increased Bcl-2 levels. In addition, ET-1 promoted cell survival after UV irradiation through activation of the PI3K pathway. Inhibition of PI3K/Akt signaling attenuated the anti-apoptotic effect of ET-1 on irradiated melanocytes [46]. ET-1 was also demonstrated to be responsible for phosphorylation of Mitf, a helix-loop-helix transcription factor that is central to melanogenesis and survival of melanocytes [46]. Mitf phosphorylation is effected through ET-1-dependent activation of the mitogen-activated protein (MAP) kinases ERK1/2, which in turn phosphorylate the transcription factor CREB, upstream of Mitf [47, 48].

More importantly, when human epidermal keratinocytes were exposed to 6-hour UVB irradiation, a dual transcriptional response was observed involving upregulation of several apoptosis-related and DNA repair factors. TRAF-interacting protein (hTRIP), CD40 receptor- associated factor-1 (CRAF), cytotoxic ligand TRAIL receptor, death-associated protein kinase 1 (DAPK1) [49-51], but also ERCC1 (NER) and XRCC1 (BER) [52–54] were all found to be upregulated. These changes were in parallel with reduced expression of ET-2 at 6 h post-irradiation. Therefore, it might be that the final cellular fate after exposure to genotoxic stress by UV irradiation is determined by a balance between DNA repair and apoptotic processes, in both of which ET signaling seems to play a role [55].

Another important observation regarding the association between the ET axis and DNA repair is that ET-1 reduces UV-induced DNA photoproducts, thus implying an involvement of ET-1 in enhancement of NER. Therefore, ET-1 signaling not only exerts a proliferative and anti-apoptotic effect but also reduces accumulation of DNA damage, which is indispensable for maintenance of genomic health. The implication of pro-survival signals, other than the ET family, in DNA repair of keratinocytes has also been described for interleukin-12 (IL-12) and IGF-I which were both found to accelerate the removal of DNA photoproducts thus preventing UV-induced apoptosis in these cells [56, 57].

In addition to the direct DNA damaging effects of exposure to UV radiation, the latter is also a major source of reactive oxygen species (ROS) production that can secondarily cause oxidative DNA damage, as well as lipid peroxidation and protein damage [58]. Increased production of hydrogen peroxide, which is the main representative of ROS, following UV exposure was found to be reversed by ET-1 in human melanocytes. Thus, ET-1-mediated prevention of UV-induced oxidative stress indirectly contributes to prevention of oxidative DNA damage. Overall, activation of melanocortins and ET-1 signaling constitutes an indispensable cellular mechanism to overcome cancer-promoting effects of UV irradiation through reduced generation of hydrogen peroxide-mediated DNA damage and activation of DNA repair and melanogenesis pathways [46].

http://dx.doi.org/10.5772/53977

Accumulated evidence supports that melanoma patients have lower DNA repair capacity compared to the general population. Risk of melanoma was found to be increased by loss-of-function mutations in the melanocortin-1 receptor gene, indicating that inefficient or/and aberrant DNA repair is central to the development of melanoma. UV irradiation induces upregulation of various pro-survival signaling molecules including NGF, NT-3, MSH and ACTH, and ET-1. This upregulation seems to have a double effect on skin melanocytes. An early response involves inhibition of apoptotic signaling elicited by UV-induced DNA damage in melanocytes as well as enhancement of DNA photoproducts and oxidative stress metabolites, particularly hydrogen peroxide. According to the proposed model, exposure of the skin to UV radiation stimulates the activation of a MSH-, ACTH-, and ET-1-dependent paracrine network that promotes melanocyte survival, enhances the repair of cyclobutane pyrimidine dimmers (CPD) and reduces the release of hydrogen peroxide. Collectively, these effects represent the immediate response to UV irradiation, which is followed by a delayed response of increased melanogenesis to establish photoprotection. Thus, melanocortins and ET-1 operate to maintain genomic stability of melanocytes and prevent evolution of unrepaired DNA damage to skin carcinogenesis [59].

There appears to be a direct association between ETRB signaling and expression of the BER member protein PARP-3. PARP-3 is part of a family of DNA damage surveillance factors [60]. ETRB antagonism was found to induce down-regulation of PARP-3 transcription in melanoma cell lines derived from primary tumors and metastases (cutaneous, lymph node, visceral) with the most prominent effect observed on the lines that were more sensitive to ETRB inhibition. Further, the extent of PARP-3 downregulation correlated with the level of apoptosis evidenced by histone-associated DNA fragmentation. The strongest decrease in PARP-3 expression in response to ETRB antagonism occurred in distal metastasis-derived cells, with little or no changes observed in primary tumor-derived melanoma cells [61].

A simplified schema of the role of ET axis in DNA damage response and repair in melanoma cells is depicted in Figure 2.

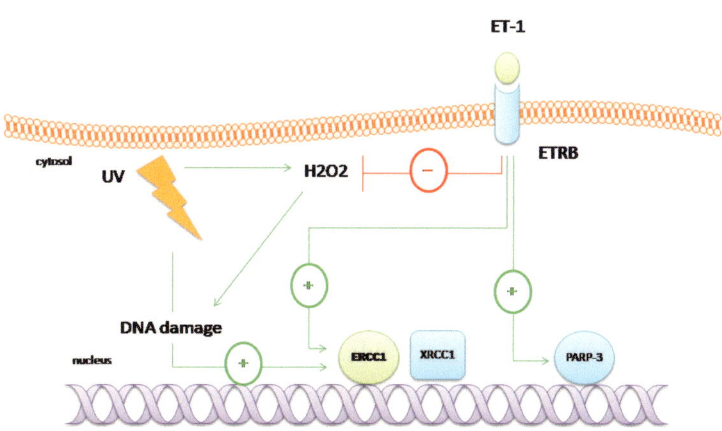

Figure 2. Simplified schema of the DNA damage control and repair transcriptional regulation by the ET axis in melanoma cells.

4. Conclusions

It is evident that the ET axis is greatly involved in the modulation of DNA repair processes. Elucidation of regulatory loops between ET family members and DNA repair factors at the transcriptional or/and post-translational level is a field of ongoing research. As expected, the use of existing or/and development of new targeted agents interfering with inhibition of ET signaling might be exploited either alone or in combination with chemotherapeutic drugs based on emerging mechanisms of action of the latter associated with DNA repair inhibition and sensitization of tumors to DNA damage.

Author details

Panagiotis J. Vlachostergios and Christos N. Papandreou

Department of Medical Oncology, University of Thessaly School of Medicine, Larissa, Greece

References

[1] Ciccia A, Elledge SJ. The DNA damage response: making it safe to play with knives. Mol. Cell 2010;40: 179–204.

[2] Lord CJ, Ashworth A. The DNA damage response and cancer therapy. Nature 2012;481(7381): 287-94.

[3] Jiricny J. The multifaceted mismatch-repair system. Nature Rev. Mol. Cell Biol 2006; 7: 335–46.

[4] Weller M, Stupp R, Reifenberger G, Brandes AA, van den Bent MJ, Wick W, Hegi ME. MGMT promoter methylation in malignant gliomas: ready for personalized medicine? Nature Rev. Neurol. 2010;6: 39–51.

[5] David SS, O'Shea VL, Kundu S. Base-excision repair of oxidative DNA damage. Nature 2007;447: 941–50.

[6] Cleaver JE, Lam ET, Revet I. Disorders of nucleotide excision repair: the genetic and molecular basis of heterogeneity. Nature Rev. Genet. 2009;10: 756–68.

[7] Moynahan ME, Jasin M. Mitotic homologous recombination maintains genomic stability and suppresses tumorigenesis. Nature Rev. Mol. Cell Biol. 2010;11: 196–207.

[8] Lieber MR. NHEJ and its backup pathways in chromosomal translocations. Nature Struct. Mol. Biol. 2010;17: 393–5.

[9] Basu B, Yap TA, Molife LR, de Bono JS. Targeting the DNA damage response in oncology: past, present and future perspectives. Curr Opin Oncol. 2012;24(3): 316-24.

[10] Rubanyi GM, Polokoff MA. Endothelins: molecular biology, biochemistry, pharmacology, physiology, and pathophysiology. Pharmacol Rev 1994;46: 325–415.

[11] Lanza V, Fadda P, Iannone C, Negri R. Low-dose ionizing radiation stimulates transcription and production of endothelin by human vein endothelial cells. Radiat Res 2007;168: 193-8.

[12] Hadj-Hamou NS, Laé M, Almeida A, de la Grange P, Kirova Y, Sastre-Garau X, Malfoy B. A transcriptome signature of endothelial lymphatic cells coexists with the chronic oxidative stress signature in radiation-induced post-radiotherapy breast angiosarcomas. Carcinogenesis 2012; 33: 1399-405.

[13] Nelson J, Bagnato A, Battistini B, Nisen P. The endothelin axis: emerging role in cancer. Nat Rev Cancer 2003;3: 110–6.

[14] Bremnes T, Paasche JD, Mehlum A, Sandberg C, Bremnes B, Attramadal H. Regulation and intracellular trafficking pathways of the endothelin receptors. J Biol Chem 2000;275: 17596–604.

[15] Abassi ZA, Tate JE, Golomb E, Keiser HR. Role of neutral endopeptidase in the metabolism of endothelin. Hypertension 1992;20: 89–95.

[16] Nelson JB, Lee W-H, Nguyen SH, Jarrard DF, Brooks JD, Magnuson SR, Opgenorth TJ, Nelson WG, Bova GS. Methylation of the 5′CpG island of the endothelin B receptor gene is common in human prostate cancer. Cancer Res 1997;57: 35–7.

[17] Pao MM, Tsutsumi M, Liang G, Uzvolgyi E, Gonzales FA, Jones PA. The endothelin receptor B (EDNRB) promoter displays heterogeneous, site specific methylation patterns in normal and tumor cells. Hum Mol Genet 2001;10: 903–10.

[18] Jerónimo C, Henrique R, Campos PF, Oliveira J, Caballero OL, Lopes C, Sidransky D. Endothelin B receptor gene hypermethylation in prostate adenocarcinoma. J Clin Pathol 2003;56: 52–5.

[19] Nelson JB. Endothelin inhibition: novel therapy for prostate cancer. J Urol 2003;170: S65–S68.

[20] Bagnato A, Rosanò L. The endothelin axis in cancer. Int J Biochem Cell Biol 2008;40: 1443–51.

[21] Bagnato A, Tecce R, Moretti C, Di Castro V, Spergel D, Catt KJ. Autocrine actions of endothelin-1 as a growth factor in human ovarian carcinoma cells. Clin Cancer Res 1995;1: 1059–66.

[22] Salani D, Di Castro V, Nicotra MR, Rosano L, Tecce R, Venuti A, Natali PG, Bagnato A. Role of endothelin-1 in neovascularization of ovarian carcinoma. Am J Pathol 2000;157: 1537–47.

[23] Bagnato A, Spinella F, Rosanò L. Emerging role of the endothelin axis in ovarian tumor progression. Endocr Relat Cancer 2005;12: 761–72.

[24] Grimshaw MJ, Hagemann T, Ayhan A, Gillett CE, Binder C, Balkwill FR. A role for endothelin-2 and its receptors in breast tumor cell invasion. Cancer Res 2004;64: 2461–8.

[25] Tanese K, Fukuma M, Ishiko A, Sakamoto M. Endothelin-2 is upregulated in basal cell carcinoma under control of Hedgehog signaling pathway. Biochem Biophys Res Commun 2010; 391: 486–91.

[26] Wiesmann F, Veeck J, Galm O, Hartmann A, Esteller M, Knuchel R, Dahl E. Frequent loss of endothelin-3 (EDN3) expression due to epigenetic inactivation in human breast cancer. Breast Cancer Res 2009;11: R34.

[27] Bagnato A, Loizidou M, Pflug BR, Curwen J, Growcott J. Role of the endothelin axis and its antagonists in the treatment of cancer. Br J Pharmacol. 2011;163(2):220-33.

[28] Imokawa G, Yada Y, Miyagishi M. Endothelins secreted from human keratinocytes are intrinsic mitogens for human melanocytes. J. Biol. Chem. 1992;267, 24675-80.

[29] Yohn JJ, Morelli JG, Walchak SJ, Rundell KB, Norris DA, Zamora MR. Cultured human keratinocytes synthesize and secrete endothelin-1. J. Invest. Dermatol. 1993;100: 23-6.

[30] Hara, M., M. Yaar and B. A. Gilchrest (1995) Endothelin-1 of keratinocyte origin is a mediator of melanocyte dendricity. J Invest Dermatol. 1995 Dec;105(6):744-8.

[31] Yada Y, Higuchi K, Imokawa G. Effects of endothelins on signal transduction and proliferation in human melanocytes. J. Biol. Chem. 1991;266: 18352-7.

[32] Imokawa G, Miyagishi M, Yada Y. Endothelin-1 as a new melanogen: coordinated expression of its gene and the tyrosinase gene in UVB-exposed human epidermis. J. Invest. Dermatol. 1996;105: 32-7.

[33] Gilchrest BA, Park HY, Eller MS, Yaar M. Mechanisms of ultraviolet light-induced pigmentation. Photochem Photobiol. 1996; 63(1): 1-10.

[34] Chambon P. The molecular and genetic dissection of the retinoid signalling pathway. Gene 1993;135: 223–8.

[35] Chambon P. A decade of molecular biology of retinoic acid receptors. FASEB J 1996; 10: 940–54.

[36] Slominski A, Paus R. Melanogenesis is coupled to murine anagen: toward new concepts for the role of melanocytes and the regulation of melanogenesis in hair growth. J Invest Dermatol 1993;101:90S–7S.

[37] Chakraborty AK, Funasaka Y, Slominski A, Ermak G, Hwang J, Pawelek JM, Ichihashi M. Production and release of proopiomelanocortin (POMC) derived peptides by

human melanocytes and keratinocytes in culture: regulation by ultraviolet B. Biochim Biophys Acta 1996;1313: 130–8.

[38] Cui R, Widlund HR, Feige E, Lin JY, Wilensky DL, Igras VE, D'Orazio J, Fung CY, Schanbacher CF, Granter SR, Fisher DE. Central role of p53 in the suntan response and pathologic hyperpigmentation. Cell 2007;128: 853–64.

[39] Murase D, Hachiya A, Amano Y, Ohuchi A, Kitahara T, Takema Y. The essential role of p53 in hyperpigmentation of the skin via regulation of paracrine melanogenic cytokine receptor signaling. J Biol Chem 2009;284: 4343–53.

[40] Hyter S, Bajaj G, Liang X Barbacid M, Ganguli-Indra G, Indra AK. Loss of nuclear receptor RXRalpha in epidermal keratinocytes promotes the formation of Cdk4-activated invasive melanomas. Pigment Cell Melanoma Res 2010;23: 635–48.

[41] Wang Z, Coleman DJ, Bajaj G, Liang X, Ganguli-Indra G, Indra AK. RXRα ablation in epidermal keratinocytes enhances UVR-induced DNA damage, apoptosis, and proliferation of keratinocytes and melanocytes. J Invest Dermatol. 2011;131(1): 177-87.

[42] Harland SP, Kuc RE, Pickard JD, Davenport AP. Expression of endothelin(A) receptors in human gliomas and meningiomas, with high affinity for the selective antagonist PD156707. Neurosurgery 1998;43(4): 890-8.

[43] Egidy G, Eberl LP, Valdenaire O, Irmler M, Majdi R, Diserens AC, Fontana A, Janzer RC, Pinet F, Juillerat-Jeanneret L. The endothelin system in human glioblastoma. Lab Invest 2000;80(11): 1681-9.

[44] Montgomery JP, Patterson PH. Endothelin receptor B antagonists decrease glioma cell viability independently of their cognate receptor. BMC Cancer 2008;8: 354.

[45] Liu Y, Ye F, Yamada K, Tso JL, Zhang Y, Nguyen DH, Dong Q, Soto H, Choe J, Dembo A, Wheeler H, Eskin A, Schmid I, Yong WH, Mischel PS, Cloughesy TF, Kornblum HI, Nelson SF, Liau LM, Tso CL. Autocrine endothelin-3/endothelin receptor B signaling maintains cellular and molecular properties of glioblastoma stem cells. Mol Cancer Res. 2011;9(12): 1668-85.

[46] Kadekaro AL, Kavanagh R, Kanto H, Terzieva S, Hauser J, Kobayashi N, Schwemberger S, Cornelius J, Babcock G, Shertzer HG, Scott G, Abdel-Malek ZA. alpha-Melanocortin and endothelin-1 activate antiapoptotic pathways and reduce DNA damage in human melanocytes. Cancer Res. 2005 May 15;65(10): 4292-9.

[47] Tada A, Pereira E, Beitner Johnson D, Kavanagh R, Abdel-Malek ZA. Mitogen and ultraviolet-B-induced signaling pathways in normal human melanocytes. J Invest Dermatol 2002;118: 316–22.

[48] Wu M, Hemesath T, Takemoto CM, Horstmann MA, Wells AG, Price ER, Fisher DZ, Fisher DE. c-Kit triggers dual phosphorylations, which couple activation and degradation of the essential melanocyte factor Mi. Genes Dev 2000; 14:301–12.

[49] Lee SY, Lee SY, Choi Y. TRAF-interacting protein (TRIP): a novel component of the tumor necrosis factor receptor (TNFR)- and CD30-TRAF signaling complexes that inhibits TRAF2-mediated NF-kappaB activation. J Exp Med 1997;185: 1275–85.

[50] Cheng G, Cleary AM, Ye ZS, Hong DI, Lederman S, Baltimore D. Involvement of CRAF1, a relative of TRAF, in CD40 signaling. Science 1995;267: 1494–8.

[51] Pan G, O'Rourke K, Chinnaiyan AM, Gentz R, Ebner R, Ni J, Dixit VM. The receptor for the cytotoxic ligand TRAIL. Science 1997;276: 111–3.

[52] Cohen O, Inbal B, Kissil JL, Raveh T, Berissi H, Spivak-Kroizaman T, Feinstein E, Kimchi A. DAP-kinase participates in TNF-alpha- and Fas-induced apoptosis and its function requires the death domain. J Cell Biol 1999;146: 141–8.

[53] Larminat F, Bohr VA. Role of the human ERCC-1 gene in gene-specific repair of cisplatin-induced DNA damage. Nucleic Acids Res 1994;22: 3005–10.

[54] Fenech M, Carr AM, Murray J, Watts FZ, Lehmann AR. Cloning and characterization of the rad4 gene of Schizosaccharomyces pombe; a gene showing short regions of sequence similarity to the human XRCC1 gene. Nucleic Acids Res 1991;19: 6737–41.

[55] Thompson LH, West MG. XRCC1 keeps DNA from getting stranded. Mutat Res 2000;459: 1–18.

[56] Decraene D, Agostinis P, Bouillon R, Degreef H, Garmyn M. Insulin-like growth factor-1-mediated AKT activation postpones the onset of ultraviolet B-induced apoptosis, providing more time for cyclobutane thymine dimer removal in primary human keratinocytes. J Biol Chem 2002;277: 32587–95.

[57] Schwarz A, Stander S, Berneburg M, Böhm M, Kulms D, van Steeg H, Grosse-Heitmeyer K, Krutmann J, Schwarz T. Interleukin-12 suppresses ultraviolet radiation-induced apoptosis by inducing DNA repair. Nat Cell Biol 2002;4: 26–31.

[58] Sander CS, Chang H, Hamm F, Elsner P, Thiele JJ. Role of oxidative stress and the antioxidant network in cutaneous carcinogenesis. Int J Dermatol 2004;43: 326–35.

[59] Kadekaro AL, Wakamatsu K, Ito S, Abdel-Malek ZA. Cutaneous photoprotection and melanoma susceptibility: reaching beyond melanin content to the frontiers of DNA repair. Front Biosci. 2006;11: 2157-73.

[60] Augustin A, Spenlehauer C, Dumond H, Ménissier-De Murcia J, Piel M, Schmit AC, Apiou F, Vonesch JL, Kock M, Bornens M, De Murcia G. PARP-3 localizes preferentially to the daughter centriole and interferes with the G1-S cell cycle progression. J Cell Sci 2003;116: 1551– 62.

[61] Lahav R, Suvà ML, Rimoldi D, Patterson PH, Stamenkovic I. Endothelin receptor B inhibition triggers apoptosis and enhances angiogenesis in melanomas. Cancer Res. 2004 Dec 15;64(24): 8945-53.

Chapter 14

DNA Repair and Telomeres — An Intriguing Relationship

Effrossyni Boutou, Dimitris Vlachodimitropoulos, Vassiliki Pappa, Horst-Werner Stürzbecher and Constantinos E. Vorgias

Additional information is available at the end of the chapter

http://dx.doi.org/10.5772/56115

1. Introduction

Recent advances in DNA repair and telomere biology further establish an intimate interrelationship between these cellular attributes, in the maintenance of genome stability under normal physiological conditions. Consequently, any pathological situation with defect in these signalling pathways may result in genome instability and related diseases. Preservation of genome integrity is depending on effective detection and repair of DNA lesions. Telomeres, the end of linear chromosomes, function to preserve chromosome integrity during each round of DNA replication, thus preventing chromosomal ends from being recognised as DNA damage and drive the cell to 'retire' when reaching specific limits. Therefore, functional telomeres are part of the genome stability maintenance machinery. Telomere dysfunction is directly related to rare diseases like pulmonary fibrosis and dyskeratosis congenita as well as to a growing list of aging related diseases and cancer. Since the pioneering work of Blackburn & Gall in 1978 [1], proving the concept of Muller (1938) that 'the terminal gene must have a special function, that of sealing the end of the chromosome' [2], numerous research publications shed light to aspects of telomere structure / function and its interrelation with DNA repair pathways and genomic stability. Moreover, many comprehensive reviews and book chapters during the recent years describe in details the wealth of information gathered [3-8]. This chapter focuses on the brief description of basics regarding telomere structure – function followed by discussion of selected recent advances, regarding telosome (functional telomere complex) interaction with DNA Damage Response (DDR) and Repair pathways, in order to restore genome information and prevent neoplastic transformation. Unsurprisingly, impairment of DNA repair – telomere function interplay is related to specific aggressive forms of cancer. Moreover, this review will hint at selected points regarding consequences of impairment of telomere integrity accompanied by cellular checkpoints abrogation. Quite interestingly, it seems that the pleiotropic effects governing a cell's decision to senesce vs. undergoing apoptosis when reaching the so-called Hayflick limit [9] (certain number of cell divisions), comprise a fertile environment for cancer formation. Cancer cells have developed numerous strategies towards bypassing these limits on the road to achieving eternal proliferation.

2. Genomic stability and telomeres

Genomic stability is the prerequisite of species survival as ensures that all required information will be passed on to the next generations. In contrast to single-cell – quickly dividing - species, higher order organisms, in order to preserve their genomic information, require more efficient DNA repair mechanisms due to later onset of reproduction. Therefore, a remarkable ability of cells to recognize and repair DNA damage and progress through the cell cycle, in a regulated and orderly manner, has been developed. A vulnerable portion of the genome, especially in eukaryotic organisms whose genome is organised in linear chromosomes, is their edges called telomeres (after the greek words '*τέλος*' (*télos*) and '*μέρος*' (*méros*) meaning 'the ending part'). Telomeres are nucleoprotein complexes that 'cap' the chromosomes' physical ends. In most eukaryotic organisms integral and stable telomeres guarantee the maintenance of genetic information and its accurate transfer to the next generation. In case telomeres are impaired, abnormal ends are recognised by the DNA damage detection machinery as double-strand DNA (dsDNA) breaks, the DDR is activated and the lesion is healed by Non-Homologous-End-Joining (NHEJ) repair activities. The result of this type of repair may be the fusion of chromosomes and the formation of dicentric /polycentric chromosomes leading in turn to further genomic instability. For this reason a number of telomere-binding protein complexes are associated with telomeres to ensure the formation of a proper secondary structure and a capping function. Intriguingly, a number of protein complexes implicated in DNA repair also contribute to telomere stability. The structure of telomeres is intrinsically dynamic, as chromosome ends should relax during genome replication and then re-establish their 'capped' state after replication. Consequently, telomeres may switch between closed (protected) and open (replication-competent) states during the cell cycle. Each state is governed by a number of interactions with specific factors and can lead the cell to either cell division or senescence / apoptosis under normal conditions, or to disorders / cancer in abnormal cases (processes still poorly understood in a large extent) [10-11]. Moreover, during development and in certain cell types in adults, telomere length should be preserved. Thus, multiple physiological processes guarantee functional and structural heterogeneity of telomeres concerning their length and nucleoprotein composition. A functional chromosome end structure is essential for genome stability, as it must prevent chromosome shortening and chromosome end fusion as well as degradation by the DNA repair machinery. Hence, structure and function of telomeres are highly conserved throughout evolution [12]. The cell's inability to properly maintain its telomeres can lead to diseases such as dyskeratosis congenita, pulmonary fibrosis, atheromatosis and cancer. On the other hand, telomere gradual shortening during the cell's life span functions among other things as a protective mechanism against cancer. These characteristics make telomeres an attractive target for specific anti-cancer therapies. Therefore, analysis of telomere structure-function biology is crucial in order to clarify how telomere length and structure are preserved, together with telomere – DNA repair intercommunication.

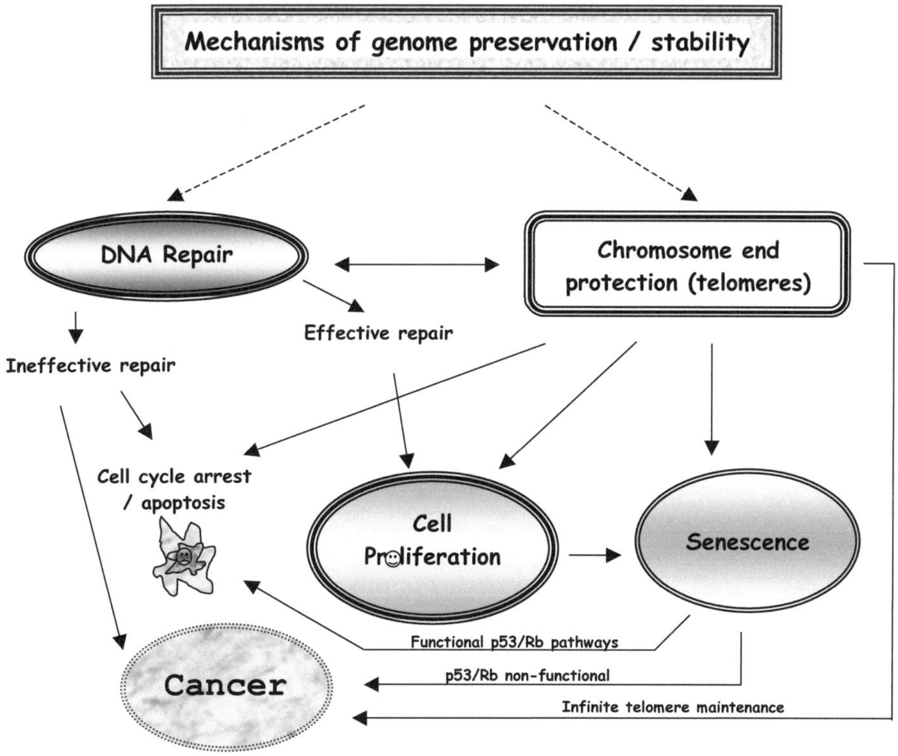

Figure 1. Scheme of Genome preservation mechanisms. Details in the text.

3. Telomere features and replication

Telomeres are long tracts of DNA at the linear chromosome's ends composed of tandem repeats of a Guanine rich sequence motif that vary in length from 2 to 20 kb, according to species. This motif is conserved in lower eukaryotes and in mammalian cells [13]. Exceptionally, the chromosome ends of a few insect species (Drosophila and some dipterans), instead of telomeric motifs, possess tandem arrays of retrotransposons [14]. Telomeric DNA is double stranded with a single – stranded terminus that is on average 130-210nt long in human cells [15]. Under normal conditions, in most somatic cells of an adult organism, telomeres shorten in each cell division (i.e. in humans by about 50–150 nucleotides (nt)). The basic telomere DNA repeat unit in vertebrates is the hexamer TTAGGG, in which the strand running 5′→ 3′ outwards the centromere is usually guanine-rich and referred to as G-tail. In order not to leave exposed a single stranded overhang this G-rich strand protrudes its complementary DNA-strand and by bending on itself it folds back to form a telomere DNA loop (t-loop), while the G-tail 3′end invades into the double strand forming a D-loop inside the t-loop (Figure3) [16]. As a result, the t-loop protects the G-tail from being recognized as a double-stranded break by sequestering the 3′-overhang into a higher order DNA structure. Inability of telomeres to form a t-loop, for example due to a very short length, results in DDR triggering and /or exonuclease degradation, chromosome fusion and further genomic instability. Despite t-loop, the G-tail is also able to form, at least *in vitro,* a secondary DNA structure of intra and intermolecular G-quadruplexes [17-18]. G-quadruplexes are piles of G-quartets, planar assemblies of four Hoogsteen-bonded guanines, with the guanines derived from one or more nucleic acid

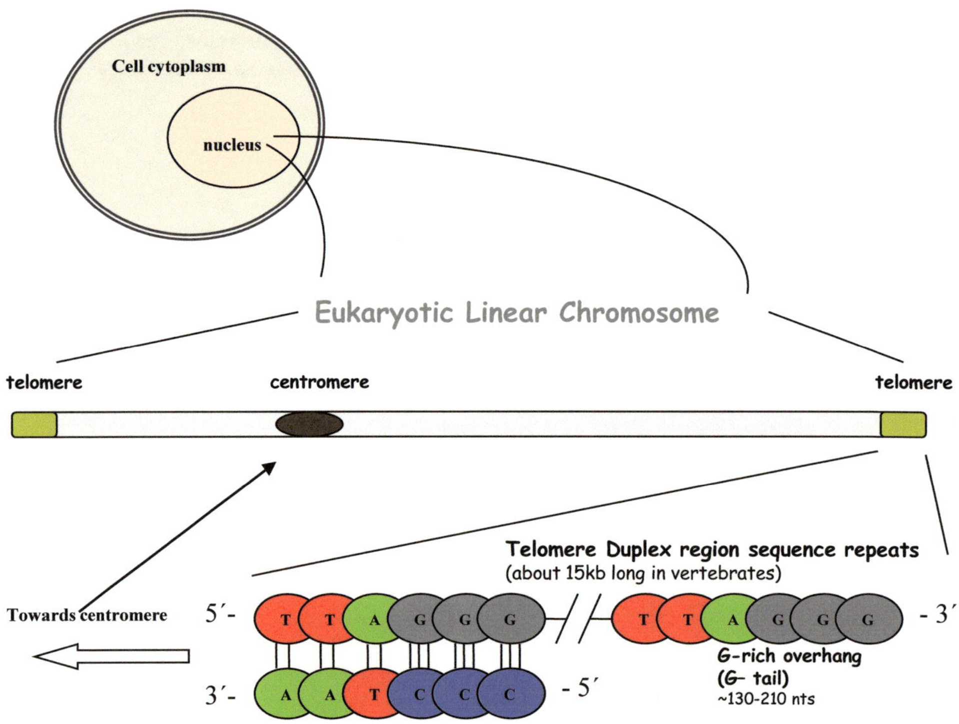

Figure 2. Telomere primary structure scheme. Details in the text.

Such secondary structures of the telomere G-tail, as the t-loop and the quadruplexes, may contribute to telomere stability and chromosome-end protection as they prohibit access of nucleases and DDR detection enzymes. On the other hand, these structures should relax to allow telomere replication. Telomeres, in the absence of any compensation mechanism, become shortened during every cell cycle due to incomplete replication of the lagging strand (referred to as the "end replication problem"), resulting in cumulative telomere attrition during aging. In addition, loss of telomere DNA also occurs due to post-replicative degradation of the 5′strand that generates long 3′G-rich overhangs [22].

Telomere replication is a multi-step process combining the classical semi-conservative and telomere-specific replication, which necessitates dynamic opening of the telomeric DNA. During genome duplication, replication of the telomere duplex occurs via the conventional replication machinery. As a next step, nucleases cleave the C-strand to generate a G-tail. G-tail then serves as an anchor for a telomere-specific reverse transcriptase (TERT), also termed as telomerase, a nucleoprotein enzyme responsible for telomere end replication. Telomerase function compensates for the inability of DNA polymerases to replicate the 5′ends of eukaryotic chromosomes [1, 23]). This remarkable and unique feature of telomerase is attributed to its specific RNA subunit termed TER. TER sequence is complementary to the G-tail DNA sequence, specifically recognises and binds to two sequential telomeric motifs, with the aid of telomerase and serves as a template [24]. Telomere G-overhang is then elongated by additions of sequence repeats by telomerase leading to the telomere loss counteraction [25, 26, 27]. The complementary C-rich strand is then synthesized by conventional RNA-primed DNA replication [28,29]. Following replication, the telomeres created by the synthesis of the leading strand are either blunt-ended or left carrying a small 50 nt overhang whereas those created by the lagging-strand synthesis have a 3′ overhang with a length determined by the position of the outermost RNA primer [30]. This fact underlines the importance of telomerase activity for genome integrity, especially during development and in certain adult cell types, where telomere shortening during each cell division should at least partially be restored. Many excellent recent reviews extensively cover telomerase structure-function in health and disease [31, 32].

Following telomere synthesis, the created G-tail reforms the t-loop structure and the telomeres are re-bound by shelterin, a specific multi-tasked protein complex (figure 3). Since the role of telomere protection is vital for cell viability, shelterin complex and interacting proteins have evolved to specifically interact with these chromosome end structures and survey proper telomere protection / preservation, depending on the cell's status [3]. The shelterin complex is formed by a core of six proteins including the Sab/Myb-type homeodomain TRF proteins in mammals which bind the duplex form of the telomere repeats, the OB-fold containing protein POT1 in mammals which binds the single-stranded telomere 3′overhang and by other proteins associated via protein–protein interactions with them [33]. The main roles of shelterins are to repress the DNA repair machinery at telomeres, and regulate telomere length [3, 35, 36] therefore they are evolutionary conserved to a great extent [4].

In addition, telomeres are also associated with a large number of non-telomere specific proteins mainly factors and enzymes involved in DNA double strand signalling and repair. Obviously, intact telomeres are essential for chromosome integrity [37-39]. Therefore, telomere associated proteins protect the ends of eukaryotic chromosomes from being recognized as double strand breaks, and avoid chromosome end degradation by nucleases and non-canonical chromosome-end fusions.

Another intrinsic feature of telomeres is their transcriptional activity, despite their heterochromatin-like structure, giving rise to a long non-coding G-rich RNA (lncRNA) termed TERRA (telomere repeat-containing RNA), which forms an integral component of telomere heterochromatin [4, 5, 40 - 44]. TERRA associates with telomeres and is suggested to be involved in telomere structure and the state of telomeric chromatin during development and differentiation [41, 45, 46]. TERRA transcription occurs at most or all chromosome ends and is regulated by RNA surveillance factors and in response to changes in telomere length. The accumulation of TERRA at telomeres may also interfere with telomere replication [40, 41, 43].

4. Telomere maintenance / impairment consequences

Telomeres are able to counterbalance incomplete replication of terminal DNA by conventional DNA polymerase and overcome the so-called 'end replication problem' as during each genome replication, due to inability of the DNA polymerase to extend a 5' DNA end, the lagging strand, after removal of the RNA primer, is not copied completely. As a result telomeres gradually shorten with each round of genome replication [47, 48]. Consequently, a mechanism was required to get through this obstacle. Upon each genome duplication, cells would otherwise keep loosing genetic material, eventually resulting in premature cell death, a critical problem for both the species and an individual's survival. This issue is even more prominent especially in multi-cellular organisms with late onset of reproduction. During ontogenesis, eukaryotic organisms solved this problem by preventing telomere attrition in dividing cells, through recruitment of the specialized and unique reverse transcriptase that replicates telomeric DNA sequences (telomerase), thereby maintaining them at a 'constant' length, as a limited telomere length is a prerequisite for cell replication [49]. Telomerase is routinely active only during embryogenesis and development, while in adults is expressed only to rapidly dividing cells (i.e. proliferative skin and gastrointestinal cells, activated lymphocytes, specific bone marrow stem cells and dividing male germ cell lineages [50].

In most adult cells telomerase is not expressed. Consequently, after a number of cell divisions, telomeres reach a critical length and chromosomes become uncapped. This leads, depending on the cellular context in which the uncapping occurs, either to a permanent cell cycle arrest (termed cellular senescence) or to apoptosis (programmed cell death) [51,52]. Extreme telomere shortening leads to chromosome instability, end-to-end fusions, and checkpoint-mediated cell cycle arrest and/or apoptosis [for review see 52 - 53]. All these processes are related in mammals not only to aging, but also to several age associated diseases such as cancer, coronary artery disease, and heart failure [54-57]. Cells programmed to enter senescence may escape this procedure due to checkpoint dysfunction and instead continue infinite proliferation, leading to oncogenesis. In such cases genomic stability has to be re-established and telomere length has to be restored by a Telomere Maintenance Mechanism (TMM). In most of tumor cells telomere maintenance is achieved by re-expression of telomerase. Interestingly, tumors have been described where telomerase could not be detected. Further studies revealed that in addition to the role of telomerase in maintaining telomere length, homologous recombination (HR) constitute an alternative method (ALT "alternative lengthening of telomeres") to maintain telomere DNA in telomerase- deficient cells. ALT TMM, in contrast to telomerase dependent TMM, results in telomeres with high heterogeneity in length and at least in the well-studied model of S. cerevisiae, consists of two pathways. While the bulk of cancer and

http://dx.doi.org/10.5772/56115

immortalized cells utilize telomerase re-expression to maintain telomere length, about 10-15% of tumors described operate using the ALT mechanism [58-60].

5. Telomere structure — Function relationship

As aforementioned, in the absence of telomerase, telomeres become non-functional, shorten with successive cell divisions, and chromosome termini can fuse as a consequence of de-protection. Telomere fusions are the result of non-homologous-end-joining (NHEJ) which is one of the prevailing mechanisms of a double strand break (DSB) healing. The outcome of such events could be the creation of chromosomes bearing more than one centromeres, which will likely be pooled to opposite poles during mitosis, resulting in chromosome breakage and further genomic instability through repeated fusion – breakage events. In vertebrates, the role of chromosome end protection in order to be distinguished from chromosome breaks is attributed to a specific complex of proteins collectively referred to as shelterin. Shelterin complex is basically composed by six proteins. Two members of the shelterin complex, TRF1 and TRF2 (from Telomere Repeat-binding Factor 1 and 2) bind directly to double stranded telomeric sequence, while POT1 binds ssDNA. TRF2 interacts with and recruits RAP1, while TIN2 mediates TPP1 – POT1 binding to the TIRF1 / TIRF2 core complex. POT1 binds to and protects the 3' single-stranded DNA overhang of telomeres (G-tail), while TIN2 likely links the single and double-stranded DNA binding complexes, especially in the area of the telomeric D-loop formation (figure 3) [5]. It seems that this core shelterin complex is mainly located at the telomere end (also referred to as telosome) and serves both in stabilizing t-loop structure, protecting it at the same time from being recognized as DNA damage and repaired by NHEJ. Additionally, shelterin regulates access to restoration processes of telomeric DNA after each genome replication. In general, shelterin complex seems to function as a platform regulating recruitment of a growing list of factors involved in chromatin remodelling, DNA replication, DNA damage repair, recombination and telomerase function, thus regulating telomere access / modification by diverse cellular processes (figure 4), recently reviewed in [61].

Interestingly, it appears that more than one type of core shelterin complex exists and not all of them are necessarily part of the telosome. Complexes containing only TRF1-TIN2-TPP1-POT1 or TRF2-RAP1 have been detected. Recent data measuring the absolute and relative amounts of TRF1 and TRF2 in the cell revealed that TRF2 is about twice as abundant as TRF1 [62] and this is consistent with TRF2 being detected in spatially directed DNA damage induced foci in non-telomeric chromosome regions. TRF2 recruitment to sites of DNA damage is consistent with it playing a critical role in the DNA damage response [63]. The complexity of the telosome created network is practically based on the unique structural features of the shelterin members. TRF1 and 2 bear a SAB/MYB domain by which they both recognise a TTAGGGTTA motif on telomere ds DNA, an acidic rich (D/E) terminal region and a specific docking motif referred to as TRF homology (TRFH) motif [64]. The TRFH domain mediates homo-dimerization of TRF1 or TRF2 [65, 66] but prohibits heterodimerization due to structural constraints [67]. A FxLxP motif and a Y/FxLxP motif are required for TRF1 and TRF2 binding, respectively. These domains are re-

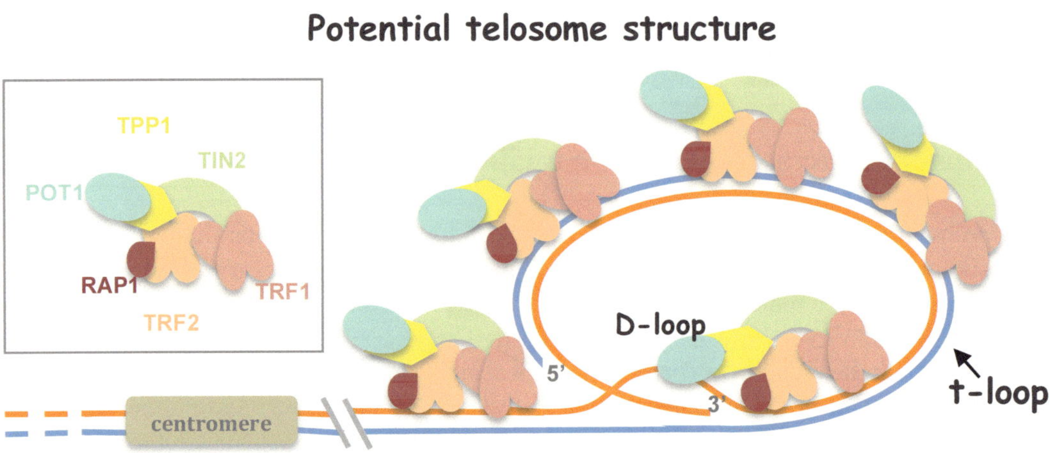

Figure 3. Schematic model of potential telomere capping arrangement by the shelterin complex. Proteins of the shelterin complex participate in telomere protection, replication and length regulation. TRF1 and TRF2 proteins bind specifically to telomeric ds DNA, while POT1 (TPP1) recognizes ssDNA (stabilizing D-loop). TIN2 interconnects ssDNA to dsDNA binding complexes, stabilizing telosome structure. Telomeric DNA consists of repetitive DNA sequence, a duplex region and a ssDNA G-strand overhang (G-strand, orange; C-strand, blue). The shelterin complex binds to both the duplex and ssDNA regions through specific protein–DNA interactions. Formation of the t-loop involves strand invasion of the G-overhang to create a displacement-loop (D-loop). The t-loop is proposed to mask the chromosome end from DNA damage sensors. For simplicity reasons the shelterin complex is depicted as a six-protein complex homogeneously dispersed onto telomere. See text for further details.

ferred to as TRFH Binding Motifs (TBM). The Phe 142 amino acid residue in TRF1-TRFH motif is responsible for TIN2 binding through its TBM region. TIN2-TBM has significantly lower affinity for the corresponding region of TRF2 (Phe 120) due to structural differences in the vicinity of Phe 120 and finally is attached to TRF2 via a unique TRF2 region near the N-terminus of the protein. Nevertheless, Phe 120 residue is crucial for specific interaction with other telomere associated factors like Apollo nuclease, a TRF2 binding partner. Complex formation between shelterin core members and associated factors with TBM like motifs [68] are likely to be also directed by changes in binding affinities due to post-translational modifications. A nice example is the TRF1 parsylation by tankyrase, resulting in significant decrease of the DNA-TRF1 affinity, allowing telomere lengthening and sister telomeres separation by specifically relieving cohesion complex from TRF1 and TIN2 [4, 5, 69-72]. Misbalance of such interactions could be detrimental for genome integrity as shown by elevated levels of TIFS formed in cells overexpressing an isolated TBM as a tandem YRL repeat. Analogous deleterious results were obtained when expressing a TRF2-F120 substitution allele [68].

Recent structural studies of one of the two OB (Oligonucleotide/oligosaccharide-binding) folds of S. pombe Pot1, that comprise the binding site of ssDNA, revealed that non-specific nucleotide recognition of ssDNA is achieved by hitherto unidentified binding modes that thermodynamically compensate for base-substitutions through alternate stacking interactions and new H-bonding networks [73]. Thus, delineating in detail the structure of shelterin members and associated factors is expected to geometrically improve our understanding of the networks consisted and the way quantity vs. quality changes interfere with structural modifications leading to functional alterations, finely tuning genome stability. Undoubtedly, the wealth of information gathered has already paved the way of using anti-telomerase agents in clinical trials, with robust expected outcome.

Apart from shelterin and interacting partners, another significant complex has recently emerged to be also involved in telomere biology, the CST complex. The CST complex is composed of CTC1, STN1 (OBFC1) and TEN1, and has been attributed the rescue of stalled replication forks during replication stress. The CST complex interconnects telomeres to genome replication and protection independently of the Pot1 pathway [5, 74].

Accumulating evidence by numerous publications quite unexpectedly demonstrated that DNA damage response (DDR) and repair pathways, despite seeming a paradox, share common features with telomere maintenance strategies. DDR early response proteins are recruited to telomeres and proteins believed to function in telomere maintenance have been also evidenced to be involved in DDR. Paradoxically, DDR factors in telomeres, in normal conditions, seem to interfere with telomere restoration and length preservation. This distinct phenomenon is attributed to shelterin co-ordination of DDR factors access and function at telomeres. TRF2 can bind to and suppress ATM, while POT1, when bound to the G-tail through TPP1, inhibits ATR. Suppression of TRF2 activity elicits p53 and ATM activation, leading to telomere dysfunction induced foci (TIFs). TIFs result in end-to-end telomere fusions via the NHEJ pathway and their appearance is correlated with the induction of senescence [75]. The interplay seems to be based on shelterin quantity and telomere length, two parameters directly related to each other, as when telomeres are critically short they are less likely to form a t-loop, a reaction catalysed by TRF2 *in vitro*, and in turn less shelterin is bound on [75]. Consequently, two major telomere maintenance structures are significantly reduced (t-loop and shelterin coating), allowing DDR activation. Yet, quite intriguingly, NHEJ machinery may also exert a protective role at telomeres through the enzymatic activity of Tankyrase related to the promotion of DNA-PKcs stability and prevention of the formation of telomere sister chromatid exchanges (T-SCEs) as a product of inter-telomere recombination [76]

Another intriguing paradigm is the MRN complex (a protein complex of meiotic recombination 11 (MRE11) – RAD50 and NBS1 proteins), where a single NBS1 molecule is associated with two dimers of MRE11 and RAD50 [77]. The MRE11 and RAD50 proteins form a heterotetramer that contains two DNA-binding and processing domains that can bridge free DNA ends [8, 77]. The MRN complex localizes to telomeres during the S and G2 phases of the cell cycle through direct interaction of NBS1 with TRF2, presumably contributing to the G-tail formation on the leading telomeric strand and thus to telomere stability [46, 77-81]. In humans, mutation in the NBS1 gene leads to the chromosomal instability disorder, Nijmegen breakage syndrome 1, associated with enhanced sensitivity to ionizing radiation and chromosomal instability and early developing cancer even in NBS1$^{+/-}$ heterozygotes. NBS1 contains a forkhead-associated (FHA), a BRCT (BRCA1 C Terminus) domain, an MRE11-binding domain, and an ATM-interacting domain. Accumulating evidence demonstrates that NBS1 interacts with telomeres and contributes to their stability, at least in human and mouse cells. Indirect immuno-fluorescence experiments revealed that NBS1 co-localizes with TRF2 during the S phase in cultured HeLa cells [64, 78], possibly by modulating t- loop formation. As TRF2 has also been found on non-telomeric sequences the impact of NBS1 co-localization with TRF2 requires further clarification. Similarly, in mouse embryonic fibroblasts, active recruitment of NBS1 to dysfunctional telomeres has been observed [46, 79, 81]. The MRN complex appears to play a dual role in telomere biology. One is to mediate, at least in part, the ATM response leading to TIF formation after TRF2 deletion [81]. Secondly, by its nuclease activity, it is required for normal telomere formation, as MRN is implicated in the processing of damaged telomeres by influencing the production of the overhang from a blunt end telomere created after telomere replication [46, 79, 81]. Such acceleration of the G-tail formation, following telomere dysfunction / de-protection prevents the fusion of leading blunt-ended strands of de-protected telomeres during S phase. Apollo nuclease may be also recruited and be involved in this process. Direct interaction of NBS1 with telomere repeat-binding factor 1 (TRF1) has been shown for immortalized telomerase negative cells [13] implying that this interaction might be involved in the alternative lengthening of telomeres. Furthermore, in telomerase expressing cells, MRN complex, through downregulation and removal of TRF1 (NBS1-dependent phosphorylation of TRF1 by ATM) may also promote accessibility of telomerase to the 3' end of telomeres [82, 83]. DNA repair intercommunication with telomere stability is a relationship established quite early in evolution as indicated by the fact that MRE11 and RAD50 together with protein kinases ATM and ATR, are also essential for proper telomere maintenance in plants [4,5].

Recently, another protein phosphatase, PNUTS (phosphatase 1 nuclear-targeting subunit), which interacts with TRF2, inserts another piece in the puzzle of the DDR and telomere relation [68]. In addition, detected by genome-wide searching for TBM containing proteins, the three BRCT domain bearing MCPH1 proximal DDR factor also interacts with TRF2. MCPH1 mutations are associated with developmental defects and increased tumor incidence [84]. MCPH1 depleted cells present decreased levels of BRCA1 and Chk1 and are defective in the G2/M checkpoint [85].

An essential role in telomere integrity is also attributed to BRCA2, a key component of the HR DNA repair pathway. BRCA2 associates with telomeres during the S/G2 cell cycle phases and appears to facilitate RAD51 recombinase loading [86]. Therefore, BRCA2-mediated HR activity is required for telomere length maintenance. These findings may explain, at least in part, the shorter telomeres found in BRCA2 mutated human breast tumors. Therefore, telomere dysfunction may be also implicated in the genomic instability observed in BRCA2-deficient breast and ovarian cancers [86].

In total, a number of DNA repair molecules, which are collectively part of the HR, NHEJ, NER and Fanconi Anemia pathways have been found to be recruited at telomeres, with TRF2 mainly functioning as a protein hub. In normal conditions, ATM/ATR signalling, upon de-protection due to short telomere length and subsequent 'retirement' of the cell (senescence / apoptosis) is part of the normal, tumor-initiation protective mechanism against genome-destabilized cells. In cells bearing normal telomere length there are inhibitory relationships between these different DNA repair systems, preventing each other's activation.

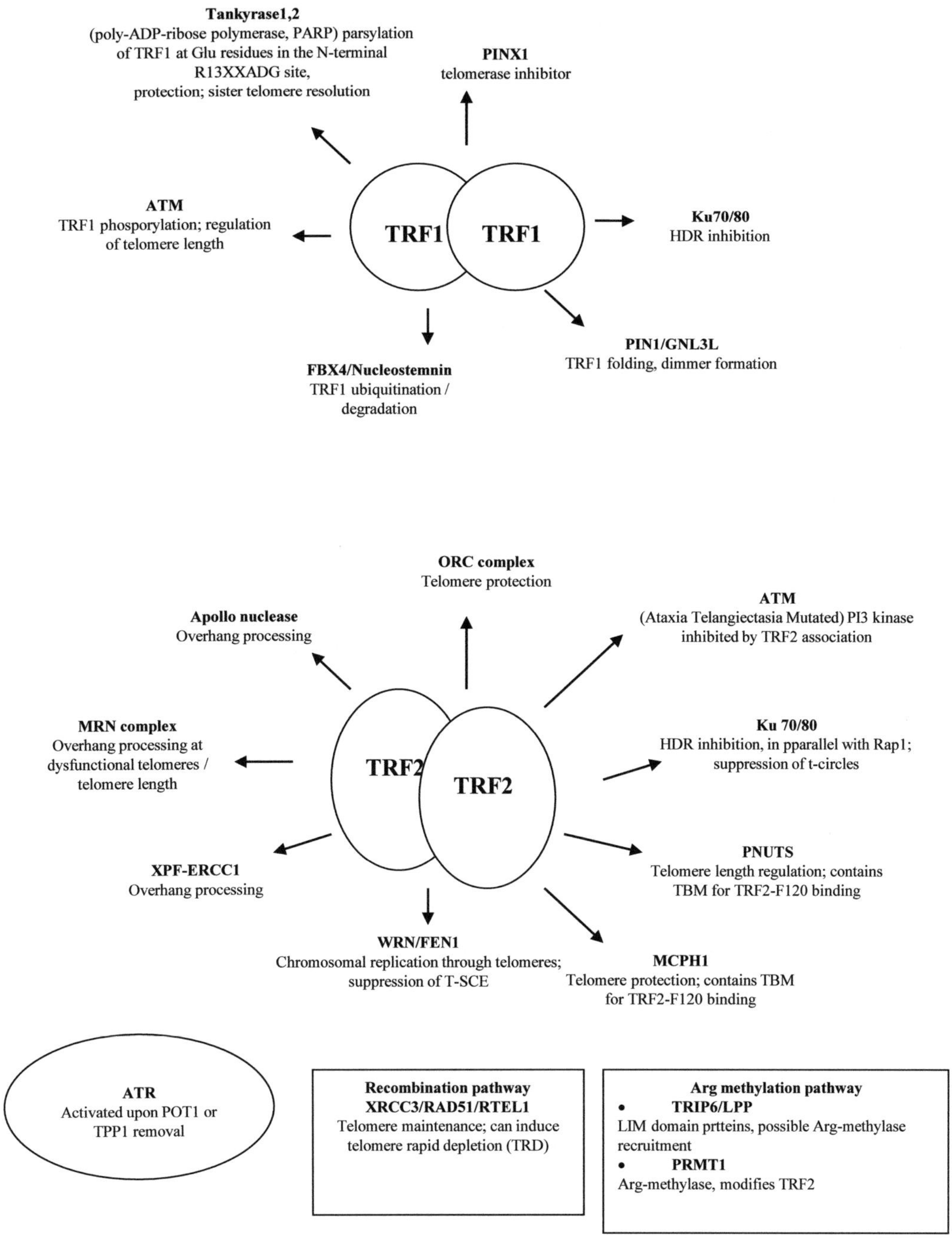

Figure 4. Shelterin associated factors also involved in DNA Damage Response. Details in the text

Telomeres are part of heterochromatin structure meaning that specific signals define their location in the nucleus. Although the fact that telomeres are expected to be by definition stable and inert chromosome ends, nevertheless appear to be dynamic nucleoprotein complexes also involved in chromatin remodelling. Recruitment of heterochromatin binding protein HP1 [87, 88], enriched tri-methylation of histone H3 lysine 9 (H3K9) and H4K20 [89], as well as methylation of CpG dinucleotides in subtelomeric DNA repeats [90] support this notion. These heterochromatic marks are replaced by characteristics of open chromatin (increased acetylation on histone tails, etc.) when telomeres become shorter. Such changes imply that a minimum telomere length is required to maintain heterochromatin–like conformation at chromosome ends, a structure that may change following telomere attrition. Moreover, telomeres and the shelterin complex should loosen their tight structure during chromosome replication and re-establish their compact form after completion of DNA duplication. An analogous loosening of telomere structure should be required in cases of telomere restoration by either telomerase or DNA repair mechanisms, although possibly through distinct procedures. In order to achieve this plasticity, chromatin should be remodelled through a number of enzymes, according to a local histone code [91]. A number of histone modifications are implicated where distinct histone tail-protein interactions promote telomere complex structure relaxation or compression [92]. As an example, SIRT6 (a histone H3K9 deacetylase that modulates telomeric chromatin) depletion experiments by RNA interference provided evidence of increased nuclear DNA damage and the formation of telomere dysfunction-induced foci. These experiments suggested that SIRT6 protects endothelial cells from telomere and genomic DNA damage, thus preventing a decrease in replicative capacity and the onset of premature senescence, in this particular case implicated in maintaining endothelial homeostatic functions and delay vascular ageing.

Another important set of factors implicating in telomere biology is the products of ATRX and DAXX genes, which are implicated in chromatin remodelling along with histone H3.3 [93-95]. Mutations or deletions in these genetic loci have been directly correlated with ALT+ status on cell lines or tumors per se [93,95]. According to these findings, screening for ATRX/DAXX mutations/expression may represent the most - up to date - reliable marker for tumors that have chosen the ALT TMM pathway.

Collectively, it is the proper assembly of shelterins in telomeres that is essential for chromosome stability (differentiates chromosome ends from DNA ds breaks and prevents loss of genetic information through either nucleolytic attack (exonuclease-mediated degradation) or aberrant chromosome fusions and undesirable recombination, during a cell's life span. Together with proper structure, functional co-ordination controlling TMM and telomerase activity are strictly regulated throughout the cell cycle by a number of implicated accessory factors, transiently recruited by the shelterin complexes / subcomplexes [75].

Apart from their protective role, proper interaction of shelterins with components of DNA repair machinery as well as telomerase components and telomerase recruitment, allows telomere restoration when appropriate. The importance of the correct structure – function of shelterin components in telomere biology and cancer formation, together with telomere-associated diseases, are depicted by association of mutation detection in i.e. TIN2 in many of these cases [96].

6. Telomeres and diseases

Telomere function is directly implicated in cellular senescence and therefore is expected to play a fundamental role in aging processes. Indeed, numerous publications the recent years reveal a correlation of telomere maintenance and retardation of aging in both cellular and animal models. Moreover, large epidemiological studies have reported an association between shorter telomere length in peripheral leukocytes and several inflammatory diseases of the elderly including diabetes, atherosclerosis and, recently, periodontitis [97].

To the present, leukocyte telomere length (LTL) serves in many cases as a predictor of age-related diseases and mortality. The potential role of telomere attrition in the onset or evolution of chronic inflammatory diseases, although requiring further investigation, could serve as a monitor of disease progression and effectiveness of treatment schemes. Furthermore, recent work of Entriger et al., provides preliminary evidence in humans, supporting a correlation of maternal psychological stress during pregnancy with the setting of newborn leukocyte telomere length. [98].

Apart from aging and specific syndromes (dyskeratosis congenita, pulmonary fibrosis) directly related to telomere dysfunction, abnormal telomere biology critically interferes with cancer [99-102]. One of the hallmarks of cancer is unlimited cell proliferation therefore tumour cells require a telomere maintenance mechanism (TMM) in order to retain the ability of infinite propagation. This issue will be more extensively discussed in the next paragraphs.

7. Telomere maintenance in non-physiological situations — ALT pathway

In adult vertebrates telomere length is –in most of the cell types - normally reduced during each cell division, while a limited telomere length is a prerequisite for cell replication. Following a certain number of replication cycles, telomere length is gradually shortened and this shortening during cell life span functions among others as a protective mechanism against both organismal ageing and neoplasia development. When telomere length reaches a critical value it triggers DNA Damage Response (DDR) followed by replicative senescence and / or check point-driven cell death, thereby prohibiting cellular aging and the capability of continuous proliferation. On the other hand, critical telomere length causes telomere uncapping and may result in the fusion of chromosomes by the NHEJ mechanism. Random telomere fusions mean either random fusions of various replicated chromosomes or fusion of sister chromatids of the same chromosome. [3,5,103]. In every case the consequences are fatal for genome integrity and normal cell well-being. In case that either senescence or apoptosis will be bypassed by deregulated cell fate control mechanisms, as for example mutated Rb or p53 proteins, then carcinogenesis might occur. Cancer cells depend on extensive cell proliferation and thus intact telomeres of a minimal length are also required for tumour survival and expansion. Telomere maintenance in cancer is achieved by two major mechanisms. In most of the cases telomere attrition in cancer cells is counteracted by telomerase upregulation [104] but in about 10-15% of tumour telomeres are preserved by telomerase independent mechanisms referred to as the Alternative Lengthening of Telomeres (ALT) pathways which are based on homologous recombination [105,106]. ALT has been detected in many tumour types but is most prevalent in tumours of mesenchymal origin like glioblastomas, osteosarcomas, soft tissue sarcomas, all of which tend to present particularly poor prognosis (table 1). The list includes 20-65% of sarcomas (in approximately half of osteosarcomas and in about one third of soft tissues sarcomas, one fourth of the primary brain tumor, glioblastoma multiforma and 10% of neuroblastomas) and 5-15% carcinomas (approximately half of which is gastric carcinoma and an about 15% adrenocortical & ovarian carcinoma) [94,107-115].

Genetic or epigenetic changes that unleash ALT are not yet deciphered. It seems that human mesenchymal stem cells might have a particular tendency to activate ALT [116]. ALT process has not been detected in normal cells although it might be part of a physiological process with or without modifications, since most, if not all, of the molecules implicated in ALT seem to be present also in normal cells, raising the question what inhibits / prevents ALT under physiological conditions. The Rb family member p130 seems to play a role in ALT inhibition as p130 forms a complex with the RAD50 interacting protein RINT-1, possibly blocking RAD50 from binding to MRE11 towards formation of a functional MRN complex postulated to prevent telomerase independent telomere lengthening in normal cells [117]. A recent report [118] provides evidence possibly explaining how ALT is upregulated in Human Papiloma Virus (HPV) induced cervical cancer. The mechanism involves E7 viral protein, which degrades p130 and by this way ALT TMM is used to prolong telomeres. This observation renders p130 a potential suppressor of ALT pathway, paving the way of using p130 in gene therapy approaches against cervical cancers. ALT is characterized by a number of phenotypic characteristics (figure 5) that have been observed in tumour cells and certain immortalized cell lines. In ALT cells many characteristics of normal telomere biology have been detected as duplex TTAGGG repeats with single stranded G-tails, shelterin complex together with other telomere associated proteins and the ability of t-loop formation. Besides these features, ALT cells present a number of exceptional characteristics with the most prominent being extrachromosomal telomeric sequences detected in many forms. Double stranded telomeric circles (t-circles) [106,119,120] are mainly detected, while partially single stranded circles (either C- or G- circles) are also abundant [121,122]. Moreover, linear ds-DNA [123,124] and very high molecular weight 't-complex' DNA that is likely to contain abnormal, highly branched structures are also been detected [122]. Another quite common but not universal characteristic of ALT cells is the formation of ALT-associated Promyelocytic Leukaemia (PML) nuclear bodies referred to as APBS [125]. APBS are quite interesting macromolecular structures that are considered to represent locations of ALT activity, as they contain telomeric DNA, associated telomere binding, DNA repair and recombination proteins like MRE11 complex, Mus81 and the SMC5/6 sumoylation pathway, [5,6,106,125-136], despite a number of inconsistencies. Moreover APBs might also function in sequestering of extrachromosomal DNA and are also related to cell cycle

Soft tissue sarcomas	• Chondrosarcoma • Undifferentiated pleomorphic sarcomas (including malignant fibrous histiocytoma • Leiomyorsarcoma • Epithelioid sarcoma • Liposarcoma • Fibrosarcoma (and variants) • Angiosarcoma and neurofibroma
Central Nervous System cancer subtypes	• Grade 2 diffuse astrocytoma • Grade 3 anaplastic astrocytoma • Grade 4 paediatric glioblastoma multiforme (GBM) • Oligodendroglioma • Anaplastic medulloblastoma • Other embryonal tumours • Grade 1 pilocytic astrocytoma, nonaplastic medduloblastoma, mengingioma, schwannoma etc
Urinary bladder subsets	• Small cell carcinoma • Invasive urothelial carcinoma
Adrenal gland / peripheral nervous system subtypes	• ganglioneuroblastoma • neuroblastoma • pheochromocytoma
Neuroendocrine neoplasms	• paraganglioma
Kidney subsets	• Chromophobe carcinoma • Sarcomatoid carcinoma • Clear cell and papillary carcinoma
Lung and pleural subtypes	• Malignant mesothelioma • Large cell carcinoma • Small cell carcinoma
Skin	• Malignant melanoma
Liver	• Hepatocellular carcinoma
Testis	• Nonseminomatous germ cell tumour
Breast	• Lobular carcinoma • Ductal carcinoma • Medullary carcinoma
Uterus	• Serous endometrial carcinoma • Squamous carcinoma
Ovary	• Clear cell carcinoma • Endometrioid carcinoma
Gall bladder	• adenocarcinoma
Oesophagus	• adenocarcinoma

Table 1. ALT + tumour types listed in descending order of prevalence [94].

arrest and senescence. Cesare & Reddel propose a model consistent with more than one type of APBs, depending on the cell cycle stage and the telomere status. According to this hypothesis and in conjunction to the published experimental data there might be two major classes of APBs: large APBs that contain compacted chromatin and accumulated under conditions of cell cycle arrest, including senescence and others that are the sites of ALT activity [106]. As APBs seem to be dynamic structures interacting with PML bodies, chromatin and DNA repair machinery (and also have been detected in many cell cycle stages), it is likely that APBs consist of a core basic domain and interact with the above referred components depending on / sensing telomere dysfunction status. In the latter case DDR may be elicited and lead cell to senescence. Of course, more experimental approaches are required in order to elucidate APBs' puzzle. Nevertheless, APBs formation, although common, does not appear to be a universal characteristic of the ALT pathway or a prerequisite for ALT activity.

Among ALT features t-circles seem to be involved in both ALT and physiological telomere biology [136]. t-circles could be the by-product of telomere-loop junctions (t-loop) resolution performed by recombination enzymes. This process could result in free t-circles and truncated telomeres [120], although in ALT cells t-circles are detected in significantly higher numbers than normal cells [119,120]. This reaction is dependent on the recombination factors Nijmegen breakage syndrome 1 (NBS1) and X-ray repair cross-complementing 3 (XRCC3) in human cells, while it is suppressed by the basic domain of TRF2 [120,133,137]. t-circles, although found to be more abundant in ALT cells compared to non-ALT cells [119,120], are also detected in telomerase – positive human cell lines with artificially elongated telomeres due to increased expression of telomerase components [138]. Experimental data suggest that human cells have a 'telomere trimming' mechanism that shortens telomeres through telomere-loop junction resolution (t-loop junction resolution). Therefore, abundant t-circles detected in ALT cells may represent the by-product of trimming of overlengthened telomeres and not a direct player in the ALT pathway per se.

On the other hand C-circles (telomeric circles consisting of an essentially complete C-rich strand and an incomplete G-rich strand) [121] seem to be involved in a more direct way with ALT mechanism. A quantitative relationship between the amount of ALT activity and the number of partially ds telomeric C-circles was observed [121], with an estimation of approximately 1,000 C-circles present per ALT cell. C-circles are possibly generated by nucleolytic degradation of the G-rich strand of t-circles, a hypothesis requiring further investigation. G-circles are also detected in ALT cells but reduced by 100-fold. Another result supportive of C-circles being characteristic of ALT cells is their detection in cell lines maintaining telomere length in the absence of telomerase without bearing any other ALT features [121]. Supportive to that is the observation that in immortalized cultured cells onset of ALT activity was temporary correlated with the appearance of C-circles. In accordance, ALT inhibition was accompanied by C-circles disappearance within 24 hours [121]. Taken together, the above reported data together with the fact that C-circles are also detected in blood samples from patients with ALT-positive osteosarcomas, it may be concluded that assaying C-circles may represent one of the most reliable marker of ALT activity. This notion is under validation for use at patient diagnosis level.

Epigenetic changes may also interfere with telomere biology and turn the balance towards the TMM selection. Concomitant with this hypothesis is the increasing evidence that depletion of chromatin remodelling complex ATRX/DAXX has been directly correlated with ALT phenotype, presumably repressing ALT under normal conditions [94,95]. Screening for ATRX/DAXX and the related histone variant H3.3 may therefore represent part of the signature of tumours replenishing their telomeres by homologous recombination pathways. ATRX/DAXX manipulation experiments suggest that their expression deficiency and the concomitant lack of H3.3 deposition into telomeric chromatin, is not sufficient to launch TMM choice in favour of ALT

http://dx.doi.org/10.5772/56115

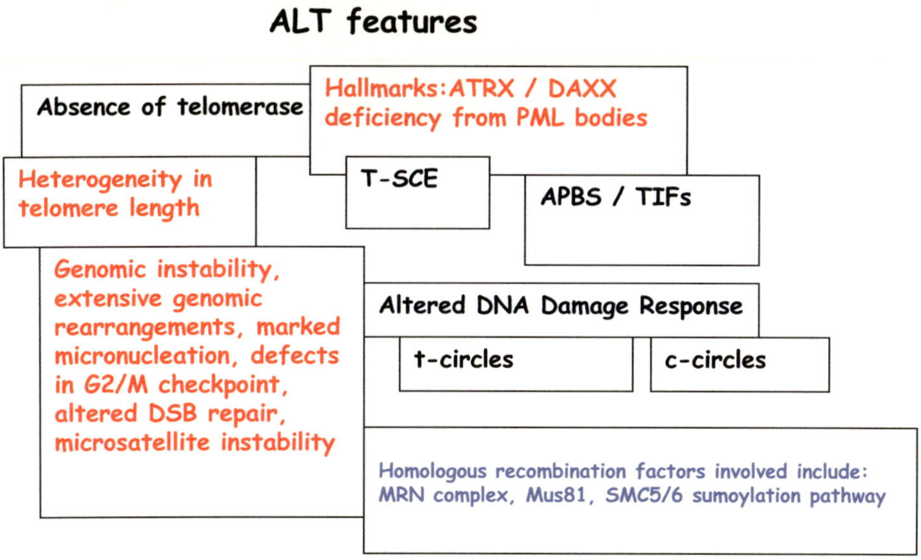

Figure 5. Basic ALT features. Telomere length heterogeneity, ARTX/DAXX lack of expression and extensive genomic instability seem to be universal characteristics, whereas APBs and c-circles have not been found in some telomerase negative cases.

pathway, pointing to the need to identify additional co-operating (epi-)genetic changes. ALT cells exhibit a high degree of ongoing genomic instability, including frequent micronuclei, high basal levels of DNA damage foci, and elevated checkpoint signalling in absence of exogenous damage, implying that ATRX/DAXX may interfere with repressing genes involved in telomere recombination, a hypothesis requiring further clarification [95]. Extensive genome instability, accompanied by G2/M checkpoint deficiencies detected in many ALT+ cells may explain how these cells keep on proliferating overcoming DNA damage events. Based on these findings, G2/M checkpoint inhibitors are currently developed and evaluated in clinical trials under the concept of enhancing the efficacy of clastogenic therapies [139].

Taken together, current hypotheses support a model where multiple steps, including loss of ATRX/DAXX function together with defects in the G2/M checkpoint in a high level of spontaneous DNA damage environment, are required for ALT-mediated immortalization. Thus, ALT tumours may present unique vulnerabilities [95] offering the potential for development of selective targeting agents towards personalized treatment schemes. A promising example might be targeting topoisomerase (Topo) IIIα, which associates with BLM helicase, an important player allowing telomere recombination in the absence of telomerase. Repression of Topo IIIα resulted in reduced ALT cells survival, decreased levels of TRF2 and BLM proteins, significant increase in the formation of anaphase bridges, degradation of the G-tail signal and TIF formation while telomerase expressing cells were unaffected [140]. Quite strikingly, Telomestatin, a natural compound functioning as a G-quadruplex ligand, impairs Topo IIIα binding to telomeres. Consequently, the Topo III/BLM/TRF2 complex is depleted from telomeres, APBs are disrupted and uncapped telomeres seem to trigger DDR [141].

In accordance to the multi-step process assumed to be required for activation of ALT TMM, major defects in DNA repair were observed to occur between preneoplasia and breast cancer, as monitored by ATM activation and subsequent significant repression, respectively [142]. Such defects are associated with changes in telomere length between the preneoplastic and the cancer stage.

8. ALT-mediated telomere elongation

Cumulative evidence supports a telomerase-independent, recombination-dependent, telomere length maintenance mechanism (TMM) [110]. Such an ALT process has been found to depend on the function of the homologous recombination gene RAD52 in telomerase-null mutant yeast [143], followed by numerous studies reporting detection of ALT pathways in human cell lines [144-146]. Further evidence established the existence of ALT mechanism as a telomerase maintenance process involving recombination events between non-sister telomeres or extrachromosomal sequences [119-121]. Such TMM activities may also explain the high heterogeneity of telomere length found in ALT cells in contrast to telomerase re-expressing cells. Telomere sister chromatid exchanges (T-SCEs) were also detected in much higher frequencies in ALT cells compared to normal or telomerase-expressing cells [148,149]. A model based on this observation attempted to explain TMM by ALT cells. Normally, SCEs may result from recombinational repair of broken replication forks [151] and therefore the detection of nicks and gaps in telomeric DNA [152] may result in T-SCEs. By this way unequal T-SCE may lead to cells with inherited elongated telomeres, resulting in a prolonged proliferative capacity, while other cells bearing shortened telomeres were characterized by decreased proliferative capacity [153]. Moreover, although there was no increase in SCE frequency detected elsewhere in the genome [148,149], overall recombination activity may be upregulated in ALT cells and not restricted only to telomeres. This could explain the poor outcome of ALT positive cancers as hyper-recombination events might confer to chemoresistance and further genomic instability leading to more aggressive cancer types. Despite data further supporting that ALT mechanism requires DNA recombination processes, the exact mechanism / mechanisms are still under investigation.

A theory consistent with the unequal T-SCE model would be that the same cell would inherit all lengthened telomeres, which would lead to unlimited proliferation of the given cell's descendants, a rather unlikely assumption, despite a few opposing evidences [154]. Such a hypothesis would require a specific telomere length based segregation mechanism, a theory necessitating further exploitation. Such an example is the case of copying of a DNA tag of a single telomere to other chromosome ends only in ALT-positive and not in telomerase-positive cells [147]. Therefore, ALT cells may use the unequal T-SCE model and the homologous recombination (HR) - dependent replication model. It is possible that the two suggested mechanisms are not mutually exclusive.

On the other hand, the HR – dependent telomere replication model, based on the hypothesis that recombination – mediated synthesis of new telomeric DNA occurs using an existing telomere sequence, is supported by more evidence. In this model telomeres from adjacent chromosomes could serve as templates [147,155], resulting in a net increase in telomeric DNA. In support of the view that ALT TMM functions through homology-directed recombination, an elevated frequency of sequence exchanges between telomeres has been observed in ALT cells [122, 147-149]. Furthermore, ALT cells contain extrachromosomal linear and circular telomeric DNA [119] and often exhibit heterogeneously-sized telomeres. These features, summarized in figure 5, are consistent with hyperactive HR activities, probably by a Break Induced Replication (BIR) – like mechanism [155,156]. In normal cells entering telomere crisis, cellular senescence and apoptosis, in a functional p53 or Rb pathway dependent processes, will occur. Most of the ALT cell lines and tumours lack normal p53 and Rb tumour suppressor functions and they are therefore tolerating persistent DSBs [157-159]. Many DNA repair proteins involved in HR are particularly active in ALT, like Rad52 and MRN complex. Especially, the MRN complex has been found to be necessary for ALT mediated telomere elongation [106,127]. This makes sense as MRN facilitates 5' to 3' resection of the DNA ends to create 3' overhangs for strand invasion, a prerequisite for HR [160]. In ALT cells MRN has been detected in APBs, which in turn recruits BRCA1. As previously mentioned, MRN is also necessary for ATM phoshorylation of TRF1 and its dissociation from telomeres regardless which TMM pathway is active. Therefore, MRN functions in order to facilitate HR events at shortened telomeres [83]. MRN does not seem to be absolutely vital for ALT TMM, as it's depletion did not result in unstable telomeres, implying the existence of related redundant pathways [127,161]. On the other hand, the formation of ALT characteristic c-circles depends on active recombination proteins like XRCC3, NBS1 and Ku70/80 [162], implying that t-circle formation requires NHEJ activity in ALT cells. In the context of HR, BLM RecQ helicase, an ATPase-driven helicase possessing 3'-5' unwinding activity, Holliday junction branch migration and ssDNA annealing function, is particularly active in ALT and may have a crucial involvement in ALT-TMM. Along comes the WRN helicase, possessing exonuclease activity and interacting with DNA-PKcs, RPA, MRN and Rad51 in response to DSBs. WRN has been detected in APBs together with TRF1 and TRF2 in S-phase, presumably resolving T-loops in order to facilitate telomere elongation. Depletion of HR components like Rad51D, MUS81, BLM or FANCA/D2 in ALT+ cells results in extremely shortened telomeres and reduced cell survival [105,106,135,163,164]. These results strongly suggest that HR is a major mechanism of TMM in ALT cells and targeting specific HR components may drive to specific and effective anti-ALT therapies.

As previously mentioned, telomere dysfunction and the resulting genomic instability comprise a fertile environment for carcinogenesis. Most of the cancer types manage to restore telomere length by upregulating telomerase and based on that observation an anti-telomerase oligonucleotide- based therapy (Imetelstat) showed promising results in CLL, MM, breast cancer and NSCLC patients in the context of Phase I clinical trials. Recently, a more advanced vaccine designed to raise immunity against a 16mer peptide from the active sites of human TERT has already entered Phase I & II clinical trials in cases of NSCLC (Non-Small Cell Lung Carcinoma), hepatocellular carcinoma and non-resectable pancreativ carcinoma. Moreover, there is an ongoing randomized Phase III clinical trial in patients with locally advanced or metastatic pancreatic cancer (ClinicalTrials.gov Identifier: NCT00425360) [165-166]. Never-

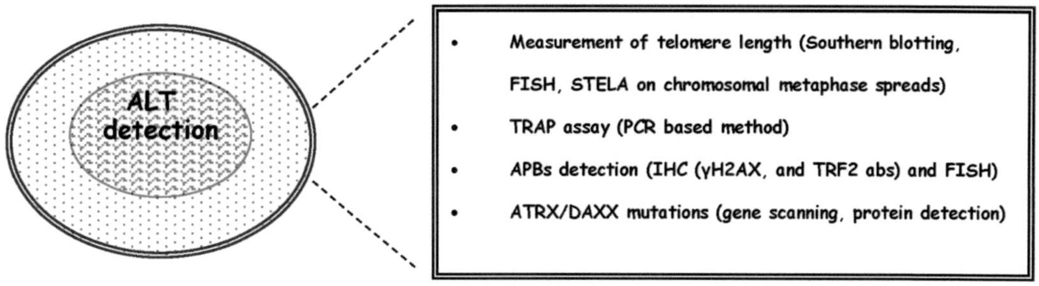

Figure 6. ALT detections approaches based on ALT features and biomarkers.

theless, anti-telomerase therapies are obviously of no value in telomerase non-expressing tumours, not to mention potential toxicity due to off-target effects. Furthermore, anti-telomerase treatment can always drive to selection for resistant cells that may activate an ALT mechanism [167]. These data render ALT an attractive target for anti-tumour therapies based on a personalized treatment approach. Recent reports support this notion, as repression of ALT in ALT-dependent immortal cell lines resulted in selective senescence and cell death [106], while ALT inhibition by siRNA-targeting of ALT components appear to result in more rapid telomere dysfunction [105,106,135,163,164] increasing therapeutic efficacy. Quite fascinatingly, preliminary results from the use of Telomestatin (a macrocyclic compound binding to G4-quadruplexes) exhibited effective elimination of both telomerase-expressing and ALT+ cell lines [141]. Of course there is a scepticism raised here as except of telomeres a significant portion of gene promoters also tend to adopt a G-quadruplex structure [168]. In addition, the puzzle becomes more complicated as transition of TMM pathway from telomerase upregulation to ALT and vice versa has been observed, especially in cases of secondary tumours and cases where both TMM pathways appear to co-exist, although not necessarily in the same tumour cell [169-172].

In conclusion, more extensive analysis of the detailed molecular mechanisms underlying TMM pathways and the structure-function relationship of the components involved is a prerequisite towards individualized treatment schemes with higher efficacy and lower toxicity. Unravelling of the detailed mechanisms incorporated in order to restore a minimum telomere length along with elucidation of the escape pathways that ALT+ cells are thought to use may ultimately lead to design of specific ALT-component directed compounds conferring high selectivity in targeting tumour against normal surrounding tissue cells.

Acknowledgments

This work is co-financed by the European Union (European Social Fund – ESF) and Greek national funds through the Operational Program "Education and Lifelong Learning" of the National Strategic Reference Framework (NSRF) - Research Funding Program: THALIS –

UOA- 'Analysis of genotoxic resistance mechanisms of breast cancer stem cells: applications in prognosis – diagnosis & treatment'.

Author details

Effrossyni Boutou[1], Dimitris Vlachodimitropoulos[2], Vassiliki Pappa[3], Horst-Werner Stürzbecher[4] and Constantinos E. Vorgias[1]

1 Dept of Biochemistry & Molecular Biology, Faculty of Biology, School of Sciences, National and Kapodistrian University of Athens, Greece

2 Lab of Toxicology & Forensic Medicine, Medical School, National and Kapodistrian University of Athens, Greece

3 nd Propaedeutic Pathology Clinic, Medical School, National and Kapodistrian University of Athens, Greece

4 Molecular Cancer Biology Group, Institute of Pathology, Lübeck University, Germany

References

[1] Blackburn, E. H, & Gall, J. G. A tandemly repeated sequence at the termini of the extrachromosomal ribosomal RNA genes in Tetrahymena. *J Mol Biol.* (1978). http://www.sciencedirect.com/science/article/pii/0022283678902942, 120(1), 33-53.

[2] Muller HJ: The remaking of chromosomes. (1938). *The Collecting Net-Woods Hole,* 13, 181-198.

[3] Palm, W, & De Lange, T. How shelterin protects mammalian telomeres. *Annu Rev Genet.* (2008). doi:annurev.genet.41.110306.130350., 42, 301-34.

[4] Linger, B. R, & Price, C. M. Conservation of telomere protein complexes: shuffling through evolution. *Crit Rev Biochem Mol Biol.* (2009). doi:, 44(6), 434-46.

[5] Stewart JA, Chaiken MF, Wang F, Price CM. Maintaining the end: roles of telomere proteins in end-protection, telomere replication and length regulation. *Mutat Res.* 2012;730(1-2):12-9. doi: 10.1016/j.mrfmmm.2011.08.011.

[6] Murnane JP. Telomere dysfunction and chromosome instability. *Mutat Res.* 2012;730(1-2):28-36. doi: 10.1016/j.mrfmmm.2011.04.008.

[7] Lin J, Epel E, Blackburn E. Telomeres and lifestyle factors: roles in cellular aging. *Mutat Res.* 2012;730(1-2):85-9. doi: 10.1016/j.mrfmmm.2011.08.003.

[8] Oeseburg H, de Boer RA, van Gilst WH, van der Harst P. Telomere biology in healthy aging and disease. *Pflugers Arch.* 2010;459(2):259-68. doi: 10.1007/s00424-009-0728-1.

[9] Hayflick L. The cell biology of aging. *J Invest Dermatol.* 1979;73(1):8-14. PMID: 448179

[10] Harley CB, Futcher AB, Greider CW. Telomeres shorten during ageing of human fibroblasts. *Nature.* 1990;345(6274):458-60. http://www.nature.com/nature/journal/v345/n6274/abs/345458a0.html

[11] d'Adda di Fagagna F, Reaper PM, Clay-Farrace L, Fiegler H, Carr P, Von Zglinicki T, Saretzki G, Carter NP, Jackson SP. A DNA damage checkpoint response in telomere-initiated senescence. *Nature.* 2003;426(6963):194-8. http://www.nature.com/nature/journal/v426/n6963/full/nature02118.html

[12] Silvestre DC, Londoño-Vallejo A. Telomere dynamics in mammals. *Genome Dyn.* 2010;7:29-45. doi: 10.1159/000337128.

[13] Greider CW. Telomeres and senescence: the history, the experiment, the future. *Curr Biol.* 1998;8(5):R178-81. http://www.cell.com/current-biology/retrieve/pii/S0960982298701058

[14] Abad JP, De Pablos B, Osoegawa K, De Jong PJ, Martín-Gallardo A, Villasante A. Genomic analysis of Drosophila melanogaster telomeres: full-length copies of HeT-A and TART elements at telomeres. *Mol Biol Evol.* 2004;21(9):1613-9. http://mbe.oxfordjournals.org/content/21/9/1613.long

[15] Makarov VL, Hirose Y, Langmore JP. Long G tails at both ends of human chromosomes suggest a C strand degradation mechanism for telomere shortening. *Cell.* 1997;88(5):657-66. http://www.cell.com/retrieve/pii/S009286740081908X

[16] Griffith JD, Comeau L, Rosenfield S, Stansel RM, Bianchi A, Moss H, de Lange T. Mammalian telomeres end in a large duplex loop. *Cell.* 1999;97(4):503-14. http://www.cell.com/retrieve/pii/S0092867400807606

[17] Maizels N. Dynamic roles for G4 DNA in the biology of eukaryotic cells. *Nat Struct Mol Biol.* 2006;13(12):1055-9. http://www.nature.com/nsmb/journal/v13/n12/full/nsmb1171.html

[18] Fry M. Tetraplex DNA and its interacting proteins. *Front Biosci.* 2007;12:4336-51. http://www.bioscience.org/2007/v12/af/2391/fulltext.htm

[19] De Cian A, Gros J, Guédin A, Haddi M, Lyonnais S, Guittat L, Riou JF, Trentesaux C, Saccà B, Lacroix L, Alberti P, Mergny JL. DNA and RNA quadruplex ligands. *Nucleic Acids Symp Ser (Oxf).* 2008;(52):7-8. doi: 10.1093/nass/nrn004.

[20] De Cian A, Lacroix L, Douarre C, Temime-Smaali N, Trentesaux C, Riou JF, Mergny JL. Targeting telomeres and telomerase. *Biochimie.* 2008;90(1):131-55. http://www.sciencedirect.com/science/article/pii/S0300908407001873

[21] Johnson JE, Smith JS, Kozak ML, Johnson FB. In vivo veritas: using yeast to probe the biological functions of G-quadruplexes. *Biochimie.* 2008;90(8):1250-63. doi: 10.1016/j.biochi.2008.02.013.

[22] Wellinger RJ, Ethier K, Labrecque P, Zakian VA. Evidence for a new step in telomere maintenance. *Cell.* 1996;85(3):423-33. http://www.cell.com/retrieve/pii/S0092867400811204

[23] Podlevsky JD, Chen JJ. It all comes together at the ends: telomerase structure, function, and biogenesis. *Mutat Res.* 2012;730(1-2):3-11. doi: 10.1016/j.mrfmmm.2011.11.002.

[24] Chan SR, Blackburn EH. Telomeres and telomerase. *Philos Trans R Soc Lond B Biol Sci.* 2004;359(1441):109-21. http://www.ncbi.nlm.nih.gov/pmc/articles/PMC1693310/

[25] Morin GB. The human telomere terminal transferase enzyme is a ribonucleoprotein that synthesizes TTAGGG repeats. *Cell.* 1989;59(3):521-9. http://www.cell.com/retrieve/pii/0092867489900354

[26] Masutomi K, Yu EY, Khurts S, Ben-Porath I, Currier JL, Metz GB, Brooks MW, Kaneko S, Murakami S, DeCaprio JA, Weinberg RA, Stewart SA, Hahn WC. Telomerase maintains telomere structure in normal human cells. *Cell.* 2003;114(2):241-53. http://www.cell.com/retrieve/pii/S0092867403005506

[27] Zhao Y, Sfeir AJ, Zou Y, Buseman CM, Chow TT, Shay JW, Wright WE. Telomere extension occurs at most chromosome ends and is uncoupled from fill-in in human cancer cells. *Cell.* 2009;138(3):463-75. doi: 10.1016/j.cell.2009.05.026.

[28] Gilson E, Géli V. How telomeres are replicated. *Nat Rev Mol Cell Biol.* 2007;8(10):825-38. http://www.nature.com/nrm/journal/v8/n10/full/nrm2259.html

[29] Verdun RE, Karlseder J. Replication and protection of telomeres. *Nature.* 2007;447(7147):924-31. http://www.nature.com/nature/journal/v447/n7147/full/nature05976.html

[30] de Lange T. How telomeres solve the end-protection problem. *Science.* 2009;326(5955):948-52. doi: 10.1126/science.1170633.

[31] Wu P, de Lange T. Human telomerase caught in the act. *Cell.* 2009;138(3):432-4. doi: 10.1016/j.cell.2009.07.018.

[32] Gomez DE, Armando RG, Farina HG, Menna PL, Cerrudo CS, Ghiringhelli PD, Alonso DF. Telomere structure and telomerase in health and disease. *Int J Oncol.* 2012;41(5):1561-9. doi: 10.3892/ijo.2012.1611.

[33] Rhodes D, Fairall L, Simonsson T, Court R, Chapman L. Telomere architecture. *EMBO Rep.* 2002;3(12):1139-45. http://www.nature.com/embor/journal/v3/n12/full/embor012.html

[34] Vega LR, Mateyak MK, Zakian VA. Getting to the end: telomerase access in yeast and humans. *Nat Rev Mol Cell Biol.* 2003;4(12):948-59. http://www.nature.com/nrm/journal/v4/n12/full/nrm1256.html

[35] de Lange T. Shelterin: the protein complex that shapes and safeguards human telomeres. *Genes Dev.* 2005;19(18):2100-10. http://genesdev.cshlp.org/content/19/18/2100.long

[36] Martínez P, Blasco MA. Telomeric and extra-telomeric roles for telomerase and the telomere-binding proteins. *Nat Rev Cancer.* 2011;11(3):161-76. doi: 10.1038/nrc3025.

[37] Zakian VA. Telomeres: beginning to understand the end. *Science.* 1995;270(5242):1601-7. http://www.sciencemag.org/content/270/5242/1601.long

[38] Hande MP. DNA repair factors and telomere-chromosome integrity in mammalian cells. *Cytogenet Genome Res.* 2004;104(1-4):116-22. http://www.karger.com/Article/FullText/77475

[39] Paeschke K, McDonald KR, Zakian VA. Telomeres: structures in need of unwinding. *FEBS Lett.* 2010;584(17):3760-72. doi: 10.1016/j.febslet.2010.07.007.

[40] Azzalin CM, Reichenbach P, Khoriauli L, Giulotto E, Lingner J. Telomeric repeat containing RNA and RNA surveillance factors at mammalian chromosome ends. *Science.* 2007;318(5851):798-801. http://www.sciencemag.org/content/318/5851/798.long

[41] Luke B, Lingner J. TERRA: telomeric repeat-containing RNA. *EMBO J.* 2009;28(17):2503-10. doi: 10.1038/emboj.2009.166.

[42] Luke B, Panza A, Redon S, Iglesias N, Li Z, Lingner J. The Rat1p 5' to 3' exonuclease degrades telomeric repeat-containing RNA and promotes telomere elongation in Saccharomyces cerevisiae. *Mol Cell.* 2008;32(4):465-77. doi: 10.1016/j.molcel.2008.10.019.

[43] Schoeftner S, Blasco MA. Developmentally regulated transcription of mammalian telomeres by DNA-dependent RNA polymerase II. *Nat Cell Biol.* 2008;10(2):228-36. http://www.nature.com/ncb/journal/v10/n2/full/ncb1685.html

[44] Sánchez-Alonso P, Guzman P. Predicted elements of telomere organization and function in Ustilago maydis. *Fungal Genet Biol.* 2008;45 Suppl 1:S54-62. doi: 10.1016/j.fgb.2008.04.009.

[45] Maicher A, Kastner L, Luke B. Telomeres and disease: enter TERRA. *RNA Biol.* 2012;9(6):843-9. doi: 10.4161/rna.20330.

[46] Deng Z, Norseen J, Wiedmer A, Riethman H, Lieberman PM. TERRA RNA binding to TRF2 facilitates heterochromatin formation and ORC recruitment at telomeres. *Mol Cell.* 2009;35(4):403-13. doi: 10.1016/j.molcel.2009.06.025.telomeres.

[47] Watson JD. Origin of concatemeric T7 DNA. *Nat New Biol.* 1972;239(94):197-201. PMID: 4507727

[48] Olovnikov AM. A theory of marginotomy. The incomplete copying of template margin in enzymic synthesis of polynucleotides and biological significance of the phenomenon. *J Theor Biol.* 1973;41(1):181-90. http://www.sciencedirect.com/science/article/pii/0022519373901987

[49] Blackburn EH, Greider CW, Szostak JW. Telomeres and telomerase: the path from maize, Tetrahymena and yeast to human cancer and aging. *Nat Med.* 2006;12(10):1133-8. http://www.nature.com/nm/journal/v12/n10/full/nm1006-1133.html

[50] Ulaner GA, Giudice LC. Developmental regulation of telomerase activity in human fetal tissues during gestation. *Mol Hum Reprod.* 1997;3(9):769-73. http://molehr.oxfordjournals.org/content/3/9/769.long

[51] Blasco MA. Telomeres and human disease: ageing, cancer and beyond. *Nat Rev Genet.* 2005;6(8):611-22. http://www.nature.com/nrg/journal/v6/n8/full/nrg1656.html

[52] Galati A, Micheli E, Cacchione S. Chromatin structure in telomere dynamics. *Front Oncol.* 2013;3:46. doi: 10.3389/fonc.2013.00046.

[53] Shore D, Bianchi A. Telomere length regulation: coupling DNA end processing to feedback regulation of telomerase. *EMBO J.* 2009;28(16):2309-22. doi: 10.1038/emboj.2009.195.

[54] Sherr CJ, McCormick F. *The RB and p53 pathways in cancer. Cancer Cell.* 2002;2(2):103-12. http://www.cell.com/cancer-cell/retrieve/pii/S1535610802001022

[55] Ogami M, Ikura Y, Ohsawa M, Matsuo T, Kayo S, Yoshimi N, Hai E, Shirai N, Ehara S, Komatsu R, Naruko T, Ueda M. Telomere shortening in human coronary artery diseases. *Arterioscler Thromb Vasc Biol.* 2004;24(3):546-50. http://atvb.ahajournals.org/content/24/3/546.long

[56] Starr JM, McGurn B, Harris SE, Whalley LJ, Deary IJ, Shiels PG. Association between telomere length and heart disease in a narrow age cohort of older people. *Exp Gerontol.* 2007;42(6):571-3. http://www.sciencedirect.com/science/article/pii/S0531556506004505

[57] Donate LE, Blasco MA. Telomeres in cancer and ageing. *Philos Trans R Soc Lond B Biol Sci.* 2011;366(1561):76-84. doi: 10.1098/rstb.2010.0291.

[58] Lundblad V, Blackburn EH. An alternative pathway for yeast telomere maintenance rescues est1- senescence. *Cell.* 1993;73(2):347-60. http://www.cell.com/retrieve/pii/009286749390234H

[59] Teng SC, Zakian VA. Telomere-telomere recombination is an efficient bypass pathway for telomere maintenance in Saccharomyces cerevisiae. *Mol Cell Biol.* 1999;19(12):8083-93. http://mcb.asm.org/content/19/12/8083.long

[60] Teng SC, Chang J, McCowan B, Zakian VA. Telomerase-independent lengthening of yeast telomeres occurs by an abrupt Rad50p-dependent, Rif-inhibited recombination-

al process. *Mol Cell.* 2000;6(4):947-52. http://www.cell.com/molecular-cell/retrieve/pii/S1097276505000948

[61] Diotti R, Loayza D. Shelterin complex and associated factors at human telomeres. Nucleus. 2011;2(2):119-35. doi: 10.4161/nucl.2.2.15135.

[62] Takai KK, Hooper S, Blackwood S, Gandhi R, de Lange T. In vivo stoichiometry of shelterin components. *J Biol Chem.* 2010;285(2):1457-67. doi: 10.1074/jbc.M109.038026.

[63] Huda N, Abe S, Gu L, Mendonca MS, Mohanty S, Gilley D. Recruitment of TRF2 to laser-induced DNA damage sites. *Free Radic Biol Med.* 2012;53(5):1192-7. doi: 10.1016/j.freeradbiomed.2012.07.024.

[64] Chen Y, Yang Y, van Overbeek M, Donigian JR, Baciu P, de Lange T, Lei M. A shared docking motif in TRF1 and TRF2 used for differential recruitment of telomeric proteins. *Science.* 2008;319(5866):1092-6. doi:10.1126/science.1151804.

[65] Bianchi A, Smith S, Chong L, Elias P, de Lange T. TRF1 is a dimer and bends telomeric DNA. *EMBO J.* 1997;16(7):1785-94. http://www.nature.com/emboj/journal/v16/n7/full/7590167a.html

[66] Broccoli D, Smogorzewska A, Chong L, de Lange T. Human telomeres contain two distinct Myb-related proteins, TRF1 and TRF2. *Nat Genet.* 1997;17(2):231-5. http://www.nature.com/ng/journal/v17/n2/abs/ng1097-231.html

[67] Fairall L, Chapman L, Moss H, de Lange T, Rhodes D. Structure of the TRFH dimerization domain of the human telomeric proteins TRF1 and TRF2. *Mol Cell.* 2001;8(2):351-61. http://www.cell.com/molecular-cell/retrieve/pii/S1097276501003215

[68] Kim H, Lee OH, Xin H, Chen LY, Qin J, Chae HK, Lin SY, Safari A, Liu D, Songyang Z. TRF2 functions as a protein hub and regulates telomere maintenance by recognizing specific peptide motifs. *Nat Struct Mol Biol.* 2009;16(4):372-9. doi: 10.1038/nsmb.1575.

[69] Smith S, de Lange T. Tankyrase promotes telomere elongation in human cells. *Curr Biol.* 2000;10(20):1299-302. http://www.cell.com/current-biology/retrieve/pii/S0960982200007521

[70] Canudas S, Houghtaling BR, Kim JY, Dynek JN, Chang WG, Smith S. Protein requirements for sister telomere association in human cells. *EMBO J.* 2007;26(23):4867-78. http://www.nature.com/emboj/journal/v26/n23/full/7601903a.html

[71] Hsiao SJ, Smith S. Tankyrase function at telomeres, spindle poles, and beyond. *Biochimie.* 2008;90(1):83-92. http://www.sciencedirect.com/science/article/pii/S0300908407001885

[72] Ha GH, Kim HS, Go H, Lee H, Seimiya H, Chung DH, Lee CW. Tankyrase-1 function at telomeres and during mitosis is regulated by Polo-like kinase-1-mediated phosphorylation. *Cell Death Differ.* 2012;19(2):321-32. doi: 10.1038/cdd.2011.101.

[73] Dickey TH, McKercher MA, Wuttke DS. Nonspecific recognition is achieved in Pot1pC through the use of multiple binding modes. *Structure.* 2013;21(1):121-32. doi: 10.1016/j.str.2012.10.015.

[74] Miyake Y, Nakamura M, Nabetani A, Shimamura S, Tamura M, Yonehara S, Saito M, Ishikawa F. RPA-like mammalian Ctc1-Stn1-Ten1 complex binds to single-stranded DNA and protects telomeres independently of the Pot1 pathway. *Mol Cell.* 2009;36(2): 193-206. doi: 10.1016/j.molcel.2009.08.009.

[75] Oganesian L, Karlseder J. Telomeric armor: the layers of end protection. *J Cell Sci.* 2009;122(Pt 22):4013-25. doi: 10.1242/jcs.050567.

[76] Dregalla RC, Zhou J, Idate RR, Battaglia CL, Liber HL, Bailey SM. Regulatory roles of tankyrase 1 at telomeres and in DNA repair: suppression of T-SCE and stabilization of DNA-PKcs. *Aging (Albany NY).* 2010;2(10):691-708. http://www.impactaging.com/papers/v2/n10/full/100210.html

[77] Lamarche BJ, Orazio NI, Weitzman MD. The MRN complex in double-strand break repair and telomere maintenance. *FEBS Lett.* 2010;584(17):3682-95. doi: 10.1016/j.febslet.2010.07.029.

[78] Zhu XD, Küster B, Mann M, Petrini JH, de Lange T. Cell-cycle-regulated association of RAD50/MRE11/NBS1 with TRF2 and human telomeres. *Nat Genet.* 2000;25(3): 347-52. http://www.nature.com/doifinder/10.1038/77139

[79] Dimitrova N, de Lange T. Cell cycle-dependent role of MRN at dysfunctional telomeres: ATM signaling-dependent induction of nonhomologous end joining (NHEJ) in G1 and resection-mediated inhibition of NHEJ in G2. *Mol Cell Biol.* 2009;29(20): 5552-63. doi: 10.1128/MCB.00476-09.

[80] Verdun RE, Crabbe L, Haggblom C, Karlseder J. Functional human telomeres are recognized as DNA damage in G2 of the cell cycle. *Mol Cell.* 2005;20(4):551-61. http://www.cell.com/molecular-cell/retrieve/pii/S109727650501645X

[81] Attwooll CL, Akpinar M, Petrini JH. The mre11 complex and the response to dysfunctional telomeres. *Mol Cell Biol.* 2009;29(20):5540-51. doi: 10.1128/MCB.00479-09.

[82] Chai W, Sfeir AJ, Hoshiyama H, Shay JW, Wright WE. The involvement of the Mre11/Rad50/Nbs1 complex in the generation of G-overhangs at human telomeres. *EMBO Rep.* 2006;7(2):225-30. http://www.nature.com/embor/journal/v7/n2/full/7400600.html

[83] Wu Y, Xiao S, Zhu XD. MRE11-RAD50-NBS1 and ATM function as co-mediators of TRF1 in telomere length control. *Nat Struct Mol Biol.* 2007;14(9):832-40. http://www.nature.com/nsmb/journal/v14/n9/full/nsmb1286.html

[84] Mohammad DH, Yaffe MB. 14-3-3 proteins, FHA domains and BRCT domains in the DNA damage response. *DNA Repair (Amst).* 2009;8(9):1009-17. doi: 10.1016/j.dnarep.2009.04.004.

[85] Gavvovidis I, Pöhlmann C, Marchal JA, Stumm M, Yamashita D, Hirano T, Schindler D, Neitzel H, Trimborn M. MCPH1 patient cells exhibit delayed release from DNA damage-induced G2/M checkpoint arrest. *Cell Cycle.* 2010;9(24):4893-9. http://www.landesbioscience.com/journals/cc/article/14157/

[86] Badie S, Escandell JM, Bouwman P, Carlos AR, Thanasoula M, Gallardo MM, Suram A, Jaco I, Benitez J, Herbig U, Blasco MA, Jonkers J, Tarsounas M. BRCA2 acts as a RAD51 loader to facilitate telomere replication and capping. *Nat Struct Mol Biol.* 2010;17(12):1461-9. doi: 10.1038/nsmb.1943.

[87] Koering CE, Pollice A, Zibella MP, Bauwens S, Puisieux A, Brunori M, Brun C, Martins L, Sabatier L, Pulitzer JF, Gilson E. Human telomeric position effect is determined by chromosomal context and telomeric chromatin integrity. *EMBO Rep.* 2002;3(11):1055-61. http://www.nature.com/embor/journal/v3/n11/full/embor043.html

[88] Sharma GG, Hwang KK, Pandita RK, Gupta A, Dhar S, Parenteau J, Agarwal M, Worman HJ, Wellinger RJ, Pandita TK. Human heterochromatin protein 1 isoforms HP1(Hsalpha) and HP1(Hsbeta) interfere with hTERT-telomere interactions and correlate with changes in cell growth and response to ionizing radiation. *Mol Cell Biol.* 2003;23(22):8363-76. http://mcb.asm.org/content/23/22/8363.long

[89] García-Cao M, O'Sullivan R, Peters AH, Jenuwein T, Blasco MA. Epigenetic regulation of telomere length in mammalian cells by the Suv39h1 and Suv39h2 histone methyltransferases. *Nat Genet.* 2004;36(1):94-9. http://www.nature.com/ng/journal/v36/n1/full/ng1278.html

[90] Gonzalo S, Jaco I, Fraga MF, Chen T, Li E, Esteller M, Blasco MA. DNA methyltransferases control telomere length and telomere recombination in mammalian cells. *Nat Cell Biol.* 2006;8(4):416-24. http://www.nature.com/ncb/journal/v8/n4/full/ncb1386.html

[91] Misri S, Pandita S, Kumar R, Pandita TK. Telomeres, histone code, and DNA damage response. *Cytogenet Genome Res.* 2008;122(3-4):297-307. doi: 10.1159/000167816.

[92] Michishita E, McCord RA, Berber E, Kioi M, Padilla-Nash H, Damian M, Cheung P, Kusumoto R, Kawahara TL, Barrett JC, Chang HY, Bohr VA, Ried T, Gozani O, Chua KF. SIRT6 is a histone H3 lysine 9 deacetylase that modulates telomeric chromatin. *Nature.* 2008 Mar 27;452(7186):492-6. doi: 10.1038/nature06736.

[93] Heaphy CM, de Wilde RF, Jiao Y, Klein AP, Edil BH, Shi C, Bettegowda C, Rodriguez FJ, Eberhart CG, Hebbar S, Offerhaus GJ, McLendon R, Rasheed BA, He Y, Yan H, Bigner DD, Oba-Shinjo SM, Marie SK, Riggins GJ, Kinzler KW, Vogelstein B, Hruban RH, Maitra A, Papadopoulos N, Meeker AK. Altered telomeres in tumors with ATRX and DAXX mutations. *Science.* 2011;333(6041):425. doi: 10.1126/science.1207313.

[94] Durant ST. Telomerase-independent paths to immortality in predictable cancer subtypes. *J Cancer.* 2012;3:67-82. doi: 10.7150/jca.3965.

[95] Lovejoy CA, Li W, Reisenweber S, Thongthip S, Bruno J, de Lange T, De S,Petrini JH, Sung PA, Jasin M, Rosenbluh J, Zwang Y, Weir BA, Hatton C, Ivanova E, Macconaill L, Hanna M, Hahn WC, Lue NF, Reddel RR, Jiao Y, Kinzler K, Vogelstein B, Papadopoulos N, Meeker AK; ALT Starr Cancer Consortium. Loss of ATRX, genome instability, and an altered DNA damage response are hallmarks of the alternative lengthening of telomeres pathway. *PLoS Genet.* 2012;8(7):e1002772. http://www.plosgenetics.org/article/info%3Adoi%2F10.1371%2Fjournal.pgen.1002772

[96] Walne AJ, Vulliamy T, Beswick R, Kirwan M, Dokal I. TINF2 mutations result in very short telomeres: analysis of a large cohort of patients with dyskeratosis congenita and related bone marrow failure syndromes. *Blood.* 2008;112(9):3594-600. doi: 10.1182/blood-2008-05-153445.

[97] Steffens JP, Masi S, D'Aiuto F, Spolidorio LC. Telomere length and its relationship with chronic diseases - New perspectives for periodontal research. *Arch Oral Biol.* 2012 (Epub). doi: 10.1016/j.archoralbio.2012.09.009.

[98] Entringer S, Epel ES, Lin J, Buss C, Shahbaba B, Blackburn EH, Simhan HN, Wadhwa PD. Maternal psychosocial stress during pregnancy is associated with newborn leukocyte telomere length. *Am J Obstet Gynecol.* 2013;208(2):134.e1-7. doi: 10.1016/j.ajog.2012.11.033.

[99] Armanios M. Telomerase and idiopathic pulmonary fibrosis. *Mutat Res.* 2012;730(1-2):52-8. doi: 10.1016/j.mrfmmm.2011.10.013.

[100] Nelson ND, Bertuch AA. Dyskeratosis congenita as a disorder of telomere maintenance. *Mutat Res.* 2012;730(1-2):43-51. doi: 10.1016/j.mrfmmm.2011.06.008.

[101] Prescott J, Wentzensen IM, Savage SA, De Vivo I. Epidemiologic evidence for a role of telomere dysfunction in cancer etiology. *Mutat Res.* 2012;730(1-2):75-84. doi: 10.1016/j.mrfmmm.2011.06.009.

[102] Lin J, Epel E, Blackburn E. Telomeres and lifestyle factors: roles in cellular aging. *Mutat Res.* 2012;730(1-2):85-9. doi: 10.1016/j.mrfmmm.2011.08.003.

[103] Gallego ME, White CI. DNA repair and recombination functions in Arabidopsis telomere maintenance. *Chromosome Res.* 2005;13(5):481-91. http://link.springer.com/article/10.1007%2Fs10577-005-0995-4

[104] Shay JW. Molecular pathogenesis of aging and cancer: are telomeres and telomerase the connection? *J Clin Pathol.* 1997;50(10):799-800. http://jcp.bmj.com/content/50/10/799.long

[105] Royle NJ, Méndez-Bermúdez A, Gravani A, Novo C, Foxon J, Williams J, Cotton V, Hidalgo A. The role of recombination in telomere length maintenance. *Biochem Soc Trans.* 2009;37(Pt 3):589-95. doi: 10.1042/BST0370589.

[106] Cesare AJ, Reddel RR. Alternative lengthening of telomeres: models, mechanisms and implications. *Nat Rev Genet.* 2010;11(5):319-30. doi: 10.1038/nrg2763.

[107] Hakin-Smith V, Jellinek DA, Levy D, Carroll T, Teo M, Timperley WR, McKay MJ, Reddel RR, Royds JA. Alternative lengthening of telomeres and survival in patients with glioblastoma multiforme. *Lancet.* 2003;361(9360):836-8. http://linkinghub.elsevier.com/retrieve/pii/S0140673603126815

[108] Henson JD, Hannay JA, McCarthy SW, Royds JA, Yeager TR, Robinson RA, Wharton SB, Jellinek DA, Arbuckle SM, Yoo J, Robinson BG, Learoyd DL, Stalley PD, Bonar SF, Yu D, Pollock RE, Reddel RR. A robust assay for alternative lengthening of telomeres in tumors shows the significance of alternative lengthening of telomeres in sarcomas and astrocytomas. *Clin Cancer Res.* 2005;11(1):217-25. http://clincancerres.aacrjournals.org/content/11/1/217.long

[109] Costa A, Daidone MG, Daprai L, Villa R, Cantù S, Pilotti S, Mariani L, Gronchi A, Henson JD, Reddel RR, Zaffaroni N. Telomere maintenance mechanisms in liposarcomas: association with histologic subtypes and disease progression. *Cancer Res.* 2006;66(17):8918-24. http://cancerres.aacrjournals.org/content/66/17/8918.long

[110] Bryan TM, Englezou A, Dalla-Pozza L, Dunham MA, Reddel RR. Evidence for an alternative mechanism for maintaining telomere length in human tumors and tumor-derived cell lines. *Nat Med.* 1997;3(11):1271-4. PMID: 9359704

[111] Jeyapalan JN, Mendez-Bermudez A, Zaffaroni N, Dubrova YE, Royle NJ. Evidence for alternative lengthening of telomeres in liposarcomas in the absence of ALT-associated PML bodies. *Int J Cancer.* 2008;122(11):2414-21. doi: 10.1002/ijc.23412.

[112] Villa R, Daidone MG, Motta R, Venturini L, De Marco C, Vannelli A, Kusamura S, Baratti D, Deraco M, Costa A, Reddel RR, Zaffaroni N. Multiple mechanisms of telomere maintenance exist and differentially affect clinical outcome in diffuse malignant peritoneal mesothelioma. *Clin Cancer Res.* 2008;14(13):4134-40. doi: 10.1158/1078-0432.CCR-08-0099.

[113] Subhawong AP, Heaphy CM, Argani P, Konishi Y, Kouprina N, Nassar H, Vang R, Meeker AK. The alternative lengthening of telomeres phenotype in breast carcinoma is associated with HER-2 overexpression. *Mod Pathol.* 2009 Nov;22(11):1423-31. doi: 10.1038/modpathol.2009.125.

[114] Henson JD, Reddel RR. Assaying and investigating Alternative Lengthening of Telomeres activity in human cells and cancers. *FEBS Lett.* 2010;584(17):3800-11. doi: 10.1016/j.febslet.2010.06.009.

[115] Plantinga MJ and Broccoli D. Telomere Maintenance Mechanisms in Soft Tissue Sarcomas, Soft Tissue Tumors, Prof. Fethi Derbel (Ed.), ISBN: 978-953-307-862-5, InTech; 2011 http://www.intechopen.com/books/soft-tissue-tumors/telomere-maintenance-mechanisms-in-soft-tissuesarcomas

[116] Lafferty-Whyte K, Cairney CJ, Will MB, Serakinci N, Daidone MG, Zaffaroni N, Bilsland A, Keith WN. A gene expression signature classifying telomerase and ALT immortalization reveals an hTERT regulatory network and suggests a mesenchymal stem cell origin for ALT. *Oncogene.* 2009;28(43):3765-74. doi: 10.1038/onc.2009.238.

[117] Kong LJ, Meloni AR, Nevins JR. The Rb-related p130 protein controls telomere lengthening through an interaction with a Rad50-interacting protein, RINT-1. *Mol Cell.* 2006;22(1):63-71. http://www.cell.com/molecular-cell/retrieve/pii/S1097276506001183

[118] Zhang W, Tian Y, Chen JJ, Zhao W, Yu X. A postulated role of p130 in telomere maintenance by human papillomavirus oncoprotein E7. *Med Hypotheses.* 2012;79(2): 178-80. doi: 10.1016/j.mehy.2012.04.028.

[119] Cesare AJ, Griffith JD. Telomeric DNA in ALT cells is characterized by free telomeric circles and heterogeneous t-loops. *Mol Cell Biol.* 2004;24(22):9948-57. http://mcb.asm.org/content/24/22/9948.long

[120] Wang RC, Smogorzewska A, de Lange T. Homologous recombination generates T-loop-sized deletions at human telomeres. *Cell.* 2004;119(3):355-68. http://www.cell.com/retrieve/pii/S0092867404009924

[121] Henson JD, Cao Y, Huschtscha LI, Chang AC, Au AY, Pickett HA, Reddel RR. DNA C-circles are specific and quantifiable markers of alternative-lengthening-of-telomeres activity. *Nat Biotechnol.* 2009;27(12):1181-5. doi: 10.1038/nbt.1587.

[122] Nabetani A, Ishikawa F. Alternative lengthening of telomeres pathway: recombination-mediated telomere maintenance mechanism in human cells. *J Biochem.* 2011;149(1):5-14. doi: 10.1093/jb/mvq119.

[123] Ogino H, Nakabayashi K, Suzuki M, Takahashi E, Fujii M, Suzuki T, Ayusawa D. Release of telomeric DNA from chromosomes in immortal human cells lacking telomerase activity. *Biochem Biophys Res Commun.* 1998;248(2):223-7. http://www.sciencedirect.com/science/article/pii/S0006291X98988751

[124] Tokutake Y, Matsumoto T, Watanabe T, Maeda S, Tahara H, Sakamoto S, Niida H, Sugimoto M, Ide T, Furuichi Y. Extra-chromosomal telomere repeat DNA in telomerase-negative immortalized cell lines. *Biochem Biophys Res Commun.* 1998;247(3):765-72. http://www.sciencedirect.com/science/article/pii/S0006291X98988763

[125] Yeager TR, Neumann AA, Englezou A, Huschtscha LI, Noble JR, Reddel RR. Telomerase-negative immortalized human cells contain a novel type of promyelocytic leukemia (PML) body. *Cancer Res.* 1999;59(17):4175-9. http://cancerres.aacrjournals.org/content/59/17/4175.long

[126] Perrem K, Colgin LM, Neumann AA, Yeager TR, Reddel RR. Coexistence of alternative lengthening of telomeres and telomerase in hTERT-transfected GM847 cells. *Mol Cell Biol.* 2001;21(12):3862-75. http://mcb.asm.org/content/21/12/3862.long

[127] Jiang WQ, Zhong ZH, Henson JD, Neumann AA, Chang AC, Reddel RR. Suppression of alternative lengthening of telomeres by Sp100-mediated sequestration of the MRE11/RAD50/NBS1 complex. *Mol Cell Biol.* 2005 Apr;25(7):2708-21. Erratum in: Mol Cell Biol. 2005;25(10):4334. http://mcb.asm.org/content/25/7/2708.long

[128] Jiang WQ, Ringertz N. Altered distribution of the promyelocytic leukemia-associated protein is associated with cellular senescence. *Cell Growth Differ.* 1997;8(5):513-22. http://cgd.aacrjournals.org/cgi/reprint/8/5/513

[129] Wu G, Lee WH, Chen PL. NBS1 and TRF1 colocalize at promyelocytic leukemia bodies during late S/G2 phases in immortalized telomerase-negative cells. Implication of NBS1 in alternative lengthening of telomeres. *J Biol Chem.* 2000;275(39):30618-22. http://www.jbc.org/content/275/39/30618.long

[130] Nabetani A, Yokoyama O, Ishikawa F. Localization of hRad9, hHus1, hRad1, and hRad17 and caffeine-sensitive DNA replication at the alternative lengthening of telomeres-associated promyelocytic leukemia body. *J Biol Chem.* 2004;279(24):25849-57. http://www.ncbi.nlm.nih.gov/pubmed/?term=PMID%3A+15075340

[131] Grobelny JV, Godwin AK, Broccoli D. ALT-associated PML bodies are present in viable cells and are enriched in cells in the G(2)/M phase of the cell cycle. *J Cell Sci.* 2000 Dec;113 Pt 24:4577-85. http://jcs.biologists.org/content/113/24/4577.long

[132] Wang RC, Smogorzewska A, de Lange T. Homologous recombination generates T-loop-sized deletions at human telomeres. *Cell.* 2004;119(3):355-68. http://www.cell.com/retrieve/pii/S0092867404009924

[133] Compton SA, Choi JH, Cesare AJ, Ozgür S, Griffith JD. Xrcc3 and Nbs1 are required for the production of extrachromosomal telomeric circles in human alternative lengthening of telomere cells. *Cancer Res.* 2007;67(4):1513-9. http://cancerres.aacrjournals.org/content/67/4/1513.long

[134] Potts PR, Yu H. The SMC5/6 complex maintains telomere length in ALT cancer cells through SUMOylation of telomere-binding proteins. *Nat Struct Mol Biol.* 2007;14(7):581-90. http://www.nature.com/nsmb/journal/v14/n7/full/nsmb1259.html

[135] Zeng S, Xiang T, Pandita TK, Gonzalez-Suarez I, Gonzalo S, Harris CC, Yang Q. Telomere recombination requires the MUS81 endonuclease. *Nat Cell Biol.* 2009;11(5):616-23. doi: 10.1038/ncb1867.

[136] Tomaska L, Nosek J, Kramara J, Griffith JD. Telomeric circles: universal players in telomere maintenance? *Nat Struct Mol Biol.* 2009;16(10):1010-5. doi: 10.1038/nsmb.1660.

[137] Cesare AJ, Reddel RR. Telomere uncapping and alternative lengthening of telomeres. *Mech Ageing Dev.* 2008;129(1-2):99-108. doi: 10.1016/j.mad.2007.11.006.

[138] Pickett HA, Cesare AJ, Johnston RL, Neumann AA, Reddel RR. Control of telomere length by a trimming mechanism that involves generation of t-circles. *EMBO J.* 2009;28(7):799-809. doi: 10.1038/emboj.2009.42.

[139] Bucher N, Britten CD. G2 checkpoint abrogation and checkpoint kinase-1 targeting in the treatment of cancer. *Br J Cancer.* 2008;98(3):523-8. doi: 10.1038/sj.bjc.6604208.

[140] Temime-Smaali N, Guittat L, Wenner T, Bayart E, Douarre C, Gomez D, Giraud-Panis MJ, Londono-Vallejo A, Gilson E, Amor-Guéret M, Riou JF. Topoisomerase IIIalpha is required for normal proliferation and telomere stability in alternative lengthening of telomeres. *EMBO J.* 2008;27(10):1513-24. doi: 10.1038/emboj.2008.74.

[141] Temime-Smaali N, Guittat L, Sidibe A, Shin-ya K, Trentesaux C, Riou JF. The G-quadruplex ligand telomestatin impairs binding of topoisomerase IIIalpha to G-quadruplex-forming oligonucleotides and uncaps telomeres in ALT cells. *PLoS One.* 2009;4(9):e6919. doi: 10.1371/journal.pone.0006919.

[142] Raynaud CM, Hernandez J, Llorca FP, Nuciforo P, Mathieu MC, Commo F, Delaloge S, Sabatier L, André F, Soria JC. DNA damage repair and telomere length in normal breast, preneoplastic lesions, and invasive cancer. *Am J Clin Oncol.* 2010;33(4):341-5. doi: 10.1097/COC.0b013e3181b0c4c2.

[143] Lundblad V, Blackburn EH. An alternative pathway for yeast telomere maintenance rescues est1- senescence. *Cell.* 1993 Apr 23;73(2):347-60. http://www.cell.com/retrieve/pii/009286749390234H

[144] Bryan TM, Englezou A, Gupta J, Bacchetti S, Reddel RR. Telomere elongation in immortal human cells without detectable telomerase activity. *EMBO J.* 1995;14(17):4240-8. http://www.ncbi.nlm.nih.gov/pmc/articles/PMC394507/

[145] Murnane JP, Sabatier L, Marder BA, Morgan WF. Telomere dynamics in an immortal human cell line. *EMBO J.* 1994;13(20):4953-62. http://www.ncbi.nlm.nih.gov/pmc/articles/PMC395436/

[146] Rogan EM, Bryan TM, Hukku B, Maclean K, Chang AC, Moy EL, Englezou A, Warneford SG, Dalla-Pozza L, Reddel RR. Alterations in p53 and p16INK4 expression and telomere length during spontaneous immortalization of Li-Fraumeni syndrome fibroblasts. *Mol Cell Biol.* 1995;15(9):4745-53. http://mcb.asm.org/content/15/9/4745.long

[147] Dunham MA, Neumann AA, Fasching CL, Reddel RR. Telomere maintenance by recombination in human cells. *Nat Genet.* 2000;26(4):447-50. http://www.nature.com/ng/journal/v26/n4/full/ng1200_447.html

[148] Bechter OE, Shay JW, Wright WE. The frequency of homologous recombination in human ALT cells. *Cell Cycle.* 2004;3(5):547-9. http://www.landesbioscience.com/journals/cc/article/850/

[149] Londoño-Vallejo JA, Der-Sarkissian H, Cazes L, Bacchetti S, Reddel RR. Alternative lengthening of telomeres is characterized by high rates of telomeric exchange. *Cancer Res.* 2004;64(7):2324-7. http://cancerres.aacrjournals.org/content/64/7/2324.long

[150] Varley H, Pickett HA, Foxon JL, Reddel RR, Royle NJ. Molecular characterization of inter-telomere and intra-telomere mutations in human ALT cells. *Nat Genet.* 2002;30(3):301-5. http://www.nature.com/ng/journal/v30/n3/full/ng834.html

[151] Wilson DM 3rd, Thompson LH. Molecular mechanisms of sister-chromatid exchange. *Mutat Res.* 2007;616(1-2):11-23. http://www.sciencedirect.com/science/article/pii/S0027510706003174

[152] Nabetani A, Ishikawa F. Unusual telomeric DNAs in human telomerase-negative immortalized cells. *Mol Cell Biol.* 2009;29(3):703-13. doi: 10.1128/MCB.00603-08.

[153] Bailey SM, Brenneman MA, Goodwin EH. Frequent recombination in telomeric DNA may extend the proliferative life of telomerase-negative cells. *Nucleic Acids Res.* 2004;32(12):3743-51. http://nar.oxfordjournals.org/content/32/12/3743.long

[154] Falconer E, Chavez EA, Henderson A, Poon SS, McKinney S, Brown L, Huntsman DG, Lansdorp PM. Identification of sister chromatids by DNA template strand sequences. *Nature.* 2010;463(7277):93-7. doi: 10.1038/nature08644.

[155] Henson JD, Neumann AA, Yeager TR, Reddel RR. Alternative lengthening of telomeres in mammalian cells. *Oncogene.* 2002;21(4):598-610. http://www.nature.com/onc/journal/v21/n4/full/1205058a.html

[156] Groff-Vindman C, Cesare AJ, Natarajan S, Griffith JD, McEachern MJ. Recombination at long mutant telomeres produces tiny single- and double-stranded telomeric circles. *Mol Cell Biol.* 2005;25(11):4406-12. http://mcb.asm.org/content/25/11/4406.long

[157] Vousden KH, Lane DP. p53 in health and disease. *Nat Rev Mol Cell Biol.* 2007;8(4): 275-83. http://www.nature.com/nrm/journal/v8/n4/full/nrm2147.html

[158] Jansson M, Durant ST, Cho EC, Sheahan S, Edelmann M, Kessler B, La Thangue NB. Arginine methylation regulates the p53 response. *Nat Cell Biol.* 2008;10(12):1431-9. doi: 10.1038/ncb1802.

[159] Durant ST, Cho EC, La Thangue NB. p53 methylation--the Arg-ument is clear. *Cell Cycle.* 2009;8(6):801-2. http://www.landesbioscience.com/journals/cc/article/7850/

[160] Lee JH, Paull TT. Activation and regulation of ATM kinase activity in response to DNA double-strand breaks. *Oncogene.* 2007;26(56):7741-8. http://www.nature.com/onc/journal/v26/n56/full/1210872a.html

[161] Zhong ZH, Jiang WQ, Cesare AJ, Neumann AA, Wadhwa R, Reddel RR. Disruption of telomere maintenance by depletion of the MRE11/RAD50/NBS1 complex in cells that use alternative lengthening of telomeres. *J Biol Chem.* 2007;282(40):29314-22. http://www.jbc.org/content/282/40/29314.long

[162] Li B, Reddy S, Comai L. Depletion of Ku70/80 reduces the levels of extrachromosomal telomeric circles and inhibits proliferation of ALT cells. *Aging (Albany NY).* 2011;3(4):395-406. http://www.impactaging.com/papers/v3/n4/full/100308.html

[163] Saharia A, Stewart SA. FEN1 contributes to telomere stability in ALT-positive tumor cells. *Oncogene.* 2009;28(8):1162-7. doi: 10.1038/onc.2008.458.

[164] Zeng S, Yang Q. The MUS81 endonuclease is essential for telomerase negative cell proliferation. *Cell Cycle.* 2009;8(14):2157-60. http://www.landesbioscience.com/journals/cc/article/9149/

[165] Röth A, Harley CB, Baerlocher GM. Imetelstat (GRN163L)--telomerase-based cancer therapy. *Recent Results Cancer Res.* 2010;184:221-34. doi: 10.1007/978-3-642-01222-8_16.

[166] Ouellette MM, Wright WE, Shay JW. Targeting telomerase-expressing cancer cells. *J Cell Mol Med.* 2011;15(7):1433-42. doi: 10.1111/j.1582-4934.2011.01279.x.

[167] Siddiqa A, Cavazos DA, Marciniak RA. Targeting telomerase. *Rejuvenation Res.* 2006;9(3):378-90. http://online.liebertpub.com/doi/abs/10.1089/rej.2006.9.378

[168] Huppert JL. Structure, location and interactions of G-quadruplexes. *FEBS J.* 2010;277(17):3452-8. doi: 10.1111/j.1742-4658.2010.07758.x.

[169] Hiyama E, Hiyama K, Yokoyama T, Matsuura Y, Piatyszek MA, Shay JW. Correlating telomerase activity levels with human neuroblastoma outcomes. *Nat Med.* 1995;1(3):249-55. PMID: 7585042

[170] Cerone MA, Londono-Vallejo JA, Bacchetti S. Telomere maintenance by telomerase and by recombination can coexist in human cells. *Hum Mol Genet.* 2001;10(18): 1945-52. http://hmg.oxfordjournals.org/content/10/18/1945.long

[171] Hiyama E, Hiyama K, Nishiyama M, Reynolds CP, Shay JW, Yokoyama T. Differential gene expression profiles between neuroblastomas with high telomerase activity and low telomerase activity. *J Pediatr Surg.*;38(12):1730-4. http://www.jpedsurg.org/article/S0022-3468(03)00640-7/abstract

[172] Cerone MA, Autexier C, Londoño-Vallejo JA, Bacchetti S. A human cell line that maintains telomeres in the absence of telomerase and of key markers of ALT. *Oncogene.* 2005;24(53):7893-901. http://www.nature.com/onc/journal/v24/n53/full/1208934a.html

Section 3

Interface with Clinical Medicine

Chapter 15

Genetic Polymorphisms of DNA Repair Genes and DNA Repair Capacity Related to Aflatoxin B1 (AFB1)-Induced DNA Damages

Qiang Xia, Xiao-Ying Huang, Feng Xue,
Jian-Jun Zhang, Bo Zhai, De-Chun Kong,
Chao Wang, Zhao-Quan Huang and Xi-Dai Long

Additional information is available at the end of the chapter

http://dx.doi.org/10.5772/53967

1. Introduction

Aflatoxin B1 (AFB1) is an important aflatoxin produced by some strains of the moulds Aspergillus parasiticus and Aspergillus flavus [1-3]. This aflatoxin was discovered as a contaminant of human and animal food, especially peanuts (ground nuts), core, soya sauce, and fermented soy beans in tropical areas such as the Southeastern China as a result of fungal contamination during growth and after harvest which under hot and humid conditions in the late 1950s and early 1960s [1-4]. Increasing evidences have shown that AFB1 exposure levels are consistent with hepatocellular carcinoma (HCC) risk values [1, 2, 4-7]. DNA damage by AFB1 plays the central role of carcinogenesis of HCC-related to this toxin in the toxic studies [2, 8-10]. Today, AFB1 has been classified as a known human carcinogen by the International Agency for Research on Cancer [1, 2, 5, 10, 11]. However, more and more epidemiological evidence has exhibited that although many people are exposed to the same levels of AFB1, only a relatively small proportion of exposure person develop HCC [6, 12-23]. This indicates individual DNA repair capacity related to AFB1-induced DNA damage might be associated with HCC carcinogenesis [4].

This study attempts to briefly review currently available data on genetic polymorphisms of DNA repair genes and DNA repair capacity related to AFB1-induced DNA Damages, with emphasis on: (1) DNA damage types, (2) DNA repair pathways, (3) the role of DNA repair genetic polymorphisms in the repair process of DNA damage by AFB1, and (4) the elucidation of corresponding DNA repair capacity. Additionally, we summarized the association between genetic polymorphisms of DNA repair genes and AFB1-related DNA repair capacity via a meta-analysis based on published data.

2. AFB1's chemistry

In 1963, Asao *et al.* accomplished the structural elucidation of AFB1 and found AFB1 was a member of aflatoxins family (AFF) highly substituted coumarins containing a fused dihydrofurofuran moiety [24]. AFF consists of four members: AFB1, aflatoxin B2 (AFB2), aflatoxin G1 (AFG1), and aflatoxin G2 (AFG2). Among of these members, AFB1 is the most important toxin and structurally is characterized by fusion of a cyclopentenone ring to the lactone ring of the coumarin moiety [24]. AFB1 is so named because of its strong blue fluorescence in ultraviolet light. These properties facilitated the very rapid development in the early 1960s of methods for monitoring peanuts, cores, grains, and other food commodities for the presence of the toxins (Fig. 1) [1]. This type AFF possesses an unsaturated bond at the 8,9 position on the terminal furan ring, and subsequent studies have demonstrated that AFB1 may be metabolized by cytochrome P450 (CYP) enzymes to its reactive form at this position, also called AFB1-8,9-epoxide (AFB1-epoxide) [2, 10]. AFB1-epoxide can covalently bind to DNA and induce DNA damage, thus this epoxidation at at the 8,9 position is critical for AFB1's DNA genotoxic and carcinogenic potency [2]. Noticeably, another important chemiatric feature of AFB1 is the attraction of liver organ, possibly because the metabolic enzymes CYPs are mainly produced by liver [2, 10, 25].

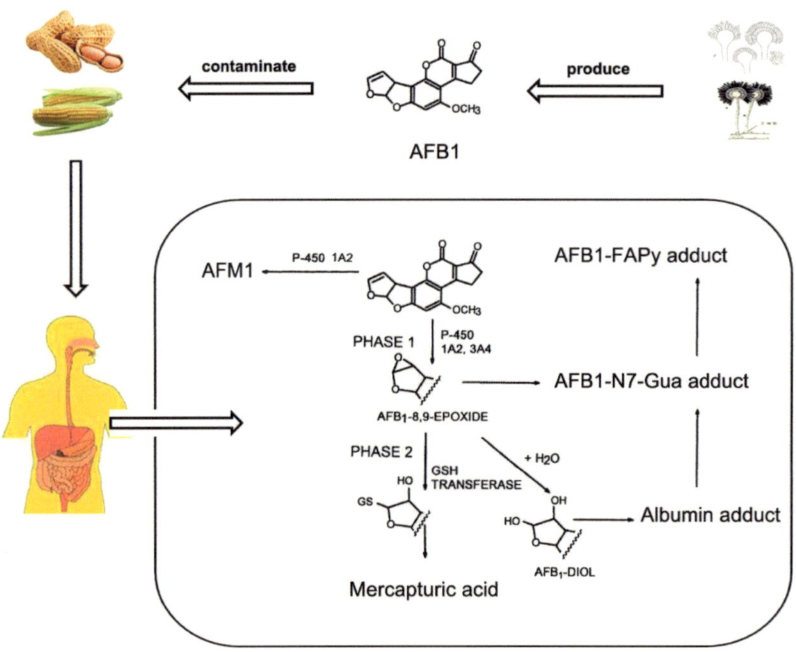

Figure 1. Biotransformation pathways for AFB1. AFB1, mainly produced by the moulds Aspergillus parasiticus (right upper figure) and Aspergillus flavus (right under figure), is metabolized by cytochrome P450 enzymes to its reactive form, AFB1-8,9-epoxide (AFB1-epoxide). AFB1-epoxide covalently binds to DNA strands and results in the formation of AFB1-DNA adducts (including AFB1-N7-Gua adduct and AFB1-FAPy adduct).

3. DNA damage by AFB1

Several previous reviews have significantly summarized the DNA toxicity of AFB1 [1, 2, 8]. Generally, the severity of DNA toxic effects in human or animals vary with exposure levels, exposure years and nutritional status [1, 2, 26]. For large doses of exposure, this agent can induce acute damage of DNA such as inhabiting DNA synthesis, decreasing DNA-dependent RNA polymerase activity, and restraining messenger RNA (mRNA) and protein synthesis, and subsequently resulting in the lethal changes of liver cells: hepatocellular severe degeneration and necrosis [1, 2].

For long-times and low-levels exposure mainly induces chronic DNA damage [1, 2]. This damage can result in neoplasia, primarily HCC, in many animals or human. Chronic DNA damages induced by AFB1 include AFB1-DNA adducts, oxidative DNA damage, DNA strand break damage, and gene mutation [1, 2, 4].

3.1. AFB1-DNA adducts

AFB1-DNA adducts, including 8,9-di-hydro-8-(N7-guanyl)-9-hydroxy–AFB1 (AFB1-N7-Gua) adduct and formamidopyridine AFB1 (AFB1-FAPy) adduct (Fig. 1), is the main type of AFB1-induced DNA damage [1-4, 25-39]. Among these AFB1-DNA adducts, AFB1-N7-Gua adduct is the most common type identified and confirmed in vivo researches [2, 25]. This type adduct is formed from two pathways: (1) Binding reaction of AFB1-epoxide with DNA; and (2) enzymatic oxidation of AFP1, AFM1, and others with unsaturated in the 8,9-position [2, 25]. In the first pathway, the formations of AFB1-N7-Gua adduct proceeds by a precovalent intercalation complex between double-stranded DNA and the highly electrophilic, unstable AFB1-epoxide isomer. After that, the induction of a positive charge on the imidazole portion of the formed AFB1-N^7-Gua adduct gives rise to another important a DNA adduct, a ring-opened AFB1-FAPy adduct. Accumulation of AFB1-FAPy adduct is characterized by time-dependence, non-enzyme, and may be of biological basis of genes mutation because of its apparent persistence in DNA. Another pathway only gives rise to minor AFB1-DNA adducts [1, 2, 25]. Additionally, some other DNA-adducts types, ex. covalent binding of AFB1 to adenosine or cytosine in DNA, has also been reported, however, needing more evidences to support this adducts [2].

Although AFB1-DNA adducts are mainly produced in liver cells, they are also found in the peripheral blood white cells [2]. Recent studies have shown that the levels of AFB1-DNA adduct of the peripheral blood white cells are positively and lineally correlated with that of liver cells, implying analysis of AFB1-DNA adducts in the peripheral blood white cells may substitute for the elucidation of tissular levels of adducts [40].

3.2. Oxidative DNA damage

In the process of agent AFB1 metabolism, this agent can induced reactive oxygen species (ROS) [2]. Especially, the metabolic particulate phases, including I and II phase involved by detoxicate enzymes such as CYP and glutathione S-transferase (GST), is postulated to contain long-lived ROS that can lead to oxidative DNA damage [2, 4]. Nowadays, ROS have also been suggested to be involved in the progression of chronic liver disease and the occurrence of HCC; whereas its' subsequent Oxidative DNA damage is generally regarded as a significant contributory cause of cancer from environmental exposures such as AFB1 exposure [41]. Of oxidative DNA damage, 8-oxodeoxyguanosine (8-oxodG), a kind of especial DNA adduct, is found as a sensitive marker of the DNA damage due to hydroxyl radical attack at the C8 of guanine [2, 4, 25, 42]. This adduct, different from the aforementioned AFB1-DNA adducts, is the most abundant endogenous DNA lesion caused by ROS, and has been classified as a biomarker of oxidative DNA damage [2, 10, 43, 44].

Previous studies have shown that in vitro treatment of hepatocytes with AFB1 resulted in a dose-dependent increase in ROS formation [45]; whereas exposure of rats to AFB1 produced a time- and dose-dependent increase in 8-oxodG in hepatic DNA [46, 47]. In 2007, Wu, *et al.* investigated the association between AFB1 exposure levels and oxidative damage levels in high AFB1 areas from Taiwan, China [48]. In this case–control study nested within a community-based cohort (74 HCC cases and 290), researchers tested the levels of urinary excretion of 8-oxodG, a biomarker of oxidative DNA damage and urinary AFB1 metabolites, a biomarker of AFB1 exposure, through enzyme-linked immunosorbent assays (ELISA). Results showed 8-oxodG levels were significantly positive correlated with AFB1 exposure, suggesting AFB1 exposure should induce oxidative DNA damage [48]. Together, these data suggest that AFB1-induced oxidative DNA damage may constitute an important pathway in AFB1 toxicity.

3.3. DNA strand break damage

Previous reviewed adducts are capable of forming subsequent repair-resistant adducts, depurination, or lead to error-prone DNA repair resulting in single-strand breaks (SSBs) and double-strand breaks (DSBs). SSBs and DSBs are two kinds of important DNA damage types by AFB1 exposure. For SSBs, there are three pathways to produce this type DNA damage under the AFB1 exposure conditions: direct attack by ROS, through base hydrolysis, and enzymatic consequence of the repair of spontaneous base damage and base loss (such as resulting from abasic AP. sites arising spontaneously or from the action of glycosylases in the process of BER pathway) [49-51]. As the most abundant lesion occurring in cellular DNA, SSBs can play havoc with replication and transcription if not efficiently eliminated. However, they might cause other DNA damage such as genic mutations, DSBs, or carcinogenesis of cells [51, 52]. While DSBs is rare and severe DNA damage type among DNA damage induced by AFB1 exposure [25], mainly produced under the high-dose AFB1 exposure conditions. This damage can lead to chromosomal rearrangements at the first mitosis after exposure to the DNA strand-breaking agent [53].

3.4. Gene mutations

For genes mutations induced by AFB1 exposure, the experimental and theoretical researches are briefly on the p53 gene [54-56]. Reaction with DNA at the N^7 position of guanine preferentially causes a G:C > T:A mutation in codon 249 of this gene, leading to an amino acid sub-

http://dx.doi.org/10.5772/53967

stitution of arginine to serine [54-56]. In high AFB1-exposure areas, this mutation is present in more than 40% of HCC and can be detected in serum DNA of patients with preneoplastic lesions and HCC. While codon 249 transversion mutations are either very rare or absent in low or no AFB1-exposure areas [4]. Using the human p53 gene in an in vitro assay, codon 249 has been exhibited to be a preferential site for formation of AFB1-N^7-Gua adducts evidence consistent with a role for AFB1 in the mutations observed in HCC [57-65]. Therefore, the codon 249 mutation of p53 gene has been defined as the hot-spot mutation of p53 gene (TP53M) resulting from AFB1 and has become the molecular symbol of HCC induced by AFB1 exposure. The frequency of TP53M is also regarded as the molecular biomarker of AFB1-related DNA repair capacity [4].

4. DNA repair pathways of AFB1-related DNA damage

A wide diversity of DNA damage induced by AFB1 exposure, if not repaired, may cause chromosomal aberrations, micronuclei, sister chromatid exchange, unscheduled DNA synthesis, and chromosomal strand breaks, and can be converted into gene mutations and genomic instability, which in turn results in cellular malignant transformation [4]. Nevertheless, human cells have evolved surveillance mechanisms that monitor the integrity of genome to minimize the consequences of detrimental mutations [9]. AFB1-induced DNA damage can be repaired through the following pathways: nucleotide excision repair (NER), base excision repair (BER), single-strand break repair (SSBR), and double-strand break repair (DSBR) [4, 25].

4.1. NER pathway

NER pathway, a major DNA repair pathways in human cells featuring genomic DNA damage, can remove structurally such diverse lesions as pyrimidine dimers, irradiative damage, and bulky chemical adducts, and DNA damage from carcinogens and some chemotherapeutic drugs [66]. To date, the mechanism of this pathway is well understood and has been reconstituted in vitro. It consists of several sequential steps: lesion sensing, opening of a denaturation bubble, incision of the damaged strand, displacement of the lesion-containing oligonucleotide, gap filling, and ligation [66, 67]. In the fibroblast cells with the deficiency of xeroderma pigmentosum A (XPA) gene, conversion of the initial AFB1-N7-Gua adduct to the AFB1-FAPy adduct has been found to be more extensive. This suggests that NER should be a major mechanism for enzymatic repair of AFB1 adducts. Its defects lead to severe diseases related AFB1 exposure, including liver injury and HCC [4].

4.2. BER

Of the oxidative DNA damage resulting from AFB1 exposure, the formation of 8-oxodG is thought to be important due to being abundant and highly mutagenic and hepatocarcinogenesis [4, 25]. The 8-oxodG lesions are repaired primarily through the BER pathway. The BER pathway facilitates DNA repair through two general pathways: a. the short-patch BER pathway, leading to a repair tract of a single nucleotide; b. the long-patch BER pathway, producing a repair tract of at least two nucleotides [68, 69]. In these two repair sub-pathways, DNA glycosylases play a central role because they can recognize and catalyze the removal of damaged bases [68, 69]. This suggests that the defect of DNA glycosylases should be related to the decreasing capacity of the BER pathway and might increase the risk of such toxicity as AFB1 [4, 25].

4.3. SSBR

SSB is a relative severe type of DNA damage produced by AFB1 exposure. If not repaired, it can disrupt transcription and replication and can be converted into potentially clastogenic and/or lethal DSBs [51]. This DNA damage is repaired via SSBR pathway. SSBR pathway includes four basic steps: a. SSB detection and signaling, through poly (ADP-ribose) polymerase (PARP); b. DNA break end processing, through the role of polynucleotide kinase (PNK), AP endonuclease-1 (APE1), DNA polymerase β (Pol β), tyrosyl phosphodiesterase 1 (TDP1), and flap endonuclease-1 (FEN-1); c. gap filling, involving in multiple DNA polymerases; d. DNA ligation, involving in multiple DNA ligases [49, 50, 52]. This pathway mainly plays an important role in the repair process of SSBs induced AFB1.

4.4. DSBR

DSBs, although only make up a very small proportion of AFB1-induced DNA damage, are critical lesions that can result in cell death or a wide variety of genetic alterations including large- or small-scale deletions, loss of heterozygosity, translocations, and chromosome loss [70]. This type damage is repaired DSBR consisting of non-homologous end-joining (NHEJ) and homologous recombination (HR) [71, 72]. There are several decades DNA repair genes involve in DSBR pathway and the defects in these genes cause genome instability and promote tumorigenesis [71-77]. During the process of damage removed by aforementioned repair pathways, DNA repair genes play a central role, because their function determines DNA repair capacity [4]. It has been shown that reduction in DNA repair capacity related to DNA repair genes is associated with increasing frequency of genic mutation, levels of DNA adducts, and risk of cancers [8, 78]. Thus, genetic polymorphisms in DNA repair genes might be correlated with AFB1-related DNA repair capacity.

5. The elucidation of DNA repair capacity related to AFB1-induced DNA damage

As shown in the previous review, two main characteristics of AFB1-induced DNA damage are AFB1-DNA adducts and the hot-spot mutation of tumor suppressor gene p53 at codon 249 (TP53M) [4, 25]. Thus, DNA repair capacity related to this type DNA damage might be elucidated using the analysis of AFB1-DNA-adducts levels and TP53M frequency in the liver tissues or other tissues. For AFB1-DNA adducts, many researchers in the relative fields regard AFB1-FAPy adduct as a validated biomarker of AFB1 exposure based on as following reasons: (1) that AFB1-FAPy adduct is the imidazole ring-opened product of AFB1-N7-Gua adduct, also the stable of form of the later adduct, and may play an important role in the development of HCC. Moreover, the accumulation of this adduct is time-dependent and non-enzymatic, and may have potential biological importance because of its apparent persistence in DNA; (2) that AFB1-N7-Gua adduct is unstable and easily lost from DNA. Increasing evidences have exhibited that AFB1-FAPy-adducts levels in the liver or placenta tissues are lineally correlated with AFB1 exposure levels and HCC risk [79, 80], suggesting this adduct should be regarded as a biomarker for DNA repair capacity related to AFB1-induced DNA damage. Remarkably, the monoclonal antibodies recognizing AFB1-FAPy adduct have been developed by several research groups. These types of antibodies are not only used to orientationally and semi-quantitatively test AFB1-DNA adduct information in the tissue specimens through immunochemistry (IHC), but to quantitatively analyze the levels of this adduct using a competitive enzyme-linked immunosorbent assay (ELISA) in human liver and placenta tissue specimens. Additionally, a quantitative indirect immunofluorescence method using monoclonal antibody 6A10 has also been developed to measure AFB1-DNA adducts in liver tissues. In 2009, Long *et al.* evaluated the validation of AFB1-FAPy adduct in DNA samples from peripheral blood leukocytes representing AFB1 exposure levels [40]. Through linear regression analysis of the adduct levels in DNA samples from peripheral blood leukocytes and from liver tissue specimens, they found peripheral blood leukocytes' adduct levels were positively and linearly related to AFB1-DNA adduct levels of the HCC cancerous tissue. These data suggested that the levels of peripheral blood leukocytes' DNA adducts were representative of the tissues' DNA-adduct levels and might be regard as a biomarker for AFB1 exposure [4, 25, 40, 78]. Together, AFB1-FAPy adduct in DNA from such tissues as liver and placenta or from such as blood leukocytes should be potential biological importance in the elucidation of DNA repair capacity related to AFB1-caused DNA damage.

As regard of the mutations of p53 gene, because AFB1 exposure results in G to T transversion in both bacteria and human cells and AFB1 preferentially binds to codon 249 of p53 gene, as previous mentioned, AFB1 mainly induces the transversion of G → T in the third position at codon 249 of TP53M. The frequent value of TP53M is more persistent biomarker and more directly represents DNA repair capacity compared with AFB1-DNA adducts. In the studies from higher AFB1 exposure areas, researchers have found TP53M frequency associates with AFB1 exposure levels and HCC risk. Thus, this mutation is the selective elucidative marker for DNA repair capacity correlated with AFB1-induced DNA damage as well as AFB1-DNA adducts.

Additionally, HCC is the most common malignant tumors caused by AFB1 exposure. More and more epidemiological studies have shown AFB1-related HCC risk is related to different DNA repair capacity [4, 8, 15, 22, 40, 78, 81-90], suggesting that tumor risk value might be regard as a selective elucidative marker for DNA repair capacity correlated with AFB1-induced DNA damage.

6. Genetic polymorphisms of DNA repair genes involved in NER pathway for AFB1-related DNA damage repair

Accumulating evidences have implied that genetic polymorphisms in NER genes are associated with DNA repair capacity related to AFB1-induced DNA damage. Molecular epidemiology studies in this field are mainly from high AFB1 exposure areas such as in China. To date, two genes involved in NER pathway, namely xeroderma pigmentosum C (XPC) and xeroderma pigmentosum D (XPD), have been investigated in the DNA repair capacity analysis.

6.1. XPC

XPC gene (Genbank accession NO. AC090645), consisting of 16 exons and 15 introns, spans 33kb on chromosome 3p25. This gene encodes a 940-amino acid protein, an important DNA damage recognition molecule which plays an important role in NER pathway. XPC protein binds tightly with another important NER protein HR23B to form a stable XPC-HR23B complex, the first protein component that recognizes and binds to the DNA damage sites [91-98]. XPC-HR23B complex can recognize a variety of DNA adducts formed by exogenous carcinogens such as AFB1 and binds to the DNA damage sites [4, 91, 99]. Therefore, it may play a role in the process of DNA repair of DNA damage related to AFB1 exposure.

Some recent studies have showed that defects in XPC have been related to many types of malignant tumors [99-114]. Transgenic mice researches have also exhibited predisposition to many kinds of neoplasms in mice model with XPC gene knockout [115]. Moreover, pathological and cellular studies have shown that increasing expression of this gene is associated with hepatocarcinogenesis [116]. Together, these studies suggest the genetic polymorphisms localizing at conserved sites of XPC gene might modify the risk of HCC induced by AFB1 exposure and decrease DNA repair capacity related to AFB1-related DNA damage. Recently, four studies from high AFB1-exposure areas have supported abovementioned hypothesis [84, 89, 101, 117].

The first study conducted by Cai *et al.*[117] is from Shunde area, Guangdong Province which is characterized by high AFB1 exposure and high incidence rate of HCC. Researchers analyzed the association between two common polymorphisms—Ala499Val and Lys939Gln—of XPC gene and risk of HCC via an 1-1 case-control study (including 78 HCC patients and 78 age- and sex-matching controls) method, and found these two polymorphisms modified HCC risk [adjusted odds ratios (ORs) were 3.77 with 95% confidence interval (CI) 1.34-12.89 for Ala499Val and 6.78 with 95% CI 2.03-22.69]. Although they did not directly evaluated the effects of genetic polymorphisms of XPC gene and DNA repair capacity related to AFB1-caused DNA damage, study population in their study is from high AFB1 exposure areas and.

The other three studies, from Guangxi Zhuang Autonomous Region which is the most common of high AFB1 exposure area all over the world [4, 118], directly investigated the modifying effects of genetic polymorphisms XPC on AFB1-related DNA repair capacity and HCC risk based on hospitals via molecular epidemiological studies [84, 89, 101]. Their results showed XPC codon 939 Gln alleles increased about 2-times risk of HCC and decreased AFB1-related DNA repair capacity. Furthermore, Wu, *et al.*[89] and Long, *et al.* [84] quantitatively elucidated AFB-exposure time and levels and their interactive effects with the genetic polymorphisms of XPC gene and found some evidence of AFB1 exposure-risk genotypes of XPC codon 939 on AFB1-related DNA repair capacity (HCC risk: XPC risk genotypes and $18.38 > 1.11 \times 4.62$ for the interaction of AFB1-exposure levels and XPC risk genotypes; $22.33 > 1.88 \times 8.69$ for the interaction of AFB1-exposure time).

Additionally, Long, *et al.* [84] also observed that Gln alleles at codon 939 of XPC gene was associated with the decrease of XPC expression levels in cancerous tissues ($r = -0.369$, $P < 0.001$) and with the poorer overall survival of HCC patients (the median survival times are 30, 25, and 19 months for patients with XPC gene codon 939 Lys/Lys, Lys/Gln, and Gln/Gln respectively). Interestingly, this decreasing 5-years survival rates would be noticeable under high AFB1 exposure conditions (the median survival times are 17 month for the joint of XPC gene codon 939 Gln/Gln and high AFB1-exposure level and 15 months for the joint of XPC gene codon 939 Gln/Gln and long-term AFB1-exposure time) [84].

As a result, these data suggest that genetic polymorphism at codon 939 of XPC gene is not only a genetic determinant in the DNA repair process of DNA damage induced by AFB1 exposure, and a risk and prognostic factor influencing HCC developing, but also is an independent genetic factor of evaluating DNA repair capacity related to AFB1-caused DNA damage. A possible reason is that this genetic polymorphism down-regulates XPC expression [84] and decrease the repair function of XPC protein [116].

However, Li *et al.* [101] reported that the proportional distribution of the Val/Val genotype at codon 499 of XPC gene did not differ between HCC cases and controls in Guangxi Zhuang Autonomous Region, China ($P > 0.05$), dissimilar to the data from another high AFB1 exposure area of China, Guangdong Province, suggesting this genetic polymorphism might not modify AFB1-related DNA repair capacity. Possible explanations for these inconsistent finding may be either due to unknown confounders or due to small sample size.

6.2. XPD

XPD protein, a DNA-dependent ATPase/helicase encoded by DNA repair gene XPD (also called excision repair cross-complementing rodent repair deficiency complementation group 2 (ERCC2), COFS2, EM9, or TTD.) (Genbank ID. 2068) which spans about 20 kb on chromosome 19q13.3 and contains 23 exons and 22 introns is one of seven central proteins in the NER pathway [119-122]. This protein is associated with the TFIIH transcription-factor complex, and plays a role in NER pathway [66, 67, 119-121, 123-125]. During NER, XPD participates in the opening of the DNA helix to allow the excision of the DNA fragment containing the damaged base [119-122].

There are four described polymorphisms that induce amino acid changes in the protein: at codons 199 (Ile to Met), at codon 201 (His to Tyr), at codon 312 (Asp to Asn) and at codon 751 (Lys to Gln) [123]. To date, the first two polymorphisms have not investigated because they are quite rare (~0.04%) in most population, whereas the latter two polymorphisms in conserved region of XPD have been extensively studied [123]. Several groups have done genotype-phenotype analyses with these two polymorphisms and have shown that the variant allele genotypes are associated with low DNA repair ability [126, 127]. Recent studies have showed the polymorphisms at codon 312 and 751 of XPD are correlated with DNA-adducts levels, p53 gene mutation, and cancers risk [86, 123, 128-131]. In a hospital-based case-control study conducted in a high AFB1 exposure area [40], Long, *et al.* found that the variant XPD codon 751 genotypes (namely Lys/Gln and Gln/Gln) detected by TaqMan-MGB PCR was significantly different between HCC cases (35.9% and 20.1% for Lys/Gln and Gln/Gln, respectively) and controls (26.3% for Lys/Gln and 8.6% for Gln/Gln, $P < 0.001$). Individuals having variant alleles had about 1.5- to 2.5-fold risk of developing the cancer (adjusted OR 1.75 and 95% CI 1.30-2.37 for Lys/Gln; adjusted OR 2.47 and 95% CI 1.62-3.76 for Gln/Gln). Based on relative large sample size (including 618 HCC cases and 712 controls), researchers stratified genotypes of XPD codon 751 according to matching factors and observed some evidence of interaction between XPD codon 751 Gln alleles and sex. These female with Gln alleles featured increasing HCC risk compared with those without these alleles. Moreover, the multiple interactive effects of between mutant genotypes of XPD gene codon 751 environment variant AFB1 or another NER gene XPC on HCC risk were also found, with interactive value 0.85, 1.04, and 1.71 for AFB1-exposure years, AFB1-exposure levels, and XPC gene codon 939 risk genotypes ($P_{interaction} < 0.05$).

Together, these results suggest the genetic polymorphisms at conserved sequence of XPD gene such as at codon 751 may have potential effect on AFB1-related HCC susceptibility. This supports different AFB1-related DNA repair capacity might be modified by genetic polymorphisms at codon 751 in DNA repair gene XPD. However, the study from AFB1-exposure areas shows that the genetic polymorphism at codon 312 in XPD polymorphism is not significantly correlated with DNA repair capacity related AFB1-induced DNA damage [4, 40].

7. Genetic polymorphisms of DNA repair genes involved in BER pathway for AFB1-related DNA damage repair

As previous described, DNA glycosylases play a central role in the BER pathway because they can recognize and catalyze the removal of damaged bases [68, 69]. Among having been reported genetic polymorphisms of DNA glycosylases, only human 8-oxoguanine DNA glycosylase (hOGG1) correlates with DNA repair capacity [132-143]. This gene (Genbank ID# 4968), also called HMMH, OGG1, MUTM, OGH1, 8-hydroxyguanine DNA glycosylase, AP lyase, DNA-apurinic or apyrimidinic site lyase, and N-glycosylase/DNA lyase, consisting of 7 exons and 6 introns, spans 17 kb on chromosome 3p26.2 (PubMed). This gene encodes a 546-amino acid protein, a specific DNA glycosylase that catalyzes the release of 8-$_{oxod}$G and the cleavage of DNA at the AP site [142]. Genetic structure study has shown the presence of several polymorphisms within hOGG1 locus [136]. Among these polymorphisms, the polymorphism at position 1245 in exon 7 causes an amino acid substitution (namely Ser to Cys) at codon 326, suggesting this polymorphism may glycosylase function and decrease DNA repair capacity [136].

In the past twenty years, increasing epidemiological evidences have validated aforementioned the hypothesis [132-144]. In 2003, Peng, *et al.* [138] analyzed the correlation among 8-$_{oxod}$G levels, hOGG1 expression, and hOGG1 Cys326Ser polymorphism in the high AFB1 exposure areas Guangxi Autonomous Region. They found that individuals having genotypes with hOGG1 codon 326 Cys alleles faced lower level of hOGG1 expression and higher 8-$_{oxod}$G levels. Supporting their results, Cheng, *et al.* [141] reported that hOGG1 expression was significantly linear correlated with HCC. Recently, using the molecular epidemiological methods, Zhang, *et al.* [134] found that the distribution of Cys alleles at codon 326 of hOGG1 in HCC cases (43.0%) significantly differed from in controls (33.1%). Logistic regression analysis next showed that the genotypes with Cys alleles, compared to without this alleles, increased HCC risk of Chinese population, with adjusted OR-value (95% CI) 1.5 (0.79-2.93) for Cys/Ser and 1.9 (0.83-4.55) for Cys/Cys. Similar results are also observed in the study from low AFB1 exposure areas of China [144]. A functional complementation activity assay exhibited that hOGG1 protein encoded by the 326 Cys allele had substantially lower DNA repair activity than that encoded by the 326 Ser allele [140]. Similar results were observed in human cells in vivo [137, 139]. Therefore, low capacity of 8-$_{oxod}$G repair resulting from hOGG1 326 Cys polymorphism might contribute to the persistence of 8-$_{oxod}$G in genomic DNA in vivo, which, in turn, could be associated with increased cancer risk [4, 137, 138].

As a result, these findings suggested the genetic polymorphism at codon 326 of DNA repair gene hOGG1 should modify AFB1-related DNA repair capacity. However, another case-control study from Japan shows this genetic polymorphism is not associated with HCC risk. This might result from lower AFB1 exposure in this area and not showing the relative low DNA repair capacity related to AFB1-induced DNA damage.

8. Genetic polymorphisms of DNA repair genes involved in SSBR pathway for AFB1-related DNA damage repair

SSBR pathway involves in several central DNA repair genes such as XRCC1, poly (ADP-ribose) polymerase-1 (PARP-1), APE (or DNA glycosylase), DNA ligase III, Pol β, and so on [49-51]. Of these DNA repair genes, only XRCC1 is investigated to correlate with AFB1-related DNA repair capacity. This gene, also called RCC, spans about 32 kb on chromosome 19q13.2 and contains 17 exons and 16 introns is one of three submits of DNA repair complex in the SSBR pathway (Gene dbase from PubMed). Its' encoding protein (633 amino acids), consists of three functional domains: N-terminal domain (NTD), central breast cancer susceptibility protein-1 homology C-terminal (BRCT I), and C-terminal breast cancer susceptibility protein-1 homology C-terminal (BRCT II) [4, 51, 145-151]. This protein is directly associated with Pol β, DNA ligase III, and PARP, via their three functional domains and is implicated in the core processes in SSBR and BER pathway [4, 51, 145, 150-152]. Mutant hamster ovary cell lines that lack XRCC1 genes are hypersensitive to DNA damage agents such as ionizing radiation, hydrogen peroxide, and alkylating agents [4, 51]. Furthermore, this kind of cells usually faces increasing frequency of spontaneous chromosome aberrations and deletions. Three single nucleotide polymorphisms in the coding region of XRCC1 gene that lead to amino acid substitution have been described and investigated [25]. Among these polymorphisms, the codon 399 polymorphism is of special concern, because this polymorphism resides in functionally significant regions (BRCT II) and may be related to decreasing DNA repair capacity [85, 153-179].

In 2008, Long, *et al.* [85] investigated the effects of genetic polymorphism at codon 399 in DNA repair gene XRCC1 based on the analysis of 501 AFB1-related HCC samples. They found that the HCC patients with XRCC1 genotypes with 399 Gln alleles (namely: XRCC1 codon 399 Arg/Gln or Gln/Gln) faced a significantly higher frequency of TP53M than those with the wild-type homozygote of XRCC1 [namely: XRCC1 codon 399 Arg/Arg, adjusted odds ratio (OR) = 6.13, 95% confidence interval (CI) = 3.87-9.72 for Arg/Gln; OR = 13.66, 95% CI = 4.44-42.08 for Gln/Gln, respectively]. Additionally, another study from high AFB1 areas Taiwan in China exposure showed the XRCC1 codon 399 Gln alleles were significantly associated with higher levels of AFB1-DNA adducts. Individuals with these alleles were at risk for detectable adducts (OR, 2.4; 95% CI, 1.1–5.4; $P = 0.03$) [80].

As regards of risk biomarker for DNA repair capacity namely AFB1-related HCC risk, a total of fourteen molecular epidemiological studies involving genetic polymorphism at codon 399 of DNA repair gene XRCC1 were found in PubMed database, Sprinker database, Ovid database, Wangfang Database, and Weipu database [22, 81, 83, 162, 164, 175, 180-186], summarized in Table 1. However, associations between this genetic polymorphism and DNA repair capacity have been reported in these case-control studies with the results being contradictory [172, 187]. Possible reasons are as follows: different study population, non-scientific design, the loss of matching methods or improper match, the loss of stratified analysis based on AFB1 exposure information, repeated data, and so on. To avoid above error and achieve more scientific results, we analyzed the possible causes of contradictory using meta-analysis method (Comprehensive Meta-Analysis Version 2, http://www.meta-analysis.com/). Fig. 2, 3, and 4 showed the meta-analysis results of the modifying effects of genetic polymorphism at codon 399 of XRCC1 gene on AFB1-related DNA repair capacity. Based on meta-analysis of overall studies including known published literature (Fig. 2), we found contradictive results; whereas we would observe significant modifying effects of genetic polymorphism at codon 399 of XRCC1 gene on DNA repair capacity related to AFB1-caused DNA damage if these possible repeated studies from the same researchers (Fig. 3) or adding these studies from low/no AFB1 exposure areas (Fig. 4) were excluded. Actually, although Yang, *et al.* [162] and Ren, *et al.* [173] did not observed significantly modifying effects of XRCC1 gene codon 399 polymorphism in crude logistic regression, they found Gln alleles would decrease DNA repair capacity in stratified analysis with susceptive environment variants. A individually matching case-controls demonstrated that subjects having codon 399 Gln alleles might feature remarkably increasing risk of HCC under longer-term AFB1-exposure years or higher AFB1-exposure levels conditions (adjusted OR > 10) [22]. This suggests that the genotypes with codon 399 Gln alleles of XRCC1 should be a risk biomarker of low DNA repair ability related DNA damage by AFB1 exposure.

NO.	Ref.	Year	Population	AFB1 exposure[a]	Methods	Matching Factor	Cases (n)	Controls (n)	Risk value[b] (OR)
1	Yu *et al.* (2003)	2003	Taiwanese	high	case-control	age, sex	577	389	1.54 ($P = 0.129$)
2	Han et al. (2004)	2004	Qidongese	high	case-control	age, sex	69	136	about 1 ($P > 0.05$)
3	Kirk et al. (2005)	2005	Gimbia	high	case-control	age, sex	149	294	2.66 ($P < 0.05$)
4	Long et al.(2005)	2005	Guangxiese	high	case-control	age, sex, HBV, HCV, race	140	536	2.18 ($P = 0.0001$)
5	Long et al.(2006)	2006	Guangxiese	high	case-control	age, sex, HBV, HCV, race	257	649	2.47 ($P = 0.0001$)
6	Ren et al. (2008)	2008	Beijingese	low	case-control	age, sex	50	92	0.49 ($P < 0.05$)
7	Borentain et al. (2007)	2007	French	low	case-control	age, sex	56	61	1.84 ($P = 0.015$)
8	Kiran et al.(2009)	2009	Indian	low	case-control	no	63	142	0.33-0.63 ($P < 0.05$)
9	Kiran et al.(2009)	2009	Indian	low	case-control	no	63	142	0.33-0.63 ($P < 0.05$)
10	Su et al. (2008)	2008	Liaoningese	low	case-control	age, sex	100	111	2.95 ($P < 0.001$)
11	Yang et al.(2004)	2004	Qidongese	high	case-control	age, sex	69	136	about 1 ($P > 0.05$)
12	Pan et al. (2012)	2012	Shangdongese	medium	case-control	age, sex	202	236	1.35-1.55 ($P > 0.05$)
13	Li et al. (2012)	2012	Shangdongese	medium	case-control	age, sex	150	158	1.69-1.78 ($P < 0.05$)
14	Chen et al.(2005)	2005	Taiwanese	high	case-control	age, sex	577	389	1.57 ($P > 0.05$)

[a] Defined by means of Ref Henry, *et al.* (Science, 1999).

[b] AFB1-related DNA repair capacity is evaluated using risk biomarker AFB1-related HCC risk (*see "DNA repair capacity elucidation related to AFB1-induced DNA damage" section*). Based on this thesis, AFB1-related DNA repair capacity will decrease if OR > 1 and corresponding *P*-value < 0.05; will increase if OR < 1 and corresponding *P*-value < 0.05; and will not change if OR is about 1 and/or corresponding *P*-value > 0.05.

Table 1. Characteristics of studies about genetic polymorphism at codon 399 of DNA repair gene XRCC1 and risk biomarker for DNA repair capacity (namely HCC risk)

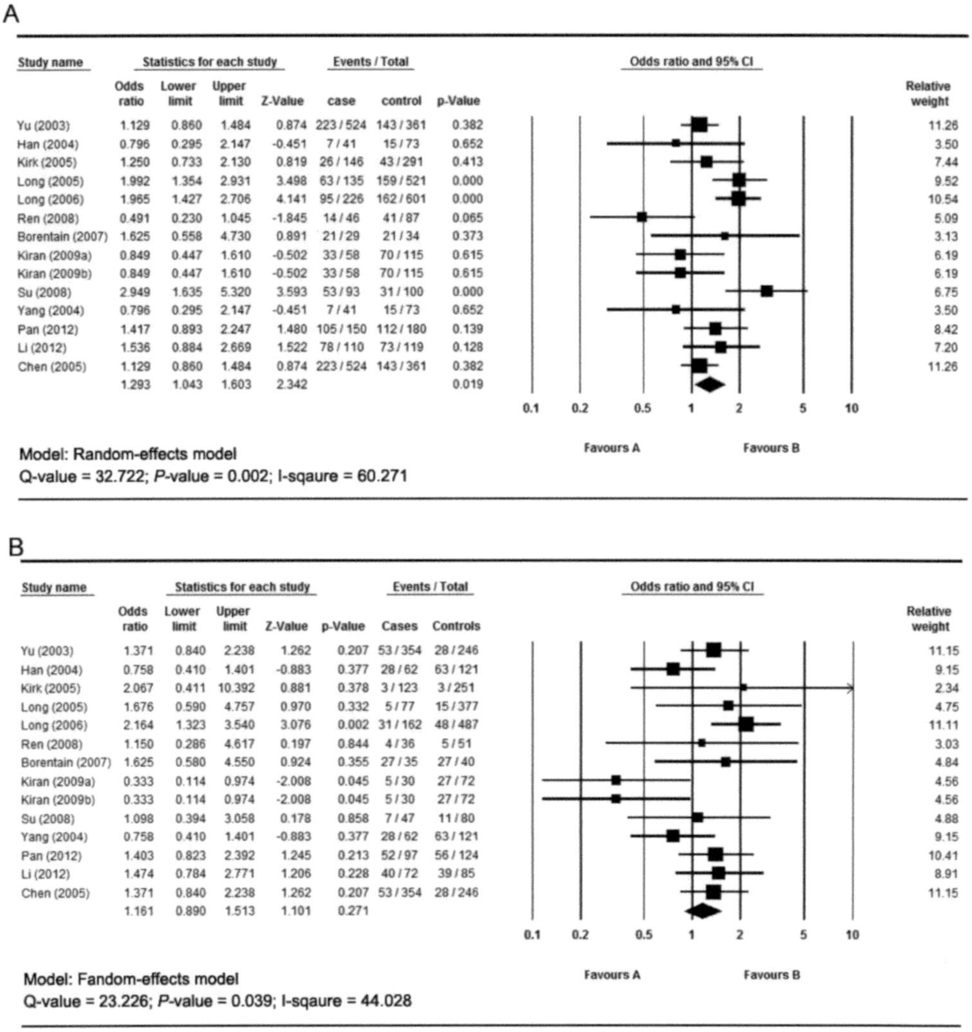

Figure 2. The meta-analysis of the relationship between genetic polymorphism at codon 399 (Arg/Gln) XRCC1 and AFB1-related HCC risk, a biomarker for DNA repair capacity correlated with AFB1-induced DNA damage, based on overall studies size. Compared with Arg/Arg genotype, Arg/Gln (A) genotype decreased AFB1-related DNA repair capacity. This effect was not observed in Gln/Gln genotype (B).

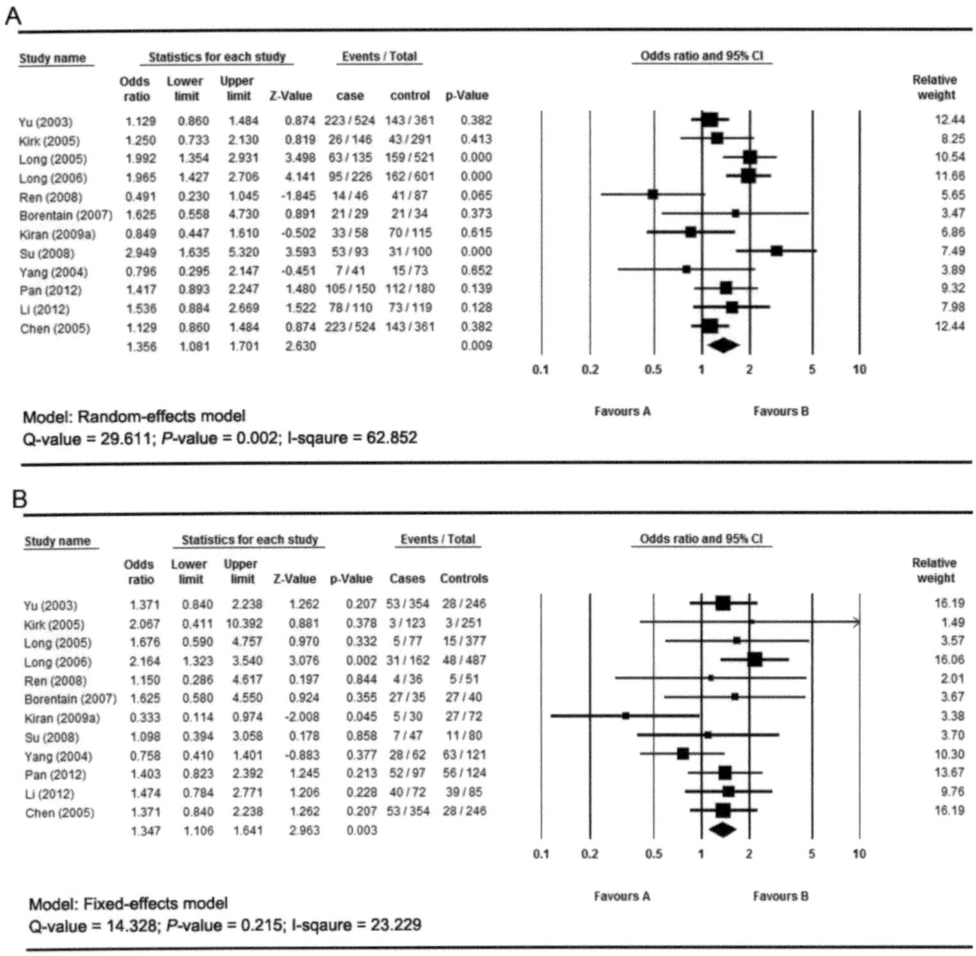

Figure 3. The meta-analysis of the relationship between genetic polymorphism at codon 399 (Arg/Gln) XRCC1 and AFB1-related HCC risk, a biomarker for DNA repair capacity correlated with AFB1-induced DNA damage, based on overall studies size excluded possible repeated studies. Compared with Arg/Arg genotype, Arg/Gln (A) and Gln/Gln (B) genotype decreased AFB1-related DNA repair capacity.

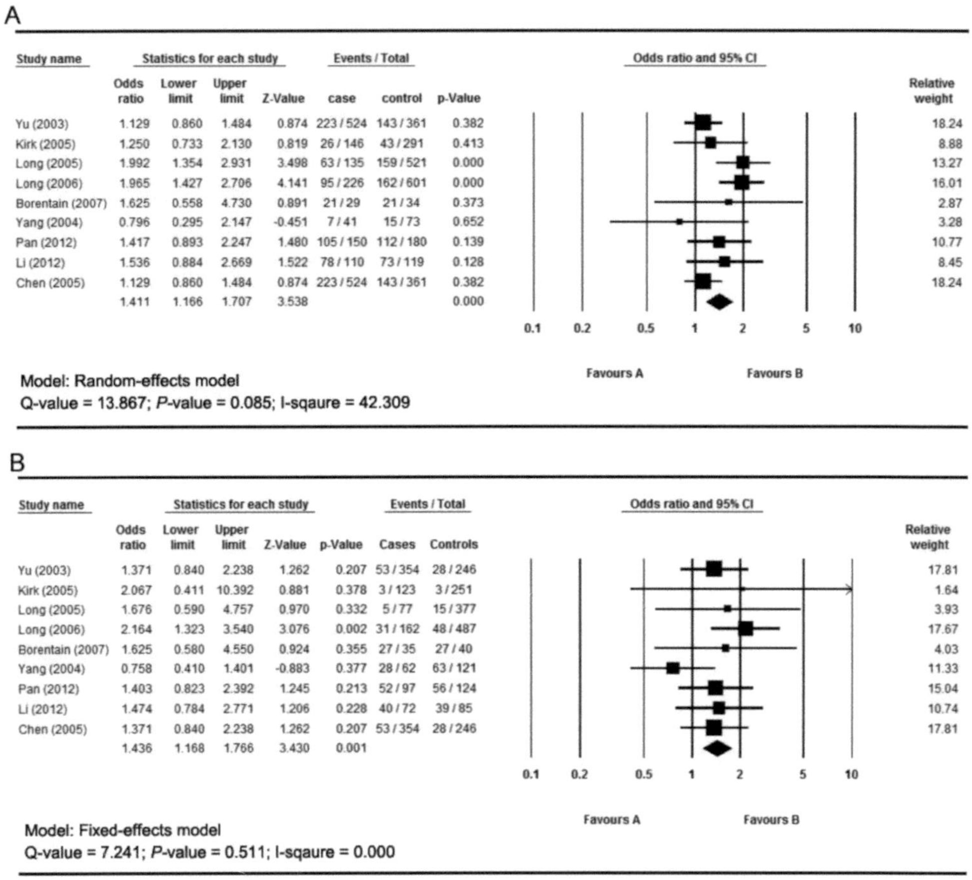

Figure 4. The meta-analysis of the relationship between genetic polymorphism at codon 399 (Arg/Gln) XRCC1 and AFB1-related HCC risk, a biomarker for DNA repair capacity correlated with AFB1-induced DNA damage, based on overall studies size excluded possible repeated studies and studies from low AFB1 exposure areas. Compared with Arg/Arg genotype, Arg/Gln (A) and Gln/Gln (B) genotype decreased AFB1-related DNA repair capacity.

These data support XRCC1 codon 399 Gln alleles decrease AFB1-related DNA repair capacity. Additionally, several studies have shown that the other two genetic polymorphisms (at codon 194 and codon 280) of XRCC1 also decrease DNA repair capacity related AFB1-induced DNA damage, with adjusted value 2.25-2.27 for codon 194 polymorphism and 4.95-6.27 for codon 280 polymorphism ($P < 0.05$) [175]. Furthermore, this decreasing DNA repair ability might more noticeable under the haplotypes with both codon 194 Arg alleles and codon codon 280 His alleles conditions [183].

9. Genetic polymorphisms of DNA repair genes involved in DSBR pathway for AFB1-related DNA damage repair

DSBR pathway involves a series of DNA repair genes. In published molecular epidemiological studies, only XRCC3 gene codon Thr241Met polymorphism and XRCC7 rs#7003908 polymorphism affect AFB1-related DNA repair capacity [8, 15, 78].

9.1. XRCC3

The product of the XRCC3 gene is one of identified paralogs of the strand-exchange protein RAD51 in human beings [188-192]. This protein correlates directly with DNA breaks and facilitates of the formation of the RAD51 nucleoprotein filament, which is crucial both for homologous recombination and HRR [188-192]. Previous studies have shown that a common polymorphism at codon 241 of XRCC3 gene (Thr to Met) modifies the function of this gene [193-205]. Two reports from high AFB1-exposure areas all of world supported above-mentioned conclusions [15, 90].

In the first frequent case-control study in Guangxiese [90], we observed that the genotypes with XRCC3 codon 241 Met alleles (namely Thr/Met and Met/Met) was significantly different between controls (33.01%) and HCC cases (61.48%, $P < 0.001$). Met alleles increases about 2- to 10-fold risk of HCC and this running-up risk is modulated by the number of Met alleles (adjusted OR 2.48 and 10.06 for one and two this alleles). Considering small sample size in this study, we recruited, in another independent frequent case-control study [15], a relatively larger sample size to compare the results. Subjects included in this study, 491 HCC cases and 862 age-, sex, race, hepatitis virus infection information-matching controls, were permanent residents of Guangxi areas. Similar to the results of the first report, the distribution of XRCC3 codon 241 Met allele frequencies was found to be significantly different between cases (59.7%) and controls (32.1%). Individuals having the Thr/Met or Met/Met were at a 2.22-fold or 7.19 fold increased risk of developing HCC cancer. Above two studies showed this allele multiplicatively interacted with AFB1 exposure in the process of hepato-tumorigenesis. These results exhibits that the polymorphism at codon 241 of XRCC3 gene is a genetic determinant in AFB1-related DNA repair ability for DSBR pathway.

9.2. XRCC7

DNA repair gene XRCC7, called DNA-dependent protein kinase catalytic subunit (DNA-PKcs), DNAPK, DNPK1, HYRC, HYRC1, or p350) (Genbank ID. 5591), spans about 197 kb on chromosome 8q11 and contains 85 exons and 86 introns (Gene dBase in PubMed). This gene encodes DNA-PKcs that constitutes the large catalytic subunit of the DNA-PK complex. When DNA-PKcs is recruited to the site of DSBs by the Ku70/Ku80 heterodimer, DNA-PK complex changes into its active form and subsequently initiates the non-homologous end joining (NHEJ) repair, an important DSBR pathway [206-213]. Murine mutants defective in the XRCC7 have non-detectable DNA-PK activity, suggesting that XRCC7 is required for NHEJ pathway protein. More than 20 polymorphisms have been reported in the XRCC7 gene, some of which are correlated with malignant tumors such as bladder cancer (dbSNP in NCBI Database). Of these genetic polymorphisms in XRCC7 gene, only two loci (rs7003908 and rs10109984) are investigated their modifying effects on AFB1-related DNA repair capacity [8].

In this hospital-based case-control study conducted by Long, *et al.* [8], they found that these individuals with XRCC7 rs7003908 G alleles increased HCC risk compared the homozygote of XRCC7 rs7003908 T alleles (XRCC7-TT), with OR value 3.45 (2.40–4.94) for XRCC7-TG and 5.04 (3.28–7.76) for XRCC7-GG, respectively. Additionally, they also found this genetic polymorphism was correlated with higher the levels of AFB1-DNA adducts (r = 0.142, $P <$ 0.001). However, another polymorphism rs10109984 did not modify AFB1-related HCC risk ($P >$ 0.05). As a result, these data explore that genetic polymorphism of XRCC7 rs7003908 but not rs10109984 might decrease AFB1-related DSBR capacity, inquiring more studies to support this conclusion.

10. Future directions

Recently, great progress has been made in understanding the molecular mechanisms of the genetic susceptibility to DNA repair capacity related to AFB1-induced DNA damages. However, we are still far from a comprehensive view of the issue. The molecular mechanism about genetic polymorphisms in the DNA repair genes modifying DNA repair capacity related AFB1-induced DNA damages remains largely unknown. Although several reports have shown the spot mutation resulting from genetic polymorphisms may decrease DNA repair capacity via changing the structure of DNA repair proteins, downregulating expression of DNA repair genes or decreasing the function of DNA repair genes, more direct evidence is lost. Disclosing the roles of different genetic types of DNA repair genes in the different toxicity of AFB1 will greatly benefit our understanding of pathological mechanisms of the genetic polymorphisms in the DNA repair genes affecting DNA repair capacity related to AFB1-induced DNA damage, and will shed important light on the clinical therapy for these patients with risk types.

11. Summary

AFB1 is an important environment variation of DNA damage. This toxic variation is characterized by: (1) the attraction of specific organs, especially liver; (2) genotoxicity, mainly inducing the formation of AFB1-DNA adducts and the hot-spot mutation of p53 gene; and (3) carcinogenicity, primarily causing HCC. Among these chronic DNA damage characteristics, AFB1-DNA adducts play a central role because of their genotoxicity and interactions with genetic susceptive factors. In human, there are several repair pathways, including NER, BER, SSBR, and DSBR, is able to repair this type damage. Genetic polymorphisms in DNA repair genes might modify the expression and the functions of

DNA repair proteins encoded by the relative genes and decrease the AFB1-correlated DNA repair capacity. Based on this knowledge, DNA repair capacity related to AFB1-induced DNA damage can be elucidated via the following three methods: testing the levels of AFB1-DNA adducts (mainly AFB1-FAPy adduct), analyzing the frequency of TP53M, and evaluating the risk of HCC by AFB1 exposure.

Numerous studies reviewed in this paper have demonstrated that the hereditary variations in DNA repair genes are associated with DNA repair capacity of DNA damage induced by AFB1. These molecular epidemiological studies have significantly contributed to our knowledge of the importance of genetic polymorphisms in DNA repair genes in the individual's susceptibility to AFB1 exposure. It would be expected that genetic susceptibility factors involved in DNA repair genes for AFB1-induced DNA damage repair could serve as useful biomarkers for identifying at-low-DNA-repair-capacity individuals by AFB1 exposure and, therefore, targeting prevention of this toxicity-related malignant tumor.

However, there are several issues to be noted. The conclusions should first be drawn carefully, because of conflicting data existing in the same ethnic population in view of between some genotypes of DNA repair genes and the AFB1-related DNA damage repair capacity. Second, because of the fact that AFB1-related DNA repair is polygenic, no single genetic marker may sufficiently predict DNA repair capacity. Therefore, a panel of susceptive biomarkers is warranted to define individuals at low DNA repair capacity. Last, the corresponding molecular mechanisms of risk types modifying DNA repair capacity correlated with AFB1-induced DNA damages should be paid close attention.

Acknowledgments

We are grateful to Yuan-Feng Zhou for the collection and management of data. This study is partly supported by the National Nature & Science Foundation of China (NO. 81160255), the Science Foundation of Youjiang Medical College for Nationalities (NO. 2005 and 2008), and Guangxi Key Construction Project of Laboratory Room (NO. 2009).

Abbreviations

AFB1, Aflatoxin B1; AFB1-epoxide, AFB1-8,9-epoxide; AFB1-N^7-Gua, 8,9-di-hydro-8-(N^7-guanyl)-9-hydroxy–AFB1; AFB1-FAPy, ring-opened formamidopyridine AFB1; AFF, aflatoxins family; APE1, AP endonuclease-1; BER, base excision repair; CI, confidence interval; DNA-PKcs, DNA-dependent protein kinase catalytic subunit; DSB, double-strand break; DSBR, double-strand break repair; HBV, hepatitis virus B; HCV, hepatitis virus C; HCC, hepatocellular carcinoma; hOGG1, Human oxoguanine glycosylase 1; NER, nucleotide excision repair; OR, odds ratio; 8-$_{oxod}$G, 8-oxodeoxyguanosine; PARP, poly (ADP-ribose) polymerase; PLC, Primary liver cancer; PNK, polynucleotide kinase; Pol β, DNA polymerase β; ROS, reactive oxygen species; SSB, single-strand break; SSBR, single-strand break repair;

XPA, xeroderma pigmentosum A; XPC, xeroderma pigmentosum C; XPD, xeroderma pigmentosum D; XRCC1, x-ray repair cross complementary 1; XRCC3, x-ray repair cross complementary 3; XRCC4, x-ray repair cross complementary 4; XRCC7, x-ray repair cross complementary 7.

Author details

Qiang Xia[1*], Xiao-Ying Huang[2], Feng Xue[1], Jian-Jun Zhang[1], Bo Zhai[1], De-Chun Kong[3], Chao Wang[2], Zhao-Quan Huang[2] and Xi-Dai Long[1*]

*Address all correspondence to: xiaqiang@medmail.com.cn

*Address all correspondence to: xiaolonglong200166@yahoo.com.cn

1 Department of Liver Surgery, the Affiliated Renji Hospital, Shanghai Jiao Tong University School of Medicine, Shanghai, P.R. China

2 Department of Pathology, the Affiliated Hospital, Youjiang Medical College for Nationalities, Baise, P.R. China

3 Department of Physiology, the Basic Medicine, Shanghai Jiao Tong University School of Medicine, Shanghai, P.R. China

References

[1] Kensler TW, Roebuck BD, Wogan GN, et al. Aflatoxin: a 50-year odyssey of mechanistic and translational toxicology. Toxicological sciences : an official journal of the Society of Toxicology, 2011; 120(Suppl 1):(S28-48.

[2] Wang JS, Groopman JD. DNA damage by mycotoxins. Mutat Res, 1999; 424(1-2): 167-181.

[3] Groopman JD, Croy RG, Wogan GN. In vitro reactions of aflatoxin B1-adducted DNA. Proc Natl Acad Sci U S A, 1981; 78(9): 5445-5449.

[4] Long XD, Yao JG, Zeng Z, et al. DNA repair capacity-related to genetic polymorphisms of DNA repair genes and aflatoxin B1-related hepatocellular carcinoma among Chinese population. In: Kruman I (ed)). DNA Repair (Amst). Rijeka: InTech, 2011; 505-524.

[5] Jemal A, Bray F, Center MM, et al. Global cancer statistics. CA: a cancer journal for clinicians, 2011; 61(2): 69-90.

[6] Yu MC, Yuan JM, Lu SC. Alcohol, cofactors and the genetics of hepatocellular carcinoma. J Gastroenterol Hepatol, 2008; 23(Suppl 1): (S92-97.

[7] Yeh FS, Mo CC, Yen RC. Risk factors for hepatocellular carcinoma in Guangxi, People's Republic of China. Natl Cancer Inst Monogr, 1985; 69:47-48.

[8] Long XD, Yao JG, Huang YZ, et al. DNA repair gene XRCC7 polymorphisms (rs#7003908 and rs#10109984) and hepatocellular carcinoma related to AFB1 exposure among Guangxi population, China. Hepatology research : the official journal of the Japan Society of Hepatology, 2011; 41(11): 1085-1093.

[9] Wilson DM, 3rd, Thompson LH. Life without DNA repair. Proc Natl Acad Sci U S A, 1997; 94(24): 12754-12757.

[10] Guengerich FP, Johnson WW, Shimada T, et al. Activation and detoxication of aflatoxin B1. Mutat Res, 1998; 402(1-2): 121-128.

[11] Parkin DM, Bray F, Ferlay J, et al. Global cancer statistics, 2002. CA Cancer J Clin, 2005; 55(2): 74-108.

[12] Long XD, Ma Y, Zhou YF, et al. XPD codon 312 and 751 polymorphisms, and AFB1 exposure, and hepatocellular carcinoma risk. BMC Cancer, 2009; 9(1):400.

[13] Wang F, Chang D, Hu FL, et al. DNA repair gene XPD polymorphisms and cancer risk: a meta-analysis based on 56 case-control studies. Cancer Epidemiol Biomarkers Prev, 2008; 17(3): 507-517.

[14] Sreeja L, Syamala VS, Syamala V, et al. Prognostic importance of DNA repair gene polymorphisms of XRCC1 Arg399Gln and XPD Lys751Gln in lung cancer patients from India. J Cancer Res Clin Oncol, 2008; 134(6): 645-652.

[15] Long XD, Ma Y, Qu de Y, et al. The polymorphism of XRCC3 codon 241 and AFB1-related hepatocellular carcinoma in Guangxi population, China. Ann Epidemiol, 2008; 18(7): 572-578.

[16] Yuan JM, Lu SC, Van Den Berg D, et al. Genetic polymorphisms in the methylenetetrahydrofolate reductase and thymidylate synthase genes and risk of hepatocellular carcinoma. Hepatology, 2007; 46(3): 749-758.

[17] Suarez-Martinez EB, Ruiz A, Matias J, et al. Early-onset of sporadic basal-cell carcinoma: germline mutations in the TP53, PTCH, and XPD genes. P R Health Sci J, 2007; 26(4): 349-354.

[18] Shao J, Gu M, Xu Z, et al. Polymorphisms of the DNA gene XPD and risk of bladder cancer in a Southeastern Chinese population. Cancer Genet Cytogenet, 2007; 177(1): 30-36.

[19] Yin J, Vogel U, Ma Y, et al. Polymorphism of the DNA repair gene ERCC2 Lys751Gln and risk of lung cancer in a northeastern Chinese population. Cancer Genet Cytogenet, 2006; 169(1): 27-32.

[20] Stern MC, Conway K, Li Y, et al. DNA repair gene polymorphisms and probability of p53 mutation in bladder cancer. Mol Carcinog, 2006; 45(9): 715-719.

[21] Manuguerra M, Saletta F, Karagas MR, et al. XRCC3 and XPD/ERCC2 single nucleotide polymorphisms and the risk of cancer: a HuGE review. Am J Epidemiol, 2006; 164(4): 297-302.

[22] Long XD, Ma Y, Wei YP, et al. The polymorphisms of GSTM1, GSTT1, HYL1*2, and XRCC1, and aflatoxin B1-related hepatocellular carcinoma in Guangxi population, China. Hepatol Res, 2006; 36(1): 48-55.

[23] Chen G, Luo DZ, Liu L, et al. Hepatic local micro-environmental immune status in hepatocellular carcinoma and cirrhotic tissues. West Indian Med J, 2006; 55(6): 403-408.

[24] Carnaghan RB, Hartley RD, O'Kelly J. Toxicity and Fluorescence Properties of the Aflatoxins. Nature, 1963; 200: 1101.

[25] Long XD, Tang YH, Qu DY, et al. The toxicity and role of aflatoxin B1 and DNA repair (corresponding DNA repair enzymes) Youjiang Medical College for Nationalities Xue Bao, 2006; 28(2): 278-280.

[26] Wild CP, Turner PC. The toxicology of aflatoxins as a basis for public health decisions. Mutagenesis, 2002; 17(6): 471-481.

[27] Wild CP, Montesano R. A model of interaction: aflatoxins and hepatitis viruses in liver cancer aetiology and prevention. Cancer Lett, 2009; 286(1): 22-28.

[28] Ben Rejeb I, Arduini F, Arvinte A, et al. Development of a bio-electrochemical assay for AFB1 detection in olive oil. Biosens Bioelectron, 2009; 24(7): 1962-1968.

[29] Hsu CY, Chen YH, Chao PY, et al. Naturally occurring chlorophyll derivatives inhibit aflatoxin B1-DNA adduct formation in hepatoma cells. Mutat Res, 2008; 657(2): 98-104.

[30] Scholl PF, McCoy L, Kensler TW, et al. Quantitative analysis and chronic dosimetry of the aflatoxin B1 plasma albumin adduct Lys-AFB1 in rats by isotope dilution mass spectrometry. Chem Res Toxicol, 2006; 19(1): 44-49.

[31] Habib SL, Said B, Awad AT, et al. Novel adenine adducts, N7-guanine-AFB1 adducts, and p53 mutations in patients with schistosomiasis and aflatoxin exposure. Cancer Detect Prev, 2006; 30(6): 491-498.

[32] Giri I, Stone MP. Wobble dC.dA pairing 5' to the cationic guanine N7 8,9-dihydro-8-(N7-guanyl)-9-hydroxyaflatoxin B1 adduct: implications for nontargeted AFB1 mutagenesis. Biochemistry, 2003; 42(23): 7023-7034.

[33] Wang JS, Shen X, He X, et al. Protective alterations in phase 1 and 2 metabolism of aflatoxin B1 by oltipraz in residents of Qidong, People's Republic of China. Journal of the National Cancer Institute, 1999; 91(4): 347-354.

[34] Johnson WW, Guengerich FP. Reaction of aflatoxin B1 exo-8,9-epoxide with DNA: kinetic analysis of covalent binding and DNA-induced hydrolysis. Proc Natl Acad Sci U S A, 1997; 94(12): 6121-6125.

[35] Chou MW, Chen W. Food restriction reduces aflatoxin B1 (AFB1)-DNA adduct formation, AFB1-glutathione conjugation, and DNA damage in AFB1-treated male F344 rats and B6C3F1 mice. The Journal of nutrition, 1997; 127(2): 210-217.

[36] Croy RG, Wogan GN. Temporal patterns of covalent DNA adducts in rat liver after single and multiple doses of aflatoxin B1. Cancer Res, 1981; 41(1): 197-203.

[37] Croy RG, Essigmann JM, Reinhold VN, et al. Identification of the principal aflatoxin B1-DNA adduct formed in vivo in rat liver. Proc Natl Acad Sci U S A, 1978; 75(4): 1745-1749.

[38] Martin CN, Garner RC. Aflatoxin B -oxide generated by chemical or enzymic oxidation of aflatoxin B1 causes guanine substitution in nucleic acids. Nature, 1977; 267(5614): 863-865.

[39] Lin JK, Miller JA, Miller EC. 2,3-Dihydro-2-(guan-7-yl)-3-hydroxy-aflatoxin B1, a major acid hydrolysis product of aflatoxin B1-DNA or -ribosomal RNA adducts formed in hepatic microsome-mediated reactions and in rat liver in vivo. Cancer Res, 1977; 37(12): 4430-4438.

[40] Long XD, Ma Y, Zhou YF, et al. XPD Codon 312 and 751 Polymorphisms, and AFB1 Exposure, and Hepatocellular Carcinoma Risk. BMC Cancer, 2009; 9(1): 400.

[41] Collins AR, Dusinska M, Gedik CM, et al. Oxidative damage to DNA: do we have a reliable biomarker? Environ Health Perspect, 1996; 104(Suppl 3): 465-469.

[42] Katafuchi A, Nohmi T. DNA polymerases involved in the incorporation of oxidized nucleotides into DNA: their efficiency and template base preference. Mutat Res, 2010; 703(1): 24-31.

[43] Kohda K, Tada M, Kasai H, et al. Formation of 8-hydroxyguanine residues in cellular DNA exposed to the carcinogen 4-nitroquinoline 1-oxide. Biochemical and biophysical research communications, 1986; 139(2): 626-632.

[44] Kasai H, Crain PF, Kuchino Y, et al. Formation of 8-hydroxyguanine moiety in cellular DNA by agents producing oxygen radicals and evidence for its repair. Carcinogenesis, 1986; 7(11): 1849-1851.

[45] Shen HM, Shi CY, Shen Y, et al. Detection of elevated reactive oxygen species level in cultured rat hepatocytes treated with aflatoxin B1. Free radical biology & medicine, 1996; 21(2): 139-146.

[46] Shen HM, Ong CN, Lee BL, et al. Aflatoxin B1-induced 8-hydroxydeoxyguanosine formation in rat hepatic DNA. Carcinogenesis, 1995; 16(2): 419-422.

[47] Shen HM, Ong CN, Shi CY. Involvement of reactive oxygen species in aflatoxin B1-induced cell injury in cultured rat hepatocytes. Toxicology, 1995; 99(1-2): 115-123.

[48] Wu HC, Wang Q, Wang LW, et al. Urinary 8-oxodeoxyguanosine, aflatoxin B1 exposure and hepatitis B virus infection and hepatocellular carcinoma in Taiwan. Carcinogenesis, 2007; 28(5): 995-999.

[49] Fortini P, Dogliotti E. Base damage and single-strand break repair: mechanisms and functional significance of short- and long-patch repair subpathways. DNA Repair (Amst), 2007; 6(4): 398-409.

[50] Caldecott KW. Mammalian single-strand break repair: mechanisms and links with chromatin. DNA Repair (Amst), 2007; 6(4): 443-453.

[51] Thompson LH, West MG. XRCC1 keeps DNA from getting stranded. Mutat Res, 2000; 459(1): 1-18.

[52] Fortini P, Ferretti C, Pascucci B, et al. DNA damage response by single-strand breaks in terminally differentiated muscle cells and the control of muscle integrity. Cell death and differentiation, 2012.

[53] Morgan WF, Corcoran J, Hartmann A, et al. DNA double-strand breaks, chromosomal rearrangements, and genomic instability. Mutat Res, 1998; 404(1-2): 125-128.

[54] Bressac B, Kew M, Wands J, et al. Selective G to T mutations of p53 gene in hepatocellular carcinoma from southern Africa. Nature, 1991; 350(6317): 429-431.

[55] Aguilar F, Hussain SP, Cerutti P. Aflatoxin B1 induces the transversion of G-->T in codon 249 of the p53 tumor suppressor gene in human hepatocytes. Proc Natl Acad Sci U S A, 1993; 90(18): 8586-8590.

[56] Coursaget P, Depril N, Chabaud M, et al. High prevalence of mutations at codon 249 of the p53 gene in hepatocellular carcinomas from Senegal. Br J Cancer, 1993; 67(6): 1395-1397.

[57] Liu YP, Lin Y, Ng ML. Immunochemical and genetic analysis of the p53 gene in liver preneoplastic nodules from aflatoxin-induced rats in one year. Ann Acad Med Singapore, 1996; 25(1): 31-36.

[58] Shen HM, Ong CN. Mutations of the p53 tumor suppressor gene and ras oncogenes in aflatoxin hepatocarcinogenesis. Mutat Res, 1996; 366(1): 23-44.

[59] Soini Y, Chia SC, Bennett WP, et al. An aflatoxin-associated mutational hotspot at codon 249 in the p53 tumor suppressor gene occurs in hepatocellular carcinomas from Mexico. Carcinogenesis, 1996; 17(5): 1007-1012.

[60] Hainaut P, Vahakangas K. p53 as a sensor of carcinogenic exposures: mechanisms of p53 protein induction and lessons from p53 gene mutations. Pathol Biol (Paris), 1997; 45(10): 833-844.

[61] Lunn RM, Zhang YJ, Wang LY, et al. p53 mutations, chronic hepatitis B virus infection, and aflatoxin exposure in hepatocellular carcinoma in Taiwan. Cancer Res, 1997; 57(16): 3471-3477.

[62] Mace K, Aguilar F, Wang JS, et al. Aflatoxin B1-induced DNA adduct formation and p53 mutations in CYP450-expressing human liver cell lines. Carcinogenesis, 1997; 18(7): 1291-1297.

[63] Deng ZL, Ma Y. Aflatoxin sufferer and p53 gene mutation in hepatocellular carcinoma. World J Gastroenterol, 1998; 4(1): 28-29.

[64] Ghebranious N, Sell S. The mouse equivalent of the human p53ser249 mutation p53ser246 enhances aflatoxin hepatocarcinogenesis in hepatitis B surface antigen transgenic and p53 heterozygous null mice. Hepatology, 1998; 27(4): 967-973.

[65] Ghebranious N, Sell S. Hepatitis B injury, male gender, aflatoxin, and p53 expression each contribute to hepatocarcinogenesis in transgenic mice. Hepatology, 1998; 27(2): 383-391.

[66] Nouspikel T. DNA repair in mammalian cells : Nucleotide excision repair: variations on versatility. Cellular and molecular life sciences : CMLS, 2009; 66(6): 994-1009.

[67] Rechkunova NI, Lavrik OI. Nucleotide excision repair in higher eukaryotes: mechanism of primary damage recognition in global genome repair. Sub-cellular biochemistry, 2010; 50: 251-277.

[68] Robertson AB, Klungland A, Rognes T, et al. DNA repair in mammalian cells: Base excision repair: the long and short of it. Cellular and molecular life sciences : CMLS, 2009; 66(6): 981-993.

[69] Donigan KA, Sweasy JB. Sequence context-specific mutagenesis and base excision repair. Molecular Carcinogenesis, 2009; 48(4): 362-368.

[70] Mills KD, Ferguson DO, Alt FW. The role of DNA breaks in genomic instability and tumorigenesis. Immunological reviews, 2003; 194: 77-95.

[71] Sonoda E, Hochegger H, Saberi A, et al. Differential usage of non-homologous end-joining and homologous recombination in double strand break repair. DNA Repair (Amst), 2006; 5(9-10): 1021-1029.

[72] Cahill D, Connor B, Carney JP. Mechanisms of eukaryotic DNA double strand break repair. Front Biosci, 2006; 11: 1958-1976.

[73] Iliakis G, Wu W, Wang M. DNA double strand break repair inhibition as a cause of heat radiosensitization: re-evaluation considering backup pathways of NHEJ. Int J Hyperthermia, 2008; 24(1): 17-29.

[74] van den Bosch M, Lohman PH, Pastink A. DNA double-strand break repair by homologous recombination. Biol Chem, 2002; 383(6): 873-892.

[75] Kanaar R, Hoeijmakers JH, van Gent DC. Molecular mechanisms of DNA double strand break repair. Trends Cell Biol, 1998; 8(12): 483-489.

[76] Pastwa E, Blasiak J. Non-homologous DNA end joining. Acta Biochim Pol, 2003; 50(4): 891-908.

[77] Shrivastav M, De Haro LP, Nickoloff JA. Regulation of DNA double-strand break repair pathway choice. Cell Res, 2008; 18(1): 134-147.

[78] Long XD, Ma Y, Deng ZL. GSTM1 and XRCC3 polymorphisms: Effects on levels of aflatoxin B1-DNA adducts. Chinese Journal of Cancer Research, 2009; 21(3): 177-184.

[79] Hsieh LL, Hsieh TT. Detection of aflatoxin B1-DNA adducts in human placenta and cord blood. Cancer Res, 1993; 53(6): 1278-1280.

[80] Lunn RM, Langlois RG, Hsieh LL, et al. XRCC1 polymorphisms: effects on aflatoxin B1-DNA adducts and glycophorin A variant frequency. Cancer Res, 1999; 59(11): 2557-2561.

[81] Long XD, Ma Y, Wei YP, et al. X-RAY REPAIR CROSS-COMPLEMENTING GROUP 1 (XRCC1) Arg 399 Gin POLYMORPHISM AND AFLATOXIN B1 (AFB1)-RELATED HEPATOCELLULAR CARCINOMA (HCC) IN GUANGXI POPULATION. 2005.

[82] Zhao L, Long XD, Yao JG, et al. Genetic polymorphism of XRCC3 codon 241 and Helicobacter pylori infection-related gastric antrum adenocarcinoma in Guangxi Population, China: A hospital-based case-control study. Cancer epidemiology, 2011; 35(6): 564-568.

[83] Long XD, Ma Y, Wei YP, et al. X-ray repair cross-complementing group 1 (XRCC1) Arg 399 Gln polymorphism and aflatoxin B1 (AFB1)-related hepatocellular carcinoma (HCC) in Guangxi population. Chinese Journal of Cancer Research, 2005; 17(1): 17-21.

[84] Long XD, Ma Y, Zhou YF, et al. Polymorphism in xeroderma pigmentosum complementation group C codon 939 and aflatoxin B1-related hepatocellular carcinoma in the Guangxi population. Hepatology, 2010; 52(4): 1301-1309.

[85] Long XD, Ma Y, Huang HD, et al. Polymorphism of XRCC1 and the frequency of mutation in codon 249 of the p53 gene in hepatocellular carcinoma among Guangxi population, China. Mol Carcinog, 2008; 47(4): 295-300.

[86] Long XD, Ma Y, Huang YZ, et al. Genetic polymorphisms in DNA repair genes XPC, XPD, and XRCC4, and susceptibility to Helicobacter pylori infection-related gastric antrum adenocarcinoma in Guangxi population, China. Mol Carcinog, 2010; 49(6): 611-618.

[87] Long XD, Ma Y, Wei YP, et al. [A study about the association of detoxication gene GSTM1 polymorphism and the susceptibility to aflatoxin B1-related hepatocellular carcinoma]. Zhonghua Gan Zang Bing Za Zhi, 2005; 13(9): 668-670.

[88] Long XD, Ma Y, Wei YP, et al. [Study on the detoxication gene gstM1-gstT1-null and susceptibility to aflatoxin B1 related hepatocellular carcinoma in Guangxi]. Zhonghua Liu Xing Bing Xue Za Zhi, 2005; 26(10): 777-781.

[89] X.M. W, Ma Y, Deng ZL, et al. The polymorphism at codon 939 of xeroderma pigmentosum C gene and hepatocellular carcinoma among Guangxi population. Zhonghua Xiaohua Zazhi, 2010; 30(11): 846-848.

[90] Long XD, Ma Y, Deng ZL, et al. [Association of the Thr241Met polymorphism of DNA repair gene XRCC3 with genetic susceptibility to AFB1-related hepatocellular

carcinoma in Guangxi population]. Zhonghua Yi Xue Yi Chuan Xue Za Zhi, 2008; 25(3): 268-271.

[91] Sugasawa K. XPC: its product and biological roles. Adv Exp Med Biol, 2008; 637: 47-56.

[92] Khan SG, Yamanegi K, Zheng ZM, et al. XPC branch-point sequence mutations disrupt U2 snRNP binding, resulting in abnormal pre-mRNA splicing in xeroderma pigmentosum patients. Hum Mutat, 2010; 31(2): 167-175.

[93] van der Spek PJ, Eker A, Rademakers S, et al. XPC and human homologs of RAD23: intracellular localization and relationship to other nucleotide excision repair complexes. Nucleic Acids Res, 1996; 24(13): 2551-2559.

[94] Wang XW, Vermeulen W, Coursen JD, et al. The XPB and XPD DNA helicases are components of the p53-mediated apoptosis pathway. Genes Dev, 1996; 10(10): 1219-1232.

[95] Yokoi M, Masutani C, Maekawa T, et al. The xeroderma pigmentosum group C protein complex XPC-HR23B plays an important role in the recruitment of transcription factor IIH to damaged DNA. J Biol Chem, 2000; 275(13): 9870-9875.

[96] Boulikas T. Xeroderma pigmentosum and molecular cloning of DNA repair genes. Anticancer Res, 1996; 16(2): 693-708.

[97] Araujo SJ, Wood RD. Protein complexes in nucleotide excision repair. Mutat Res, 1999; 435(1): 23-33.

[98] Bohr VA. Preferential DNA repair in active genes. Dan Med Bull, 1987; 34(6): 309-320.

[99] Qiu L, Wang Z, Shi X, et al. Associations between XPC polymorphisms and risk of cancers: A meta-analysis. Eur J Cancer, 2008; 44(15): 2241-2253.

[100] Sakano S, Matsumoto H, Yamamoto Y, et al. Association between DNA repair gene polymorphisms and p53 alterations in Japanese patients with muscle-invasive bladder cancer. Pathobiology, 2006; 73(6): 295-303.

[101] Li LM, Zeng XY, Ji L, et al. [Association of XPC and XPG polymorphisms with the risk of hepatocellular carcinoma]. Zhonghua gan zang bing za zhi = Zhonghua ganzangbing zazhi = Chinese journal of hepatology, 2010; 18(4): 271-275.

[102] Zhou RM, Li Y, Wang N, et al. [Correlation of XPC Ala499Val and Lys939Gln polymorphisms to risks of esophageal squamous cell carcinoma and gastric cardiac adenocarcinoma]. Ai Zheng, 2006; 25(9): 1113-1119.

[103] Ryk C, Kumar R, Sanyal S, et al. Influence of polymorphism in DNA repair and defence genes on p53 mutations in bladder tumours. Cancer Lett, 2006; 241(1): 142-149.

[104] Zhang D, Chen C, Fu X, et al. A meta-analysis of DNA repair gene XPC polymorphisms and cancer risk. J Hum Genet, 2008; 53(1): 18-33.

[105] Kazimirova A, Barancokova M, Dzupinkova Z, et al. Micronuclei and chromosomal aberrations, important markers of ageing: possible association with XPC and XPD polymorphisms. Mutat Res, 2009; 661(1-2): 35-40.

[106] Laczmanska I, Gil J, Karpinski P, et al. Polymorphism in nucleotide excision repair gene XPC correlates with bleomycin-induced chromosomal aberrations. Environ Mol Mutagen, 2007; 48(8): 666-671.

[107] De Ruyck K, Szaumkessel M, De Rudder I, et al. Polymorphisms in base-excision repair and nucleotide-excision repair genes in relation to lung cancer risk. Mutat Res, 2007; 631(2): 101-110.

[108] Mechanic LE, Millikan RC, Player J, et al. Polymorphisms in nucleotide excision repair genes, smoking and breast cancer in African Americans and whites: a population-based case-control study. Carcinogenesis, 2006; 27(7): 1377-1385.

[109] Shore RE, Zeleniuch-Jacquotte A, Currie D, et al. Polymorphisms in XPC and ERCC2 genes, smoking and breast cancer risk. Int J Cancer, 2008; 122(9): 2101-2105.

[110] Dong Z, Guo W, Zhou R, et al. Polymorphisms of the DNA repair gene XPA and XPC and its correlation with gastric cardiac adenocarcinoma in a high incidence population in North China. J Clin Gastroenterol, 2008; 42(8): 910-915.

[111] Zhang L, Zhang Z, Yan W. Single nucleotide polymorphisms for DNA repair genes in breast cancer patients. Clin Chim Acta, 2005; 359(1-2): 150-155.

[112] Hansen RD, Sorensen M, Tjonneland A, et al. XPA A23G, XPC Lys939Gln, XPD Lys751Gln and XPD Asp312Asn polymorphisms, interactions with smoking, alcohol and dietary factors, and risk of colorectal cancer. Mutat Res, 2007; 619(1-2): 68-80.

[113] Liang J, Gu A, Xia Y, et al. XPC gene polymorphisms and risk of idiopathic azoospermia or oligozoospermia in a Chinese population. Int J Androl, 2009; 32(3): 235-241.

[114] Francisco G, Menezes PR, Eluf-Neto J, et al. XPC polymorphisms play a role in tissue-specific carcinogenesis: a meta-analysis. Eur J Hum Genet, 2008; 16(6): 724-734.

[115] Cheo DL, Burns DK, Meira LB, et al. Mutational inactivation of the xeroderma pigmentosum group C gene confers predisposition to 2-acetylaminofluorene-induced liver and lung cancer and to spontaneous testicular cancer in Trp53-/- mice. Cancer Res, 1999; 59(4): 771-775.

[116] Fautrel A, Andrieux L, Musso O, et al. Overexpression of the two nucleotide excision repair genes ERCC1 and XPC in human hepatocellular carcinoma. J Hepatol, 2005; 43(2): 288-293.

[117] Cai XL, Gao YH, Yu ZW, et al. [A 1:1 matched case-control study on the interaction between HBV, HCV infection and DNA repair gene XPC Ala499Val, Lys939Gln for primary hepatocellular carcinoma]. Zhonghua Liu Xing Bing Xue Za Zhi, 2009; 30(9): 942-945.

[118] Henry SH, Bosch FX, Troxell TC, et al. Reducing Liver Cancer--Global Control of Aflatoxin. Science, 1999; 286(5449): 2453-2454.

[119] Aloyz R, Xu ZY, Bello V, et al. Regulation of cisplatin resistance and homologous recombinational repair by the TFIIH subunit XPD. Cancer Res, 2002; 62(19): 5457-5462.

[120] Bienstock RJ, Skorvaga M, Mandavilli BS, et al. Structural and functional characterization of the human DNA repair helicase XPD by comparative molecular modeling and site-directed mutagenesis of the bacterial repair protein UvrB. J Biol Chem, 2003; 278(7): 5309-5316.

[121] Keriel A, Stary A, Sarasin A, et al. XPD mutations prevent TFIIH-dependent transactivation by nuclear receptors and phosphorylation of RARalpha. Cell, 2002; 109(1): 125-135.

[122] Sturgis EM, Castillo EJ, Li L, et al. XPD/ERCC2 EXON 8 Polymorphisms: rarity and lack of significance in risk of squamous cell carcinoma of the head and neck. Oral Oncol, 2002; 38(5): 475-477.

[123] Benhamou S, Sarasin A. ERCC2/XPD gene polymorphisms and cancer risk. Mutagenesis, 2002; 17(6): 463-469.

[124] Qiao Y, Spitz MR, Shen H, et al. Modulation of repair of ultraviolet damage in the host-cell reactivation assay by polymorphic XPC and XPD/ERCC2 genotypes. Carcinogenesis, 2002; 23(2): 295-299.

[125] Kobayashi T, Uchiyama M, Fukuro S, et al. Mutations in the XPD gene in xeroderma pigmentosum group D cell strains: confirmation of genotype-phenotype correlation. Am J Med Genet, 2002; 110(3): 248-252.

[126] Rzeszowska-Wolny J, Polanska J, Pietrowska M, et al. Influence of polymorphisms in DNA repair genes XPD, XRCC1 and MGMT on DNA damage induced by gamma radiation and its repair in lymphocytes in vitro. Radiat Res, 2005; 164(2): 132-140.

[127] Spitz MR, Wu X, Wang Y, et al. Modulation of nucleotide excision repair capacity by XPD polymorphisms in lung cancer patients. Cancer Res, 2001; 61(4): 1354-1357.

[128] Stern MC, Johnson LR, Bell DA, et al. XPD codon 751 polymorphism, metabolism genes, smoking, and bladder cancer risk. Cancer Epidemiol Biomarkers Prev, 2002; 11(10 Pt 1): 1004-1011.

[129] Tang D, Cho S, Rundle A, et al. Polymorphisms in the DNA repair enzyme XPD are associated with increased levels of PAH-DNA adducts in a case-control study of breast cancer. Breast Cancer Res Treat, 2002; 75(2): 159-166.

[130] Terry MB, Gammon MD, Zhang FF, et al. Polymorphism in the DNA repair gene XPD, polycyclic aromatic hydrocarbon-DNA adducts, cigarette smoking, and breast cancer risk. Cancer epidemiology, biomarkers & prevention : a publication of the American Association for Cancer Research, cosponsored by the American Society of Preventive Oncology, 2004; 13(12): 2053-2058.

[131] Mechanic LE, Marrogi AJ, Welsh JA, et al. Polymorphisms in XPD and TP53 and mutation in human lung cancer. Carcinogenesis, 2005; 26(3): 597-604.

[132] Zhang H, He BC, He FC. [Impact of DNA repair gene hOGG1 Ser326Cys polymorphism on the risk of hepatocellular carcinoma]. Shijie Huaren xiaohua zazhi, 2006; 14(23): 2311-2314.

[133] Zhang H, Hao BT, He FC. [Impact of DNA repair gene hOGG1 Ser326Cys polymorphism on the risk of hepatocellular carcinoma]. 2006, 2006; 23(

[134] Zhang H, HAO B, HE F. Studies on Association between Susceptibility of Hepatocellular Carcinoma and Genetic Polymorphism Ser326Cys of DNA Repair Gene hOGG1. CHINESE JOURNAL OF CLINICAL ONCOLOGY, 2005; 32(15): 841-843.

[135] Ye X, Peng T, Li L. Study on polymorphisms in metabolic enzyme genes, DNA repair genes and individual susceptibility to hepatocellular carcinoma. Weisheng Yanjiu, 2006; 35(6): 805-807.

[136] Weiss JM, Goode EL, Ladiges WC, et al. Polymorphic variation in hOGG1 and risk of cancer: a review of the functional and epidemiologic literature. Molecular Carcinogenesis, 2005; 42(3): 127-141.

[137] Sakamoto T, Higaki Y, Hara M, et al. hOGG1 Ser326Cys polymorphism and risk of hepatocellular carcinoma among Japanese. Journal of epidemiology / Japan Epidemiological Association, 2006; 16(6): 233-239.

[138] Peng T, Shen HM, Liu ZM, et al. Oxidative DNA damage in peripheral leukocytes and its association with expression and polymorphisms of hOGG1: a study of adolescents in a high risk region for hepatocellular carcinoma in China. World J Gastroenterol, 2003; 9(10): 2186-2193.

[139] Nishimura S. Involvement of mammalian OGG1(MMH) in excision of the 8-hydroxyguanine residue in DNA. Free radical biology & medicine, 2002; 32(9): 813-821.

[140] Kohno T, Shinmura K, Tosaka M, et al. Genetic polymorphisms and alternative splicing of the hOGG1 gene, that is involved in the repair of 8-hydroxyguanine in damaged DNA. Oncogene, 1998; 16(25): 3219-3225.

[141] Cheng B, Jungst C, Lin J, et al. [Potential role of human DNA-repair enzymes hMTH1, hOGG1 and hMYHalpha in the hepatocarcinogenesis]. Journal of Huazhong University of Science and Technology Medical sciences, 2002; 22(3): 206-211, 215.

[142] Boiteux S, Radicella JP. The human OGG1 gene: structure, functions, and its implication in the process of carcinogenesis. Archives of biochemistry and biophysics, 2000; 377(1): 1-8.

[143] Aizhong W, CONG W, HE X, et al. [A hOGGl gene polymorphism and genetic susceptibility to colorectal cancer and hepatocellular carcinoma]. China J Gastroenterol, 2008; 17(10): 854-857.

[144] Yuan T, Wei J, Luo J, et al. Polymorphisms of Base-Excision Repair Genes hOGG1 326cys and XRCC1 280His Increase Hepatocellular Carcinoma Risk. Dig Dis Sci, 2012; 57(9): 2451-2457.

[145] Lakshmipathy U, Campbell C. Mitochondrial DNA ligase III function is independent of Xrcc1. Nucleic Acids Res, 2000; 28(20): 3880-3886.

[146] Marintchev A, Robertson A, Dimitriadis EK, et al. Domain specific interaction in the XRCC1-DNA polymerase beta complex. Nucleic Acids Res, 2000; 28(10): 2049-2059.

[147] Taylor RM, Moore DJ, Whitehouse J, et al. A cell cycle-specific requirement for the XRCC1 BRCT II domain during mammalian DNA strand break repair. Mol Cell Biol, 2000; 20(2): 735-740.

[148] Yamane K, Katayama E, Tsuruo T. The BRCT regions of tumor suppressor BRCA1 and of XRCC1 show DNA end binding activity with a multimerizing feature. Biochem Biophys Res Commun, 2000; 279(2): 678-684.

[149] Bhattacharyya N, Banerjee S. A novel role of XRCC1 in the functions of a DNA polymerase beta variant. Biochemistry, 2001; 40(30): 9005-9013.

[150] Dulic A, Bates PA, Zhang X, et al. BRCT domain interactions in the heterodimeric DNA repair protein XRCC1-DNA ligase III. Biochemistry, 2001; 40(20): 5906-5913.

[151] Vidal AE, Boiteux S, Hickson ID, et al. XRCC1 coordinates the initial and late stages of DNA abasic site repair through protein-protein interactions. EMBO J, 2001; 20(22): 6530-6539.

[152] Yacoub A, Park JS, Qiao L, et al. MAPK dependence of DNA damage repair: ionizing radiation and the induction of expression of the DNA repair genes XRCC1 and ERCC1 in DU145 human prostate carcinoma cells in a MEK1/2 dependent fashion. Int J Radiat Biol, 2001; 77(10): 1067-1078.

[153] Abdel-Rahman SZ, El-Zein RA. The 399Gln polymorphism in the DNA repair gene XRCC1 modulates the genotoxic response induced in human lymphocytes by the tobacco-specific nitrosamine NNK. Cancer Lett, 2000; 159(1): 63-71.

[154] Matullo G, Palli D, Peluso M, et al. XRCC1, XRCC3, XPD gene polymorphisms, smoking and (32)P-DNA adducts in a sample of healthy subjects. Carcinogenesis, 2001; 22(9): 1437-1445.

[155] Ratnasinghe D, Yao SX, Tangrea JA, et al. Polymorphisms of the DNA repair gene XRCC1 and lung cancer risk. Cancer Epidemiol Biomarkers Prev, 2001; 10(2): 119-123.

[156] Nelson HH, Kelsey KT, Mott LA, et al. The XRCC1 Arg399Gln polymorphism, sunburn, and non-melanoma skin cancer: evidence of gene-environment interaction. Cancer Res, 2002; 62(1): 152-155.

[157] Park JY, Lee SY, Jeon HS, et al. Polymorphism of the DNA repair gene XRCC1 and risk of primary lung cancer. Cancer Epidemiol Biomarkers Prev, 2002; 11(1): 23-27.

[158] Hsieh LL, Chien HT, Chen IH, et al. The XRCC1 399Gln polymorphism and the frequency of p53 mutations in Taiwanese oral squamous cell carcinomas. Cancer Epidemiol Biomarkers Prev, 2003; 12(5): 439-443.

[159] Shu XO, Cai Q, Gao YT, et al. A population-based case-control study of the Arg399Gln polymorphism in DNA repair gene XRCC1 and risk of breast cancer. Cancer Epidemiol Biomarkers Prev, 2003; 12(12): 1462-1467.

[160] Kelsey KT, Park S, Nelson HH, et al. A population-based case-control study of the XRCC1 Arg399Gln polymorphism and susceptibility to bladder cancer. Cancer Epidemiol Biomarkers Prev, 2004; 13(8): 1337-1341.

[161] Matsuo K, Hamajima N, Suzuki R, et al. Lack of association between DNA base excision repair gene XRCC1 Gln399Arg polymorphism and risk of malignant lymphoma in Japan. Cancer Genet Cytogenet, 2004; 149(1): 77-80.

[162] Yang JL, Han YN, Zheng SG. Influence of human XRCC1-399 single nucleotide polymorphism on primary hepatocytic carcinoma. Zhongliu, 2004; 24(4): 322-324.

[163] Jeon YT, Kim JW, Park NH, et al. DNA repair gene XRCC1 Arg399Gln polymorphism is associated with increased risk of uterine leiomyoma. Hum Reprod, 2005; 20(6): 1586-1589.

[164] Kirk GD, Turner PC, Gong Y, et al. Hepatocellular carcinoma and polymorphisms in carcinogen-metabolizing and DNA repair enzymes in a population with aflatoxin exposure and hepatitis B virus endemicity. Cancer epidemiology, biomarkers & prevention : a publication of the American Association for Cancer Research, cosponsored by the American Society of Preventive Oncology, 2005; 14(2): 373-379.

[165] Chung HH, Kim MK, Kim JW, et al. XRCC1 R399Q polymorphism is associated with response to platinum-based neoadjuvant chemotherapy in bulky cervical cancer. Gynecol Oncol, 2006; 103(3): 1031-1037.

[166] Kocabas NA, Karahalil B. XRCC1 Arg399Gln genetic polymorphism in a Turkish population. Int J Toxicol, 2006; 25(5): 419-422.

[167] Long XD, Ma Y, Wei YP, et al. The polymorphisms of GSTM1, GSTT1, HYL1*2, and XRCC1, and aflatoxin B1-related hepatocellular carcinoma in Guangxi population, China. Hepatology research : the official journal of the Japan Society of Hepatology, 2006; 36(1): 48-55.

[168] Bau DT, Hsieh YY, Wan L, et al. Polymorphism of XRCC1 codon arg 399 Gln is associated with higher susceptibility to endometriosis. Chin J Physiol, 2007; 50(6): 326-329.

[169] Deligezer U, Akisik EE, Dalay N. Lack of association of XRCC1 codon 399Gln polymorphism with chronic myelogenous leukemia. Anticancer Res, 2007; 27(4B): 2453-2456.

[170] Monaco R, Rosal R, Dolan MA, et al. Conformational effects of a common codon 399 polymorphism on the BRCT1 domain of the XRCC1 protein. Protein J, 2007; 26(8): 541-546.

[171] Sobti RC, Singh J, Kaur P, et al. XRCC1 codon 399 and ERCC2 codon 751 polymorphism, smoking, and drinking and risk of esophageal squamous cell carcinoma in a North Indian population. Cancer Genet Cytogenet, 2007; 175(2): 91-97.

[172] Geng J, Zhang YW, Huang GC, et al. XRCC1 genetic polymorphism Arg399Gln and gastric cancer risk: A meta-analysis. World J Gastroenterol, 2008; 14(43): 6733-6737.

[173] Ren y, Wang DS, Li Z, et al. Study on the Relationship between Gene XRCC1 Codon 399 Single Nucleotide Polymorphisms and Primary Hepatic Carcinoma in Han Nationality. Linchuang Gandang Bing Zazhi, 2008; 24(5): 361-364.

[174] Geng J, Zhang Q, Zhu C, et al. XRCC1 genetic polymorphism Arg399Gln and prostate cancer risk: a meta-analysis. Urology, 2009; 74(3): 648-653.

[175] Kiran M, Saxena R, Chawla YK, et al. Polymorphism of DNA repair gene XRCC1 and hepatitis-related hepatocellular carcinoma risk in Indian population. Mol Cell Biochem, 2009; 327(1-2): 7-13.

[176] Li Y, Long C, Lin G, et al. Effect of the XRCC1 codon 399 polymorphism on the repair of vinyl chloride metabolite-induced DNA damage. J Carcinog, 2009; 8(14.

[177] Saadat M, Ansari-Lari M. Polymorphism of XRCC1 (at codon 399) and susceptibility to breast cancer, a meta-analysis of the literatures. Breast Cancer Res Treat, 2009; 115(1): 137-144.

[178] Zeng X, Yu H, Qiu X, et al. [A case-control study of polymorphism of XRCC1 gene and the risk of hepatocellular carcinoma]. Chin J Dis Contr ol Pr ev, 2010; 14(8): 760-763.

[179] Qiu Y, Zhu S, Liu J, et al. [Study of susceptibility of chromosomal damage induced by vinyl chloride monomer associated with genetic polymorphism in APE1, XRCC1]. Wei Sheng Yan Jiu, 2007; 36(2): 132-136.

[180] Yu MW, Yang SY, Pan IJ, et al. Polymorphisms in XRCC1 and glutathione S-transferase genes and hepatitis B-related hepatocellular carcinoma. Journal of the National Cancer Institute, 2003; 95(19): 1485-1488.

[181] Pan HZ, Liang J, Yu Z, et al. Polymorphism of DNA repair gene XRCC1 and hepatocellular carcinoma risk in Chinese population. Asian Pacific journal of cancer prevention : APJCP, 2011; 12(11): 2947-2950.

[182] Liu F, Li B, Wei Y, et al. XRCC1 genetic polymorphism Arg399Gln and hepatocellular carcinoma risk: a meta-analysis. Liver international : official journal of the International Association for the Study of the Liver, 2011; 31(6): 802-809.

[183] Kiran M, Chawla YK, Jain M, et al. Haplotypes of microsomal epoxide hydrolase and x-ray cross-complementing group 1 genes in Indian hepatocellular carcinoma patients. DNA and cell biology, 2009; 28(11): 573-577.

[184] Han X, Xing Q, Li Y, et al. Study on the DNA Repair Gene XRCC1 and XRCC3 Polymorphism in Prediction and Prognosis of Hepatocellular Carcinoma Risk. Hepatogastroenterology, 2012; 59(119).

[185] Chen CC, Yang SY, Liu CJ, et al. Association of cytokine and DNA repair gene polymorphisms with hepatitis B-related hepatocellular carcinoma. Int J Epidemiol, 2005; 34(6): 1310-1318.

[186] Borentain P, Gerolami V, Ananian P, et al. DNA-repair and carcinogen-metabolising enzymes genetic polymorphisms as an independent risk factor for hepatocellular carcinoma in Caucasian liver-transplanted patients. European journal of cancer, 2007; 43(17): 2479-2486.

[187] Chen BP, Long XD, Fu GH. Meta-analysis of XRCC1 Codon 399 polymorphism and susceptibility to hepatocellular carcinoma. Shanghai Jiao Tong Xaxue Xuebao (Medical Version), 2011; 31(11): 1588-1591.

[188] Liu Y, Tarsounas M, O'Regan P, et al. Role of RAD51C and XRCC3 in genetic recombination and DNA repair. J Biol Chem, 2007; 282(3): 1973-1979.

[189] Xu ZY, Loignon M, Han FY, et al. Xrcc3 induces cisplatin resistance by stimulation of Rad51-related recombinational repair, S-phase checkpoint activation, and reduced apoptosis. J Pharmacol Exp Ther, 2005; 314(2): 495-505.

[190] Forget AL, Bennett BT, Knight KL. Xrcc3 is recruited to DNA double strand breaks early and independent of Rad51. J Cell Biochem, 2004; 93(3): 429-436.

[191] Bishop DK, Ear U, Bhattacharyya A, et al. Xrcc3 is required for assembly of Rad51 complexes in vivo. J Biol Chem, 1998; 273(34): 21482-21488.

[192] Brenneman MA, Weiss AE, Nickoloff JA, et al. XRCC3 is required for efficient repair of chromosome breaks by homologous recombination. Mutat Res, 2000; 459(2): 89-97.

[193] Wang J, Zhao Y, Jiang J, et al. Polymorphisms in DNA repair genes XRCC1, XRCC3 and XPD, and colorectal cancer risk: a case-control study in an Indian population. J Cancer Res Clin Oncol, 2010; 136(10): 1517-1525.

[194] Jiang Z, Li C, Xu Y, et al. A meta-analysis on XRCC1 and XRCC3 polymorphisms and colorectal cancer risk. Int J Colorectal Dis, 2010; 25(2): 169-180.

[195] Fang F, Wang J, Yao L, et al. Relationship between XRCC3 T241M polymorphism and gastric cancer risk: a meta-analysis. Med Oncol, 2010.

[196] Economopoulos KP, Sergentanis TN. XRCC3 Thr241Met polymorphism and breast cancer risk: a meta-analysis. Breast Cancer Res Treat, 2010; 121(2): 439-443.

[197] Zhang ZQ, Yang L, Zhang Y, et al. [Relationship between NQO1C(609T), RAD51(G135C), XRCC3(C241T) single nucleotide polymorphisms and acute lymphoblastic leukemia]. Zhongguo Shi Yan Xue Ye Xue Za Zhi, 2009; 17(3): 523-528.

[198] Sobczuk A, Romanowicz-Makowska H, Fiks T, et al. XRCC1 and XRCC3 DNA repair gene polymorphisms in breast cancer women from the Lodz region of Poland. Pol J Pathol, 2009; 60(2): 76-80.

[199] Krupa R, Synowiec E, Pawlowska E, et al. Polymorphism of the homologous recombination repair genes RAD51 and XRCC3 in breast cancer. Exp Mol Pathol, 2009; 87(1): 32-35.

[200] Andreassi MG, Foffa I, Manfredi S, et al. Genetic polymorphisms in XRCC1, OGG1, APE1 and XRCC3 DNA repair genes, ionizing radiation exposure and chromosomal DNA damage in interventional cardiologists. Mutat Res, 2009; 666(1-2): 57-63.

[201] Yen CY, Liu SY, Chen CH, et al. Combinational polymorphisms of four DNA repair genes XRCC1, XRCC2, XRCC3, and XRCC4 and their association with oral cancer in Taiwan. J Oral Pathol Med, 2008; 37(5): 271-277.

[202] Tekeli A, Isbir S, Ergen A, et al. APE1 and XRCC3 polymorphisms and myocardial infarction. In Vivo, 2008; 22(4): 477-479.

[203] Mateuca RA, Roelants M, Iarmarcovai G, et al. hOGG1(326), XRCC1(399) and XRCC3(241) polymorphisms influence micronucleus frequencies in human lymphocytes in vivo. Mutagenesis, 2008; 23(1): 35-41.

[204] Liu L, Yang L, Zhang Y, et al. [Polymorphisms of RAD51(G135C) and XRCC3(C241T) genes and correlations thereof with prognosis and clinical outcomes of acute myeloid leukemia]. Zhonghua Yi Xue Za Zhi, 2008; 88(6): 378-382.

[205] Jacobsen NR, Raaschou-Nielsen O, Nexo B, et al. XRCC3 polymorphisms and risk of lung cancer. Cancer Lett, 2004; 213(1): 67-72.

[206] Sakata K, Someya M, Matsumoto Y, et al. Ability to repair DNA double-strand breaks related to cancer susceptibility and radiosensitivity. Radiation medicine, 2007; 25(9): 433-438.

[207] Fujimoto M, Matsumoto N, Tsujita T, et al. Characterization of the promoter region, first ten exons and nine intron-exon boundaries of the DNA-dependent protein kinase catalytic subunit gene, DNA-PKcs (XRCC7). DNA Res, 1997; 4(2): 151-154.

[208] Blunt T, Finnie NJ, Taccioli GE, et al. Defective DNA-dependent protein kinase activity is linked to V(D)J recombination and DNA repair defects associated with the murine scid mutation. Cell, 1995; 80(5): 813-823.

[209] van der Burg M, van Dongen JJ, van Gent DC. DNA-PKcs deficiency in human: long predicted, finally found. Current opinion in allergy and clinical immunology, 2009; 9(6): 503-509.

[210] Smider V, Chu G. The end-joining reaction in V(D)J recombination. Semin Immunol, 1997; 9(3): 189-197.

[211] Jolly CJ, Cook AJ, Manis JP. Fixing DNA breaks during class switch recombination. The Journal of experimental medicine, 2008; 205(3): 509-513.

[212] Sipley JD, Menninger JC, Hartley KO, et al. Gene for the catalytic subunit of the human DNA-activated protein kinase maps to the site of the XRCC7 gene on chromosome 8. Proc Natl Acad Sci U S A, 1995; 92(16): 7515-7519.

[213] Johnston PJ, MacPhail SH, Stamato TD, et al. Higher-order chromatin structure-dependent repair of DNA double-strand breaks: involvement of the V(D)J recombination double-strand break repair pathway. Radiat Res, 1998; 149(5): 455-462.

Chapter 16

DNA Damage, DNA Repair and Cancer

Carol Bernstein, Anil R. Prasad,
Valentine Nfonsam and Harris Bernstein

Additional information is available at the end of the chapter

http://dx.doi.org/10.5772/53919

1. Introduction

DNA damage appears to be a fundamental problem for life. In this chapter we review evidence indicating that DNA damages are a major primary cause of cancer. DNA damages give rise to mutations and epimutations that, by a process of natural selection, can cause progression to cancer. First, we describe the distinguishing characteristics of DNA damage, mutation and epimutation.

DNA damage is a change in the basic structure of DNA that is not itself replicated when the DNA is replicated. A DNA damage can be a chemical addition or disruption to a base of DNA (creating an abnormal nucleotide or nucleotide fragment) or a break in one or both chains of the DNA strands. When DNA carrying a damaged base is replicated, an incorrect base can often be inserted opposite the site of the damaged base in the complementary strand, and this can become a mutation in the next round of replication. Also DNA double-strand breaks may be repaired by an inaccurate repair process leading to mutations. In addition, a double strand break can cause rearrangements of the chromosome structure (possibly disrupting a gene, or causing a gene to come under abnormal regulatory control), and, if such a change can be passed to successive cell generations, it is also a form of mutation. Mutations, however, can be avoided if accurate DNA repair systems recognize DNA damages as abnormal structures, and repair the damages prior to replication. As illustrated in Figure 1, when DNA damages occur, DNA repair is a crucial protective process blocking entry of cells into carcinogenesis.

We note that DNA damages occur in both replicating, proliferative cells (e.g. those forming the internal lining of the colon or blood forming "hematopoietic" cells), and in differentiated, non-dividing cells (e.g. neurons in the brain or myocytes in muscle). Cancers occur primarily in proliferative tissues. If DNA damages in proliferating cells are not repaired due to inadequate expression of a DNA repair gene, this increases the risk of cancer. In contrast, when DNA damages occur in non-proliferating cells and are not repaired due to inadequate expression of a DNA repair gene, the damages can accumulate and cause premature aging. As examples, deficiencies in DNA repair genes *ERCC1* or *XPF* [1] or in *WRN* [2, 3] cause both increased risk of cancer as well as premature aging. In Figure 1, DNA repair is indicated as a crucial process impeding both cancer and premature aging.

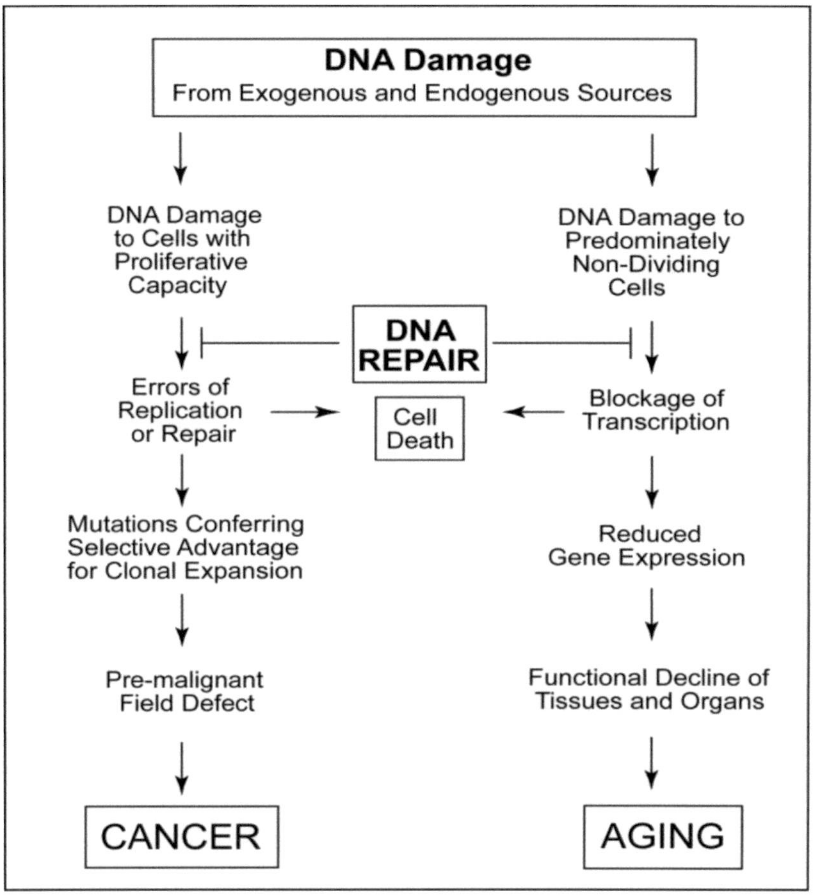

Figure 1. The roles of DNA damage and DNA repair in cancer and aging.

A mutation is a change in the DNA sequence in which normal base pairs are substituted, added, deleted or rearranged. The DNA containing a mutation still consists of a sequence of standard base pairs, and the altered DNA sequence can be copied when the DNA is replicated. A mutation can prevent a gene from carrying out its function, or it can cause a gene to be translated into a protein that functions abnormally. Mutations can activate oncogenes, inactivate tumor suppressor genes or cause genomic instability in replicating cells, and an assemblage of such mutations, together in the same cell, can lead to cancer. Cancers usually arise from an assemblage of mutations conferring a selective advantage that leads to clonal expansion (Figure 1). Colon cancers, for example, have an average of 15 "driver" mutations (mutations occurring repeatedly in different colon cancers) and about 75 "passenger" mutations (mutations occurring infrequently in colon cancers) [4, 5]. Colon cancers also were found to have an average of 9 duplications or deletions of chromosome segments [6] or, more recently, 17 focal amplifications, 28 recurrent deletions and up to 10 translocations [5]. Since mutations have normal DNA structure, they cannot be recognized or removed by DNA repair processes in living cells. Removal of a mutation only occurs if it is sufficiently deleterious to cause the death of the cell.

Another type of inheritable alteration, similar in some ways to a mutation, is an epigenetic change. An epigenetic change refers to a functionally relevant modification of the DNA, or of the histone proteins controlling the relaxation or tightened winding of the DNA within their nucleosome structures. Some epigenetic changes involve specific alterations of the DNA nucleotides. Examples of such changes include methylation of the DNA at particular sites (CpG islands) where the DNA starts to be transcribed into RNA. These changes may inhibit transcription. Other epigenetic changes involve modification of histones associated with particular regions of the DNA. These may inhibit or promote the ability of these regions to be transcribed into mRNA. Methylation of CpG islands or modification of histones can directly alter transcription of gene-encoded mRNAs but they can also occur in parts of the genome that code for microRNAs (miRNAs). MiRNAs are endogenous short non-protein coding RNAs (~22 nucleotides long) that post-transcriptionally regulate mRNA expression in a sequence specific manner. miRNAs either cause degradation of mRNAs or block their translation. Epigenetic modifications can play a role similar to mutation in carcinogenesis, and about 280 cancer prone epigenetic alterations are listed by Schnekenburger and Diederich [7]. Epigenetic alterations are usually copied onto the daughter chromosomes when the parental chromosome replicates.

Although epigenetic changes can be passed down from one cell generation to the next, they are not regarded as true mutations. Most epigenetic changes appear to be part of the differentiation program of the cell and are necessary to allow different types of cells to carry out different functions. In most cells of a human body, only about 5% of genes are active at any one time, often due to epigenetic modifications. However, abnormal unprogrammed epigenetic changes may also occur that alter the functioning of a cell and these changes are referred to as "epimutations." Programmed epigenetic changes can be reversed. During development, as daughter cells of a stem cell differentiate, some epigenetic changes are programmed for reversal. However, a double strand break in DNA (a type of DNA damage) can initiate unprogrammed epigenetic gene silencing both by causing methylation of a CpG island as well as by promoting silencing types of histone modifications [8]. Another form of epigenetic silencing may occur during DNA repair. The enzyme Parp1 (poly(ADP)-ribose polymerase) and its product poly(ADP)-ribose (PAR) accumulate at sites of DNA damage as part of a repair process [9]. This, in turn, directs recruitment and activation of the chromatin remodeling protein ALC1 that may cause nucleosome remodeling [10]. Nucleosome remodeling has been found to cause, for instance, epigenetic silencing of DNA repair gene *MLH1* [11]. Chemicals previously identified as DNA damaging agents, including benzene, hydroquinone, styrene, carbon tetrachloride and trichloroethylene, were shown to cause considerable hypomethylation of DNA, some through the activation of oxidative stress pathways [12]. Dietary agents also have been shown to affect DNA methylation or histone modification by numerous pathways [13]. Recent evidence indicates that epimutations occur in DNA repair genes that reduce their function. Epimutations in DNA repair genes allow DNA damages to accumulate, and are a cause of progression to cancer [14].

2. DNA damages are frequent, and DNA repair processes can be overwhelmed

Tens of thousands of DNA damages occur per day per cell, on average, in humans, due to reactive molecules produced by metabolism or by hydrolytic reactions in the warm aqueous cellular media. Some types of such endogenous damages, and their rates of occurrence, are shown in Table 1.

A considerable number of other types of endogenous DNA damages have been identified, many of which are mutagenic. These include propano-, etheno- and malondialdehyde-derived DNA adducts, base propenals, estrogen-DNA adducts, alkylated bases, deamination of each of cytosine, adenine and guanine (to form uracil, hypoxanthine and xanthine, respectively) and adducts formed with DNA by reactive carbonyl species [15].

While there are repair pathways that act on these DNA damages, the repair processes are not 100% efficient, and further damages occur even as current DNA damages are being repaired. Thus there is a steady state level of many DNA damages, reflecting the efficiencies of repair and the frequencies of occurrence. For instance, Helbock et al. [16] estimated the steady state level of oxidative adducts in rat liver as 24, 000 adducts per cell in young rats and 66, 000 adducts per cell in old rats. Nakamura and Swenberg [17] determined the number of AP sites (apurinc and apyrimidinic sites) in normal tissues of the rat (i.e. in lung, kidney, liver, testis, heart, colon and brain). The data indicated that the number of AP sites ranged from about 50, 000 per cell in liver, kidney and lung to about 200, 000 per cell in the brain. These steady state numbers of AP sites in genomic DNA were considered to represent the balance between formation and repair of AP sites.

DNA damages	Reported rate of occurrence	Ref.
Oxidative	86,000 per cell per day in rats	[18]
	10,000 per cell per day in humans 100,000 per cell per day in rats	[19]
	11,500 per cell per day for humans 74,000 per cell per day for rats	[16]
Specific oxidative damage products 8-hydroxyguanine, 8-hydroxydeoxyguanosine, 5-(hydroxymethyl) uracil	2,800 per cell per day in humans 34,800 per cell per day in mice	[20]
Depurinations	10,000 per cell during 20-hour generation period	[21]
	13,920 per cell per day (580/cell/hr)	[22]
	2,000 to 10,000 per cell per day	[23,24]
	9,000 per cell per day	[25]
Depyrimidinations	500 pyrimidines per cell during 20-hour generation period	[21]
	696 per cell per day (29/cell/hr)	[22]
Single-strand breaks	55,200 per cell per day (2,300/cell/hr)	[22]
Double-strand breaks	~10 per cell cycle in humans	[26]
	~50 per cell cycle in humans	[27]
O^6-methylguanine	3,120 per cell per day (130/cell/hr)	[22]
Cytosine deamination	192 per cell per day (8/cell/hr)	[22]

Table 1. DNA damages due to natural endogenous causes in mammalian cells

DNA repair pathways are usually able to keep up with the endogenous damages in replicating cells, in part by halting DNA replication at the site of damage until repair can occur [28, 29]. In contrast, non-replicating cells have a build-up of DNA damages, causing aging [30, 31].

However, some exogenous DNA damaging agents, such as those in tobacco smoke, discussed below, may overload the repair pathways, either with higher levels of the same type of DNA damages as those occurring endogenously or with novel types of damage that are repaired more slowly. In addition, if DNA repair pathways are deficient, due to inherited mutations or sporadic somatic epimutations in DNA repair genes in replicating somatic cells, unrepaired endogenous and exogenous damages will increase due to insufficient repair. Increased DNA damages would likely give rise to increased errors of replication past the damages (by trans-lesion synthesis) or increased error prone repair (e.g. by non-homologous end-joining), causing mutations. Increased mutations that activate oncogenes, inactivate tumor suppressor genes, cause genomic instability or give rise to other driver mutations in replicating cells would increase the risk of cancer.

3. Cancers are often caused by exogenous DNA damaging agents

Cancer incidence, in different areas of the world, varies considerably. Thus, the incidence of colon cancer among Black Native-Africans is less than 1 person out of 100, 000, while among male Black African-Americans it is 72.9 per 100, 000, and this difference is likely due to differences in diet [32, 33]. Rates of colon cancer incidence among populations migrating from lower-incidence to higher-incidence countries change rapidly, and within one generation can reach the rate in the higher-incidence country. This is observed, for instance, in migrants from Japan to Hawaii [34].

The most common cancers for men and women and their rates of incidence per 100, 000, averaged over the more developed areas and less developed areas of the world, are shown in Table 2 (from [35]). Overall, worldwide, cancer incidence in all organs combined is 300.1 per 100, 000 per year in more developed areas and 160.3 per 100, 000 per year in less developed areas [35]. The differences in cancer incidence between more developed areas of the world and less developed areas are likely due, in large part, to differences in exposure to exogenous carcinogenic factors. The lowest rates of cancers in a given organ (Table 2) may be due, at least in part, to endogenous DNA damages (as described in the previous section) that cause errors of replication (trans-lesion synthesis) or error prone repair (e.g. non-homologous end-joining), leading to carcinogenic mutations. The higher rates (Table 2) are likely largely attributable to exogenous factors, such as higher rates of tobacco use or diets higher in saturated fats that directly, or indirectly, increase the incidence of DNA damage.

It is interesting to note in Table 2 that, in cases where cancers occur in the same organs of men and women, men consistently have a higher rate of cancer than women. The basis for this is currently unknown.

http://dx.doi.org/10.5772/53919

	More developed areas		Less developed areas	
	Incidence	*Mortality*	*Incidence*	*Mortality*
Breast (women)	66.4	15.3	27.3	10.8
Prostate (men)	62.0	10.6	12.0	5.6
Lung (men)	47.4	39.4	27.8	24.6
Lung (women)	18.6	13.6	11.1	9.7
Colorectum (men)	37.6	15.1	12.1	6.9
Colorectum (women)	24.2	9.7	9.4	5.4
Esophagus (men)	6.5	5.3	11.8	10.1
Esophagus (women)	1.2	1.0	5.7	4.7
Stomach (men)	16.7	10.4	21.1	16.0
Stomach (women)	7.3	4.7	10.0	8.1
Liver (men)	8.1	7.2	18.9	17.4
Liver (women)	2.7	2.5	7.6	7.2
Bladder (men)	16.6	4.6	5.4	2.6
Bladder (women)	3.6	1.0	1.4	0.7
Cervix/Uterine (women)	12.9	2.4	5.9	1.7
Kidney (men)	11.8	4.1	2.5	1.3
Kidney (women)	5.8	1.7	1.4	0.8
Non-Hodgkin lymphoma (men)	10.3	3.6	4.2	3.0
Non-Hodgkin lymphoma (women)	7.0	2.2	2.8	1.9
Melanoma (men)	9.5	1.8	0.7	0.3
Melanoma (women)	8.6	1.1	0.6	0.3
Ovarian (women)	9.4	5.1	5.0	3.1

Table 2. Incidence and mortality rates for the most common cancers in age standardized rates per 100, 000 (excluding non-melanoma skin cancer) (Adapted from Jemal et al. [35]).

4. Exogenous DNA damaging agents in carcinogenesis

Carcinogenic exogenous factors have been identified as a major cause of many common cancers, including cancers of the lung, colorectum, esophagus, stomach, liver, cervix/uterus and melanoma. Often such exogenous factors have been shown to cause DNA damage, as described below.

5. Exogenous DNA damaging agents in lung cancer

In both developed and undeveloped countries, lung cancer is the most frequent cause of cancer mortality (Table 2, data for men and women combined). Lung cancer is largely caused by tobacco smoke, since risk estimates for lung cancer indicate that, in the United States, tobacco smoke is responsible for 90% of lung cancers. Also implicated in lung cancer (and somewhat overlapping with smoking) are occupational exposure to carcinogens (approximately 9 to 15%), radon (10%) and outdoor air pollution (perhaps 1 to 2%) [36].

Acrolein	122.4
Formaldehyde	60.5
Acrylonitrile	29.3
1,3-butadiene	105.0
Acetaldehyde	1448.0
Ethylene oxide	7.0
Isoprene	952.0
Benzo[a]pyrene	0.014

Table 3. Weight, in μg per cigarette, of several likely carcinogenic DNA damaging agents in tobacco smoke (from [37] Cunningham et al., 2011])

Tobacco smoke is a complex mixture of over 5, 300 identified chemicals, of which 150 are known to have specific toxicological properties (see partial summary by Cunningham [37]). A "Margin of Exposure" approach has recently been established to determine the most important exogenous carcinogenic factors in tobacco smoke [37]. This quantitative-type of measurement is based on published dose response data for mutagenicity or carcinogenicity and the concentrations of these components in tobacco smoke (Table 3). Using the "Margin of Exposure" approach, Cunningham et al. [37] found the most important tumorigenic compounds in tobacco smoke to be, in order of importance, acrolein, formaldehyde, acrylonitrile, 1, 3-butadiene, acetaldehyde, ethylene oxide and isoprene.

Acrolein, the first agent in Table 3, is the structurally simplest α, β-unsaturated aldehyde (Figure 2). It can rapidly penetrate through the cell membrane and bind to the nucleophilic N^2-amine of deoxyguanine (dG) followed by cyclization of N1, to give the exocyclic DNA adduct α-hydroxy-1, N^2-propano-2′-deoxyguanine (α-HOPdG) (shown in Figure 2) and another product designated γ-HOPdG. The adducts formed by acrolein are a major type of DNA damage caused by tobacco smoke, and acrolein has been found to be mutagenic [38].

In tobacco smoke, acrolein has a concentration >8, 000 fold higher than benzo[a]pyrene (reviewed in [38]), with 122.4 μg of acrolein per cigarette. Benzo[a]pyrene has long been thought to be an important carcinogen in tobacco smoke [39]. As reviewed by Alexandrov et al. [39], benzo[a]pyrene damages DNA by forming DNA adducts at the N^2 position of guanine (similar to where acrolein forms adducts). However, by the "Margin of Exposure" approach, based on published dose response data and its concentration in cigarette smoke of 0.014 μg per cigarette, benzo[a]pyrene is thought to be a much less important mutagen for lung tissue than acrolein and the other six highly likely carcinogens in tobacco smoke listed in Table 3 [37].

The other agents in Table 3 cause DNA damages in different ways. Formaldehyde, the second agent in Table 3, primarily causes DNA damage by introducing DNA-protein cross-links. These cross-links, in turn, cause mutagenic deletions or other small-scale chromosomal rearrangements [40] and may also cause mutations through single-nucleotide insertions [41]. Acrylonitrile, the third agent in Table 3, appears to cause DNA damage indirectly by increasing oxidative stress, leading to increased levels of 8′-hydroxyl-2-deoxyguanosine (8-OHdG) in DNA [42]. Oxidative stress also causes lipid peroxidation that generates malondialdehyde (MDA), and MDA forms DNA adducts with guanine, adenine and cytosine [43]. The fourth agent in Table 3, 1, 3-butadiene, causes genotoxicity both directly by forming a DNA adduct as well as indirectly by causing global loss of DNA methylation and histone methylation leading to epigenetic alterations [44]. The fifth agent in Table 3, acetaldehyde, reacts with 2′-deoxyguanosine in DNA to form DNA adducts [45]. The sixth agent in Table 3, ethylene oxide, forms mutagenic hydroxyethyl DNA adducts with adenine and guanine [46]. The seventh agent in Table 3, isoprene, is normally produced endogenously by humans, and is the main hydrocarbon of non-smoking human breath [47]. However, smoking one cigarette causes an increase of breath isoprene levels by an average of 70% [48]. Isoprene, after being metabolized to mono-epoxides, causes DNA damage measured as single and double strand breaks in DNA [49].

A large number of studies have been published in which the levels and characteristics of DNA adducts in the lung and bronchus of smokers and non-smokers have been compared, as reviewed by Phillips [50]. In most of these studies, significantly elevated levels of DNA adducts were detected in the peripheral lung, bronchial epithelium or bronchioalveolar lavage cells of the smokers, especially for total bulky DNA adducts. As further discussed by Phillips [50], mean levels of DNA adducts in ex-smokers (usually with at least a 1 year interval since smoking cessation) are found generally to be intermediate between the levels of smokers and life-long non-smokers. From these comparisons, the half-life of some DNA adducts in lung tissue are estimated to be ~1–2 years.

6. Exogenous DNA damaging agents in colorectal cancer

Up to 20% of current colorectal cancers in the United States may be due to tobacco smoke [51]. Presumably tobacco smoke causes colon cancer due to the DNA damaging agents described above for lung cancer. These agents may be taken up in the blood and carried to organs of the body.

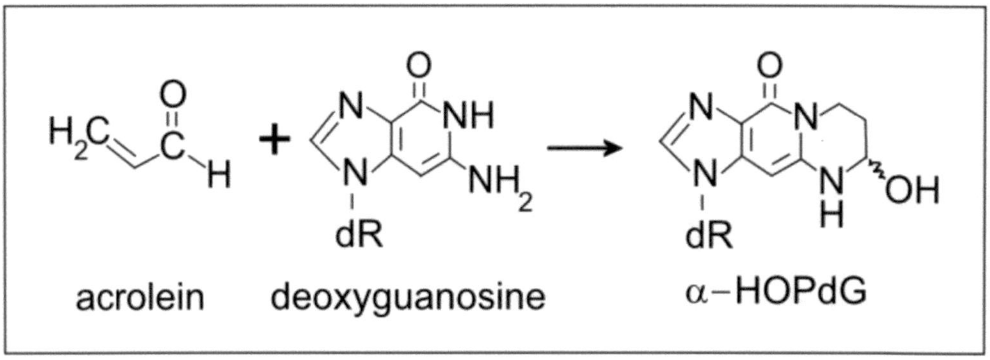

Figure 2. Reaction of acrolein with deoxyguanosine

The human colon is exposed to many compounds that are either of direct dietary origin or result from digestive and/or microbial processes. Four different classes of colonic mutagenic compounds were analysed by de Kok and van Maanen [52] and evaluated for fecal mutagenicity. These included (1) pyrolysis compounds from food (heterocyclic aromatic amines and polycyclic aromatic hydrocarbons), (2) *N*-nitroso-compounds (from high meat diets, from drinking water with high nitrates or produced during ulcerative colitis), (3) fecapentaenes (produced by the colonic bacteria *Bacteriodes* in the presence of bile acids) and (4) bile acids (increased in the colon in response to a high fat diet and metabolized to genotoxic form by bacteria in the colon). Many of these diet-related mutagenic compounds were analysed by Pearson et al. [53] in terms of their presence in fecal water, and their effect on the cytotoxic or genotoxic activity of fecal water. Evidence in both of these studies was insufficient to evaluate the colorectal cancer risk as a result of specific exposures in quantitative terms.

However, substantial evidence implicates bile acids (the 4th possibility above) in colon caner. Bernstein et al. [54], summarized 12 studies indicating that the bile acids deoxycholic acid (DCA) and/or lithocholic acid (LCA) induce production of DNA damaging reactive oxygen species and/or reactive nitrogen species in colon cells of animal or human origin. They also tabulated 14 studies showing that DCA and LCA induce DNA damage in colon cells. In addition to causing DNA damage, bile acids may also generate genomic instability by causing mitotic perturbations and reduced expression of spindle checkpoint proteins, giving rise to micro-nuclei, chromosome bridges and other structures that are precursors to aneuploidy [55]. Furthermore, at high physiological concentrations, bile acids cause frequent apoptosis, and those cells in the exposed populations with reduced apoptosis capability tend to survive and selectively proliferate [54, 56]. Cells with reduced ability to undergo apoptosis in response to DNA damage would tend to accumulate mutations when replication occurs past those damages, and such cells may give rise to colon cancers. In addition, 7 epidemiological studies between 1971 and 1990 (reviewed by Bernstein et al. [54]), found that fecal bile acid concentrations are increased in populations with a high incidence of colorectal cancer. A similar 2012 epidemiological study showed that concentrations of fecal LCA and DCA, respectively, were 4-fold and 5-fold higher in a population at 65-fold higher risk of colon cancer compared to a population at lower risk of colon cancer [32]. This evidence points to bile acids DCA and LCA as centrally important DNA-damaging carcinogens in colon cancer.

Dietary total fat intake and dietary saturated fat intake is significantly related to incidence of colon cancer [57]. Increasing total fat or saturated fat in human diets results in increases in DCA and LCA in the feces [58, 59], indicating increased contact of the colonic epithelium with DCA and LCA. Bernstein et al. [60] added the bile acid DCA to the standard diet of wild-type mice. This supplement raised the level of DCA in the feces of mice from the standard-diet fed mouse level of 0.3 mg DCA/g dry weight to 4.6 mg DCA/g dry weight, a level similar to that for humans on a high fat diet of 6.4 mg DCA/g dry weight. After 8 or 10 months on the DCA-supplemented diet, 56% of the mice developed invasive colon cancer. This directly indicates that DCA, a DNA damaging agent, at levels present in humans after a high fat diet, can cause colorectal cancer.

7. Exogenous DNA damaging agents implicated in other major cancers

It is beyond the scope of this chapter to detail the evidence implicating DNA damaging agents as etiologic agents in all of the significant cancers. Therefore, in Table 4 we indicate with a single reference the major DNA damaging agent in five additional prevalent cancers, in order to illustrate the generality of exogenous DNA damaging agents as causes of cancer. In particular, we point out, as reviewed by Handa et al. [61], *Helicobacter pylori* infection increases the production of reactive oxygen and reactive nitrogen species (RNS) in the human stomach, which, in turn, significantly increases DNA damage in the gastric epithelial cells. Thus, *H. pylori* infection acts as a DNA damaging agent. In the case of human papillomavirus (HPV) infection, Wei et al. [62] showed that cervical cells could resist RNS stress when not infected with HPV. However, cervical cells infected by HPV and exposed to RNS had higher levels of DNA double strand breaks as well as a higher mutation rate. This appeared to occur due to the ability of HPV to greatly reduce protein expression of the DNA damage repair/response gene *P53* when infected cells were stressed by RNS. Since reduced *P53* expression leads to greater RNS-induced DNA damage, HPV infection acts as a DNA damaging agent in the presence of RNS stress.

Cancer	Exogenous DNA damaging agent	Ref.
Esophagus	Bile acids	[63]
Stomach	*Helicobacter pylori* infection	[61]
Liver	*Aspergillus* metabolite aflatoxin B(1)	[64]
Cervix/Uterus	Human papillomavirus plus increased nitric oxide from tobacco smoke or other infection	[62]
Melanoma	UV light from solar radiation	[65]

Table 4. Selected cancers and relevant implicated exogenous DNA damaging agents

8. Deficient DNA repair due to a germ line mutation allows DNA damages to increase, leading to increased frequencies of mutation, epimutation and cancer

Expression of DNA repair genes may be reduced by inherited germ line mutations or genetic polymorphisms, or by epigenetic alterations or mutations in somatic cells, and these reductions may substantially increase the risk of cancer. Overall, about 30% of cancers are considered to be familial (largely due to inherited germ line mutations or genetic polymorphisms) and 70% are considered to be sporadic [66].

In 2 overlapping databases [67, 68] 167 and169 human genes (depending on the database) are listed that are directly employed in DNA repair or influence DNA repair processes. The lists were originally devised by Wood et al. [69, 70]. The genes are distributed in groups of DNA repair pathways and in related functions that affect DNA repair (Table 5). Bernstein et al. [71] illustrate many of the steps and order of action of the gene products involved for the first five DNA repair pathways listed in Table 5.

Individuals with an inherited impairment in DNA repair capability are often at considerably increased risk of cancer. If an individual has a germ line mutation in a DNA repair gene or a DNA damage response gene (that recognizes DNA damage and activates DNA repair), usually one abnormal copy of the gene is inherited from one of the parents and then the other copy is inactivated at some later point in life in a somatic cell. The inactivation may be due, for example, to point mutation, deletion, gene conversion, epigenetic silencing or other mechanisms [72]. The protein encoded by the gene will either not be expressed or be expressed in a mutated form. Consequently the DNA repair or DNA damage response function will be deficient or impaired, and damages will accumulate. Such DNA damages can cause errors during DNA replication or inaccurate repair, leading to mutations that can give rise to cancer.

Increased oxidative DNA damages also cause increased gene silencing by CpG island hypermethylation, a form of epimutation. These oxidative DNA damages induce formation and relocalization of a silencing complex that may result in cancer-specific aberrant DNA methylation and transcriptional silencing [73]. As pointed out above, the enzyme Parp1 (poly(ADP)-ribose polymerase) and its product poly(ADP)-ribose (PAR) accumulate at sites of DNA damage as part of a repair process [9], recruiting chromatin remodeling protein ALC1, causing nucleosome remodeling [10] that has been shown to direct epigenetic silencing of DNA repair gene *MLH1* [11]. If silencing of genes necessary for DNA repair occurs, the repair of further DNA damages will be deficient and more damages will accumulate. Such additional DNA damages will cause increased errors during DNA synthesis, leading to mutations that can give rise to cancer.

	Number of genes listed in the two databases
Homologous Recombinational Repair (HRR)	21,21
Non-homologous End Joining (NHEJ)	8,7
Nucleotide Excision Repair (NER)	30,29
Base Excision Repair (including PARP enzymes) (BER)	19,20
Mis-Match Repair (MMR)	11,10
Fanconi Anemia (FANC) [affects HRR (above) and translesion synthesis (TLS)]	10,16
Direct reversal of damage	3,3
DNA polymerases (act in various pathways)	17,15
Editing and processing nucleases (act in various pathways)	6,8
Ubiquitination and modification/Rad6 pathway including TLS	11,5
DNA damage response	12,14
Modulation of nucleotide pools	3,3
Chromatin structure	2,3
Defective in diseases and syndromes	4,5
DNA-topoisomerase crosslinks	2,1
Other genes	8,9

Table 5. DNA repair pathways and other processes affecting DNA repair [67, 68]

9. Inherited mutations in genes employed in DNA repair that give rise to syndromes characterized by increased risk of cancer.

Table 6 lists 36 genes for which an inherited mutation results in an increased risk of cancer. The proteins encoded by 35 of these genes are involved in DNA repair and in some cases also in other aspects of the DNA damage response such as cell cycle arrest and apoptosis. The polymerase coded for by the 36th gene, *XPV (POLH)*, is involved in bypass (rather than repair) of DNA damage, called translesion synthesis. The genes listed in Table 6, when mutated in the germ line, give rise to a considerably increased lifetime risk of cancer, of up to 100% (e.g. p53 mutations [74]). Thus defects in DNA repair cause progression to cancer.

In addition to mutations in genes that may substantially raise lifetime cancer risk, there appear to be many weakly effective genetically inherited polymorphisms [single nucleotide polymophisms (SNPs) and copy number variants (CNVs)]. By the HapMap Project, more than 3 million SNPs have been found, and by Genome Wide Association studies (GWAs), about 30 SNPs were found to increase risk of cancers. However the added risk of cancer by these SNPs is usually small, i.e. less than a factor of 2 increase [75]. A large twin study [66], involving 44, 788 pairs of twins, evaluated the risk of the same cancer before the age of 75 for monozygotic twins (identical genomes with the same polymorphisms) and dizygotic twins (having a 50% chance of the same polymorphisms). If one twin had colorectal, breast or prostate cancer, the monozygotic twin had an 11 to 18 percent chance of developing the same cancer while the dizygotic twin had only a 3 to 9% risk. The differences in monozygotic and dizygotic rates of paired cancer were not significant for the other 24 types of cancer evaluated in this study. Polymorphisms of the DNA repair gene ERCC1 will be discussed below in relation to targeted chemotherapy.

10. Epimutations may repress DNA repair gene expression, allowing DNA damages to increase, leading to increased frequency of further epimutation, mutation and cancer

While germ line (familial) mutations in DNA repair genes cause a high risk of cancer, somatic mutations in DNA repair genes are rarely found in sporadic (non-familial) cancers [4]. Much more often, DNA repair genes are found to have epigenetic alterations in cancers.

One example of the epigenetic down-regulation of a DNA repair gene in cancers comes from studies of the MMR protein MLH1. Truninger et al. [76] assessed 1, 048 unselected consecutive colon cancers. Of these, 103 were deficient in protein expression of *MLH1*, with 68 of these cancers being sporadic (the remaining *MLH1* deficient cancers were due to germ line mutations). Of the 68 sporadic MLH1 protein-deficient colon cancers, 65 (96%) were found to be deficient due to epigenetic methylation of the CpG island of the *MLH1* gene. Deficient protein expression of *MLH1* may also have been caused, in the remaining 3 sporadic MLH1 protein-deficient cancers (which did not have germ line mutations), by over expression of the microRNA miR-155. When miR-155 was transfected into cells it caused reduced expression of *MLH1* [77]. Overexpression of miR-155 was found in colon cancers in which protein expression of *MLH1* was deficient and the *MLH1* gene was neither mutated nor hypermethylated in its CpG island [77].

DNA repair gene(s)	Encoded protein	Repair pathway(s) affected	Ref.	Cancers with increased risk	Ref.
breast cancer 1 & 2	BRCA1, BRCA2	HRR of double strand breaks and daughter strand gaps	[85]	Breast, Ovarian	[86]
ataxia telangiectasia mutated	ATM	Different mutations in ATM reduce HRR, single strand annealing (SSA), NHEJ or homology directed double strand break rejoining (HDR)	[87]	Leukemia, Lymphoma, Breast	[87,88]
Nijmegen breakage syndrome	NBS	NHEJ	[89]	Lymphoid cancers	[89]
meiotic recombination 11	MRE11	HRR and NHEJ	[90]	Breast	[91]
Bloom's Syndrome (helicase)	BLM	HRR	[92]	Leukemia, Lymphoma, Colon, Breast, Skin, Auditory canal, Tongue, Esophagus, Stomach, Tonsil, Larynx, Lung, Uterus	[93]
Werner Syndrome (helicase)	WRN	HRR, NHEJ, long patch BER	[94]	Soft tissue sarcoma, Colorectal, Skin, Thyroid, Pancreatic	[95]
Rothman Thomson syndrome Rapadilino syndrome Baller Gerold syndrome	RECQ4	Helicase likely active in HRR	[96]	Basal cell carcinoma, Squamous cell carcinoma, Intraepidemial carcinoma	[97]
Fanconi's anemia gene FANC A,B,C,D1,D2,E,F,G,I,J,L,M,N	FANCA etc.	HRR and TLS	[98]	Leukemia, Liver tumors, Solid tumors many areas	[99]
xeroderma pigmentosa C, E [DNA damage binding protein 2 (DDB2)]	XPC XPE	Global genomic NER repairs damage in both transcribed and untranscribed DNA	[100, 101]	Skin cancer (melanoma and non-melanoma)	[100, 101]
xeroderma pigmentosa A, B, D, F, G	XPA XPB XPD XPF XPG	Transcription coupled NER repairs the transcribed strands of transcriptionally active genes	[102]	Skin cancer (melanoma and non-melanoma), Central nervous system cancers	[102]
xeroderma pigmentosa V (also called polymerase H)	XPV (POLH)	Translesion Synthesis (TLS)	[102]	Skin cancer (melanoma and non-melanoma)	[102]

DNA repair gene(s)	Encoded protein	Repair pathway(s) affected	Ref.	Cancers with increased risk	Ref.
mutS (E. coli) homolog 2 mutS (E. coli) homolog 6 mutL (E. coli) homolog 1 postmeiotic segregation increased 2 (S. cerevisiae)	MSH2 MSH6 MLH1 Pms2	MMR	[76]	Colorectal, endometrial. ovarian	[103]
mutY homolog (E. coli)	MUTYH	BER of A mispaired with 8OHdG, G, FapydG and C	[104]	Colon	[105]
ataxia telaniectsia and *RAD3* related	ATR	DNA damage response likely affects HRR, not NHEJ	[106]	Oropharyngeal cancer	[107]
Li Fraumeni syndrome	P53	HRR, BER, NER and DNA Damage Response for those and for NHEJ and MMR	[108]	Sarcoma, Breast, Lung, Skin, Pancreas, Leukemia, Brain	[74]

Table 6. Inherited mutations in DNA repair genes that increase the risk of cancer

Another example of the epigenetic down-regulation of a DNA repair gene in cancer comes from studies of the direct reversal of methylated guanine bases by methyl guanine methyl transferase (MGMT). In the most common form of brain cancer, glioblastoma, the DNA repair gene *MGMT* is epigenetically methylated in 29% [78] to 66% [79] of tumors, thereby reducing protein expression of MGMT. However, for 28% of glioblastomas, the MGMT protein is deficient but the *MGMT* promoter is not methylated [79]. Zhang et al. [78] found, in the glioblastomas without methylated *MGMT* promoters, that the level of microRNA miR-181d is inversely correlated with protein expression of MGMT and that the direct target of miR-181d is the MGMT mRNA 3′UTR (the three prime untranslated region of MGMT mRNA), though they indicated that other miRNAs may also be involved in the reduction of protein expression of MGMT.

Almost all DNA repair deficiencies found, so far, in sporadic cancers, and in precancerous tissues surrounding cancers (field defects) are due to epigenetic changes. Examples of such epigenetic alterations in DNA repair genes in different types of cancer are shown in Table 7. A recent review [80] lists 41 reports (mostly not overlapping with those listed in Table 7) indicating methylation of 20 DNA repair genes in various cancers. In Table 7 data are also shown on DNA repair gene deficiencies for the field defects associated with colorectal, gastric, laryngeal and non-small cell lung cancer.

As summarized above, epimutations can result from oxidative DNA damages. Such damages cause formation and relocalization of a silencing complex that in turn causes increased gene silencing by CpG island hypermethylation [73]. Epigenetic nucleosome remodeling during DNA repair can also silence gene expression [11]. When CpG island methylation or nucleosome remodeling or other types of epigenetic alterations (e.g. micro RNAs or histone modifications) inhibit DNA repair genes, more damages will accumulate. Accumulated DNA damages cause increased errors during DNA synthesis and repair. Thus epigenetic deficiencies in DNA repair genes can have a cascading effect (a mutator phenotype), leading to genomic instability and accumulation of mutations and epimutations that can give rise to cancer.

Cancer	Epigenetic changes in cancer (mechanism)	% sporadic cancers with epimutations	Epigenetic changes in field defect (mechanism)	% field defects with epi-mutations	Ref.
Breast	*BRCA1* (CGI*)	13% unselected 67% medullary 55% mucinous			[108]
	WRN (CGI)	17% unselected			[2]
Ovarian	*BRCA1* (CGI)	31% of those with loss of heterozygosity			[108]
Colorectal	*WRN* (CGI)	38%			[2]
	MGMT (CGI)	46%	*MGMT* (CGI)	23%	[109]
	MGMT (CGI)	90%			[110]
	MLH1 (CGI)	65%			
	MLH1 (CGI)	10%			[76]
	MLH1 (CGI)	2%			
	MSH2 (CGI)	13%	*MSH2*	5%	[111]
	MGMT (CGI)	47%	*MGMT*	11%	
	ERCC1	100%	*ERCC1*	40%	
	PMS2	88%	PMS2	50%	[112]
XPF	55%	XPF	40%		
Gastric	*MGMT* (CGI)	88%	*MGMT* (CGI)	29%	[113]
	WRN (CGI)	25%			[2]
Esophageal squamous cell carcininoma	*MLH1* (CGI)	49%			[114,115]
	MLH2 (CGI)	35%			
	MGMT (CGI)	41%			
Larynx	*MGMT* (CGI)	54%	*MGMT* (CGI)	38%	[116]

Cancer	Epigenetic changes in cancer (mechanism)	% sporadic cancers with epimutations	Epigenetic changes in field defect (mechanism)	% field defects with epi-mutations	Ref.
Non-small cell Lung	*WRN* (CGI)	38%			[2]
	MGMT (CGI)	70%	*MGMT* (CGI)	40%	[117]
Prostate	*WRN* (CGI)	20%			[2]
Thyroid	*WRN* (CGI)	13%			[2]
Non-Hodgkin lymphoma	*WRN* (CGI)	24%			[2]
Leukemias	*WRN* (CGI)	5-10%			[2]
Chondrosarcomas	*WRN* (CGI)	33%			[2]
Osteosarcomas	*WRN* (CGI)	11%			[2]
Brain glioblastoma	*MGMT* (CGI)	51%			[118]
	MGMT (miRNA)	28%			[78]
Liver hepatocellular carcinoma	*P53* (non-CGI promoter site specific methylation)	100%			[119]
Papillary thyroid (tested 23 DNA repair genes for CGI)	*MLH1* (CGI)	21%			[120]
	PCNA (CGI)	13%			
	OGG1 (CGI)	2%			

*CGI=CpG island methlyation

Table 7. Examples of epigenetic alterations (epimutations) of DNA repair genes in cancers and in field defects, with mechanisms indicated where known.

Deficiencies in DNA repair genes cause increased mutation rates. Mutations rates increase in MMR defective cells [81, 82] and in HRR defective cells [83]. Chromosomal rearrangements and aneuploidy also increase in HRR defective cells [84]. Thus, deficiency in DNA repair causes genomic instability and genomic instability is the likely main underlying cause of the genetic alterations leading to tumorigenesis. Deficient DNA repair permits the acquisition of a sufficient number of alterations in tumor suppressor genes and oncogenes to fuel carcinogenesis. Deficiencies in DNA repair appear to be central to the genomic and epigenomic instability characteristic of cancer.

http://dx.doi.org/10.5772/53919

Figure 3 illustrates the chain of consequences of exposure of cells to endogenous and exogenous DNA damaging agents that lead to cancer. The role of germ line defects in DNA repair genes in familial cancer are also indicated. The large role of DNA damage and consequent epigenetic DNA repair defects leading to sporadic cancer are emphasized. The roles of germ line mutation and directly induced somatic mutation in sporadic cancer are indicated as well.

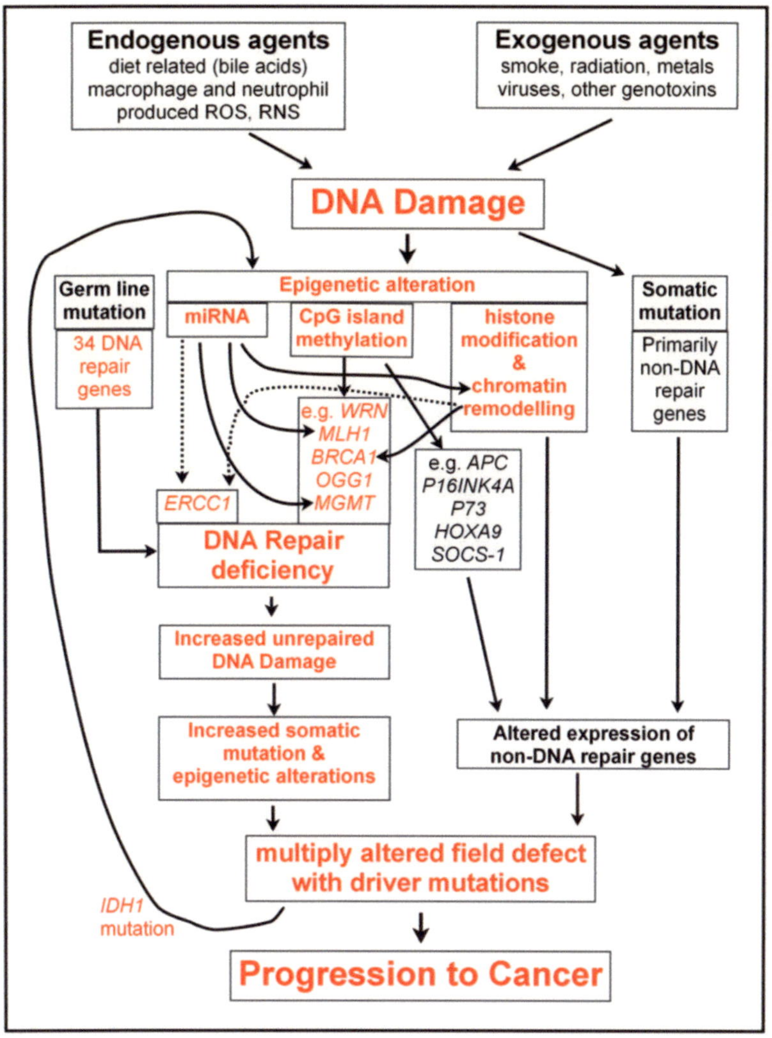

Figure 3. The roles of DNA damage, epigenetic deficiencies in DNA repair and mutation in progression to cancer.

11. Epigenetic alterations caused by micro RNAs

MicroRNAs (miRNAs) are endogenous non-coding RNAs, 19-25 nucleotides in length, that can have substantial effects on DNA repair. miRNAs can either directly or indirectly reduce expression of DNA repair or DNA damage response genes. As discussed above, over-expression of miR-155 causes reduced expression of DNA repair protein MLH1, and miR-155 is overexpressed in colon cancers [77] (curved arrow in Figure 3). Similarly, miR-181d is overexpressed in glioblastomas, causing reduced expression of DNA repair protein MGMT [78]. Although miRNAs can epigenetically regulate DNA repair gene expression, the expression levels of many miRNAs may themselves be subject to epigenetic regulation. One mechanism of epigenetic regulation of miRNA expression is hypomethylation of the promoter region of the DNA sequence that codes for the miRNA. Schnekenburger and Diederich [7] list miR-155 as one of a long list of mi-RNAs whose expression is increased by hypomythylation in colorectal cancers. In particular, hypomethylated miR-155 (the hypomethylation making it more active) targets genes *MLH1, MSH2* and *MSH6,* causing each of them to have reduced expression [7].

Wan et al. [121] referred to 6 further DNA repair genes that are directly targeted by miRNAs. *ATM, RAD52, RAD23B, MSH2, BRCA1* and *P53,* are each specifically targeted by one or two of the 8 miRNAs miR-21, miR-24, miR-125b, miR-182, miR-210, miR-373, miR-421 and miR-504, with all but miR-210, miR-421 and miR-504 among those identified by Schnekenburger and Diederich [7] as overexpressed through epigenetic hypomethylation. Overexpression of any one of these miRNAs leads to reduced expression of its target DNA repair gene. Wan et al. [121] further listed 16 DNA damage response genes targeted by specific miRNAs. Wan et al. [121] indicated miR-15a, miR-16, miR-17, miR-20a, miR-21, miR-24, miR-29, miR-34a, miR-106a, miR-93, miR-124a, miR-125b, miR-192, miR-195, miR-215, miR-182, miR-373 as among those targeting DNA damage response genes. Of these, all but miR-124a were identified by Schnekenburger and Diederich [7], (and Malumbres [122] further identified miR-34a and miR-124a) as being among miRNAs whose expression is subject to epigenetic alteration in tumors. Other miRNAs whose expression is subject to epimutation in colorectal cancers (and their target DNA repair or DNA damage response genes) include miR-17 (*E2F1*), miR-34b/c (*P53*), miR-106a (*E2F1*), miR-200a and miR-200b (*MLH1, MSH2*) and miR-675 (*Rb*) [7].

12. Epigenetic alterations caused by chromosome remodeling and histone modification

Specific miRNAs can also indirectly (and strongly) reduce protein expression of DNA repair genes through their role in repression of proteins designated High Mobility Group A1 (HMGA1) and HMGA2 (the names come from the proteins' high electrophoretic mobility on acrylamide gels). HMGA1 and HMGA2 cause chromatin remodeling at specific sites in DNA and reduce expression at those sites. In particular, these proteins appear to control

DNA repair genes *BRCA1* and *ERCC1*. BRCA1 And ERCC1 proteins have key roles in DNA repair, particularly of double-strand breaks and interstrand crosslinks. *HMGA1* and *HMGA2* genes are usually active in embryogenesis, but normally have very low expression levels in adult tissues. Their expression levels in adult tissues are kept low by the actions of specific miRNAs. If expression of these miRNAs is reduced, then the repressive HMGA1 and HMGA2 proteins become highly expressed and, in particular, can reduce expression of *BRCA1* or *ERCC1* respectively.

As reviewed by Resar [123], all HMG proteins share an acidic carboxyl terminus and associate with chromatin. As an example, HMGA1A, in particular, has three AT-hook domains that allow it to bind to AT-rich regions and recruit an "enhanceosome" that may displace histones and cause chromosome remodeling and reduce gene expression. Baldassarre et al. [124] showed that HMGA1B protein binds to the promoter region of *BRCA1* and inhibits *BRCA1* promoter activity (indicated in Figure 3 as chromatin remodeling causing reduced *BRCA1*). In 12 surgically removed human breast carcinomas, there was an inverse correlation between HGMA1 protein and *BRCA1* mRNA levels. HGMA1 was almost undetectable in normal breast tissue, highly expressed in the tumor samples, and BRCA1 protein was strongly diminished in tumor samples. Baldassarre et al. [124] suggested that while only 11% of breast tumors had hypermethylation of the *BRCA1* gene, 82% of aggressive breast cancer specimens have low BRCA1 protein, and most of these could be due to chromatin remodeling by high levels of HMGA1 protein.

Similarly, HMGA2 binds to an *ERCC1* promoter site and represses *ERCC1* promoter activity [125]. The miRNAs miR-23a, miR-26a and miR-30a inhibit *HMG2A* protein expression [126] though it has not been reported whether these miRNAs are under epigenetic control. In Figure 3, one of two dotted lines is used to indicate possible repression of *ERCC1* by epigenetically induced chromatin remodeling.

Resar [123] and Baldassarre et al. [124] summarized reports indicating that *HGMA1* is widely overexpressed in aggressive malignancies including cancers of the thyroid, head and neck, colon, lung, breast, pancreas, hematopoetic system, cervix, uterine corpus, prostate and central nervous system. Palmieri et al. [127] showed that *HGMA1* and *HMGA2* are targeted (and thus strongly reduced in expression) by miR-15, miR-16, miR-26a, miR-196a2 and Let-7a. The promoter regions associated with miR-16, miR-196a2 and Let-7a miRNAs are epimutated by hypomethylation [7, 122] while Sampath et al. [128] showed, in addition, that the coding regions for miR-15 and miR-16 were epigenetically silenced due to histone deacetylase activity. Palmieri et al. [127] further showed that these 5 miRNAs are drastically reduced in a panel of 41 pituitary adenomas, accompanied by increases in *HMGA1* and *HMGA2* specific mRNAs. In a more recent study on pituitary adenomas by D'Angelo et al. [129], reduced expression of 18 miRNAs was found, with 5 of them targeting *HMGA1* or *HMGA2*. In this recent study, among the 18 miRNAs with reduced expression, the reduced expression of miR-26b, miR-34b, miR-432 and miR-592 was known to be due to epigenetic alteration [7, 122]. Thus, epigenetic miRNA silencing, causing strong expression of *HMGA1* and *HMGA2*, occurs in many types of cancer and this may be related to reductions found in expression of DNA repair genes *BRCA1, BRCA2* and *ERCC1*.

Suzuki et al. [130], using genome wide profiling, found 174 primary transcription units for miRNAs, called "pri-miRNAs" (large precursor RNAs which may encode multiple miRNAs), of which they identified 37 as potential targets for epigenetic silencing. Of these 37 pri-miRNAs, 22 were encoded by DNA sequences with CpG islands (all of which were hypermethylated in colorectal cancer cells) while the other pri-miRNAs were subject to regulation by epigenetic "activating marks" without evidence of deregulated methylation.

Activating marks are alterations on histones that cause transcriptional activation of the genes associated with those altered histones (reviewed by Tchou-Wong et al. [131]). In particular, the nucleosome, the fundamental subunit of chromatin, is composed of 146 bp of DNA wrapped around an octamer of four core histone proteins (H3, H4, H2A, and H2B). Posttranslational modifications (i.e., acetylation, methylation, phosphorylation, and ubiquitination) of the N- and C-terminal tails of the four core histones play an important role in regulating chromatin biology. These specific histone modifications, and their combinations, are translated, through protein interactions, into distinct effects on nuclear processes, such as activation or inhibition of transcription. In eukaryotes, methylation of lysine 4 in histone H3 (H3K4), which interacts with the promoter region of genes, is linked to transcriptional activation. There is a strong positive correlation between trimethylation of H3K4, transcription rates, active polymerase II occupancy and histone acetylation. Thus trimethylation of H3K4 is an activating mark.

In addition to pri-miRNAs being regulated by activating marks, some miRNAs appear to be directly regulated by these histone modifications. As summarized by Sampath et al. [128], histone deacetylases catalyze the removal of acetyl groups on specific lysines around gene promoters to trigger demethylation of otherwise methylated lysine 4 on histones (H3K4me2/3) and this causes loss of these activating marks, promoting chromatin compaction, and leading to epigenetic silencing. Sampath et al. [128] showed that such histone deacetylase activity mediates the epigenetic silencing of miRNAs miR-15a, miR-16, and miR-29b. As indicated above, miR-15, miR-16 specifically target *HGMA1* and *HMGA2*. If miR-15 and miR-16 lose their activating marks, they have reduced expression, causing *HGMA1* and *HGMA2* to be transcriptionally activated, thus reducing expression of DNA repair genes *BRCA1* and *ERCC1*.

In Figure 3, histone modification and chromatin remodeling are indicated as epigentically altering the expression of many genes in progression to cancer, and specifically causing reduced *BRCA1* and possibly (as indicated by one dotted line) reduced expression of *ERCC1*. In addition, a second dotted line is used to indicate possible repression of *ERCC1* by an miRNA. Klase et al. [132] showed that a particular virally coded miRNA down regulates ERCC1 protein expression at the p-body level (a p-body is a cytoplasmic granule "processing body" that interacts with miRNAs to repress translation or trigger degradation of target mRNAs). A survey of human miRNA homology regions to *ERCC1* mRNA indicates at least 21 human coded miRNAs that could act to decrease *ERCC1* mRNA translation (shown in Microcosm Targets [133]). ERCC1 protein expression, assessed by immunohistochemical staining, is deficient due to an epigenetic mechanism in colon cancers [110], and this could be due to action of one or more miRNAs, acting directly on *ERCC1* mRNA.

13. Driver mutations and pathways to cancer progression

Recent research indicates a mechanism by which an early driver mutation may cause subsequent epigenetic alterations or mutations in pathways leading to cancer. Wang et al. [134] point out that isocitrate dehydrogenase genes *IDH1* and *IDH2* are the most frequently mutated metabolic genes in human cancer. A gene frequently mutated in cancer is considered to be a driver mutation [4] so that mutations in *IDH1* and *IDH2* would be driver mutations. Wang et al. [134] further point out that *IDH1* and *IDH2* mutant cells produce an excess metabolic intermediate, 2-hydroxyglutarate, which binds to catalytic sites in key enzymes that are important in altering histone and DNA promoter methylation. Thus, mutations in *IDH1* and *IDH2* generate a DNA CpG island methylator phenotype that causes promoter hypermethylation and concomitant silencing of tumor suppressor genes such as the DNA repair genes *MLH1, MGMT* and *BRCA1*. As shown in Figure 3, a driver mutation in *IDH1* can cause a feedback loop leading to increased DNA repair deficiency, further mutations and epimutations, and consequent accelerated tumor progression.

A study, involving 51 patients with brain gliomas who had two or more biopsies over time, showed that mutation in the *IDH1* gene occurred prior to the occurrence of a *p53* mutation or a 1p/19q loss of heterozygosity, indicating that *IDH1* mutation is an early driver mutation [135]. Work by Turcan et al. [136] showed that *IDH1* mutation alone is sufficient to establish the brain glioma CpG island methylator phenotype. Carillo et al. [137] showed that when an *IDH1* mutation was present in glioblastoma tumors, 64% of these were hypermethylated in the promoter regions of *MGMT*.

Other initial driver mutations can cause progression to glioblastoma as well. As pointed out above, increased levels of miR-181d also cause reduced expression of MGMT protein in glioblastoma. Nelson et al. [138] indicate that a single type of miRNA may target hundreds of different mRNAs, causing alterations in multiple pathways. Patients with a glioblastoma that does not harbor an *IDH1* mutation have an overall fairly short survival time, while patients with both mutated *IDH1* and methylated *MGMT* have a subtype of glioblastoma with a much longer survival time (implying a different pathway of cancer progression) [137].

An *IDH1* mutation that gives rise to a CpG island methylator phenotype that causes promoter hypermethylation and concomitant silencing of *MGMT* also causes promoter silencing of other genes as well. In addition to silencing of genes, the CpG island methylator phenotype can cause methylation of the promoter regions of long interspersed nuclear element-1 (LINE-1) DNA sequences. Ohka et al. [139] point out that LINE-1 is a class of retroposons that are the most successful integrated mobile elements in the human genome, and account for about 18% of human DNA. Ohka et al. [139] found that LINE-1 methylation is directly proportional to *MGMT* promoter methylation in gliomas and suggested that LINE-1 methylation could be used as a proxy to indicate the CpG island methylator phenotype status in glioblastomas. This phenotype, likely associated with methylation of the *MGMT* promoter, in turn, indicates whether treatment with the DNA alkylating agent temozolomide will be beneficial in treatment of a patient with a glioblastoma, since MGMT removes the alkyl groups added to guanine by temozolomide.

14. Field defects

Field defects have been described in many types of gastrointestinal cancers [140]. A field defect arises when an epimutation or mutation occurs in a stem cell that causes that stem cell to give rise to a number of daughter stem cells that can out-compete neighboring stem cells. These initial mutated cells form a patch of somewhat more rapidly growing cells (an initial field defect). That patch then enlarges at the expense of neighboring cells, followed by, at some point, an additional mutation or epimutation arising in one of the field defect stem cells so that this new stem cell with two advantageous mutations can generate daughter stem cells that can out-compete the surrounding field defect of cells that have just one advantageous mutation. As illustrated in Figure 4, this process of expanding sub-patches within earlier patches will occur multiple times until a particular constellation of mutations results in a cancer (represented by the small dark patch in Figure 4. It should also be noted that a cancer, once formed, continues to evolve and continues to produce sub clones. A renal cancer, sampled in 9 areas, had 40 ubiquitous mutations, 59 mutations shared by some, but not all regions, and 29 "private" mutations only present in one region [141].

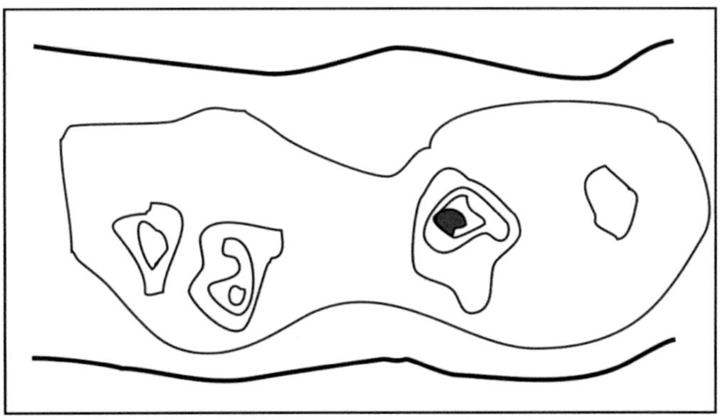

Figure 4. Schematic of a field defect in progression to cancer

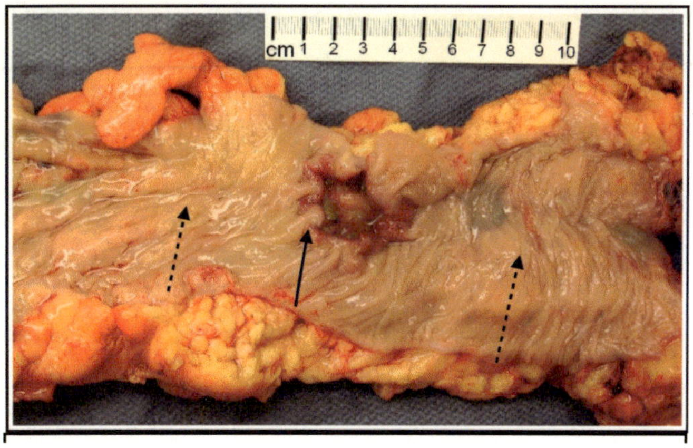

Figure 5. Colon resection including a colon cancer. Dashed arrows indicate grossly unremarkable colonic mucosa. Ulcerated hemorrhagic mass represents a moderately differentiated invasive adenocarcinoma. Solid arrow indicates the heaped up edge of the malignant ulcer

Figure 5 shows an opened resected segment of a human colon that has a colon cancer. As illustrated by Bernstein et al. [142], there are about 100 colonic microscopic epithelial crypts per sq mm in the colonic epithelium. The resection shown in Figure 5 has an area of about 6.5 cm by 23 cm, or 150 sq cm, or 15, 000 sq mm. Thus this area has about 1.5 million crypts. There are 10-20 stem cells at the base of each colonic crypt [143, 144]. Therefore there are likely about 15 million stem cells in the grossly unremarkable colonic mucosal epithelium shown in Figure 5. Evidence reported by Facista et al. [112], and listed in Table 7, indicates that in many such resections, most of the stem cells in such an area up to 10 cm distant (in each direction) from a colon cancer (such as in the grossly unremarkable area shown in Figure 5), and the majority of their differentiated daughter cells, are epigenetically deficient for protein expression of the DNA repair genes *ERCC1, PMS2* and/or *XPF,* although the epithelium is histologically normal.

The stem cells most distant from the cancer, deficient for *ERCC1, PMS2* and/or *XPF,* can be considered to constitute an outer ring, and be deficient as well in the inner rings, of a field defect schematically illustrated in Figure 4. The outer ring in Figure 4 includes, within its circumscribed area, on the order of 15 million stem cells, presumably arising from an initial progenitor stem cell deficient in DNA repair (due to epigenetic silencing). As a result of this repair deficit, the initial stem cell was genetically unstable, giving rise to an increased frequency of mutations in its decendents. One daughter stem cell among its decendents had a mutation that, by chance, provided a replicative advantage. This descendent then underwent clonal expansion because of its replicative advantage. Among the further decendents of the clone, new mutations arose frequently, since these descendents had a mutator phenotype [145], due to the repair deficiency passed down epigenetically from the original repair-defective stem cell. Among these new mutations, some would provide further replicative advantages, giving rise to a succession of more aggressively growing sub clones (inner rings), and eventually a cancer.

15. Exogenous carcinogenic agents cause reduced expression of DNA repair genes

Many known carcinogenic agents cause reduced expression of DNA repair genes or directly inhibit the actions of DNA repair proteins. Table 8 lists examples of carcinogens that have such effects. Due to space limitations, many other such carcinogens are not listed. These findings further link DNA damage to cancer.

Carcinogens	Inhibit DNA Repair Gene	Mechanism Shown	Ref.
Arsenic compounds	*PARP*		[146,147]
	XRCC1 *Ligase 3* *Ligase 4*		[146,148]
	DNA POLB, XRCC4 *DNA PKCS, TOPO2B*		[146]
	OGG1, ERCC1, XPF		[149]
	XPB, XPC, XPE		[150]
	P53	Inhibition of P53 serine 15 phosphorylation	[151]
Cadmium compounds	*MSH2, ERCC1, XRCC1* *OGG1*	Promoter methylation	[152]
	MSH2, MSH6 proteins	Cd^{2+} binds to proteins	[153]
	OGG1 protein	Oxidation of Ogg1	[154]
	DNA-PK, XPD		[155]
	XPC		[156]
Bile acids			
deoxycholate	*MUTYH, OGG1*	mRNA reduced	[157]
	BRCA1		[158]
lithocholate	*DNA POLB*		[159]
Lipid peroxidation compounds			
4-hydroxy-2-nonenal (4-HNE)	Nuc. Excision Repair	NER protein adducts	[160]
Malondialdehyde	Nuc. Excision Repair	NER protein adducts	[161]

Carcinogens	Inhibit DNA Repair Gene	Mechanism Shown	Ref.
Oxidative stress	MisMatch Repair	Oxidative damage to MMR proteins	[162]
	ERCC1 protein	Oxidative attack	[163]
	OGG1 protein	Degraded by calpain	[164]
Gamma irrad.	*OGG1, XRCC1*	mRNA reduced	[165]
Benzo(a)pyrene	*BRCA1*	miR-638 increased	[166]
Methylcholanthrene/ diethylnitrosamine	*BRCA1, ERCC1, XRCC1, MLH1*		[167]
Styrene	*XRCC1, OGG1, XPC*	mRNA reduced	[168]
Aristolochic acid	*P53, PARP1, OGG1, ERCC1, MGMT*	mRNA reduced	[169]
Antimony	*XPE*	mRNA reduced	[170]
Nickel	*MGMT*	Promoter methylation	[171]

Table 8. Examples of carcinogenic agents that cause reduced expression of DNA repair genes

16. Polyphenols can epigenetically increase expression of DNA repair genes

Some polyphenols affect expression of many genes, including DNA repair genes, through epigenetic alterations, as reviewed by Link et al. [172]. Examples of DNA repair genes expression increased by epigenetic alteration are listed in Table 9.

Phytochemical	Plant source	Mechanism	Targeted DNA Repair Genes	Ref.
Epigalocatechin-3-gallate	Green tea	Reversal of CpG island methylation	*MGMT, MLH1*	[173]
Dihydrocoumarin	Yellow sweet clover	p53 acetylation	*P53*	[174]
Genistein	Soy	Reversal of CpG island methylation	*MGMT*	[173]
Genistein	Soy	Histone acetylation	*P53*	[175]

Table 9. Examples of phytochemicals that increase expression of DNA repair genes by an epigenetic mechanism

17. Possible protection against cancer by phytochemicals that increase DNA repair by unknown mechanisms

A recent review article by Collins et al. [176] summarizes some examples of micronutrients that affect DNA repair gene expression, though by unknown mechanisms. Table 10 lists such phytochemicals, without defined mechanisms, that increase DNA repair gene expression, along with commonly known foods that are high in those phytochemicals [177, 178, 179].

Phytochemical (test system)	Examples of foods high in nutrient	Increased DNA Repair Gene Expression	Ref.
Ellagic acid (mice)	Raspberries, pomeganate	*XPA, ERCC5, DNA Ligase 3*	[180]
Silymarin (cells *in vitro*)	Artichoke, milk thistle	*MGMT*	[181]
Curcumin (cells *in vitro*)	Turmeric	*MGMT*	
Chlorogenic acid (cells *in vitro*)	Blueberries, coffee, sunflower seeds, artichoke	*PARP*	[182]
Caffeic acid (cells *in vitro*)	coffee, cranberry, carrot	*PMS2*	
m-coumaric acid (cells *in vitro*)	olives (and metabolite of caffeic acid)	*PARP, PMS2*	
3-(m-hydroxyphenyl) propionic acid (cells *in vitro*)	(major metabolite of caffeic acid and degradation product of proanthocyanidins in chocholate)	*PARP, PMS2*	

Table 10. Examples of phytochemicals that increase expression of DNA repair genes by unknown mechanisms

Bernstein et al. [182] evaluated antioxidants based on their ability to increase DNA repair proteins PARP-1 and Pms2 *in vitro*. They tested 19 anti-oxidant compounds and of these 19 compounds only chlorogenic acid and its metabolic products: chlorogenic acid, caffeic acid, *m*-coumaric acid and 3-(*m*-hydroxyphenyl) propionic acid, increased expression of the two tested DNA repair genes in HCT-116 cells (Table 10).

Chlorogenic acid (CGA) (high in blueberries, coffee, sunflower seeds, artichoke) [177, 183, 184] was then tested as a preventive agent in the recently devised diet-related mouse model of colon cancer [60]. As described above in the section Exogenous DNA damaging agents in colorectal cancer, deoxycholic acid (DCA), a DNA damaging agent, at levels present after a high fat diet, can cause colorectal cancer. When DCA is added to the diet of wild-type mice to raise the level of DCA in the mouse feces to the level in feces of humans on a high fat diet, by 10 months of feeding 94% of the mice develop tumors in their colons with 56% developing colonic adenocarcinomas [60]. This mouse model develops tumors solely in the colon, phenotypically similar to development of colon cancer in humans. When CGA, equivalent to 3 cups of coffee a day for humans, was added to the DCA supplemented diet it was dramatically protective against development of colon cancer, reducing incidence of colon cancer significantly from 56% to 18% [60].

18. Targeting of chemotherapeutic agents to cancers deficient in DNA repair

As discussed above, DNA repair deficiency often arises early in progression to cancer and can give rise to genomic instability, a general feature of cancers. If cancer cells are deficient in DNA repair they are likely to be more vulnerable than normal cells to inactivation by DNA damaging agents. This vulnerability of cancer cells can be exploited to the benefit of the patient. Some of the most clinically effective chemotherapeutic agents currently used in cancer treatment are DNA damaging agents, and their therapeutic effectiveness appears to often depend on deficient DNA repair in cancer cells.

In the next four sections we discuss repair deficiencies in cancer cells that can be effectively targeted by DNA damaging chemotherapeutic agents. In addition, deficiency in a DNA repair pathway that arises during tumor development may make cancer cells more reliant on a remaining reduced set of DNA repair pathways for survival. Recent studies indicate that drugs that inhibit one of these alternative pathways in such cancers cells can be useful in cancer therapy. Targeting cancer cells having a repair deficiency with specific DNA damaging agents, or with agents that inhibit alternative repair pathways, offers a new promising approach for treating a variety of cancers.

19. Targeting cancers deficient in BRCA1

The BRCA1 (breast cancer 1 early onset) protein is employed in an important DNA repair pathway, homologous recombinational repair (HRR). This pathway removes a variety of types of DNA damages, and is the only pathway that can accurately remove double-strand damages such as double-strand breaks and inter-strand cross-links. BRCA1 also has other functions related to preservation of genome integrity (reviewed by Yun and Hiom [185]). Individuals with a germ-line inherited defect in the *BRCA1* gene are at increased risk of breast, ovarian and other cancers. In addition to inherited germ-line defects in *BRCA1*, deficiencies in expression of this gene may arise in somatic cells either by mutation or by epimutation during progression to sporadic (non-germline) cancer.

Patients with a variety of types of cancer are treated effectively with chemotherapeutic agents that cause double-strand breaks (e.g. the topoisomerase inhibitor etoposide), or cause inter-strand cross-links (e.g. the platinum compound cisplatin). These damages can cause cancer cells to undergo apoptosis (a form of cell death). However, patients treated with these agents often prove to be intrinsically resistant, or develop resistance during treatment. Quinn et al. [186] demonstrated that BRCA1 expression is necessary for such resistance. This finding suggests that BRCA1-mediated DNA repair can protect cancer cells from therapeutic

DNA damaging drugs. Thus, although high expression of BRCA1 may be initially beneficial to the individual by reducing the risk of developing cancer, it also may be detrimental once cancer has developed by counteracting the therapeutic effect of DNA-damaging agents targeted to the cancer cells.

Patients with non-small cell lung cancer (NSLC) are often treated with DNA cross-linking platinum therapeutic compounds such as cisplatin, carboplatin or oxaliplatin. NSCLC is the leading cause of cancer deaths worldwide, and almost 70% of patients with NSCLC have locally advanced or metastatic disease at diagnosis. Improved survival after platinum-containing chemotherapy in metastatic NSCLC correlates with low BRCA1 expression in the primary tumor [187, 188]. This finding indicates that low BRCA1-mediated DNA repair is detrimental to the cancer upon treatment, and thus beneficial to the patient. BRCA1 likely protects cancer cells by participating in a pathway that removes the potentially lethal DNA cross-links introduced by the platinum drugs. Since low BRCA1 expression in the tumor appears to be beneficial to the patient, Taron et al. [187] and Papadek et al. [188] concluded that BRCA1 expression is potentially an important tool for use in cancer management and should be assessed for predicting chemosensitivity and tailoring chemotherapy in lung cancer.

Over 90% of ovarian cancers appear to arise sporadically in somatic cells and are associated with BRCA1 dysfunction. Weberpals et al. [189] showed for patients having sporadic ovarian cancer treated with platinum drugs, the median survival was longer for patients with lower expression of BRCA1 vs. higher BRCA1 expression (46 vs. 33 months).

20. Targeting cancers deficient in ERCC1

ERCC1 (Excision Repair Cross-Complementaion group 1) is a key protein needed to remove platinum adducts and repair inter- and intra-strand cross-links [190]. ERCC1 dimerizes with XPF (xeroderma pigmentosum complementation group F) protein to form a complex that can excise damaged DNA. Over-expression of ERCC1 is associated with cellular resistance to platinum compounds, whereas ERCC1 down-regulation sensitizes cells to cisplatin [191, 192].

Cisplatin has made a major impact in the chemotherapeutic treatment of testicular cancer. Over 90% of patients with newly diagnosed testicular germ cell cancer, and 70 to 80% of patients with metastatic testicular cancer, can be cured using cisplatin based combination chemotherapy [193]. Hypersensitivity of testicular cancer to cisplatin appears to be due to low levels of the three NER proteins ERCC1, XPF and XPA [194].

Simon et al. [195] evaluated ERCC1 mRNA expression in lung tumors as a predictor of survival of NSCLC patients. They found that patients with relatively low ERCC1 mRNA expression had poor overall survival. This finding suggests that low ERCC1-mediated DNA repair allows DNA damages to persist and give rise to carcinogenic mutations. However, they also noted that those NSCLC tumors with relatively low ERCC1 expression responded better to platinum based therapy. Lord et al. [196] found that low *ERCC1* mRNA expression in the primary tumor correlates with prolonged survival after cisplatin plus gemitabine chemotherapy in NSCLC. Median overall survival with low ERCC1 expression tumors was 61.6 weeks compared to 20.4 weeks for patients with high expression tumors.

Zhou et al. [197] reported that a particular genetic polymorphism that alters ERCC1 mRNA level predicts overall survival in advanced NSCLC patients treated with platinum based chemotherapy. Olaussen et al. [198] found that patients with completely resected NSCLC tumors that were ERCC1-negative benefited from adjuvant cisplatin-based chemotherapy, whereas patients with ERCC1-positive tumors did not benefit. They suggested that determination of ERCC1 expression in NSCLC cells before chemotherapy can make a contribution as an independent predictor of the effect of adjuvant chemotherapy. Papadaki et al. [188] found that *ERCC1* mRNA level in the primary tumor of patients with metastatic NSCLC could predict the effectiveness of cisplatin based chemotherapy. Low *ERCC1* mRNA level was significantly associated with higher response rate, longer median progression-free survival and median overall survival. Leng et al. [199] found that patients with ERCC1 negative expression had a longer progression free survival and overall survival than ERCC1 positive patients after receiving platinum based adjuvant therapy. Thus *ERCC1* mRNA level, like *BRCA1* mRNA level (discussed above), in the primary tumor at the time of diagnosis could be used to predict platinum sensitivity of NSCLC.

ERCC1 expression also appears to have predictive significance for ovarian cancer. Dabholkar et al. [200] found in ovarian tumor tissues that *ERCC1* mRNA expression levels were higher in patients who were resistant to platinum based therapy than in those patients who responded to such therapy. Kang et al. [201] observed that a particular polymorphism of the ERCC1 gene sequence was associated with clinical outcome of platinum based chemotherapy in patients with ovarian cancer. Weberpals et al. [189] also showed for ovarian cancer patients that higher ERCC1 mRNA level, alone, or especially in combination with higher *BRCA1* mRNA level in the tumor, predicted shorter overall patient survival after platinum therapy.

ERCC1 protein expression is often reduced within colon cancers and in a field defect surrounding these cancers [112]. For metastatic colorectal cancer patients receiving combination oxaliplatin and fluorouracil chemotherapy, lower *ERCC1* mRNA expression in the tumor predicts longer survival [202]. Viguier et al. [203] found that a particular ERCC1 genetic polymorphism predicts a better tumor response to oxaliplatin/5-fluorouracil combination chemotherapy in patients with metastatic colorectal cancer.

Low *ERCC1* mRNA levels also predict better response and survival for gastric cancer patients [204] and bladder cancer patients [205] receiving cisplatin-based chemotherapy.

Thus numerous studies involving cancer of the testis, lung, ovary, colon, stomach and bladder indicated that platinum based chemotherapy can enhance patient outcome when targeted specifically to tumors with low ERCC1 expression. Such tumors have diminished ability to repair the DNA damages, particularly the cross-links, induced in the tumors by the platinum compound.

21. Targeting cancers deficient in MGMT

Alkylating agents, including chloroethylnitrosoureas, procarbazine and temozolomide, are commonly used to treat malignant brain tumors. These agents cause DNA damage by adding alkyl groups to DNA. Such damages may then be repaired or, if unrepaired, trigger cell death. As an example, temozolomide methylates DNA at several sites generating mainly N^7-methylguanine and N^3-methyladenine adducts, which constitute nearly 90% of the total methylation events. However these adducts are efficiently removed and accurately replaced by the base excision repair pathway, and thus have low cytotoxic potential. About 5 to 10% of the methylation events caused by temozolomide produce O^6-methylguanine which is cytotoxic, and this adduct accounts for the beneficial therapeutic effect of temozolomide and other alkylating agents on malignant brain tumors.

O^6-methylguanine methyltransferase (MGMT) is a DNA repair enzyme that rapidly reverses alkylation (including methylation) at the O^6 position of guanine, thus neutralizing the cytotoxic effects of chemotherapeutic alkylating agents such as temozolomide. High MGMT activity in tumor tissue is associated with resistance to alkylating agents. MGMT activity is controlled by a promoter sequence, and methylation of the CpG island in the promoter silences the gene in cancer cells, so that these cells no longer produce MGMT. In addition, as described above, an increased level of miR-181d can also decrease MGMT expression and help the ability of temozolomide to give a beneficial therapeutic effect [78].

Esteller et al. [206] showed that methylation of the *MGMT* promoter increases the responsiveness of the gliomas (brain tumors) to chemotherapeutic alkylating agents, leading to regression of the tumors and prolonged overall and disease free survival. Paz et al. [207] showed that hypermethylation of CpG islands within the promoter sequence of the *MGMT* gene predicts a better clinical response to temozolomide in primary gliomas. They considered that their results might open up possibilities for more customized treatments of human brain tumors. Hegi et al. [208] demonstrated a significantly improved clinical outcome in patients with malignant glioma who had a methylated *MGMT* promoter and were treated with temozolomide. The 18-month survival rate was 62% among patients with a methylated *MGMT* promoter compared with only 8% in the absence of promoter methylation. Hegi et al. [209] reviewed further evidence that *MGMT* promoter methylation is associated with improved progression-free and overall survival in malignant glioma patients treated with alkylating agents. They also discussed strategies to overcome MGMT-mediated chemoresistance that are currently under investigation. Upon reviewing the relevant evidence, Weller et al. [210] concluded that *MGMT* promoter methylation is the key mechanism of *MGMT* gene silencing, and could be used as a biomarker for predicting a favorable outcome in patients with malignant glioma who are exposed to alkylating chemotherapy. They considered that this biomarker is on the verge of entering clinical decision-making.

22. Targeting cancers with a repair deficiency using a PARP inhibitor; synthetic lethality

If a tumor is deficient in an essential protein component of a DNA repair pathway, the cancer cells would likely be more reliant on remaining DNA repair pathways for survival. Drugs that inhibit one of these alternative pathways, in principle, might prove to be useful in cancer therapy by selectively killing the cancer cells. An example of such an approach is the use of poly(ADP-ribose) polymerase [PARP] inhibitors against tumors that are deficient in BRCA1 or BRCA2 [211]. This approach has provided proof-of-concept for an anticancer strategy termed "synthetic lethality." By this strategy the inhibition of a particular repair pathway in cancer cells that are already deficient in another repair pathway preferentially induces greater toxicity in repair deficient cancer cells than in normal non-cancer cells. Current research guided by this strategy is directed at finding new agents that inactivate protein components of major repair pathways, and thus could be targeted against cancers that are already deficient in another repair pathway [212].

A germ-line mutation in one *BRCA1* or *BRCA2* allele substantially increases the risk of developing several cancers, including breast, ovarian, and prostate cancer. Diploid cells heterozygous for either a *BRCA1* or a *BRCA2* mutant allele may lose expression of the remaining wild-type allele, resulting in deficient homologous recombinational repair. This loss causes an increase in unrepaired DSBs that can lead to mutations (through compensatory inaccurate repair) and chromosomal aberrations that drive carcinogenesis. Inactivation of the wild-type allele in the cell lineage leading to the tumor is thought to be an obligate step in this carcinogenesis pathway, a step that does not occur in the normal non-cancer tissues of the patient.

The deficiency in homologous recombinational repair is thus specific to the tumor, and can be exploited by employing PARP inhibitors. Ordinarily, single-strand breaks (SSBs), as distinct from DSBs, are repaired by the base excision repair pathway, in which the enzyme PARP1 plays a key role. The inhibition of PARP1 leads to the accumulation of DNA SSBs. Unrepaired SSBs can give rise to DSBs at replication forks during DNA replication. Thus PARP inhibition in tumor cells with deficient homologous recombinational repair (because of the absence of BRCA1 or BRCA2) generates unrepaired SSBs that are likely to cause an overwhelming accumulation of DSBs leading to tumor cell death. In contrast, the normal tissues of a patient consists of cells that are heterozygous for a *BRCA1* or *BRCA2* mutant allele and therefore retain homologous recombinational repair function, and have a sensitivity to PARP inhibitors similar to that of wild-type cells. Thus PARP inhibition induces selective tumor cell killing while sparing normal cells.

Fong et al. [213] conducted a preliminary clinical evaluation of the oral PARP inhibitor olaparib. They observed that 63% of patients carrying *BRCA1* or *BRCA2* mutations who had ovarian, breast or prostate cancer had a clinical benefit from treatment with olaparib with few adverse side effects. This is an example of the concept of "synthetic lethality" which occurs when there is a potent lethal synergy between two otherwise non-lethal events. The two events in this case are (1) a specific PARP inhibitor blocks repair of SSBs causing an increase in SSBs leading to an increase in DSBs; and (2) a tumor restricted genetic loss of function or homologous recombinational repair that is ordinarily needed to accurately repair these DSBs.

A subsequent trial of olaparib in BRCA mutation-associated breast cancer demonstrated objective positive response rates of 41%, again with limited toxicity [214]. About 10% of women with ovarian cancer carry a *BRCA1* or *BRCA2* mutant allele. Audeh et al. [215] showed that the oral PARP inhibitor olaparib has antitumor activity in women carriers of *BRCA1* or *BRCA2* alleles who have ovarian cancer. The objective positive response rate was 33%.

23. Overview of the role of DNA damage and repair in carcinogenesis

In this section we present a brief overview of the relationship of DNA damage and repair to carcinogenesis, and the implications of this relationship for strategies of prevention and therapy, emphasizing the evidence reviewed above. Carcinogenesis is generally viewed as a Darwinian process that occurs in a somatic cell lineage by mutation or epimutation and natural selection. Natural selection operates on the basis of the adaptive benefit to individual cells in the lineage of more rapid cell division or higher resistance to cell death (apoptosis) than occurs in neighboring cells. Most of the random mutations and epimutations that arise during progression to cancer are likely to be disadvantageous or neutral from the prospective of the emerging cancerous cells, and only those that promote more rapid overall growth are advantageous. The cell lineage that ultimately becomes a cancer probably passes through a series of evolutionary pre-cancerous stages involving sequential rounds of mutation/epimutation and selection [216]. The initial stage is probably a lineage of cells with a small selective advantage that forms an early field within a tissue. Within this defective field successive mutation and selection events occur which finally give rise to an invasive and then metastatic cell lineage. During this process the cell lineage acquires the hallmarks of cancer (summarized by Hanahan and Weinberg [217]). These include: sustaining proliferative signaling, evading growth suppressors, resisting cell death, enabling replicative immortality, inducing angiogenesis, reprogramming energy metabolism, and evading immune destruction.

Mutations arise from unrepaired DNA damages, either by translesion synthesis during DNA replication or by inaccurate repair of DNA damages, as in the inaccurate process of non-homologous end joining of double-strand breaks. Mutations may also arise by spontaneous replication errors without the intervention of DNA damage, but this source of mutation is likely less frequent than mutations caused by DNA damage. The primary cause(s) of epimutations (such as CpG island methylations) are not well understood, but evidence suggests that epimutations arise during the repair processes that remove DNA damages. The sources of DNA damage underlying carcinogenesis can be extrinsic or intrinsic. Epidemiologic evidence suggests that a large proportion of the DNA damages contributing to cancer arise from extrinsic stressful conditions, including such factors as smoking, high fat diet, certain infections and UV light exposure. The possible contribution from intrinsic causes, such as free radical production during normal metabolism, have not been assessed. A pervasive characteristic of human tumors is genomic instability [217]. A likely major source of this instability is loss of DNA repair capability. Germ line mutations in DNA repair genes generally lead to syndromes characterized by a greatly increased risk of cancer. The majority of cancers arise sporadically, i.e. are not primarily due to germ line mutations. A frequent characteristic of sporadic cancers is loss of expression of one or more DNA repair proteins through epigenetic silencing. The several different DNA repair pathways that occur in mammalian cells each specialize in removing different types of damage, but they are also partially overlapping. Thus reduction of a particular repair pathway may have different carcinogenic consequences from loss of another repair pathway [218]. However, the deleterious effect of loss of one pathway may be partially ameliorated by another functioning pathway.

This general view of the role of DNA damage and repair in carcinogenesis has implications for the prevention and treatment of cancer. Cancer incidence could be substantially reduced by a general avoidance of the known sources of DNA damage such as smoking. In addition to avoiding DNA damage, it should also be beneficial to increase DNA repair, or at least to avoid extrinsic factors that decrease repair. The factors affecting repair capability are less well studied than those causing DNA damage, but several are known, and a significant benefit may be derived from considering such factors as well.

The finding that DNA repair deficiency is a common feature of cancers, and is perhaps the underlying cause of the genetic instability of cancers, has implications for therapy. If a cancer is composed of cells deficient in DNA repair, it is, in principle, vulnerable to agents that cause DNA damage. Thus a chemotherapeutic DNA damaging agent can be targeted to cancers that lack the capability to repair the particular type of DNA damage caused by the agent. This can lead to a level of DNA damages that overwhelms the defenses of the cancer cells and causes their death. Non-cancerous cells with normal repair would not be targeted. Thus the toxicity of such DNA damaging agents to the treated patient would be limited. A dramatic example of such targeted therapy is the high cure rate of testicular cancer due to a defect in the ability of the cancer cells to repair DNA inter-strand cross-links, and the use of cross-linking platinum compounds to kill such cells.

Another strategy, which is currently the basis for numerous ongoing clinical trials, involves synthetic lethality. By this strategy cancers that are deficient in one DNA repair pathway can be made more vulnerable to DNA damage by treatment with agents that inhibit an additional repair pathway. Promising clinical results, so far, have been obtained in the treatment of patients with breast and ovarian cancer due to an inherited genetic defect in the homologous recombinational repair pathway. Such cancers are deficient in the ability to repair double-strand breaks. Treatment of these cancers with an agent that interferes with another pathway that ordinarily repairs single-strand breaks allows such breaks to accumulate and to be converted to double-strand breaks during DNA replication. The increase in double-strand breaks appears to overwhelm the cancer cells, while sparing normal cells, thus providing positive clinical benefit to the patient without much toxicity.

Author details

Carol Bernstein[1*], Anil R. Prasad[2], Valentine Nfonsam[3] and Harris Bernstein[4]

*Address all correspondence to: bernstein324@yahoo.com

1 Research Service Line, Southern Arizona Veterans Affairs Health Care System, Tucson, AZ, USA

2 Department of Pathology, University of Arizona, Tucson, AZ, USA

3 Department of Surgery, University of Arizona, Tucson, AZ, USA

4 Department of Cellular and Molecular Medicine, University of Arizona, Tucson, AZ, USA

References

[1] Gregg SQ, Robinson AR, Niedernhofer LJ. Physiological consequences of defects in ERCC1-XPF DNA repair endonuclease. DNA Repair (Amst) 2011;10(7) 781-791.

[2] Agrelo R, Cheng WH, Setien F, Ropero S, Espada J, Fraga MF, Herranz M, Paz MF, Sanchez-Cespedes M, Artiga J, Guerrero D, Castells A, von Kobbe C, Bohr VA, Esteller M. Epigenetic inactivation of the premature aging Werner syndrome gene in human cancer. Proc Natl Acad Sci U S A 2006;103(23) 8822-8827.

[3] Dreesen O, Stewart CL. Accelerated aging syndromes, are they relevant to normal human aging? Aging (Albany NY) 2011;3(9) 889-895.

[4] Wood LD, Parsons DW, Jones S, Lin J, Sjöblom T, Leary RJ, Shen D, Boca SM, Barber T, Ptak J, Silliman N, Szabo S, Dezso Z, Ustyanksky V, Nikolskaya T, Nikolsky Y, Karchin R, Wilson PA, Kaminker JS, Zhang Z, Croshaw R, Willis J, Dawson D, Shipitsin M, Willson JK, Sukumar S, Polyak K, Park BH, Pethiyagoda CL, Pant PV, Ballinger DG, Sparks AB, Hartigan J, Smith DR, Suh E, Papadopoulos N, Buckhaults P, Markowitz SD, Parmigiani G, Kinzler KW, Velculescu VE, Vogelstein B. The genomic landscapes of human breast and colorectal cancers. Science 2007;318(5853) 1108-1113.

[5] Cancer Genome Atlas Network. Comprehensive molecular characterization of human colon and rectal cancer. Nature 2012;487(7407) 330-337. doi: 10.1038/nature11252.

[6] Leary RJ, Lin JC, Cummins J, Boca S, Wood LD, Parsons DW, Jones S, Sjöblom T, Park BH, Parsons R, Willis J, Dawson D, Willson JK, Nikolskaya T, Nikolsky Y, Kopelovich L, Papadopoulos N, Pennacchio LA, Wang TL, Markowitz SD, Parmigiani G, Kinzler KW, Vogelstein B, Velculescu VE. Integrated analysis of homozygous deletions, focal amplifications, and sequence alterations in breast and colorectal cancers. Proc Natl Acad Sci USA 2008;105(42) 16224-16229.

[7] Schnekenburger M, Diederich M. Epigenetics Offer New Horizons for Colorectal Cancer Prevention. Curr Colorectal Cancer Rep 2012;8(1) 66-81.

[8] O'Hagan HM, Mohammad HP, Baylin SB. Double strand breaks can initiate gene silencing and SIRT1-dependent onset of DNA methylation in an exogenous promoter CpG island. PLoS Genet 2008;4(8) e1000155.

[9] Malanga M, Althaus FR. The role of poly(ADP-ribose) in the DNA damage signaling network. Biochem Cell Biol 2005;83(3) 354-64.

[10] Gottschalk AJ, Timinszky G, Kong SE, Jin J, Cai Y, Swanson SK, Washburn MP, Florens L, Ladurner AG, Conaway JW, Conaway RC. Poly(ADP-ribosyl)ation directs recruitment and activation of an ATP-dependent chromatin remodeler. Proc Natl Acad Sci U S A 2009;106(33) 13770-13774.

[11] Lin JC, Jeong S, Liang G, Takai D, Fatemi M, Tsai YC, Egger G, Gal-Yam EN, Jones PA. Role of nucleosomal occupancy in the epigenetic silencing of the MLH1 CpG island. Cancer Cell 2007;12(5) 432-444.

[12] Tabish AM, Poels K, Hoet P, Godderis L. Epigenetic Factors in Cancer Risk: Effect of Chemical Carcinogens on Global DNA Methylation Pattern in Human TK6 Cells. PLoS One 2012;7(4) e34674. Epub 2012 Apr 11.

[13] Stefanska B, Karlic H, Varga F, Fabianowska-Majewska K, Haslberger AG. Epigenetic mechanisms in anti-cancer actions of bioactive food components-the implications in cancer prevention. Br J Pharmacol 2012 Apr 27. doi: 10.1111/j.1476-5381.2012.02002.x. [Epub ahead of print]

[14] Jacinto FV, Esteller M. Mutator pathways unleashed by epigenetic silencing in human cancer. Mutagenesis 2007;22(4) 247-253.

[15] De Bont R, van Larebeke N. Endogenous DNA damage in humans: a review of quantitative data. Mutagenesis 2004;19(3) 169-185. http://mutage.oxfordjournals.org/content/19/3/169.full.pdf+html

[16] Helbock HJ, Beckman KB, Shigenaga MK, Walter PB, Woodall AA, Yeo HC, Ames BN. DNA oxidation matters: the HPLC-electrochemical detection assay of 8-oxo-deoxyguanosine and 8-oxo-guanine. Proc Natl Acad Sci U S A. 1998;95(1) 288-293.

[17] Nakamura J, Swenberg JA. Endogenous apurinic/apyrimidinic sites in genomic DNA of mammalian tissues. Cancer Res 1999;59(11) 2522-2526.

[18] Fraga CG, Shigenaga MK, Park JW, Degan P, Ames BN. Oxidative damage to DNA during aging: 8-hydroxy-2'-deoxyguanosine in rat organ DNA and urine. Proc Natl Acad Sci U S A 1990;87(12) 4533-4537.

[19] Ames BN, Shigenaga MK, Hagen TM. Oxidants, antioxidants, and the degenerative diseases of aging. Proc Natl Acad Sci U S A 1993;90(17) 7915-7922.

[20] Foksinski M, Rozalski R, Guz J, Ruszkowska B, Sztukowska P, Piwowarski M, Klungland A, Olinski R. Urinary excretion of DNA repair products correlates with

metabolic rates as well as with maximum life spans of different mammalian species. Free Radic Biol Med 2004;37(9) 1449-1454.

[21] Lindahl T. DNA repair enzymes acting on spontaneous lesions in DNA. In: Nichols WW and Murphy DG (eds.) DNA Repair Processes. Symposia Specialists, Miami, 1977. p225-240.

[22] Tice, R.R., and Setlow, R.B. DNA repair and replication in aging organisms and cells. In: Finch EE and Schneider EL (eds.) Handbook of the Biology of Aging. Van Nostrand Reinhold, New York. 1985. p173-224.

[23] Lindahl T, Nyberg B. Rate of depurination of native deoxyribonucleic acid. Biochemistry 1972;11(19) 3610-3618.

[24] Lindahl T. Instability and decay of the primary structure of DNA. Nature 1993;362(6422) 709-715.

[25] Nakamura J, Walker VE, Upton PB, Chiang SY, Kow YW, Swenberg JA. Highly sensitive apurinic/apyrimidinic site assay can detect spontaneous and chemically induced depurination under physiological conditions. Cancer Res 1998;58(2) 222-225.

[26] Haber JE. DNA recombination: the replication connection. Trends Biochem Sci 1999;24(7) 271-275.

[27] Vilenchik MM, Knudson AG. Endogenous DNA double-strand breaks: production, fidelity of repair, and induction of cancer. Proc Natl Acad Sci U S A 2003;100(22) 12871-12876. http://www.ncbi.nlm.nih.gov/pmc/articles/PMC240711/?tool=pubmed

[28] Nam EA, Cortez D. ATR signalling: more than meeting at the fork. Biochem J 2011;436(3) 527-536.

[29] Maher RL, Branagan AM, Morrical SW. Coordination of DNA replication and recombination activities in the maintenance of genome stability. J Cell Biochem 2011;112(10) 2672-82. doi: 10.1002/jcb.23211.

[30] Holmes GE, Bernstein C, Bernstein H. Oxidative and other DNA damages as the basis of aging: a review. Mutat Res 1992;275(3-6) 305-315.

[31] Hoeijmakers JH. DNA damage, aging, and cancer. N Engl J Med 2009;361(15) 1475-1485.

[32] Ou J, DeLany JP, Zhang M, Sharma S, O'Keefe SJ. Association between low colonic short-chain fatty acids and high bile acids in high colon cancer risk populations. Nutr Cancer 2012;64(1) 34-40.

[33] O'Keefe SJ, Kidd M, Espitalier-Noel G, Owira P. Rarity of colon cancer in Africans is associated with low animal product consumption, not fiber. Am J Gastroenterol 1999;94(5) 1373-1380.

[34] Maskarinec G, Noh JJ. The effect of migration on cancer incidence among Japanese in Hawaii. Ethn Dis 2004 Summer;14(3) 431-439.

[35] Jemal A, Bray F, Center MM, Ferlay J, Ward E, Forman D. Global cancer statistics. CA Cancer J Clin 2011;61(2) 69-90.

[36] Alberg AJ, Ford JG, Samet JM; American College of Chest Physicians. Epidemiology of lung cancer: ACCP evidence-based clinical practice guidelines (2nd edition). Chest 2007;132(3 Suppl) 29S-55S.

[37] Cunningham FH, Fiebelkorn S, Johnson M, Meredith C. A novel application of the Margin of Exposure approach: segregation of tobacco smoke toxicants. Food Chem Toxicol 2011;49(11) 2921-2933.

[38] Liu XY, Zhu MX, Xie JP. Mutagenicity of acrolein and acrolein-induced DNA adducts. Toxicol Mech Methods 2010;20(1) 36-44.

[39] Alexandrov K, Rojas M, Satarug S. The critical DNA damage by benzo(a)pyrene in lung tissues of smokers and approaches to preventing its formation. Toxicol Lett 2010;198(1) 63-68.

[40] Speit G, Merk O. Evaluation of mutagenic effects of formaldehyde in vitro: detection of crosslinks and mutations in mouse lymphoma cells. Mutagenesis 2002;17(3) 183-187.

[41] Grogan D, Jinks-Robertson S. Formaldehyde-induced mutagenesis in Saccharomyces cerevisiae: molecular properties and the roles of repair and bypass systems. Mutat Res 2012;731(1-2) 92-98.

[42] Pu X, Kamendulis LM, Klaunig JE. Acrylonitrile-induced oxidative stress and oxidative DNA damage in male Sprague-Dawley rats. Toxicol Sci 2009;111(1) 64-71.

[43] Marnett LJ. Oxy radicals, lipid peroxidation and DNA damage. Toxicology 2002;181-182 219-222.

[44] Koturbash I, Scherhag A, Sorrentino J, Sexton K, Bodnar W, Swenberg JA, Beland FA, Pardo-Manuel Devillena F, Rusyn I, Pogribny IP. Epigenetic mechanisms of mouse interstrain variability in genotoxicity of the environmental toxicant 1, 3-butadiene. Toxicol Sci. 2011;122(2) 448-456.

[45] Garcia CC, Angeli JP, Freitas FP, Gomes OF, de Oliveira TF, Loureiro AP, Di Mascio P, Medeiros MH. (13C2)-Acetaldehyde promotes unequivocal formation of 1, N2-propano-2'-deoxyguanosine in human cells. J Am Chem Soc 2011;133(24) 9140-9143.

[46] Tompkins EM, McLuckie KI, Jones DJ, Farmer PB, Brown K. Mutagenicity of DNA adducts derived from ethylene oxide exposure in the pSP189 shuttle vector replicated in human Ad293 cells. Mutat Res 2009;678(2) 129-137.

[47] Gelmont D, Stein RA, Mead JF. Isoprene-the main hydrocarbon in human breath. Biochem Biophys Res Commun 1981;99(4) 1456-1460.

[48] Senthilmohan ST, McEwan MJ, Wilson PF, Milligan DB, Freeman CG. Real time analysis of breath volatiles using SIFT-MS in cigarette smoking. Redox Rep 2001;6(3) 185-187.

[49] Fabiani R, Rosignoli P, De Bartolomeo A, Fuccelli R, Morozzi G. DNA-damaging ability of isoprene and isoprene mono-epoxide (EPOX I) in human cells evaluated with the comet assay. Mutat Res 2007;629(1) 7-13.

[50] Phillips DH. Smoking-related DNA and protein adducts in human tissues. Carcinogenesis 2002;23(12) 1979-2004.

[51] Giovannucci E, Martínez ME. Tobacco, colorectal cancer, and adenomas: a review of the evidence. J Natl Cancer Inst 1996;88(23) 1717-1730.

[52] de Kok TM, van Maanen JM. Evaluation of fecal mutagenicity and colorectal cancer risk. Mutat Res 2000; 463(1) 53-101.

[53] Pearson JR, Gill CI, Rowland IR. Diet, fecal water, and colon cancer--development of a biomarker. Nutr Rev 2009;67(9) 509-526.

[54] Bernstein H, Bernstein C, Payne CM, Dvorak K. Bile acids as endogenous etiologic agents in gastrointestinal cancer. World J Gastroenterol 2009;15(27) 3329-3340.

[55] Payne CM, Crowley-Skillicorn C, Bernstein C, Holubec H, Moyer MP, Bernstein H. Hydrophobic bile acid-induced micronuclei formation, mitotic perturbations, and decreases in spindle checkpoint proteins: relevance to genomic instability in colon carcinogenesis. Nutr Cancer 2010;62(6) 825-840.

[56] Bernstein H, Bernstein C, Payne CM, Dvorakova K, Garewal H. Bile acids as carcinogens in human gastrointestinal cancers. Mutat Res 2005;589(1) 47-65.

[57] Hursting SD, Thornquist M, Henderson MM. Types of dietary fat and the incidence of cancer at five sites. Prev Med 1990;19(3) 242-253.

[58] Reddy BS, Hanson D, Mangat S, Mathews L, Sbaschnig M, Sharma C, Simi B. Effect of high-fat, high-beef diet and of mode of cooking of beef in the diet on fecal bacterial enzymes and fecal bile acids and neutral sterols. J Nutr 1980;110(9) 1880-1887.

[59] Stadler J, Stern HS, Yeung KS, McGuire V, Furrer R, Marcon N, Bruce WR. Effect of high fat consumption on cell proliferation activity of colorectal mucosa and on soluble faecal bile acids. Gut 1988;29(10) 1326-1331.

[60] Bernstein C, Holubec H, Bhattacharyya AK, Nguyen H, Payne CM, Zaitlin B, Bernstein H. Carcinogenicity of deoxycholate, a secondary bile acid. Arch Toxicol 2011;85(8) 863-871

[61] Handa O, Naito Y, Yoshikawa T. Redox biology and gastric carcinogenesis: the role of Helicobacter pylori. Redox Rep 2011;16(1) 1-7.

[62] Wei L, Gravitt PE, Song H, Maldonado AM, Ozbun MA. Nitric oxide induces early viral transcription coincident with increased DNA damage and mutation rates in human papillomavirus-infected cells. Cancer Res 2009;69(11) 4878-4884.

[63] Goldman A, Shahidullah M, Goldman D, Khailova L, Watts G, Delamere N, Dvorak K. A novel mechanism of acid and bile acid-induced DNA damage involving Na+/H + exchanger: implication for Barrett's oesophagus. Gut 2010;59(12) 1606-1616.

[64] Smela ME, Hamm ML, Henderson PT, Harris CM, Harris TM, Essigmann JM. The aflatoxin B(1) formamidopyrimidine adduct plays a major role in causing the types of mutations observed in human hepatocellular carcinoma. Proc Natl Acad Sci U S A 2002;99(10) 6655-6660.

[65] Kanavy HE, Gerstenblith MR. Ultraviolet radiation and melanoma. Semin Cutan Med Surg 2011;30(4) 222-228

[66] Lichtenstein P, Holm NV, Verkasalo PK, Iliadou A, Kaprio J, Koskenvuo M, Pukkala E, Skytthe A, Hemminki K. Environmental and heritable factors in the causation of cancer--analyses of cohorts of twins from Sweden, Denmark, and Finland. N Engl J Med 2000;343(2) 78-85.

[67] https://dnapittcrew.upmc.com/db/orthologs.php

[68] http://sciencepark.mdanderson.org/labs/wood/dna_repair_genes.html

[69] Wood RD, Mitchell M, Sgouros J, Lindahl T. Human DNA repair genes. Science 2001;291(5507) 1284-1289.

[70] Wood RD, Mitchell M, Lindahl T. Human DNA repair genes, 2005. Mutat Res 2005;577(1-2) 275-283.

[71] Bernstein C, Bernstein H, Payne CM, Garewal H. DNA repair/pro-apoptotic dual-role proteins in five major DNA repair pathways: fail-safe protection against carcinogenesis. Mutat Res 2002;511(2) 145-178.

[72] Foulkes WD. Inherited susceptibility to common cancers. N Engl J Med 2008;359(20) 2143-2153.

[73] O'Hagan HM, Wang W, Sen S, Destefano Shields C, Lee SS, Zhang YW, Clements EG, Cai Y, Van Neste L, Easwaran H, Casero RA, Sears CL, Baylin SB. Oxidative damage targets complexes containing DNA methyltransferases, SIRT1, and polycomb members to promoter CpG Islands. Cancer Cell. 2011;20(5) 606-619.

[74] Malkin D. Li-fraumeni syndrome. Genes Cancer 2011;2(4) 475-484.

[75] Roukos DH. Genome-wide association studies: how predictable is a person's cancer risk? Expert Rev Anticancer Ther 2009;9(4) 389-392.

[76] Truninger K, Menigatti M, Luz J, Russell A, Haider R, Gebbers JO, Bannwart F, Yurtsever H, Neuweiler J, Riehle HM, Cattaruzza MS, Heinimann K, Schär P, Jiricny J, Marra G. Immunohistochemical analysis reveals high frequency of PMS2 defects in colorectal cancer. Gastroenterology 2005;128(5) 1160-1171.

[77] Valeri N, Gasparini P, Fabbri M, Braconi C, Veronese A, Lovat F, Adair B, Vannini I, Fanini F, Bottoni A, Costinean S, Sandhu SK, Nuovo GJ, Alder H, Gafa R, Calore F,

Ferracin M, Lanza G, Volinia S, Negrini M, McIlhatton MA, Amadori D, Fishel R, Croce CM. Modulation of mismatch repair and genomic stability by miR-155. Proc Natl Acad Sci U S A 2010;107(15) 6982-6987.

[78] Zhang W, Zhang J, Hoadley K, Kushwaha D, Ramakrishnan V, Li S, Kang C, You Y, Jiang C, Song SW, Jiang T, Chen CC. miR-181d: a predictive glioblastoma biomarker that downregulates MGMT expression. Neuro Oncol 2012;14(6) 712-719.

[79] Spiegl-Kreinecker S, Pirker C, Filipits M, Lötsch D, Buchroithner J, Pichler J, Silye R, Weis S, Micksche M, Fischer J, Berger W.O6-Methylguanine DNA methyltransferase protein expression in tumor cells predicts outcome of temozolomide therapy in glioblastoma patients. Neuro Oncol 2010 Jan;12(1) 28-36.

[80] Lahtz C, Pfeifer GP. Epigenetic changes of DNA repair genes in cancer. J Mol Cell Biol 2011;3(1) 51-58.

[81] Narayanan L, Fritzell JA, Baker SM, Liskay RM, Glazer PM. Elevated levels of mutation in multiple tissues of mice deficient in the DNA mismatch repair gene Pms2. Proc Natl Acad Sci U S A 1997;94(7) 3122-3127.

[82] Hegan DC, Narayanan L, Jirik FR, Edelmann W, Liskay RM, Glazer PM. Differing patterns of genetic instability in mice deficient in the mismatch repair genes Pms2, Mlh1, Msh2, Msh3 and Msh6. Carcinogenesis 2006;27(12) 2402-2408.

[83] Tutt AN, van Oostrom CT, Ross GM, van Steeg H, Ashworth A. Disruption of Brca2 increases the spontaneous mutation rate in vivo: synergism with ionizing radiation. EMBO Rep 2002;3(3) 255-260.

[84] German J. Bloom's syndrome. I. Genetical and clinical observations in the first twenty-seven patients. Am J Hum Genet 1969;21(2) 196-227.

[85] Nagaraju G, Scully R. Minding the gap: the underground functions of BRCA1 and BRCA2 at stalled replication forks. DNA Repair (Amst) 2007;6(7) 1018-1031.

[86] Lancaster JM, Powell CB, Kauff ND, Cass I, Chen LM, Lu KH, Mutch DG, Berchuck A, Karlan BY, Herzog TJ; Society of Gynecologic Oncologists Education Committee. Society of Gynecologic Oncologists Education Committee statement on risk assessment for inherited gynecologic cancer predispositions. Gynecol Oncol 2007;107(2) 159-162.

[87] Keimling M, Volcic M, Csernok A, Wieland B, Dörk T, Wiesmüller L. Functional characterization connects individual patient mutations in ataxia telangiectasia mutated (ATM) with dysfunction of specific DNA double-strand break-repair signaling pathways. FASEB J 2011;25(11) 3849-3860.

[88] Thompson LH, Schild D. Recombinational DNA repair and human disease. Mutat Res 2002;509(1-2) 49-78.

[89] Chrzanowska KH, Gregorek H, Dembowska-Bagińska B, Kalina MA, Digweed M. Nijmegen breakage syndrome (NBS). Orphanet J Rare Dis 2012;7 13.

[90] Rapp A, Greulich KO. After double-strand break induction by UV-A, homologous recombination and nonhomologous end joining cooperate at the same DSB if both systems are available. J Cell Sci 2004;117(Pt 21) 4935-4945.

[91] Bartkova J, Tommiska J, Oplustilova L, Aaltonen K, Tamminen A, Heikkinen T, Mistrik M, Aittomäki K, Blomqvist C, Heikkilä P, Lukas J, Nevanlinna H, Bartek J. Aberrations of the MRE11-RAD50-NBS1 DNA damage sensor complex in human breast cancer: MRE11 as a candidate familial cancer-predisposing gene. Mol Oncol 2008;2(4) 296-316.

[92] Nimonkar AV, Ozsoy AZ, Genschel J, Modrich P, Kowalczykowski SC. Human exonuclease 1 and BLM helicase interact to resect DNA and initiate DNA repair. Proc Natl Acad Sci U S A 2008;105(44) 16906-16911.

[93] German J. Bloom's syndrome. XX. The first 100 cancers. Cancer Genet Cytogenet 1997;93(1) 100-106.

[94] Bohr VA. Deficient DNA repair in the human progeroid disorder, Werner syndrome. Mutat Res 2005;577(1-2) 252-259.

[95] Monnat RJ Jr. Human RECQ helicases: roles in DNA metabolism, mutagenesis and cancer biology. Semin Cancer Biol 2010;20(5) 329-339.

[96] Singh DK, Ahn B, Bohr VA. Roles of RECQ helicases in recombination based DNA repair, genomic stability and aging. Biogerontology 2009;10(3) 235-252.

[97] Anbari KK, Ierardi-Curto LA, Silber JS, Asada N, Spinner N, Zackai EH, Belasco J, Morrissette JD, Dormans JP. Two primary osteosarcomas in a patient with Rothmund-Thomson syndrome. Clin Orthop Relat Res 2000;(378) 213-223.

[98] Thompson LH, Hinz JM. Cellular and molecular consequences of defective Fanconi anemia proteins in replication-coupled DNA repair: mechanistic insights. Mutat Res 2009;668(1-2) 54-72.

[99] Alter BP. Cancer in Fanconi anemia, 1927-2001. Cancer 2003;97(2) 425-440.

[100] Lehmann AR, McGibbon D, Stefanini M. Xeroderma pigmentosum. Orphanet J Rare Dis 2011;6 70.

[101] Oh KS, Imoto K, Emmert S, Tamura D, DiGiovanna JJ, Kraemer KH. Nucleotide excision repair proteins rapidly accumulate but fail to persist in human XP-E (DDB2 mutant) cells. Photochem Photobiol 2011;87(3) 729-733.

[102] Manchanda R, Menon U, Michaelson-Cohen R, Beller U, Jacobs I. Hereditary nonpolyposis colorectal cancer or Lynch syndrome: the gynaecological perspective. Curr Opin Obstet Gynecol 2009;21(1) 31-38.

[103] David SS, O'Shea VL, Kundu S. Base-excision repair of oxidative DNA damage. Nature 2007;447(7147) 941-950.

[104] Cleary SP, Cotterchio M, Jenkins MA, Kim H, Bristow R, Green R, Haile R, Hopper JL, LeMarchand L, Lindor N, Parfrey P, Potter J, Younghusband B, Gallinger S.

Germline MutY human homologue mutations and colorectal cancer: a multisite case-control study. Gastroenterology 2009;136(4) 1251-1260.

[105] López-Contreras AJ, Fernandez-Capetillo O. The ATR barrier to replication-born DNA damage. DNA Repair (Amst) 2010;9(12) 1249-1255.

[106] Tanaka A, Weinel S, Nagy N, O'Driscoll M, Lai-Cheong JE, Kulp-Shorten CL, Knable A, Carpenter G, Fisher SA, Hiragun M, Yanase Y, Hide M, Callen J, McGrath JA. Germline mutation in ATR in autosomal- dominant oropharyngeal cancer syndrome. Am J Hum Genet 2012;90(3) 511-517.

[107] Viktorsson K, De Petris L, Lewensohn R. The role of p53 in treatment responses of lung cancer. Biochem Biophys Res Commun 2005;331(3) 868-880.

[108] Esteller M, Silva JM, Dominguez G, Bonilla F, Matias-Guiu X, Lerma E, Bussaglia E, Prat J, Harkes IC, Repasky EA, Gabrielson E, Schutte M, Baylin SB, Herman JG. Promoter hypermethylation and BRCA1 inactivation in sporadic breast and ovarian tumors. J Natl Cancer Inst 2000;92(7) 564-569.

[109] Shen L, Kondo Y, Rosner GL, Xiao L, Hernandez NS, Vilaythong J, Houlihan PS, Krouse RS, Prasad AR, Einspahr JG, Buckmeier J, Alberts DS, Hamilton SR, Issa JP. MGMT promoter methylation and field defect in sporadic colorectal cancer. J Natl Cancer Inst 2005;97(18) 1330-1338.

[110] Psofaki V, Kalogera C, Tzambouras N, Stephanou D, Tsianos E, Seferiadis K, Kolios G. Promoter methylation status of hMLH1, MGMT, and CDKN2A/p16 in colorectal adenomas. World J Gastroenterol 2010;16(28) 3553-3560.

[111] Lee KH, Lee JS, Nam JH, Choi C, Lee MC, Park CS, Juhng SW, Lee JH. Promoter methylation status of hMLH1, hMSH2, and MGMT genes in colorectal cancer associated with adenoma-carcinoma sequence. Langenbecks Arch Surg 2011;396(7) 1017-1026.

[112] Facista A, Nguyen H, Lewis C, Prasad AR, Ramsey L, Zaitlin B, Nfonsam V, Krouse RS, Bernstein H, Payne CM, Stern S, Oatman N, Banerjee B, Bernstein C. Deficient expression of DNA repair enzymes in early progression to sporadic colon cancer. Genome Integr 2012;3(1): 3.

[113] Zou XP, Zhang B, Zhang XQ, Chen M, Cao J, Liu WJ. Promoter hypermethylation of multiple genes in early gastric adenocarcinoma and precancerous lesions. Hum Pathol 2009;40(11) 1534-1542.

[114] Ling ZQ, Li P, Ge MH, Hu FJ, Fang XH, Dong ZM, Mao WM. Aberrant methylation of different DNA repair genes demonstrates distinct prognostic value for esophageal cancer. Dig Dis Sci 2011;56(10) 2992-3004.

[115] Lee KH, Lee JS, Nam JH, Choi C, Lee MC, Park CS, Juhng SW, Lee JH. Promoter methylation status of hMLH1, hMSH2, and MGMT genes in colorectal cancer associated with adenoma-carcinoma sequence. Langenbecks Arch Surg 2011;396(7) 1017-1026.

[116] Paluszczak J, Misiak P, Wierzbicka M, Woźniak A, Baer-Dubowska W. Frequent hypermethylation of DAPK, RARbeta, MGMT, RASSF1A and FHIT in laryngeal squamous cell carcinomas and adjacent normal mucosa. Oral Oncol 2011;47(2) 104-107.

[117] Guo M, House MG, Hooker C, Han Y, Heath E, Gabrielson E, Yang SC, Baylin SB, Herman JG, Brock MV. Promoter hypermethylation of resected bronchial margins: a field defect of changes? Clin Cancer Res 2004;10(15) 5131-5136.

[118] Skiriute D, Vaitkiene P, Saferis V, Asmoniene V, Skauminas K, Deltuva VP, Tamasauskas A. MGMT, GATA6, CD81, DR4, and CASP8 gene promoter methylation in glioblastoma. BMC Cancer 2012;12(1) 218.

[119] Pogribny IP, James SJ. Reduction of p53 gene expression in human primary hepatocellular carcinoma is associated with promoter region methylation without coding region mutation. Cancer Lett 2002;176(2) 169-74.

[120] Guan H, Ji M, Hou P, Liu Z, Wang C, Shan Z, Teng W, Xing M. Hypermethylation of the DNA mismatch repair gene hMLH1 and its association with lymph node metastasis and T1799A BRAF mutation in patients with papillary thyroid cancer. Cancer 2008;113(2) 247-255.

[121] Wan G, Mathur R, Hu X, Zhang X, Lu X. miRNA response to DNA damage. Trends Biochem Sci 2011;36(9) 478-484.

[122] Malumbres M. miRNAs and cancer: An epigenetics view. Mol Aspects Med 2012 Jul 4 [Epub ahead of print]

[123] Resar LM. The high mobility group A1 gene: transforming inflammatory signals into cancer? Cancer Res 2010;70(2) 436-439.

[124] Baldassarre G, Battista S, Belletti B, Thakur S, Pentimalli F, Trapasso F, Fedele M, Pierantoni G, Croce CM, Fusco A. Negative regulation of BRCA1 gene expression by HMGA1 proteins accounts for the reduced BRCA1 protein levels in sporadic breast carcinoma. Mol Cell Biol 2003;23(7) 2225-2238.

[125] Borrmann L, Schwanbeck R, Heyduk T, Seebeck B, Rogalla P, Bullerdiek J, Wisniewski JR. High mobility group A2 protein and its derivatives bind a specific region of the promoter of DNA repair gene ERCC1 and modulate its activity. Nucleic Acids Res 2003;31(23) 6841-6851.

[126] Lee S, Jung JW, Park SB, Roh K, Lee SY, Kim JH, Kang SK, Kang KS. Histone deacetylase regulates high mobility group A2-targeting microRNAs in human cord blood-derived multipotent stem cell aging. Cell Mol Life Sci 2011;68(2) 325-336.

[127] Palmieri D, D'Angelo D, Valentino T, De Martino I, Ferraro A, Wierinckx A, Fedele M, Trouillas J, Fusco A. Downregulation of HMGA-targeting microRNAs has a critical role in human pituitary tumorigenesis. Oncogene 2011 Dec 5. doi: 10.1038/onc.2011.557.

[128] Sampath D, Liu C, Vasan K, Sulda M, Puduvalli VK, Wierda WG, Keating MJ. Histone deacetylases mediate the silencing of miR-15a, miR-16, and miR-29b in chronic lymphocytic leukemia. Blood 2012;119(5) 1162-1172.

[129] D'Angelo D, Palmieri D, Mussnich P, Roche M, Wierinckx A, Raverot G, Fedele M, Croce CM, Trouillas J, Fusco A. Altered MicroRNA Expression Profile in Human Pituitary GH Adenomas: Down-Regulation of miRNA Targeting HMGA1, HMGA2, and E2F1. J Clin Endocrinol Metab 2012;97(7) E1128-1138.

[130] Suzuki H, Takatsuka S, Akashi H, Yamamoto E, Nojima M, Maruyama R, Kai M, Yamano HO, Sasaki Y, Tokino T, Shinomura Y, Imai K, Toyota M. Genome-wide profiling of chromatin signatures reveals epigenetic regulation of MicroRNA genes in colorectal cancer. Cancer Res 2011;71(17) 5646-5658.

[131] Tchou-Wong KM, Kiok K, Tang Z, Kluz T, Arita A, Smith PR, Brown S, Costa M. Effects of nickel treatment on H3K4 trimethylation and gene expression. PLoS One 2011;6(3) e17728.

[132] Klase Z, Winograd R, Davis J, Carpio L, Hildreth R, Heydarian M, Fu S, McCaffrey T, Meiri E, Ayash-Rashkovsky M, Gilad S, Bentwich Z, Kashanchi F: HIV-1 TAR miRNA protects against apoptosis by altering cellular gene expression. Retrovirology 2009;6 18.

[133] http://www.ebi.ac.uk/enright-srv/microcosm/htdocs/targets/v5/

[134] Wang P, Dong Q, Zhang C, Kuan PF, Liu Y, Jeck WR, Andersen JB, Jiang W, Savich GL, Tan TX, Auman JT, Hoskins JM, Misher AD, Moser CD, Yourstone SM, Kim JW, Cibulskis K, Getz G, Hunt HV, Thorgeirsson SS, Roberts LR, Ye D, Guan KL, Xiong Y, Qin LX, Chiang DY. Mutations in isocitrate dehydrogenase 1 and 2 occur frequently in intrahepatic cholangiocarcinomas and share hypermethylation targets with glioblastomas. Oncogene 2012 Jul 23. doi: 10.1038/onc.2012.315. [Epub ahead of print]

[135] Watanabe T, Nobusawa S, Kleihues P, Ohgaki H. IDH1 mutations are early events in the development of astrocytomas and oligodendrogliomas. Am J Pathol 2009;174(4) 1149-1153.

[136] Turcan S, Rohle D, Goenka A, Walsh LA, Fang F, Yilmaz E, Campos C, Fabius AW, Lu C, Ward PS, Thompson CB, Kaufman A, Guryanova O, Levine R, Heguy A, Viale A, Morris LG, Huse JT, Mellinghoff IK, Chan TA. IDH1 mutation is sufficient to establish the glioma hypermethylator phenotype. Nature 2012;483(7390) 479-483.

[137] Carrillo JA, Lai A, Nghiemphu PL, Kim HJ, Phillips HS, Kharbanda S, Moftakhar P, Lalaezari S, Yong W, Ellingson BM, Cloughesy TF, Pope WB. Relationship between Tumor Enhancement, Edema, IDH1 Mutational Status, MGMT Promoter Methylation, and Survival in Glioblastoma. AJNR Am J Neuroradiol 2012;33(7) 1349-1355.

[138] Nelson PT, Kiriakidou M, Mourelatos Z, Tan GS, Jennings MH, Xie K, Wang WX. High-throughput experimental studies to identify miRNA targets directly, with special focus on the mammalian brain. Brain Res 2010;1338 122-130.

[139] Ohka F, Natsume A, Motomura K, Kishida Y, Kondo Y, Abe T, Nakasu Y, Namba H, Wakai K, Fukui T, Momota H, Iwami K, Kinjo S, Ito M, Fujii M, Wakabayashi T. The global DNA methylation surrogate LINE-1 methylation is correlated with MGMT promoter methylation and is a better prognostic factor for glioma. PLoS One 2011;6(8) e23332.

[140] Bernstein C, Bernstein H, Payne CM, Dvorak K, Garewal H. Field defects in progression to gastrointestinal tract cancers. Cancer Lett 2008;260(1-2) 1-10.

[141] Gerlinger M, Rowan AJ, Horswell S, Larkin J, Endesfelder D, Gronroos E, Martinez P, Matthews N, Stewart A, Tarpey P, Varela I, Phillimore B, Begum S, McDonald NQ, Butler A, Jones D, Raine K, Latimer C, Santos CR, Nohadani M, Eklund AC, Spencer-Dene B, Clark G, Pickering L, Stamp G, Gore M, Szallasi Z, Downward J, Futreal PA, Swanton C. N Engl J Med 2012;366(10) 883-892.

[142] Bernstein C, Facista A, Nguyen H, Zaitlin B, Hassounah N, Loustaunau C, Payne CM, Banerjee B, Goldschmid S, Tsikitis VL, Krouse R, Bernstein H. Cancer and age related colonic crypt deficiencies in cytochrome c oxidase I. World J Gastrointest Oncol 2010;2(12) 429-442.

[143] Nicolas P, Kim KM, Shibata D, Tavaré S: The stem cell population of the human colon crypt: analysis via methylation patterns. PLoS Comput Biol 2007;3 e28.

[144] Willis ND, Przyborski SA, Hutchison CJ, Wilson RG: Colonic and colorectal cancer stem cells: progress in the search for putative biomarkers. J Anat 2008;213 59-65.

[145] Loeb LA. Human cancers express mutator phenotypes: origin, consequences and targeting. Nat Rev Cancer 2011;11(6) 450-457.

[146] Roy M, Sinha D, Mukherjee S, Biswas J. Curcumin prevents DNA damage and enhances the repair potential in a chronically arsenic-exposed human population in West Bengal, India. Eur J Cancer Prev 2011;20(2) 123-131.

[147] Qin XJ, Liu W, Li YN, Sun X, Hai CX, Hudson LG, Liu KJ. Poly(ADP-ribose) polymerase-1 inhibition by arsenite promotes the survival of cells with unrepaired DNA lesions induced by UV exposure. Toxicol Sci 2012;127(1) 120-129.

[148] Ebert F, Weiss A, Bültemeyer M, Hamann I, Hartwig A, Schwerdtle T. Arsenicals affect base excision repair by several mechanisms. Mutat Res 2011;715(1-2) 32-41.

[149] Andrew AS, Karagas MR, Hamilton JW. Decreased DNA repair gene expression among individuals exposed to arsenic in United States drinking water. Int J Cancer 2003;104(3) 263-268.

[150] Nollen M, Ebert F, Moser J, Mullenders LH, Hartwig A, Schwerdtle T. Impact of arsenic on nucleotide excision repair: XPC function, protein level, and gene expression. Mol Nutr Food Res 2009;53(5) 572-582.

[151] Shen S, Lee J, Weinfeld M, Le XC. Attenuation of DNA damage-induced p53 expression by arsenic: a possible mechanism for arsenic co-carcinogenesis. Mol Carcinog 2008;47(7) 508-518.

[152] Zhou ZH, Lei YX, Wang CX. Analysis of aberrant methylation in DNA repair genes during malignant transformation of human bronchial epithelial cells induced by cadmium. Toxicol Sci 2012;125(2) 412-417.

[153] Wieland M, Levin MK, Hingorani KS, Biro FN, Hingorani MM. Mechanism of cadmium-mediated inhibition of Msh2-Msh6 function in DNA mismatch repair. Biochemistry 2009;48(40) 9492-9502.

[154] Bravard A, Vacher M, Gouget B, Coutant A, de Boisferon FH, Marsin S, Chevillard S, Radicella JP. Redox regulation of human OGG1 activity in response to cellular oxidative stress. Mol Cell Biol 2006;26(20) 7430-7436.

[155] Viau M, Gastaldo J, Bencokova Z, Joubert A, Foray N. Cadmium inhibits non-homologous end-joining and over-activates the MRE11-dependent repair pathway. Mutat Res 2008;654(1) 13-21.

[156] Schwerdtle T, Ebert F, Thuy C, Richter C, Mullenders LH, Hartwig A. Genotoxicity of soluble and particulate cadmium compounds: impact on oxidative DNA damage and nucleotide excision repair. Chem Res Toxicol 2010;23(2) 432-442.

[157] Burnat G, Majka J, Konturek PC. Bile acids are multifunctional modulators of the Barrett's carcinogenesis. J Physiol Pharmacol 2010;61(2) 185-192.

[158] Romagnolo DF, Chirnomas RB, Ku J, Jeffy BD, Payne CM, Holubec H, Ramsey L, Bernstein H, Bernstein C, Kunke K, Bhattacharyya A, Warneke J, Garewal H. Deoxycholate, an endogenous tumor promoter and DNA damaging agent, modulates BRCA-1 expression in apoptosis-sensitive epithelial cells: loss of BRCA-1 expression in colonic adenocarcinomas. Nutr Cancer 2003;46(1) 82-92.

[159] Ogawa A, Murate T, Suzuki M, Nimura Y, Yoshida S. Lithocholic acid, a putative tumor promoter, inhibits mammalian DNA polymerase beta. Jpn J Cancer Res 1998;89(11) 1154-1159.

[160] Feng Z, Hu W, Tang MS. Trans-4-hydroxy-2-nonenal inhibits nucleotide excision repair in human cells: a possible mechanism for lipid peroxidation-induced carcinogenesis. Proc Natl Acad Sci U S A 2004;101(23) 8598-8602.

[161] Feng Z, Hu W, Marnett LJ, Tang MS. Malondialdehyde, a major endogenous lipid peroxidation product, sensitizes human cells to UV- and BPDE-induced killing and mutagenesis through inhibition of nucleotide excision repair. Mutat Res 2006;601(1-2) 125-136.

[162] Chang CL, Marra G, Chauhan DP, Ha HT, Chang DK, Ricciardiello L, Randolph A, Carethers JM, Boland CR. Oxidative stress inactivates the human DNA mismatch repair system. Am J Physiol Cell Physiol 2002;283(1) C148-154.

[163] Langie SA, Knaapen AM, Houben JM, van Kempen FC, de Hoon JP, Gottschalk RW, Godschalk RW, van Schooten FJ. The role of glutathione in the regulation of nucleotide excision repair during oxidative stress. Toxicol Lett 20075;168(3) 302-309.

[164] Hill JW, Hu JJ, Evans MK. OGG1 is degraded by calpain following oxidative stress and cisplatin exposure. DNA Repair (Amst) 2008;7(4) 648-654.

[165] Sudprasert W, Navasumrit P, Ruchirawat M. Effects of low-dose gamma radiation on DNA damage, chromosomal aberration and expression of repair genes in human blood cells. Int J Hyg Environ Health. 2006;209(6) 503-511.

[166] Li D, Wang Q, Liu C, Duan H, Zeng X, Zhang B, Li X, Zhao J, Tang S, Li Z, Xing X, Yang P, Chen L, Zeng J, Zhu X, Zhang S, Zhang Z, Ma L, He Z, Wang E, Xiao Y, Zheng Y, Chen W. Aberrant expression of miR-638 contributes to benzo(a)pyrene-induced human cell transformation. Toxicol Sci 2012;125(2) 382-391.

[167] Liu WB, Ao L, Cui ZH, Zhou ZY, Zhou YH, Yuan XY, Xiang YL, Cao J, Liu JY. Molecular analysis of DNA repair gene methylation and protein expression during chemical-induced rat lung carcinogenesis. Biochem Biophys Res Commun 2011;408(4) 595-601.

[168] Hanova M, Stetina R, Vodickova L, Vaclavikova R, Hlavac P, Smerhovsky Z, Naccarati A, Polakova V, Soucek P, Kuricova M, Manini P, Kumar R, Hemminki K, Vodicka P. Modulation of DNA repair capacity and mRNA expression levels of XRCC1, hOGG1 and XPC genes in styrene-exposed workers. Toxicol Appl Pharmacol 2010;248(3) 194-200.

[169] Chen YY, Chung JG, Wu HC, Bau DT, Wu KY, Kao ST, Hsiang CY, Ho TY, Chiang SY. Aristolochic acid suppresses DNA repair and triggers oxidative DNA damage in human kidney proximal tubular cells. Oncol Rep 2010;24(1) 141-153.

[170] Grosskopf C, Schwerdtle T, Mullenders LH, Hartwig A. Antimony impairs nucleotide excision repair: XPA and XPE as potential molecular targets. Chem Res Toxicol 2010;23(7) 1175-1183.

[171] Ji W, Yang L, Yu L, Yuan J, Hu D, Zhang W, Yang J, Pang Y, Li W, Lu J, Fu J, Chen J, Lin Z, Chen W, Zhuang Z. Epigenetic silencing of O6-methylguanine DNA methyltransferase gene in NiS-transformed cells. Carcinogenesis 2008;29(6) 1267-1275.

[172] Link A, Balaguer F, Goel A. Cancer chemoprevention by dietary polyphenols: promising role for epigenetics. Biochem Pharmacol 2010;80(12) 1771-1792.

[173] Fang M, Chen D, Yang CS. Dietary polyphenols may affect DNA methylation. J Nutr 2007;137(1 Suppl) 223S-228S.

[174] Olaharski AJ, Rine J, Marshall BL, Babiarz J, Zhang L, Verdin E, Smith MT. The flavoring agent dihydrocoumarin reverses epigenetic silencing and inhibits sirtuin deacetylases. PLoS Genet 2005;1(6) e77.

[175] Kikuno N, Shiina H, Urakami S, Kawamoto K, Hirata H, Tanaka Y, Majid S, Igawa M, Dahiya R. Genistein mediated histone acetylation and demethylation activates tumor suppressor genes in prostate cancer cells. Int J Cancer 2008;123(3) 552-560.

[176] Collins AR, Azqueta A, Langie SA. Effects of micronutrients on DNA repair. Eur J Nutr 2012;51(3) 261-279.

[177] http://www.phenol-explorer.eu

[178] http://www.ajcn.org/content/93/6/1220.full.pdf+html

[179] http://www.hmdb.ca/search/search?query=caffeic+acid

[180] Aiyer HS, Vadhanam MV, Stoyanova R, Caprio GD, Clapper ML, Gupta RC. Dietary berries and ellagic acid prevent oxidative DNA damage and modulate expression of DNA repair genes. Int J Mol Sci 2008;9(3) 327-341.

[181] Niture SK, Velu CS, Smith QR, Bhat GJ, Srivenugopal KS. Increased expression of the MGMT repair protein mediated by cysteine prodrugs and chemopreventative natural products in human lymphocytes and tumor cell lines. Carcinogenesis 2007;28(2) 378-389.

[182] Bernstein H, Crowley-Skillicorn C, Bernstein C, Payne CM, Dvorak K, Garewal H. Dietary Compounds that Enhance DNA Repair and their Relevance to Cancer and Aging. In: BR Landseer (ed.) New Research on DNA Repair. New York: Nova Science Publishers, Inc.; 2007. p99-113.

[183] Clifford MN. Chlorogenic acids and other cinnamates --- nature, occurrence and dietary burden. J Sci Food Agric 1999;79(3) 362-372.

[184] Mattila P, Kumpulainen J. Determination of free and total phenolic acids in plant-derived foods by HPLC with diode-array detection. J Agric Food Chem 2002;50(13) 3660-3667.

[185] Yun MH, Hiom K. Understanding the functions of BRCA1 in the DNA-damage response. Biochem Soc Trans 2009;37(Pt 3) 597-604.

[186] Quinn JE, Kennedy RD, Mullan PB, Gilmore PM, Carty M, Johnston PG, Harkin DP. BRCA1 functions as a differential modulator of chemotherapy-induced apoptosis. Cancer Res 2003;63(19) 6221-6228.

[187] Taron M, Rosell R, Felip E, Mendez P, Souglakos J, Ronco MS, Queralt C, Majo J, Sanchez JM, Sanchez JJ, Maesire J. BRCA1 mRNA expression levels as an indicator of chemoresistance in lung cancer. Human Molecular Genetics 2004;13(20) 2443-2449.

[188] Papadaki C, Sfakianaki M, Ioannidis G, Lagoudaki E, Trypaki M, Tryfonidis K, Mavroudis D, Stathopoulos E, Georgoulias V, Souglakos J. ERCC1 and BRCA1 mRNA expression levels in the primary tumor could predict the effectiveness of the second-line cisplatin-based chemotherapy in pretreated patents with metastatic non-small cell lung cancer. J Thorac Oncol 2012;7(4) 663-671.

[189] Weberpals J, Garbuio K, O'Brien A, Clark-Knowles K, Doucette S, Antoniouk O, Goss G, Dimitroulakos J. The DNA repair proteins BRCA1 and ERCC1 as predictive markers in sporadic ovarian cancer. Int J Cancer 2009;124(4) 806-815.

[190] Reed E. Platinum-DNA adduct, nucleotide excision repair and platinum based anticancer chemotherapy. Cancer Treat Rev 1998;24(5) 331-344.

[191] Kelland L. The resurgence of platinum-based cancer chemotherapy. Nat Rev Cancer 2007;7(8) 573-584.

[192] Martin LP, Hamilton TC, Schilder RJ. Platinum Resistance: The role of DNA repair pathways. Clin Cancer Res 2008;14(5) 1291-1295.

[193] Bosl GJ, Motzer RJ. Testicular germ-cell cancer. N Engl J Med 1997;337(4) 242-253.

[194] Welsh C, Day R, McGurk C, Masters JRW, Wood RD, Koberle B. Reduced levels of XPA, ERCC1 and XPF DNA repair proteins in testis tumor cell lines. Int J Cancer 2004;110(3) 352-361.

[195] Simon GR, Sharma S, Cantor A, Smith P, Bepler G. ERCC1 expression is a predictor of survival in resected patients with non-small cell lung cancer. Chest 2005;127(3) 978-983.

[196] Lord RVN, Brabender J, Gandara D, Alberola V, Camps C, Domine M, Cardenal F, Sanchez JM, Gumerlock PH, Taron M, Sanchez JJ, Danenberg KD, Danenberg PV, Rosell R. Low ERCC1 expression correlates with prolonged survival after cisplatin plus gemcitabine chemotherapy in non-small cell lung cancer. Clin Cancer Res 2002;8(7) 2286-2291.

[197] Zhou W, Gurubhagavatula S, Liu G, Park S, Neuberg DS, Wain JC, Lynch TJ, Su L, Christiani DC. Excision repair cross-complementation group 1 polymorphism predicts overall survival in advanced non-small cell lung cancer patients treated with platinum-based chemotherapy. Clin Cancer Res 2004;10(15) 4939-4943.

[198] Olaussen KA, Dunant A, Fouret P, Brambilla E, Andre F, Haddad V, Taranchon E, Filipits M, Pirker R, Popper HH, Stahel R, Sabatier L, Pignon J-P, Tursz T, Le Chavalier T, Soria, J-C. DNA repair by ERCC1 in non-small-cell lung cancer and cisplatin-based adjuvant chemotherapy. N Engl J Med 2006;355(10) 983-991.

[199] Leng XF, Chen MW, Xian L, Dai L, Ma GY, Li MH. Combined analysis of mRNA expression of ERCC1, BAG-1, BRCA1, RRM1 and TUBB3 to predict prognosis in patients with non-small cell lung cancer who received adjuvant chemotherapy. J Exp Clin Cancer Res 2012;23 31:25.

[200] Dabholkar M, Bostick-Bruton F, Weber C, Bohr VA, Egwuagu C, Reed E. ERCC1 and ERCC2 expression in malignant tissues from ovarian cancer patients. J Natl Cancer Inst 1992;84(19) 1512-1517.

[201] Kang S, Ju W, Kim JW, Park N-H, Song Y-S, Kim SC, Park S-Y, Kang S-B, Lee H-P. Association between excision repair cross-complementation group 1 polymorphism

and clinical outcome of platinum based chemotherapy in patients with epithelial ovarian cancer. Exp Mol Med 2006;8(3) 320-324.

[202] Shirota Y, Stoehlmacher J, Brabender J, Xiong Y-P, Uetake H, Danenberg KD, Groshen S, Tsao-Wei DD, Danenberg PV, Lenz H-J. ERCC1 and thymidylate synthase mRNA levels predict survival for colorectal cancer patients receiving combination oxaliplatin and fluorouracil chemotherapy. J Clin Oncol 2001;19(23) 4298-4304.

[203] Viguier J, Boige V, Miquel C, Pocard M, Giraudeau B, Sabourin J-C, Ducreux M, Sarasin A, Praz F. ERCC1 codon 118 polymorphism is a predictive factor for the tumor response to oxaliplatin/5-fluorouracil combination chemotherapy in patients with advanced colorectal cancer. Clin Cancer Res 2005;11(17) 6212-6217.

[204] Metzger R, Leichman CG, Danenberg KD, Danenberg PV, Lenz H-J, Hayashi K, Groshen S, Salonga D, Cohen H, Laine L, Crookes P, Silberman H, Barando J, Konda B, Leichman L. ERCC1 mRNA levels complement thymidylate synthase mRNA levels in predicting response and survival for gastric cancer patients receiving combination cisplatin and fluorouracil chemotherapy. J Clin Oncol 1998;16(1) 309-316.

[205] Bellmunt J, Paz-Ares L, Cuello M, Cecere FL, Albiol S, Guillem V, Gallardo E, Carles J, Mendez P, de la Cruz JJ, Taron M, Rosell R, Baselga J; Spanish Oncology Genitourinary Group. Gene expression of ERCC1 as a novel prognostic marker in advanced bladder cancer patients receiving cisplatin-based chemotherapy. Ann Oncol 2007;18(3) 522-528.

[206] Esteller M, Garcia-Foncillas J, Andion E, Goodman SN, Hidalgo OF, Vanaclocha V, Baylin SB, Herman JG. Inactivation of the DNA-repair gene MGMT and the clinical response of gliomas to alkylating agents. N Engl J Med 2000;343(19) 1350-1354.

[207] Paz MF, Yaya-Tur R, Rojas-Marcos I, Reynes G, Pollan M, Aguirre-Cruz L, Garcia-Lopez JL, Piquer J, Safont M-J, Balana C, Sanchez-Cespedes M, Garcia-Villanueva M, Arribas L, Esteller M. CpG island hypermethylation of the DNA repair enzyme methyltransferase predicts response to temozolomide in primary gliomas. Clin Cancer Res 2004;10(15) 4933-4938.

[208] Hegi ME, Diserens A-C, Godard S, Dietrich P-Y, Regli L, Ostermann S, Otten P, Van Melle G, de Tribolet N, Stupp R. Clinical trial substantiates the predictive value of O-6-methylguanine-DNA methyltransferase promoter methylation in glioblastoma patients treated with temozolomide. Clin Cancer Res 2004;10(6) 1871-1874.

[209] Hegi ME, Liu L, Herman JG, Stupp R, Wick W, Weller M, Mehta MP, Gilbert MR. Correlation of O^6-methylguanine methyltransferase (MGMT) promoter methylation with clinical outcomes in glioblastoma and clinical strategies to modulate MGMT activity. J Clin Oncol 2008;26(25) 4189-4199.

[210] Weller M, Stupp R, Reifenberger G, Brandes AA, van den Bent MJ, Wick W, Hegi ME. MGMT promoter methylation in malignant gliomas: ready for personalized medicine? Nat Rev Neurol 2010;6(1) 39-51.

[211] Leung M, Rosen D, Fields S, Cesano A, Budman DR. Poly(ADP-ribose) polymerase-1 inhibition: preclinical and clinical development of synthetic lethality. Mol Med 2011;17(7-8) 854-862. doi: 10.2119/molmed.2010.00240.

[212] Basu B, Yap TA, Molife LR, de Bono JS. Targeting the DNA damage response in oncology: past, present and future perspectives. Curr Opin Oncol 2012;24(3) 316-324.

[213] Fong PC, Boss DS, Yap TA, Tutt A, Wu P, Roelvink, MM, Mortimer P, Swaisland H, Lau A, O'Connor MJ, Ashworth A, Carmichael J, Kaye SB, Schellens JHM, de Bono JS. Inhibition of poly(ADP-ribose) polymerase in tumors from BRCA mutation carriers. N Engl J Med 2009;361(2) 123-134.

[214] Tutt A, Robson M, Garber JE, Domchek SM, Audeh MW, Weitzel JN, Friedlander M, Arun B, Loman N, Schmutzler RK, Wardley A, Mitchell G, Earl H, Wickens M, Carmichael J. Oral poly(ADP-ribose) polymerase inhibitor olaparib in patients with BRCA1 or BRCA2 mutations and advanced breast cancer: a proof-of-concept trial. Lancet 2010;376(9737) 235-244.

[215] Audeh MW, Carmichael J, Penson RT, Friedlander M, Powell B, Bell-McGuinn KM, Scott C, Weitzel JN, Oaknin A, Loman N, Lu K, Schmutzler RK, Matulonis U, Wickens M, Tutt A. Oral poly(ADP-ribose) polymerase inhibitor olaparib in patients with BRCA1 or BRCA2 mutations and recurrent ovarian cancer: a proof-of-concept trial. Lancet 2010;376(9737) 245-251.

[216] Stratton MR. Exploring the genomes of cancer cells: progress and promise. Science 2011;331(6024) 1553-1558.

[217] Hanahan D, Weinberg RA. Hallmarks of cancer: the next generation. Cell 2011;144(5) 646-674.

[218] Lord CJ, Ashworth A. The DNA damage response and cancer therapy. Nature 2012;481(7382) 287-294.

Chapter 17

New Potential Therapeutic Approaches by Targeting Rad51-Dependent Homologous Recombination

Axelle Renodon-Cornière, Pierre Weigel,
Magali Le Breton and Fabrice Fleury

Additional information is available at the end of the chapter

http://dx.doi.org/10.5772/53973

1. Introduction

Cellular DNA is constantly exposed to the effects of endogenous or environmental agents such as free radicals, radiation and chemicals. In higher organisms, these nucleic alterations are estimated at several thousands of lesions per cell [1] which can correspond to the loss of bases and also to the breaking of one or both strands of the DNA double helix. Among these DNA breaks, the double-strand break (DSB) is the most harmful because it is the most difficult to repair. A human cell can accumulate up to 50 DSBs per cell cycle [2]. Unrepaired DSBs can have serious consequences such as permanent cell cycle arrest or cell death by apoptosis. Imperfect repair can also lead to major syndromes such as genetic disorders, premature aging or malignant cell generation.

In response to DNA damage, the cell has developed a surveillance and DNA repair network. DSBs of DNA, which are the most severe nucleic acid alterations, are repaired mainly by either non-homologous end-joining (NHEJ) or homologous recombination (HR).

NHEJ repair leads to a direct rejoining of the separated DNA ends [3]. This pathway begins by the binding of the Ku 70/80 heterodimer to DNA ends (Figure 1] which recruits and induces the activation of the DNA-dependent protein kinase catalytic subunit (DNA-PKc). Kinase activity is required for NHEJ since it causes the recruitment of other proteins and promotes the bringing together of DNA ends. Finally, ligase VI and XRCC4/XLF co-factors are involved in the final step of ligation and the generation of DNA repair. This process involves mainly the G0-G1 and S phases of the cell cycle. Its disadvantage is the possible loss of genetic information due to deletions or insertions of nucleic acids during the ligation of DNA ends and thus NHEJ repair is considered error-prone.

DNA repair by HR is more complex and needs a homologous sequence, which can be present in the homologous chromosome or in a gene in multicopy [4]. HR predominates in the S and G2 phases, when the sister chromatids are present and can also be a model for DNA repair [5]. In eukaryotic cells, DNA repair is supported by several protein complexes. Protein ATM (Ataxia Telangiectasia Mutated) has a role in DSB signaling via its activation induced by the MRN protein complex (MRE11-Rad50-NBS1 complex). MRE11 is a 5'-3' exonuclease that leads to a 3' end of DNA which is required for the process [6]. This resection of single-stranded DNA is followed by the recruitment of many proteins such as RPA, BRCA1, BRCA2, Rad51, Rad52, and Rad54. Rad52 is one of the first to settle on the DSB. BRCA1 then recruits BRCA2, Rad54 and Rad51 to form the nucleoprotein filament with ssDNA, whose role is to move the blade to the homologous sequence required for HR. Rad51 protein is the main element involved in the HR process. This recombinase catalyzes the homology search and the strand exchange with a homologous sequence and thus ensures the accurate repair of the DSB. In eukaryotes, Rad51 recombinase (RecA homolog in *Escherichia coli*) catalyzes the essential steps of homologous recombination and interacts directly with protein suppressors of breast cancer (BRCA1, BRCA2) [8] and p53 [9] which also indicates the importance of Rad51 in apoptosis.

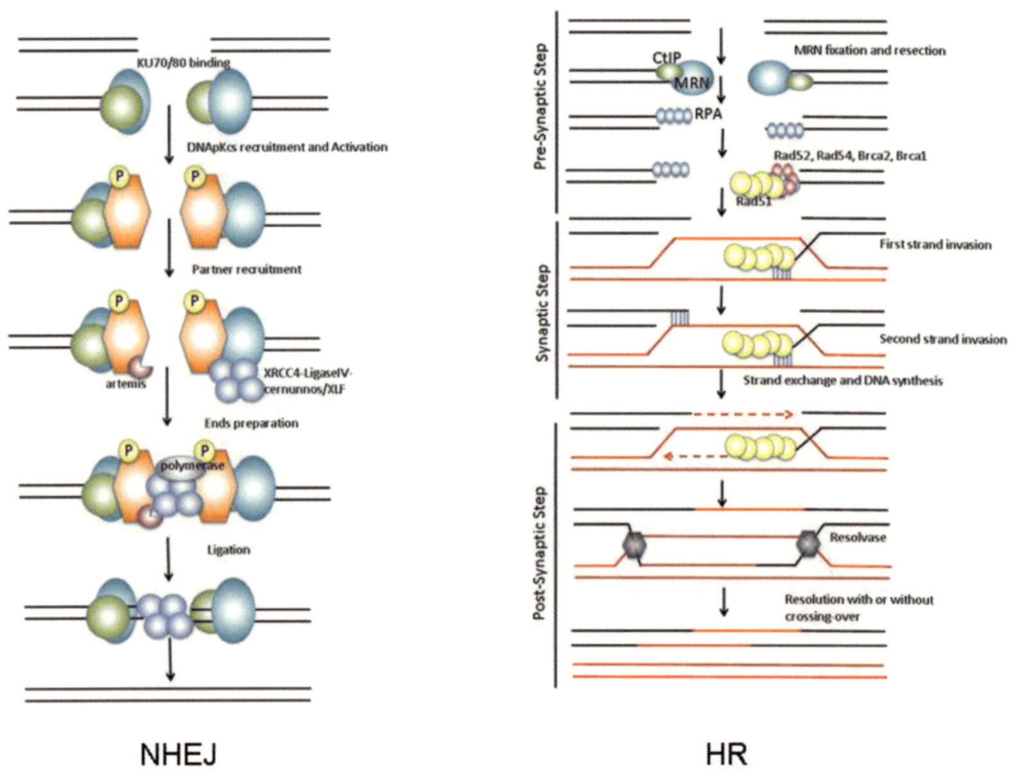

Figure 1. Schematic representation of the mechanism of DNA DSB repair by NHEJ and HR (figures taken from [7]).

HR involves a large number of protein complexes and can be divided into three main stages (Figure 1):

Formation of the HsRad51/DNA nucleofilament or pre-synaptic step. DNA DSBs are resected by nuclease to generate 3′-protruding ends. The complex MRN (MRE11-RAD50-NSB1) contributes to DNA resection which is followed by formation of the replication protein A (RPA) complex. This ssDNA-binding factor removes secondary structures of ssDNA and is subsequently replaced by Rad51. Rad51 is recruited onto ssDNA to form the nucleofilament. Protein mediators such as Rad52 and Rad51 paralogs, Rad51B-C-D, BRCA1/2, facilitate the loading of Rad51 onto the ssDNA. The DNA binding sites of Rad51 are located in the N-terminal domain of each Rad51 monomer [8].

Homologous DNA pairing or synaptic phase. The nucleofilament of Rad51 is involved in the search for homologous DNA. Once a homologous sequence is located, the Rad51 filament invades the duplex DNA and generates a displacement of the homologous DNA strand to form a D-loop.

Exchange and resolution of the DNA intermediate structure or post-synaptic phase. The second 3′ ssDNA overhang anneals to the displaced DNA strand and serves as a model strand for DNA synthesis. Two Holliday Junctions (HJ) are then formed. Their resolution is the final step and generates two dsDNA. HJ can be either resolved or dissolved resulting in crossover or non-crossover products.

It is clear that Rad51 plays an essential role at different levels of HR and several interactions are involved such as Rad51/ssDNA, Rad51/Rad51, Rad51/dsDNA, and Rad51/nucleotide. In addition, Rad51 interacts with its partners involved in HR (e.g. Rad52, Rad54).

Many cancer treatments using chemotherapy or radiotherapy target and disrupt the function of the DNA of tumor cells by inducing adducts or single- or double-strand breaks in DNA. However, these anticancer therapies are often faced with the emergence of radio- and chemoresistance, either induced or intrinsic to cancer cells. Since it was shown that some pathways of DNA repair can remove DNA damage induced by radio- or chemotherapy in cancer cells, these pathways have become potential therapeutic targets to sensitize tumors.

This observation is especially true for the Rad51 protein. A high level of HR induced by overexpression of Rad51 is frequently described in various types of cancer cell, including breast cancer, pancreatic, nonsmall-cell lung carcinoma and leukemia (AML and CML) [9-13]. In these cancer cells, this overexpression provides a degree of cancer resistance by promoting the repair of DSBs induced by cancer treatments [14]. Moreover, it has been shown that the survival of cancer patients expressing higher levels of Rad51 is shorter and that a reduced amount of Rad51, following antisense or ribozyme treatment, increases the effectiveness of cancer treatment by radiotherapy [15-17]. Modulation of HR to potentiate treatment is an option described in many publications [18]. It can be achieved by either acting directly on the recombinase activity of Rad51 or attempting to interfere with the interactions between Rad51 and some of its partners, which are not necessarily related directly to the repair of DNA.

The purpose of this chapter is to review all the chemical modulators that can act directly or indirectly on Rad51-mediated homologous recombination. First, the different steps of Rad51 activity which can be targeted will be detailed. Secondly, the chemical molecules that inhibit Rad51 activity or affect the expression level of Rad51 will be described. Finally, their applications in combination with anticancer treatments will be discussed in order to open up possibilities for counteracting chemo- and radioresistance.

2. Rad51 activity in homologous recombination

Human Rad51 (*Homo sapiens* Rad51 or HsRad51) is composed of 339 amino acids. It is the eukaryotic homolog of the RecA protein in prokaryotes. Homologs of the human recombinase are highly conserved between species: 98.8% similarity with *Mus musculus* Rad51 (MmRad51] and 81% with *Saccharomyces cerevisiae* Rad51 (ScRad51) [19,20].

To date, no complete structure of the HsRad51 protein has been determined. The crystalline structure of ScRad51 truncated at 79 N-terminal amino acids [21], one structure of *Pyrococcus furiosus* RadA [22], and five RadA of *Methanococcus voltae* [23,24] and *Sulfolobus solfataricus* [25] have been determined.

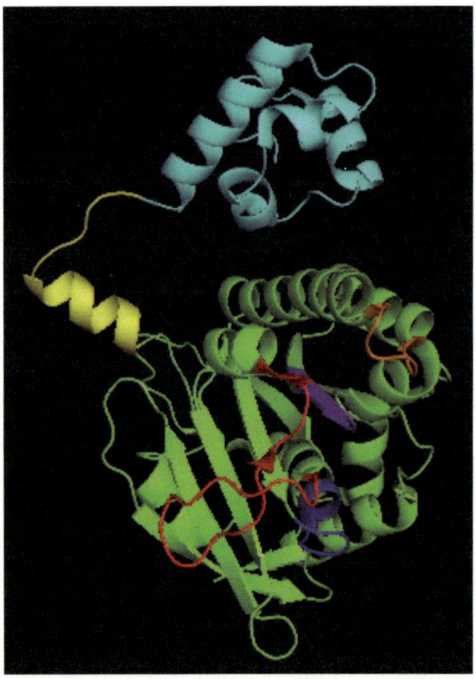

Figure 2. MvRadA subunit structure (PDB 1XU4). The N-terminal domain and the polymerization motif are colored in cyan and yellow, respectively. The putative DNA binding L1 and L2 loops are highlighted in orange and red. The Walker A and B motifs, corresponding to the ATP binding site, are labeled in blue and purple, respectively.

RadA and Rad51 are composed of two domains: a small N-terminal domain and a C-terminal domain entitled the core domain. The structures of the two HsRad51 domains were resolved by NMR [8] and crystallography [26], respectively.

The C-terminal domain of HsRad51 was crystallized in the form of a fusion protein comprising the BRC4 motif of BRCA2 protein (residues 1517-1551), a flexible linker and the central domain of HsRad51 (residues 97-339). The co-crystallization of HsRad51 with the BRC4 motif indicated the existence of a polymerization sequence located at the subunit-subunit interface of Rad51 [26]. The C-terminal domain contains an ATPase domain comprising units of Walker A (Hs: 127-134) and Walker B (Hs: 217-222) which are essential for ATP binding while loops L1 (Hs: 230-236) and L2 (Hs: 269-287) are involved in DNA binding.

The N-terminal domain of HsRad51 interacts with double-stranded DNA by a helix-hairpin-helix structure (residues 61-69). This type of protein-DNA interaction is conserved among many proteins interacting with DNA [27]. These sites of interaction, illustrated in Figure 2, are necessary for the formation of the nucleofilament, which is the key step of the recombinase activity of Rad51 (Figure 1). Nucleofilament formation is accompanied by a stretch modification of the DNA helix. The nucleofilament can adopt several conformations, only one of which is active for DNA strand exchange. The extended conformation is the functional form of the filament.

The conformation of the Rad51 filament depends on nucleotides: ATP promotes the extended conformation whereas ADP stabilizes the compressed form. Most of the structures have been solved in the presence of ATP analogs. Thus the conversion of an extended conformation to a compressed conformation accompanies the hydrolysis of ATP [28,29].

Several HsRad51 studies have also shown that ammonium sulfate [30], calcium [28,29] and AMPPNP [29] significantly increase the effectiveness of the strand exchange reaction *in vitro* by promoting the formation of an extended filament, which confirms that this structural form is the functional conformation of Rad51.

Since Rad51 protein is central to HR, all chemical molecules able to disrupt the interaction sites of Rad51 directly will also be able to modulate DNA repair by HR. Other ways of modulating HR via Rad51 are possible. Figure 3 presents the main ways and the catalytic steps of Rad51 being targeted to modulate HR.

3. Specific molecules targeting Rad51

The great majority of compounds identified as inhibitors of Rad51 have been selected by high-throughput screening from chemical libraries.

3.1. Modulators of Rad51 recombinase activity

This chemical group acts directly on the catalytic steps of Rad51 recombinase activity.

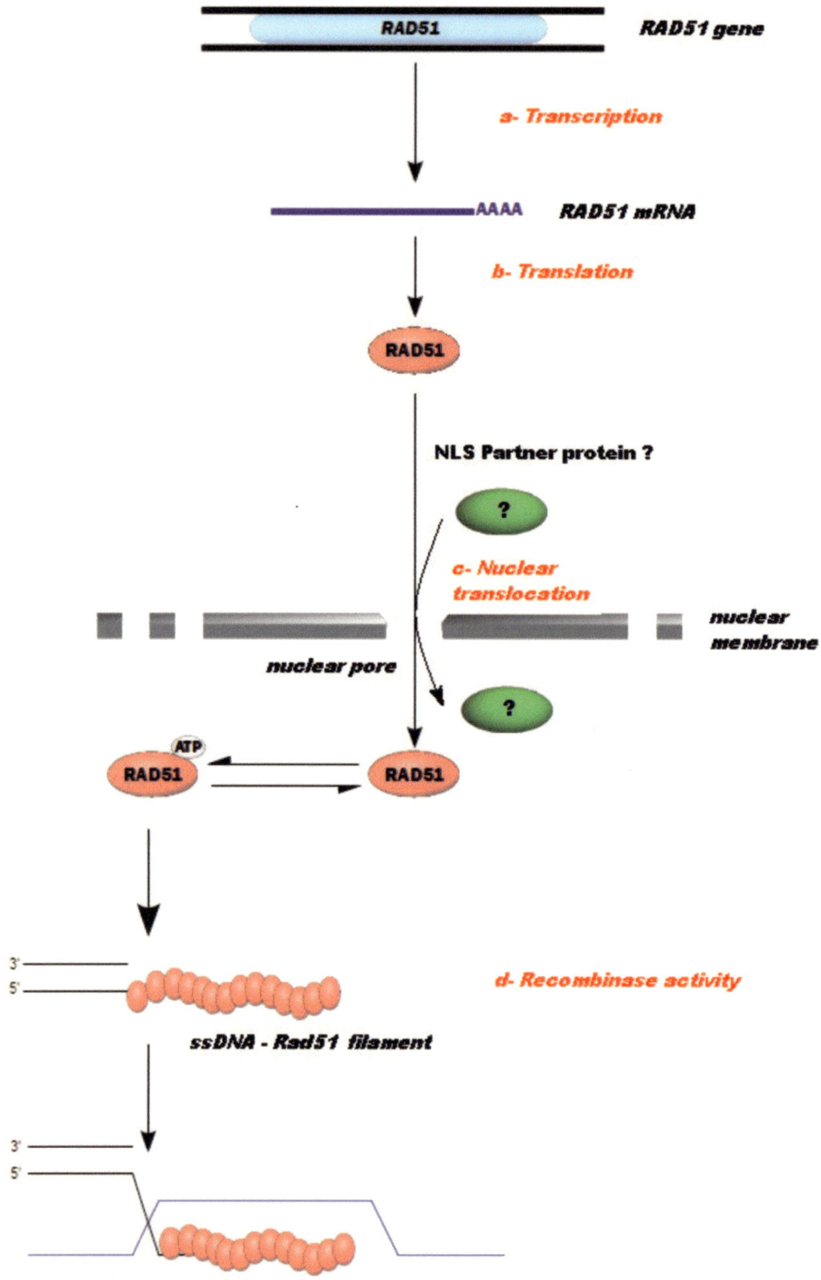

Figure 3. Intracellular pathways and catalytic steps of Rad51 as potential targets to modulate HR. (a) and (b) - The modulation of transcription and translation of Rad51 leads to changes in the recombinase activity and hence to the modification of HR repair. (c) - The intracellular localization and the delivery of Rad51 to the DNA damage sites are required for the HR process. Rad51 cellular distribution has an important regulatory role in HR and any element able to modulate the nuclear translocation of Rad51 is also able to modulate HR. (d) - Finally, molecules acting on the steps of Rad51 activity will target recombinase activity and HR-mediated DNA repair.

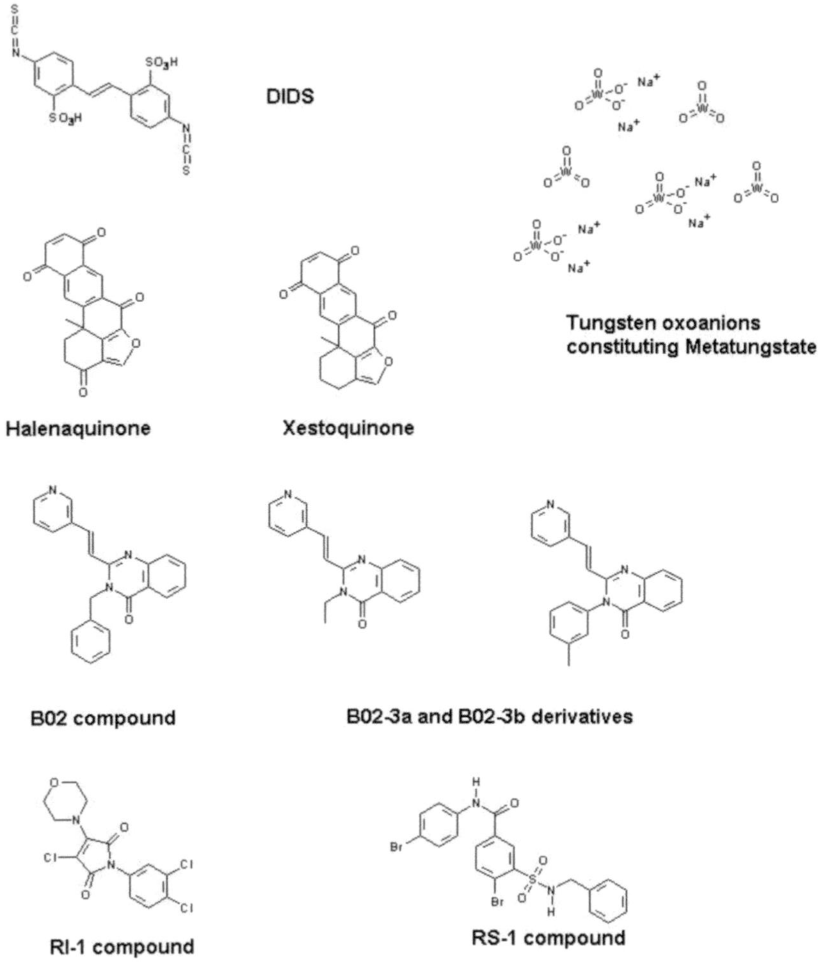

Figure 4. Structure of chemical molecules modulating the Rad51 recombinase activity.

3.1.1. *4'-Diisothiocyanostilbene-2,2'-disulfonic acid or DIDS*

DIDS (Figure 4) is a molecule known since the early 1970s for its ability to inhibit ionic channels and membrane transporters [31].

In the context of HR, Ishida T. et al. [32] have shown that DIDS can also inhibit *in vitro* the binding of Rad51 to DNA. In fact, strand exchange reactions are inhibited in the presence of DIDS. This process is dependent on salt concentration since the addition of 0.2 M KCl to the reaction medium changes the behavior of the inhibition. In the absence of KCl, increasing the concentration of DIDS gradually inhibits strand exchange with an IC50 (without KCl) close to 2 μM when the Rad51 concentration is 6 μM. In the presence of 0.2 M KCl, inhibition is considered to be shifted: the addition of DIDS has no effect up to a concentration of 1 μM. In this condition, the IC50 (with KCl) is close to 5 μM in the presence of Rad51 at 6 μM concentration. The interaction between Rad51 and DIDS probably involves electrostatic strength.

It has also been observed that the inhibition of the binding of Rad51 to ssDNA is not changed in the presence or absence of ATP. As previously described, HsRad51 contains a binding site for ATP and ATPase activity [33]. Analysis of the ATPase activity of Rad51 shows that ATP hydrolysis is greatly decreased when the protein is not bound to DNA. However, according to the results of Ishida and collaborators, Rad51 is able to hydrolyze ATP in the presence of DIDS and without DNA. The assumption is that this activation by DIDS of an asynchronous ATPase function results from the inhibition of the binding of Rad51 to DNA, which is ATP-dependent. However, Amunugama et al. [34] showed that the presence of ATP bound to Rad51 is required during strand exchange. In contrast, ATP hydrolysis does not appear to be essential for recombination. Hence, inactivation of the ATPase activity by DIDS cannot alone explain the mechanism of inhibition of Rad51.

DIDS interacts physically with Rad51 and dissociates it from ssDNA by competing with ssDNA for Rad51 binding.

3.1.2. Metatungstate

Metatungstate is a polyoxometalate (POM) consisting of 12 tungsten oxoanions (Figure 4) which dissociate into monotungstates in aqueous alkaline solution. This molecule is mainly used as a catalytic agent for chemical reactions of hydrocarbons.

Li and colleagues [35] have demonstrated that the metatungstate structure can bind *in vitro* to MvRadA protein, a homolog of Rad51 from Archaea *Methanococcus voltae* (MvRadA). The main contact zones established between the protein and metatungstate concern the L1 loop region with Arg_{218} and Arg_{230} and the L2 loop region with Arg_{224} of RadA. Both these L1 and L2 domains including Tyr_{232} and Phe_{203} are involved in DNA binding. It should be noted that the same pattern is found in HsRad51 [36]. In the MvRadA filament, these locations result in a distribution of molecules of tungstates on the longitudinal axis of rotation. It is shown that these tungsten clusters interact between the DNA-binding loops L1 and L2 stabilizing the inactive conformation of Rad51 [23,24,37].

Tungstate binding to MvRadA induces several effects on the functions of the recombinase protein activity. ATPase activity decreases by about 90% with equimolar amounts of MvRadA and metatungstate. By using gel electrophoresis *in vitro*, binding assays of MvRadA to ssDNA reveal that metatungstate inhibits ssDNA binding (IC50 = 0.13 μM for 1 μM MvRadA). The same *in vitro* assays using dsDNA also show an inhibition with a similar IC50 whereas the IC50 value of metatungstate for strand exchange activity is 0.5 μM in the presence of KCl. These observations indicate that, *in vitro*, metatungstate can inhibit the ssDNA and dsDNA binding of MvRadA, thus inactivating the functions essential for HR. As mentioned previously, the inactivation of ATPase activity does not alone explain the inhibition of Rad51 functions and probably those of RadA. It is therefore suggested that metatungstate acts as a competitive inhibitor of DNA binding by MvRadA.

Metatungstate is a potent inhibitor of ATPase and strand exchange activities of MvRadA and other experiments performed with HsRad51 have shown a significant increase in the IC50 of metatungstate for HsRad51 as compared with that for MvRadA (IC_{50}^{RadA} = 0.5 μM and IC_{50}^{Rad51} = 30 μM)[35].

3.1.3. *Halenaquinone*

Xestoquinone and halenaquinone molecules (Figure 4) are extracted from the marine sponge *Xestospongia exigua*. These molecules are similar except that xestoquinone does not contain the oxygen at the C-3 position in contrast to halenaquinone. Only halenaquinone presents inhibitory properties of phosphatidylinositol 3-kinase [38] and some anti-proliferative features [39].

Takaku et al. tested 160 crude extract fractions from marine sponge and used the D-loop formation assay to detect the homologous-pairing activity of Rad51. The authors reported that the halenaquinone inhibits HR at DNA pairing and D-loop formation stages but no inhibitory effect was observed with xestoquinone [40]. By Surface Plasmon Resonance (SPR) measurement, they showed that both halenaquinone and xestoquinone are able to bind to Rad51 but the affinity between halenaquinone and Rad51 is higher than between xestoquinone and Rad51. This result can explain the efficient inhibition of Rad51-mediated homologous pairing by halenaquinone.

Takaku and collaborators then examined whether both molecules affect ssDNA and dsDNA binding by Rad51. By an electrophoretic mobility shift approach, halenaquinone was found to inhibit Rad51-dsDNA binding specifically, but not Rad51-ssDNA binding. Interestingly, the authors showed that halenaquinone inhibits the secondary dsDNA binding by the Rad51-ssDNA complex. These results suggest that halenaquinone probably interacts near the dsDNA-binding site of Rad51. It can therefore inhibit the ternary complex formation containing ssDNA, dsDNA and Rad51 which promotes the DNA homologous pairing step during the HR process. In contrast, neither ssDNA binding nor dsDNA binding by Rad51 was affected by the presence of xestoquinone.

The authors then studied the intracellular effects of halenaquinone on the Ionizing Radiation (IR)-induced formation of Rad51 foci. When human cells were exposed to IR and treated with halenaquinone, Rad51 foci formation was significantly decreased. This result indicates that halenaquinone destabilizes the Rad51 foci, probably by inhibiting the ternary complex formation. Halenaquinone may be useful in medical research as a potential inhibitor of HR.

3.1.4. *Compound B02 and derivatives*

By high-throughput screening based on the quenching fluorescence method, Huang and colleagues have investigated the identification of specific inhibitors of the Rad51 strand exchange activity [18]. From 200,000 small molecules of the NIH repository, 174 compounds were positives and, after supplementary analyses and different controls, 13 molecules were identified as potential inhibitors of Rad51 with an inhibition higher than 30%. The IC50 values for the most potent inhibitors of Rad51-induced D-loop formation were determined.

Among these molecules, both compounds A04 and A10 were found to be inhibitors for Rad51 and RecA and their IC50 values were 5 μM and 26.6 μM, respectively. Another compound, the B02 molecule, was found to disrupt Rad51 binding to DNA and nucleoprotein filament formation. Although the B02 molecule presents an IC50 (27.4 μM) higher than A04 or A10, this molecule has a higher specificity for HsRad51.

Moreover, the study of B02 derivatives has revealed an efficient inactivation of Rad51 by both B02-3a and B02-3b, which contain an ethyl and an m-methylphenyl group, respectively (instead of the benzyl group located in the B02 molecule) (Figure 4). Modification of the pyridin radical of B02 suppresses the Rad51-induced D-loop inhibition, which demonstrates the importance of these chemical groups. The recent *in vivo* work of the same team has shown that B02 inhibits DSB-induced HR and increases cell sensitivity to the ICL agents, cisplatin and mitomycin C [41].

3.1.5. Compound RI-1 or 3-chloro-1-(3,4-dichlorophenyl)-4-(4-morpholinyl)-1H-pyrrole-2,5-dione

From a screening of 10,000 molecules of Chembridge DIVERSet™, the RI-1 compound was identified as an inhibitor of HsRad51 [42]. A first screening by fluorescence polarization (FP) enabled molecules that can bind to HsRad51 to be selected. A second screening based on the inhibition of homologous recombination in a cell line of human osteosarcoma (U20S) was used and eight molecules were identified. A final test with the human embryonic kidney cell line (HEK293) identified RI-1, whose action is the specific inactivation of HsRad51.

RI-1 is composed of a chloromaleimide moiety (Figure 4) which promotes covalent binding to the thiol group of Rad51 cysteine 319 by a Michael addition mechanism. This binding potentiates the inhibition of the polymerization of HsRad51 during nucleofilament formation. It should be noted that the binding site is located on a surface which is highly conserved among mammalian homologs of Rad51. Experiments with *Saccharomyces cerevisiae* Rad51 (ScRad51) also show a fixation on the corresponding cysteine target (C377). However, this site is not present in RecA and inhibition was not found. RI-1 is potentially a specific inhibitor for mammalian homologs of Rad51. The binding site is located on the interface between two monomers of HsRad51 so it inhibits the polymerization of Rad51 onto ssDNA [21]. It is known that cysteine 319 is located in an ATP-binding loop [23], therefore the binding of RI-1 may disrupt the interaction of Rad51 with ATP. Moreover, this interaction area is also involved in the binding of other HR repair proteins such as Rad52 and Rad54 [43]. The IC50 of RI-1 is from 5 to 30 μM depending on the HsRad51 intracellular concentration. A synergistic anticancer effect is also observed for the association of RI-1 with mitomycin C (MMC) in U20S, HeLa, MCF-7 and SH2038 cell lines.

3.1.6. Compound RS-1 (Rad51-Stimulatory-1) or 3-[(benzylamino)sulfonyl]-4-bromo-N-(4-bromophenyl)benzamide)

In contrast to inhibitors, few molecules stimulating HR have been reported. However, by screening 10,000 molecules (Chembridge DIVERSet™) using the FP method described above, Connell et al. identified a molecule, RS-1, which stimulates Rad51 binding onto ssDNA and increases the stability of the nucleofilament [44].

In the presence of RS-1 (Figure 4), the nucleofilament is in the active form characterized by the long length of the Rad51-ssDNA complex (100Å). The presence of nucleotide cofactors is also important since ATP is required for RS-1 to stimulate the formation of the active filament. However, RS-1 does not stimulate Rad51 by inhibiting its ATPase activity since it has no effect on the Rad51-dependent hydrolysis of ATP.

The RS-1-induced extension of the Rad51-ssDNA nucleofilament stimulates the exchange step of DNA strands, which can be evaluated by estimating D-loop formation. In the presence of non-hydrolyzable ATP or Ca2+, RS-1 increases D-loop formation by 5 to 11 times [28,44]. The stimulatory action of RS-1 is specific to HsRad51, since no effect with *E. coli* RecA or ScRad51 was found. This stimulation was then analyzed at the cellular level.

An analysis of cell survival (neonatal human fibroblasts) showed that the cells are more resistant to cisplatin treatment in the presence of 7.5 μM RS-1. This result is probably due to the ability of RS-1 to stimulate HR in response to DNA-damage agents like cisplatin.

3.2. Chemical modulators of Rad51 expression

3.2.1. Methotrexate drug

The structure of methotrexate (Figure 5) is similar to that of the folate metabolic precursor of coenzyme tetrahydrofolate (FH4) involved in the synthesis of nucleic bases. Methotrexate is a molecule used as an inhibitor of dihydrofolate reductase and acts in nucleic base synthesis occurring during the S phase of the cell cycle, as well as in non-restorative homologous recombination [45]. Therefore, methotrexate targets the S phase and the functions of HR by reducing the rate of repair of DNA damage, which can be shown by comet assay [46]. The study conducted by Du and colleagues [47] found that the inhibition of the formation of HsRad51 foci was effective in the presence of methotrexate in a human osteosarcoma cell line (HOS) after irradiation. This inhibition seems to be related to the Rad51 protein expression level, which is significantly decreased by the treatment. In addition, it was observed that the expression levels of BRCA2 and Rad52 were therefore not affected by methotrexate. It induces a specific downregulation of HsRad51. It should be noted that the treatment of HOS cells with 0.1 μM methotrexate causes a decrease in the transcription of 70% and > 95% of HsRad51 after 12 and 24 hours, respectively. However, these studies cannot determine the interactions involved in decreasing the mRNA levels of HsRad51.

3.2.2. Phenylhydroxamic acid or PCI-24781

Phenylhydroxamic acid (Figure 5) belongs to the inhibitory molecules of histone deacetylases (HDACs) used for their antitumor activities [48]. In particular, PCI-24781 inhibits HDAC2, which is one of the HDAC family involved in the regulation of the factors of HR. According to the work of Adimoolam et al. [49], inhibition of HDAC by PCI-24781 reduces the expression of Rad51 in the cell line derived from human colorectal carcinoma (HTC116) and thus reduces the HR response to DSBs induced by therapy. The first observation by immunofluorescence showed a complete inhibition of the formation of HsRad51 foci in the presence of PCI-24781 after irradiation and an apoptosis rate of 7% with 0.2 μM. After 24 hours, the level of protein synthesis in the absence or presence of 0.2 mM PCI-24781 showed a decrease in transcription of 60% BRCA1 and 80% for both BRCA2 and HsRad51. BRCA2 protein is also involved in the DNA repair protein complex with Rad51 [50]. The HR inhibition observed results in an additive effect of the reductions in expression levels of Rad51 and BRCA2. Moreover, the fall in BRCA2 in the nuclear compartment probably removes the inhibition of caspase-3 protease, which is able to cleave Rad51 and thus to inactivate HR DNA repair [51]. Therefore, PCI-24781 may indirectly activate the cleavage of Rad51 in addition to inducing a decrease in its synthesis. Interestingly, PCI-24781 induces the expression of the gene of the GADD45y protein which is a factor of cellular growth arrest [52]. This third effect of PCI-24781 can limit the growth of tumor cells.

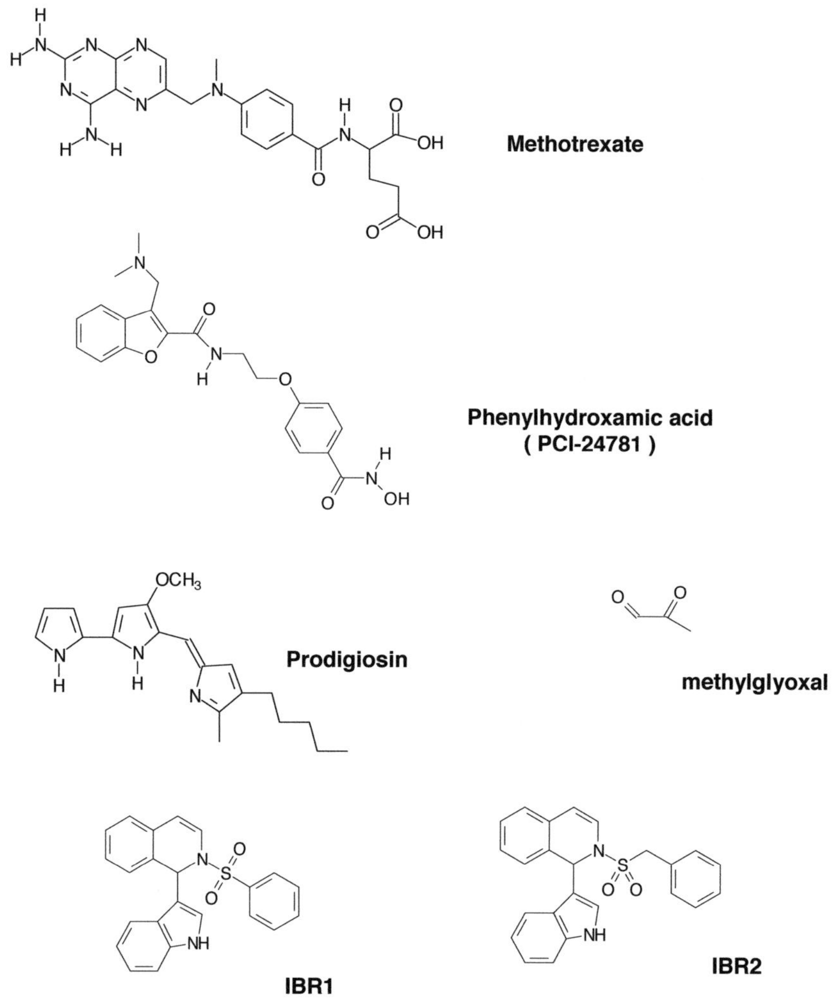

Figure 5. Structure of chemical modulators of Rad51 transcription and its nuclear translocation.

3.2.3. Prodigiosin

Prodigiosin is a tripyrrole red pigment (Figure 5) from bacteria *Serratia marcescens*. Recently, immunosuppressive and anticancer properties have been identified for this molecule [53-55]. The first action of prodigiosin is an increase in DNA DSBs, which probably results from the inhibition of both topoisomerase I and II [56]. Lu and collaborators described a significant reduction in the level of HsRad51 protein and mRNA in breast tumor cell lines (MCF-7, MDA-MB-231, T- 47D, A549, HCT116) in the presence of 50 nM prodigiosin [57]. The downregulation of Rad51 is mainly induced by lowering mRNA expression and not by proteasome-mediated Rad51 degradation. Although the tumor suppressor protein p53 is known as a repressor of Rad51 [58], prodigiosin downregulates Rad51 in a p53-independent manner. This result is an advantage for the prodigiosin-mediated therapy of cancer in which p53 is deficient compared to molecules such as flavopiridole or roscovitine, which need an activation of this protein. On the other hand, prodigiosin activates JNK and p38-MAPK signaling pathways, which are known to mediate the pro-apoptotic effect of numerous anticancer drugs [59]. By using specific inhibitors of both these signaling pathways, Lu and collaborators have shown that the level of Rad51 mRNA is restored. This result confirms the involvement of JNK and p38-MAPK signaling pathways in the prodigiosin-induced Rad51 downregulation. However, this is in contradiction with the work of Chuang et al. [60], which showed that the activation of p53-MAPK could increase the level of Rad51 protein, improving its stability and not significantly altering the level of HsRad51 mRNA. Similarly, Ko and colleagues [61] have shown a decrease in mRNA levels of HsRad51 with curcumin treatment and an inactive ERK/p38-MAPK signaling pathway. Although the Rad51 downregulation mechanism is not fully understood, prodigiosin seems to be a potent suppressor of Rad51 which may be used to overcome HR-mediated drug resistance in cancer.

4. Modulation of Rad51 by inactivation of nuclear translocation

4.1. Nuclear Localization Signal

Eukaryotic proteins are expressed in the cytoplasm. If their functions are carried out in the nucleus, they have to pass through the nuclear membrane. In contrast to small biomolecules, numerous proteins larger than 20 Kda require active transport via a signal peptide of recognition: a Nuclear Localization Signal (NLS) [62]. This signal peptide may be recognized by karyopherins [63] to form a nuclear protein complex (NPC) [64,65]. Proteins involved in HR are not exempt from this obligation for nuclear translocation. Thus, it is useful to analyze the possibility of blocking the passage of Rad51 through the nuclear membrane and thereby inhibit HR. Rad51 protein does not contain an NLS so its nuclear translocation requires an association with another protein. Interestingly, among the Rad51 paralogs, Rad51C has an NLS [66] as do Rad54 [67] and Rad52 [68] proteins. Other proteins related to DNA repair such as BRCA2 have been reported as being involved in Rad51 transport [69]. The mechanism of Rad51 transport is not clearly understood although Rad51C seems to be an interesting candidate. In particular, Gildemeister and colleagues have found that Rad51C deficiency significantly reduces the amount of Rad51 in the nucleus before and after DNA damage [69]. Another option is protein kinase B or AKT-1 protein kinase which is involved in the cytoplasmic sequestration of Rad51 [70]. The modulation of Rad51 transport offers an excellent tool to potentiate anticancer therapy through inhibition of Rad51 nuclear translocation.

4.2. AKT-1 kinase and BRCA1 proteins

Activation of AKT-1 promotes cell proliferation and the activated form is regularly found in cancer cells. In addition, to reducing malignant cell division, the inhibition of the AKT-1 signaling pathway has been investigated for the purpose of co-therapeutic approaches [71]. AKT activation occurs through a series of successive phosphorylation steps at thr-450, thr-308 and ser-473 by JNK kinases, phosphoinositide-dependent kinase 1 and by several kinases (PKD2 and others), respectively [72]. Plo and collaborators have demonstrated another aspect of the activation of AKT-1 in HR DNA repair of chemotherapy-induced DSBs [70]. This group studied the level of HsRad51 and BRCA1 in cell lines MCF7 and MDA-MB-231 and observed a decreased level in the nucleus while both these proteins accumulated in the cytoplasm. Although the HsRad51 and BRCA1 features are not modified, AKT-1 activation induces a retention signal of these proteins in the cytoplasm. Thus, their absence in the nucleus confers a deficiency of recombinase activity. The retention mechanism is still unknown, but it seems to be related to AKT-1-mediated BRCA1 NLS phosphorylation. In fact, it has been observed that AKT-1 phosphorylates BRCA1 on two sites located in the region of the NLS [73] and some mutations of these sites show a suppression of nuclear translocation of Rad51 and BRCA1, irrespective of the activated AKT-1. In this context, an activator of AKT-1 phosphorylation, such as methylglyoxal (Figure 5) [74,75] may promote the cytoplasmic sequestration of Rad51.

4.3. Modulation of the interaction between Rad51 and BRCA2

Human BRCA2 protein is constituted of 3418 amino acids (384 kDa) and contains several interaction domains. There is an interaction site with N-terminal RPA and in the central region of BRCA2 there are 8 repeated motifs called BRC motifs [76]. BRC1, BRC4, BRC7 and BRC8 motifs are able to interact with Rad51 with different affinities [77]. Pellegrini et al. [26] have shown that the BRC4 motif interacts with HsRad51 by mimicking the motif of Rad51 which is responsible for its polymerization. These BRC motifs can bind monomeric or oligomeric forms of Rad51 in a cell cycle-dependent manner and in response to DNA damage. HsRad51 regulation is also mediated by serine 3291 of the BRCA2 C-terminal domain. In the absence of DNA damage, this serine is phosphorylated by CDK1 whereas it is in a dephosphorylated form with inactivated CDK1. The ser-3291 can bind only to the oligomeric form in the nucleoprotein filament. This binding plays a role in stabilizing the Rad51-DNA complex since the phosphorylation of ser-3291 inhibits oligomerization in the absence of DSB and then synchronizes the repair mechanism [78]. It has been proposed that the BRCA2 protein is directly involved in the nuclear transport of Rad51 [50]. The pancreatic adenocarcinoma cell line CAPAN-1 is known to be defective in BRCA2 [79]. It has a deletion of the BRCA2 domains for DNA repair and the nuclear localization signals [80]. Rad51 exhibits impaired nuclear

http://dx.doi.org/10.5772/53973

translocation in CAPAN-1. Therefore, it has been proposed that Rad51 requires BRCA2 for its nuclear translocation and that C-terminally trunkated BRCA2 retains Rad51 in the cytoplasm. BRCA2-Rad51 interaction is also essential in the HR process and many works have described those derivative peptides of BRCA2 that are able to mimic and bind to this interaction site [81-83]. Small molecules have been proposed to disrupt the interaction and two patents have been deposited [84]. By using the two-hybrid system in yeast, Lee and Chen suggested several molecules from a drug screening. Two hydrophobic molecules (phenylsulfonyl indolyl isoquinoline derivatives) IBR1 and IBR2 (Figure 5) were found to be able to disrupt the interaction and can thus potentiate anticancer treatments. The authors suggest that the benzene ring of IBR2 interacts in the hydrophobic pocket of Rad51 which is involved in the subunit-subunit interaction during filament formation and also in the interaction with the BRC4 motif of BRCA2. This phenyl moiety of IBR2 may be a competitor with the Rad51 F86 or BRC4 F1524 [85].

The authors also analyzed the effect of IBR2 at cellular level. After irradiation, breast cancer cells (MCF-7) presented a lower number of Rad51 foci than when these cells were pre-treated with IBR2. Another result was the fast degradation of Rad51 in the treated cells where the HR was impaired. This work, which is ongoing, has led to the development and synthesis of other IBR2 analogs [85,86].

5. Conclusion

DNA repair by homologous recombination is now a potential target in cancer therapy. The induction of DNA damage is one of the means of action against uncontrolled cell proliferation systems, while repairs are causes of resistance to radio- and chemotherapy. DNA repair is frequently found to be deregulated in tumor cells. Rad51 is the central protein of HR and its expression level is correlated with resistance to chemotherapeutic drugs. This observation suggests that targeted inhibition of Rad51 through small chemical molecules may improve the response to drug treatment by reducing HR.

Among antitumoral strategies, several studies have proposed numerous molecules that inhibit the recombinase activity; these are described in Figure 6.

DIDS and metatungstate are molecules that deregulate the ATPase activity of Rad51. DIDS thus causes a random hydrolysis of ATP without ssDNA-bound Rad51, while metatungstate inhibits the ATPase activity. The ATPase center is located at the Rad51 subunit-subunit interface which binds and hydrolyzes ATP and regulates the conformation of the DNA binding site. Although both molecules act differently, they induce an inhibition of the binding of Rad51 onto DNA.

Inhibition of the Rad51 polymerization is also interesting since it directly affects filament formation. The compound RI-1 can bind to the thiol group of cys-319 which inhibits the interaction between monomers of Rad51.

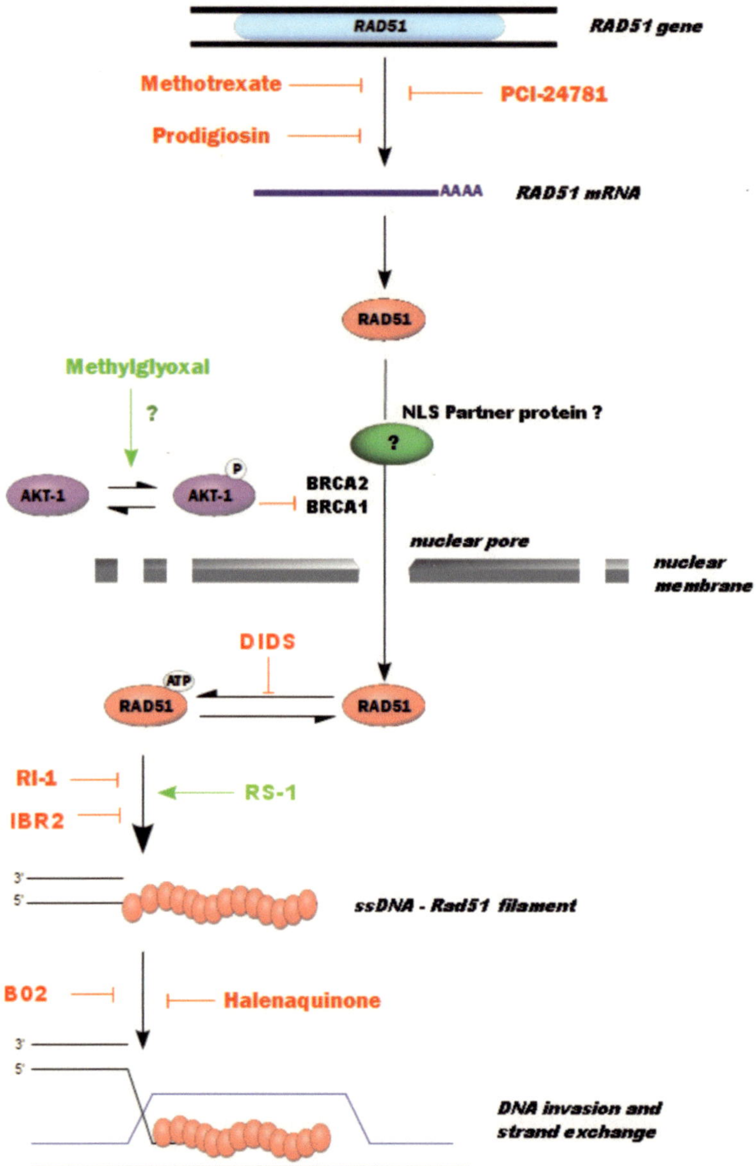

Figure 6. Potential inhibitors of Rad51-mediated HR repair: Methotrexate (100nM), Prodigiosin (100nM) and PCI-24781 (200nM) treatments reduce the levels of Rad51 mRNA between 20% and 50% in cancer cells. The decrease of Rad51 transcript level also induces an inhibition of Rad51 foci formation [47,49,57]. A 10μM concentration of DIDS significantly inhibits the binding of Rad51 to DNA, leading to the strand exchange inhibition [32]. RI-1 and B02 (20μM) decreases 50% of DNA binding by Rad51 and disrupts the formation of Rad51 foci after DNA damage in cells [18,42]. IBR2 (20μM) inhibits the Rad51 oligomerization in vitro by binding to Rad51 hydrophobic pocket [85]. 20μM of RS-1 promotes the binding of Rad51 to DNA [44]. Halenaquinone (30μM) inhibits the step of DNA homologous pairing mediated by Rad51 in vitro and the Rad51 foci formation after irradiation of cells [40]. It is noteworthy that in vitro IC50 values depend on the protein concentration and technical conditions, which makes difficult to compare them each other and to values obtained in cells.

http://dx.doi.org/10.5772/53973

Halenaquinone modulates the recombinase activity by inhibiting the binding of the Rad51-ssDNA complex with dsDNA. The hypothesis is that the presence of halenaquinone destabilizes the Rad51-ssDNA binding or the interaction between Rad51 subunits. This instability results in a disassembly of the complex, before the recognition of the homologous sequence. Compound B02 is also capable of modulating the function of Rad51 by disrupting Rad51 binding to DNA and formation of the nucleoprotein filament. Moreover, this compound increases cell sensitivity to DNA damaging agents and to PARP1 inhibitors. Thus, small molecules acting directly on the recombinase activity steps offer a potential development for new anticancer treatment associated with chemo- or radiotherapy. Another approach is to decrease the expression of the *RAD51* gene. For these purposes, several studies have demonstrated that methotrexate and molecule PCI-24781 significantly reduce the synthesis of Rad51 mRNA. Note that only the effects on mRNA levels were observed but the mechanism of transcription control remains unclear.

Prodigiosin also decreases the level of Rad51 mRNA which seems to be related to the activation of the JNK and p58-MAPK signaling pathways. Therefore, chemical compounds that up- and downregulate Rad51 production and/or activity may be useful for the suppression of tumor progression but the therapeutic applications of this strategy are currently inconceivable and unlikely. The last mode of action focuses on the transport of Rad51 from cytoplasm to nucleus. Rad51 is a protein whose nuclear functions require partners to facilitate its entry into the nucleus. It has been noted that the activation of the anti-apoptotic protein AKT-1 inactivates the nuclear translocation of Rad51 and BRCA1. The mechanism is still poorly understood but retention in the cytoplasm causes a significant decrease in HR. Several studies also suggest that BRCA2 is involved in this transport. Molecules such as IBR, which interfere with the Rad51-BRCA2 interaction, may induce cytoplasmic sequestration of Rad51 which decreases HR. These molecules capable of inhibiting the transport of Rad51 appear attractive candidates.

Most of these Rad51 inhibitors have been identified from screening libraries. These small molecules were tested in vitro and in cellular models but it will be necessary to quantify their efficacy, identify their toxicities and their potentially additional pharmacokinetic and pharmacological properties by animal assays. An understanding of toxicities, adverse effects, and special dosing considerations of existing anticancer compounds is important to the design of effective drug combinations and to the interpretation of the toxicological profile of new chemical entities.

Afterwards, a major challenge is to design new analogues to these molecules that will be more selective for Rad51 so that their efficacy will be improved and their potential toxicities will be decreased. The process of identifying and selecting these analogues has undergone a sea change in the recent decades with the development of solid-state and combinatorial chemistry and computer modeling of drug–target interactions.

By sensitizing cells to DNA damage, Rad51 inhibitors open up new perspectives in the search for agents capable of suppressing homologous recombination and thereby potentiating chemo- and radiotherapy treatments for cancer. Moreover, these molecules may be not only instrumental in the development of combination anticancer therapies but also excellent tools to analyze Rad51 activities and cellular functions.

Acknowledgements

This work was supported by grants from the Ligue contre le Cancer Comité de Loire Atlantique et de Vendée and the Région pays de la Loire (CIMath project). We thank G. Levillain for his help.

Author details

Axelle Renodon-Cornière, Pierre Weigel, Magali Le Breton and Fabrice Fleury*

*Address all correspondence to: fleury-f@univ-nantes.fr

Unité UFIP, CNRS FRE 3478, University of Nantes, France

References

[1] Jackson, S. P., and Bartek, J. (2009) *Nature* 461, 1071-1078

[2] Vilenchik, M. M., and Knudson, A. G. (2003) *Proc Natl Acad Sci U S A* 100, 12871-12876

[3] Krejci, L., Chen, L., Van Komen, S., Sung, P., and Tomkinson, A. (2003) *Prog Nucleic Acid Res Mol Biol* 74, 159-201

[4] Shinohara, A., and Ogawa, T. (1995) *Trends Biochem Sci* 20, 387-391

[5] Takata, M., Sasaki, M. S., Sonoda, E., Morrison, C., Hashimoto, M., Utsumi, H., Yamaguchi-Iwai, Y., Shinohara, A., and Takeda, S. (1998) *EMBO J* 17, 5497-5508

[6] Uziel, T., Lerenthal, Y., Moyal, L., Andegeko, Y., Mittelman, L., and Shiloh, Y. (2003) *EMBO J* 22, 5612-5621

[7] Rass, E., Grabarz, A., Bertrand, P., and Lopez, B. S. (2012) *Cancer Radiother* 16, 1-10

[8] Aihara, H., Ito, Y., Kurumizaka, H., Yokoyama, S., and Shibata, T. (1999) *J Mol Biol* 290, 495-504

[9] Bearss, D. J., Lee, R. J., Troyer, D. A., Pestell, R. G., and Windle, J. J. (2002) *Cancer Res* 62, 2077-2084

[10] Raderschall, E., Stout, K., Freier, S., Suckow, V., Schweiger, S., and Haaf, T. (2002) *Cancer Res* 62, 219-225

[11] Slupianek, A., Hoser, G., Majsterek, I., Bronisz, A., Malecki, M., Blasiak, J., Fishel, R., and Skorski, T. (2002) *Mol Cell Biol* 22, 4189-4201

[12] Maacke, H., Opitz, S., Jost, K., Hamdorf, W., Henning, W., Kruger, S., Feller, A. C., Lopens, A., Diedrich, K., Schwinger, E., and Sturzbecher, H. W. (2000) *Int J Cancer* 88, 907-913

[13] Maacke, H., Jost, K., Opitz, S., Miska, S., Yuan, Y., Hasselbach, L., Luttges, J., Kalthoff, H., and Sturzbecher, H. W. (2000) *Oncogene* 19, 2791-2795

[14] Vispe, S., Cazaux, C., Lesca, C., and Defais, M. (1998) *Nucleic Acids Res* 26, 2859-2864

[15] Ohnishi, T., Taki, T., Hiraga, S., Arita, N., and Morita, T. (1998) *Biochem Biophys Res Commun* 245, 319-324

[16] Christodoulopoulos, G., Malapetsa, A., Schipper, H., Golub, E., Radding, C., and Panasci, L. C. (1999) *Clin Cancer Res* 5, 2178-2184

[17] Collis, S. J., Tighe, A., Scott, S. D., Roberts, S. A., Hendry, J. H., and Margison, G. P. (2001) *Nucleic Acids Res* 29, 1534-1538

[18] Huang, F., Motlekar, N. A., Burgwin, C. M., Napper, A. D., Diamond, S. L., and Mazin, A. V. (2011) *ACS Chem Biol* 6, 628-635

[19] Barlow, A. L., Benson, F. E., West, S. C., and Hulten, M. A. (1997) *EMBO J* 16, 5207-5215

[20] Haaf, T., Golub, E. I., Reddy, G., Radding, C. M., and Ward, D. C. (1995) *Proc Natl Acad Sci U S A* 92, 2298-2302

[21] Conway, A. B., Lynch, T. W., Zhang, Y., Fortin, G. S., Fung, C. W., Symington, L. S., and Rice, P. A. (2004) *Nat Struct Mol Biol* 11, 791-796

[22] Shin, D. S., Pellegrini, L., Daniels, D. S., Yelent, B., Craig, L., Bates, D., Yu, D. S., Shivji, M. K., Hitomi, C., Arvai, A. S., Volkmann, N., Tsuruta, H., Blundell, T. L., Venkitaraman, A. R., and Tainer, J. A. (2003) *EMBO J* 22, 4566-4576

[23] Wu, Y., Qian, X., He, Y., Moya, I. A., and Luo, Y. (2005) *J Biol Chem* 280, 722-728

[24] Wu, Y., He, Y., Moya, I. A., Qian, X., and Luo, Y. (2004) *Mol Cell* 15, 423-435

[25] Ariza, A., Richard, D. J., White, M. F., and Bond, C. S. (2005) *Nucleic Acids Res* 33, 1465-1473

[26] Pellegrini, L., Yu, D. S., Lo, T., Anand, S., Lee, M., Blundell, T. L., and Venkitaraman, A. R. (2002) *Nature* 420, 287-293

[27] Doherty, A. J., Serpell, L. C., and Ponting, C. P. (1996) *Nucleic Acids Res* 24, 2488-2497

[28] Bugreev, D. V., and Mazin, A. V. (2004) *Proc Natl Acad Sci U S A* 101, 9988-9993

[29] Ristic, D., Modesti, M., van der Heijden, T., van Noort, J., Dekker, C., Kanaar, R., and Wyman, C. (2005) *Nucleic Acids Res* 33, 3292-3302

[30] Sigurdsson, S., Trujillo, K., Song, B., Stratton, S., and Sung, P. (2001) *J Biol Chem* 276, 8798-8806

[31] Makara, G. B., Stark, E., Karteszi, M., Palkovits, M., and Rappay, G. (1981) *Am J Physiol* 240, E441-446

[32] Ishida, T., Takizawa, Y., Kainuma, T., Inoue, J., Mikawa, T., Shibata, T., Suzuki, H., Tashiro, S., and Kurumizaka, H. (2009) *Nucleic Acids Res* 37, 3367-3376

[33] Stark, J. M., Hu, P., Pierce, A. J., Moynahan, M. E., Ellis, N., and Jasin, M. (2002) *J Biol Chem* 277, 20185-20194

[34] Amunugama, R., He, Y., Willcox, S., Forties, R. A., Shim, K. S., Bundschuh, R., Luo, Y., Griffith, J., and Fishel, R. (2011) *J Biol Chem* 287, 8724-8736

[35] Li, Y., He, Y., and Luo, Y. (2009) *Biochemistry* 48, 6805-6810

[36] Matsuo, Y., Sakane, I., Takizawa, Y., Takahashi, M., and Kurumizaka, H. (2006) *FEBS J* 273, 3148-3159

[37] Qian, X., Wu, Y., He, Y., and Luo, Y. (2005) *Biochemistry* 44, 13753-13761

[38] Fujiwara, H., Matsunaga, K., Saito, M., Hagiya, S., Furukawa, K., Nakamura, H., and Ohizumi, Y. (2001) *Eur J Pharmacol* 413, 37-45

[39] Schmitz, F. J., and Bloor, S. (1988) *J.Org.Chem* 53, 3922-3925

[40] Takaku, M., Kainuma, T., Ishida-Takaku, T., Ishigami, S., Suzuki, H., Tashiro, S., van Soest, R. W., Nakao, Y., and Kurumizaka, H. (2011) *Genes Cells* 16, 427-436

[41] Huang, F., Mazina, O. M., Zentner, I. J., Cocklin, S., and Mazin, A. V. (2012) *J Med Chem* 55, 3011-3020

[42] Budke, B., Logan, H. L., Kalin, J. H., Zelivianskaia, A. S., Cameron McGuire, W., Miller, L. L., Stark, J. M., Kozikowski, A. P., Bishop, D. K., and Connell, P. P. (2012) *Nucleic Acids Res*

[43] Krejci, L., Damborsky, J., Thomsen, B., Duno, M., and Bendixen, C. (2001) *Mol Cell Biol* 21, 966-976

[44] Jayathilaka, K., Sheridan, S. D., Bold, T. D., Bochenska, K., Logan, H. L., Weichselbaum, R. R., Bishop, D. K., and Connell, P. P. (2008) *Proc Natl Acad Sci U S A* 105, 15848-15853

[45] Mariani, B. D., Slate, D. L., and Schimke, R. T. (1981) *Proc Natl Acad Sci U S A* 78, 4985-4989

[46] Ostling, O., and Johanson, K. J. (1984) *Biochem Biophys Res Commun* 123, 291-298

[47] Du, L. Q., Du, X. Q., Bai, J. Q., Wang, Y., Yang, Q. S., Wang, X. C., Zhao, P., Wang, H., Liu, Q., and Fan, F. Y. (2012) *J Cancer Res Clin Oncol* 138, 811-818

[48] Buggy, J. J., Cao, Z. A., Bass, K. E., Verner, E., Balasubramanian, S., Liu, L., Schultz, B. E., Young, P. R., and Dalrymple, S. A. (2006) *Mol Cancer Ther* 5, 1309-1317

[49] Adimoolam, S., Sirisawad, M., Chen, J., Thiemann, P., Ford, J. M., and Buggy, J. J. (2007) *Proc Natl Acad Sci U S A* 104, 19482-19487

[50] Davies, A. A., Masson, J. Y., McIlwraith, M. J., Stasiak, A. Z., Stasiak, A., Venkitaraman, A. R., and West, S. C. (2001) *Mol Cell* 7, 273-282

[51] Brown, E. T., Robinson-Benion, C., and Holt, J. T. (2008) *Radiat Res* 169, 595-601

[52] Zhang, X., Sun, H., Danila, D. C., Johnson, S. R., Zhou, Y., Swearingen, B., and Klibanski, A. (2002) *J Clin Endocrinol Metab* 87, 1262-1267

[53] Chang, C. C., Chen, W. C., Ho, T. F., Wu, H. S., and Wei, Y. H. (2011) *J Biosci Bioeng* 111, 501-511

[54] Pandey, R., Chander, R., and Sainis, K. B. (2009) *Curr Pharm Des* 15, 732-741

[55] Perez-Tomas, R., Montaner, B., Llagostera, E., and Soto-Cerrato, V. (2003) *Biochem Pharmacol* 66, 1447-1452

[56] Montaner, B., Castillo-Avila, W., Martinell, M., Ollinger, R., Aymami, J., Giralt, E., and Perez-Tomas, R. (2005) *Toxicol Sci* 85, 870-879

[57] Lu, C. H., Lin, S. C., Yang, S. Y., Pan, M. Y., Lin, Y. W., Hsu, C. Y., Wei, Y. H., Chang, J. S., and Chang, C. C. (2012) *Toxicol Lett* 212, 83-89

[58] Lazaro-Trueba, I., Arias, C., and Silva, A. (2006) *Cell Cycle* 5, 1062-1065

[59] Fan, M., and Chambers, T. C. (2001) *Drug Resist Updat* 4, 253-267

[60] Chuang, S. M., Wang, L. H., Hong, J. H., and Lin, Y. W. (2008) *Toxicol Appl Pharmacol* 230, 290-297

[61] Ko, J. C., Tsai, M. S., Weng, S. H., Kuo, Y. H., Chiu, Y. F., and Lin, Y. W. (2011) *Toxicol Appl Pharmacol* 255, 327-338

[62] Adam, S. A., Marr, R. S., and Gerace, L. (1990) *J Cell Biol* 111, 807-816

[63] Radu, A., Blobel, G., and Moore, M. S. (1995) *Proc Natl Acad Sci U S A* 92, 1769-1773

[64] Ryan, K. J., and Wente, S. R. (2000) *Curr Opin Cell Biol* 12, 361-371

[65] Gorlich, D., and Kutay, U. (1999) *Annu Rev Cell Dev Biol* 15, 607-660

[66] French, C. A., Tambini, C. E., and Thacker, J. (2003) *J Biol Chem* 278, 45445-45450

[67] Golub, E. I., Kovalenko, O. V., Gupta, R. C., Ward, D. C., and Radding, C. M. (1997) *Nucleic Acids Res* 25, 4106-4110

[68] Shen, Z., Cloud, K. G., Chen, D. J., and Park, M. S. (1996) *J Biol Chem* 271, 148-152

[69] Gildemeister, O. S., Sage, J. M., and Knight, K. L. (2009) *J Biol Chem* 284, 31945-31952

[70] Plo, I., Laulier, C., Gauthier, L., Lebrun, F., Calvo, F., and Lopez, B. S. (2008) *Cancer Res* 68, 9404-9412

[71] Martelli, A. M., Evangelisti, C., Chiarini, F., Grimaldi, C., Manzoli, L., and McCubrey, J. A. (2009) *Expert Opin Investig Drugs* 18, 1333-1349

[72] Xiao, L., Gong, L. L., Yuan, D., Deng, M., Zeng, X. M., Chen, L. L., Zhang, L., Yan, Q., Liu, J. P., Hu, X. H., Sun, S. M., Liu, J., Ma, H. L., Zheng, C. B., Fu, H., Chen, P. C., Zhao, J. Q., Xie, S. S., Zou, L. J., Xiao, Y. M., Liu, W. B., Zhang, J., Liu, Y., and Li, D. W. (2010) *Cell Death Differ* 17, 1448-1462

[73] Altiok, S., Batt, D., Altiok, N., Papautsky, A., Downward, J., Roberts, T. M., and Avraham, H. (1999) *J Biol Chem* 274, 32274-32278

[74] Chang, T., Wang, R., Olson, D. J., Mousseau, D. D., Ross, A. R., and Wu, L. (2011) *FASEB J* 25, 1746-1757

[75] Jia, X., Chang, T., Wilson, T. W., and Wu, L. (2012) *PLoS One* 7, e36610

[76] Bork, P., Blomberg, N., and Nilges, M. (1996) *Nat Genet* 13, 22-23

[77] Wong, A. K., Pero, R., Ormonde, P. A., Tavtigian, S. V., and Bartel, P. L. (1997) *J Biol Chem* 272, 31941-31944

[78] Davies, O. R., and Pellegrini, L. (2007) *Nat Struct Mol Biol* 14, 475-483

[79] Jasin, M. (2002) *Oncogene* 21, 8981-8993

[80] Holt, J. T., Toole, W. P., Patel, V. R., Hwang, H., and Brown, E. T. (2008) *Cancer Genet Cytogenet* 186, 85-94

[81] Chen, C. F., Chen, P. L., Zhong, Q., Sharp, Z. D., and Lee, W. H. (1999) *J Biol Chem* 274, 32931-32935

[82] Nomme, J., Renodon-Corniere, A., Asanomi, Y., Sakaguchi, K., Stasiak, A. Z., Stasiak, A., Norden, B., Tran, V., and Takahashi, M. (2011) *J Med Chem* 53, 5782-5791

[83] Nomme, J., Takizawa, Y., Martinez, S. F., Renodon-Corniere, A., Fleury, F., Weigel, P., Yamamoto, K., Kurumizaka, H., and Takahashi, M. (2008) *Genes Cells* 13, 471-481

[84] Lee, W.-H. C. L. (2006) Compositions and methods for disruption of BRCA2-Rad51 interaction. USA

[85] Lee, W.-H., Chen, P.-L., Zhou, L., and Zhu, J. (2009) Compositions and methods related to Rad51 inactivation in the treatment of neoplastic diseases and especially CML. the regents of the university of California, CA, US, USA

[86] Qiu, X. L., Zhu, J., Wu, G., Lee, W. H., and Chamberlin, A. R. (2009) *J Org Chem* 74, 2018-2027

Chapter 18

DNA Repair and Resistance to Cancer Therapy

António S. Rodrigues, Bruno Costa Gomes,
Célia Martins, Marta Gromicho, Nuno G. Oliveira,
Patrícia S. Guerreiro and José Rueff

Additional information is available at the end of the chapter

http://dx.doi.org/10.5772/53952

1. Introduction

Humans are constantly exposed to diverse chemical and physical agents that have the potential to damage DNA, such as reactive oxygen species (ROS), ionizing radiation (IR), UV light, and various environmental, dietary or pollutant chemical agents. The integrity and survival of a cell is critically dependent on genome stability, and cells possess multiple pathways to repair these DNA lesions. These pathways are diverse and target different types of lesions.

The critical role played by DNA repair in the maintenance of genome stability is highlighted by the fact that many enzymes involved have been conserved through evolution [1-4]. Very rarely germ line mutations occur in several of the DNA repair genes and are the cause of cancer predisposing syndromes, such as *Xeroderma pigmentosum* (XP), [5], Fanconi anemia (FA) and ataxia telangiectasia (AT) and are associated with inherent chromosome instability [2]. One of the most well-known examples of a defect in DNA repair leading to cancer is the association of germ-line *BRCA1/2* mutations with breast, ovarian and peritoneal malignancies [6]. These rare human DNA repair syndromes have been invaluable in providing mechanistic explanations for the involvement of DNA repair system in cancer. They have also been instrumental in the translation of these findings to the clinic.

On the other hand, recent studies have shown that defective DNA damage repair is present in virtually all sporadic tumours [7]. Mutations in DNA repair genes could be either responsible for the occurrence of tumours or could arise due to random accumulation of mutations during cycling of cancer cells. The presence of incorrect DNA repair in tumour cells predisposes them to accumulate even more genetic alterations. For example, colorectal and endometrial cancers with defective DNA mismatch repair (MMR) due to mutations in the *MLH1* and *MSH2* genes exhibit increased rates of acquisition of single nucleotide changes and small insertions/deletions [8]. Thus, the presence of a "mutator phenotype" [9] could increase the evolutionary acquisition of alterations that ultimately could lead to enhanced drug resistance.

A further reminder on the importance of DNA repair is the observation that mutations in specific genes can lead not to an increase in cancer but to accelerated aging syndromes [7]. An example of this is Cockayne's syndrome (CS), which causes severe progeroid syndromes [10]. Mutations in the genes that encode two proteins in a nucleotide excision repair (NER) sub-pathway called transcription coupled repair (TCR) cause global premature cell death through apoptosis. In this case apoptosis ensures that DNA mutations are not transmitted to daughter cells, albeit at the expense of cell viability, and highlights the importance of maintaining DNA integrity.

One major problem in cancer therapy is the fact that of the 7.6 million cancer deaths that occur every year worldwide (2008 data; http://www.who.int/cancer/en/), many are due to failure of cancer therapy associated with acquired and intrinsic resistance mechanisms. These mechanisms of resistance can be classified in different ways, but the most characterized are altered cellular drug transport, increased survival or decreased cell death, altered DNA repair, and alterations in drug targets [11, 12]. Over the last years the importance of DNA repair pathways in resistance to chemotherapy has been increasingly recognized, but translation to the clinic is still scarce. Since many classical cancer therapies target DNA, the influence of DNA repair systems in response to DNA damage which primarily result from chemotherapy and radiotherapy is critical to cell survival. The use of inhibitors of DNA repair or DNA damage signalling pathways provides an interesting opportunity to target the genetic differences that exist between normal and tumour tissue [13, 14].

The rationale underlying the use of DNA damaging agents in therapeutic strategies is to kill cancer cells while sparing normal tissues, due to increased cell cycling of cancer cells. Unfortunately highly cycling normal cells (e.g. bone marrow, hair follicles and gastrointestinal epithelia) are also targeted by DNA damaging therapeutic agents, giving rise to the secondary effects normally seen after cancer therapy (e.g. diarrhoea, mouth ulcers, hair loss, anaemia and susceptibility to infections). Nevertheless, DNA-damaging chemotherapeutic agents are effective and prolong survival of cancer patients [15]. Chemotherapeutic agents commonly used in cancer treatment produce a plethora of lesions that can be targets for cellular responses. For example, DNA double strand breaks (DSBs), single-strand breaks (SSBs), and oxidized bases are induced by ionizing radiation (IR), anthracyclines, platinum compounds and taxanes. Anthracyclines are topoisomerase II inhibitors and DNA intercalating agents, which when used can lead to DSBs. Platinum compounds are bifunctional alkylating agents that induce predominantly intra- and interstrand crosslinks (ICLs) and taxanes are mitotic inhibitors. All these lesions induce cellular responses that cover a multitude of pathways, including DNA repair pathways, DNA tolerance mechanisms, coordination networks that link repair and cell cycle progression, as well as apoptotic and other cell death pathways when DNA damage is irreparable [16-19].

The DNA repair pathways that respond to these lesions include: direct repair of alkyl adducts by O6-alkylguanine DNA alkyltransferase (MGMT); repair of base damage and SSBs by base excision repair (BER); repair of bulky DNA adducts by nucleotide excision repair (NER); repair of cross-links by DNA interstrand cross-link repair and repair of mismatches and insertion/deletion loops by DNA mismatch repair (MMR); repair of DSBs by homologous recombination (HR) and non-homologous end joining (NHEJ). Detailed description of the biochemical pathways of DNA repair is beyond the scope of this chapter as several reviews on the subject have been published [1, 17, 20-23].

The observation that a variety of tumours frequently present deregulated expression of DNA repair genes (e.g. *MGMT, PARP1*) rapidly lead to the notion that DNA repair pathways could be targeted in cancer treatment and lead to personalized therapy [24, 25]. Tumours with specific DNA repair defects could be completely dependent on back-up DNA repair pathways for their survival. This dependence could be exploited therapeutically to induce cell death and apoptosis in tumour cells [26, 27]. The genetic state in which simultaneous inactivation of 2 genes (or pathways) is lethal, while loss of one or the other alone is viable is called synthetic lethality (also known as conditional genetics). The rationale for inducing synthetic lethality in cancer is that certain cancer cells lack one pathway to repair their DNA (e.g. HR) but have alternative pathways (base excision or single-strand repair) that allow them to survive. Inhibition of these alternative pathways would then impair DNA repair and induce cell death [26, 27]. Therefore it predicts that genotoxic agents leading to a particular type of DNA damage will kill cancer cells with genetic deficits in repair of that type of damage. Recently, this specific anticancer strategy has been the focus of intense investigations [28, 29].

In the case of the hereditary *BRCA1/2*-deficient breast and ovarian cancer syndromes, mentioned earlier, this strategy has been translated into the clinic, in the form of PARP inhibitors. These *BRCA1/2*$^{-}$ tumours are defective in the repair of DSBs by HR. When a replication fork in one of these tumours encounters a DNA SSB, it converts that into a DSB, but the presence of a DSB prevents progression of the replication apparatus. Since *BRCA1/2* are both required for DSB repair, the tumour cells with those mutated genes will depend on repair of SSBs to prevent DSBs from occurring. The DNA repair protein PARP1 is required for repair of SSBs, and small molecular inhibitors of PARP1 will prevent repair of SSBs, more specifically in cells that are deficient in *BRCA1/2*. Since normal cells have the ability to repair the DSBs generated at the replication fork, because they have at least one normal allele of *BRCA1/2*, the use of PARP inhibitors has the potential of targeting only tumour cells. This proof of concept proven clinically, where the PARP1 inhibitor olaparib improves the progression-free survival of familial breast cancer [30]. Following this lead several small molecule DNA repair inhibitors are being developed worldwide.

However, not all *BRCA1/2* defective tumours respond equally well to this type of therapy. Thus, in the past years evidence has accumulated that drug resistance is also linked to alterations in these pathways [31-33]. Thus, tumour cells may also acquire resistance by invoking biochemical mechanisms that reduce drug action or by acquiring additional alterations in

DNA damage response pathways [34]. Therefore, the focus has also been directed on DNA repair pathways that could be responsible for cancer drug resistance.

Resistance to chemotherapy limits the effectiveness of anti-cancer drug treatment. Tumours may be intrinsically drug-resistant or develop resistance to chemotherapy during treatment. Acquired resistance is a particular problem, as tumours not only become resistant to the drugs originally used to treat them, but may also become cross-resistant to other drugs with different mechanisms of action. Resistance to chemotherapy is believed to cause treatment failure in over 90% of patients with metastatic cancer [35]. Thus, drug resistance is clearly a major clinical problem.

The attempt to develop more targeted therapeutics has been a major objective in cancer research in last years, and more and more molecular targets are being identified (e.g. tyrosine kinase inhibitors, monoclonal antibodies targeting membrane receptor kinases). Some of these targeted therapies are in clinical use, while others are being evaluated in clinical trials to validate their efficacy. More recently, the quest for targeted therapies has also focused on DNA repair pathways. Unfortunately, resistance to these therapies is also likely to appear, as has occurred with other targeted therapies, such as the tyrosine kinase inhibitors of the fusion *BCR-ABL1* gene, responsible for most cases of chronic myeloid leukaemia (e.g. imatinib, dasatinib, nilotinib). The application of DNA repair inhibitors in the clinic has also shown to be fraught with difficulty, since they also target DNA repair pathways in normal cells. The early clinical trial with MGMT inhibitors in combination with temozolomide (TMZ) was stopped early because the combined treatments harmed bone marrow as well as cancer tissue, whereas the clinical success of PARP inhibitors transpired since PARP is not critical to cell survival. Hence, unlike past visions of a "magic bullet" towards cancer, future research on cancer therapy should more reasonably envisage cancer therapy as a "never ending story", in which novel targeted therapeutics are constantly being overcome by the evolutionary processes present in cancerous cells [36].

2. Targeting DNA repair pathways

As mentioned, DNA repair pathways include the direct reversal of lesions, essentially dealkylation of alkylated bases by *MGMT*, NER, BER, MMR and the double strand break repair by HR and NHEJ. Alterations in all these pathways have been observed in drug resistant tumour cells; however, the clinical significance of the alterations is not completely understood. Numerous genes involved in each of these pathways have been shown to be up- or down-regulated in diverse types of tumours and constitute a potential source of biomarkers to evaluate drug resistance to cancer chemotherapeutics [25, 32, 33].

3. MGMT and drug resistance

Alkylating agents are widely used to treat cancers, and one of the major DNA lesions formed occurs essentially by the alkylation of DNA at the O^6-position of guanine, which

http://dx.doi.org/10.5772/53952

subsequently can generate DNA breaks and cell death. TMZ, streptozotocin, procarbazine and dacarbazine are examples of cancer chemotherapeutics that methylate DNA [37].

Direct repair of alkylated guanine residues proceeds through the removal of the alkyl moiety by MGMT. MGMT is a conserved protein from prokaryotes through eukaryotes. The MGMT protein removes the alkyl group from O^6-alkylguanine by direct transfer to a cysteine residue in its active site to which the alkyl group becomes covalently attached, resulting in the inactivation of the protein. The MGMT protein is subsequently ubiquitinated and degraded by the proteasome [38, 39]. The O^6-alkylguanine adduct accounts for about 10% of total alkylations, but displays a strong mutagenic and cytotoxic potential, because O^6-alkylguanines exhibit distorted base pairing characteristics in pairing with thymine, thereby, resulting in G:C to A:T transitions upon DNA replication [40]. Hence the unique DNA repair mechanism which depends on the suicidal degradation of the MGMT protein.

Tumour expression of *MGMT* varies and correlates with therapeutic response to alkylating agents. Numerous studies have found a strong correlation between MGMT activity and drug resistance in primary tumours and established human tumour cell lines [16, 41, 42]. High levels of expression have also been noted in melanoma [43], pancreatic carcinoma [16] besides glioblastomas [44]. Resistance to alkylating agents such as TMZ has been linked to over-expression of *MGMT* [43]. Therefore MGMT levels are being studied as biomarkers of intrinsic chemosensitivity to alkylating agents, such as TMZ or BCNU (carmustine).

Conversely, reduced MGMT activity in cultured tumour cells and human tumours is often the result of epigenetic silencing by promoter methylation of CpG islands, which leads to the formation of inactive chromatin that limits transcription, and therefore higher chemosensitivity to alkylation. Hegi *et al.* reported that of 206 patients with glioblastoma that were treated with TMZ and radiotherapy, those with a methylated *MGMT* promoter (45%) had a significantly better survival [45]. Hence, *MGMT* promoter methylation status is emerging as a prognostic factor for tumour therapy and is currently being assessed for selecting glioblastoma chemosensitivity towards TMZ [46-48]. The mechanisms underlying increased *MGMT* promoter methylation are complex and not completely known, although it is one of the most studied DNA repair genes [38]. In normal cells *MGMT* promoter methylation is uncommon, but occurs frequently in tumours. Approximately 25% of tumours of many different types, including non-small-cell carcinoma of the lung, lymphoma, head and neck cancers, and up to 40% of glioma and colorectal tumours were found to present CpG island promoter methylation [49].

Since high *MGMT* expression results in drug resistance to alkylating agents, one strategy to overcome resistance and improve efficacy is to use pseudo substrates of MGMT, such as O^6-benzylguanine (O^6-BG) or O^6-(4-bromothenyl) guanine (O^6-BTG or lomeguatrib or PaTrin-2) which inactivate the enzyme and enhance cell death [50]. O^6-BG is a specific, potent, and nontoxic inhibitor and leads to sensitization of cancer cells to cisplatin, chloroethylating and methylating agents [51, 52]. Clinical trials are underway to test combinations of O^6-BG with carmustine or TMZ for the treatment of glioma, anaplastic glioma, lymphoma, myeloma, colon cancer, melanoma and sarcoma, among others [53]. O^6-BTG presents higher bioavailability than O^6-BG, but also presents higher haematological toxicity when co-administered with

TMZ compared to TMZ alone. Therefore full use of this inhibitor may be more distant [54, 55]. Haematological toxicity was also observed with O^6-BTG co-administered with dacarbazine in patients with advanced melanoma and other solid tumours [56]. The combination of O^6-BTG and TMZ was also evaluated in a phase I clinical trial for advanced solid tumours [57], and in a pilot study for refractory acute leukaemia [58]. A phase I clinical trial was also conducted associating O^6-BTG with Irinotecan for colorectal cancer [59]. A phase II clinical trial of O^6-BTG plus TMZ for stage IV metastatic colorectal cancer is already completed. The trial was considered completed after the recruitment of 19 patients due to the absence of responses and also because evidences from other studies suggest that the O^6-BTG dosing regimen was inappropriate [55]. These studies showed a consistent depletion of MGMT and provided non-toxic doses of O^6-BG or O^6-BTG to be used in further studies. The haematological toxicity observed with the combination of MGMT inhibitors and chemotherapeutic agents might be attributed to an effective depletion of MGMT in off-target cells [60]. Additionally, the administration of a sub-optimal dose of the MGMT inhibitor, a therapeutic dosing schedule that allows the recovery of the MGMT activity or the choice of an inadequate treatment for the type of cancer could explain the lack of effects in clinical trials. In view of this, tumour-targeted delivery of MGMT inhibitors by the development of specific formulations or local administration [61] could be adopted to improve the therapeutic efficacy of the chemotherapeutic drugs and to translate into the clinic the results obtained in preclinical studies. Nonetheless, it is not clear if clinical application of MGMT inhibitors is a viable therapy in all settings.

4. Targeting MMR in cancer drug resistance

MMR is involved in the detection and repair of base-base mispairs during DNA replication, small insertion/deletion mutations at repetitive microsatellite regions and also in the regulation of homologous recombination [62]. MMR proteins are also involved in the repair of DNA damage caused by ROS and alkylating agents. MMR proteins interact with components of other repair pathways, including NER, BER, and HR, thus signalling with other pathways in response to DNA damage.

The MMR system consists of various proteins. MSH2 heterodimerizes with MSH6 or MSH3 to form MutSα or MutSβ, respectively, both of which are ATPases that play a critical role in mismatch recognition and initiation of repair. This induces a conformational change in MutS, resulting in a clamp that translocates on DNA in a ATP dependent manner, recruits the MutL complex, which in humans is a heterodimer consisting of the MLH1 and PMS2 proteins, and displaces DNA polymerase and PCNA, thereafter recruiting an exonuclease (EXO1) that degrades the newly synthesized DNA strand [63]. Other MMR genes (*MLH1, MLH3, PMS1,* and *PMS2*) are involved in MMR. MLH1 also heterodimerizes with PMS2, PMS1, or MLH3 to form MutLα, MutLβ, or MutLγ, respectively [63]. Polymerase δ (pol δ) then polymerizes the DNA stretch and DNA Ligase I performs ligation.

MMR deficiency leads to a wide range of tumour types. Germline deficiency in MMR accounts for the Lynch syndrome (hereditary non-polyposis colorectal cancer -HNPCC), in which a large increase in frequency of insertion and deletion mutations in simple repeat (microsatellite) sequences, a phenomenon known as microsatellite instability (MSI), is observed [64]. DNA mismatch repair deficiency in sporadic tumours is seen in colonic, gastric, endometrial, and other solid tumours. MSI is also associated with a wide variety of non-HNPCC and non-colonic tumours, including endometrial, ovarian, gastric, cervical, breast, skin, lung, prostate, and bladder tumours as well as glioma, leukaemia, and lymphoma [65].

Defects in MMR are also associated with resistance to certain chemotherapeutic agents [66]. Resistance to alkylating agents such as TMZ and procarbazine occurs with inactivation of MMR in tumour cells [63]. MMR-deficient cells are relatively resistant to methylating agents (up to 100 fold), whereas cells with a functioning MMR system enter either G2 arrest or apoptosis, depending on the severity of the DNA damage [67]. Down regulation of proteins of the MMR pathway is associated with resistance to clinically important drugs including platinum-containing compounds, anthracyclines, alkylating agents, antimetabolites and epipodophyllotoxins [68].

For example, MSH2 protein deficiency by enhancing MSH2 degradation leads to substantial reduction in DNA mismatch repair and increased resistance to thiopurines. Somatic deletions of genes regulating MSH2 degradation result in undetectable levels of MSH2 protein in leukaemia cells, MMR deficiency and drug resistance [69].

Another agent, etoposide, is a topoisomerase II alpha (*TOP2A*) inhibitor, which is used in the treatment of breast cancer. Alterations in the expression of drug targets or DNA repair genes are among the important resistance mechanisms against TOP2A inhibitors. Decrease in the expression levels of *TOP2A*, and the MMR genes *MSH2* and *MLH1* may play significant roles in the development of chemotherapeutic resistance to etoposide in breast cancer. These genes may be considered for further development of new strategies to overcome resistance against topoisomerase II inhibitors [70].

MMR is also involved in repair of cross-linking agents such as platinum based chemotherapeutics. Increased tolerance to platinum-induced DNA damage can occur through loss of function of the MMR pathway. During MMR, cisplatin-induced DNA adducts are recognized by the MMR pathway, but are not repaired, giving rise to successive repair cycles, ultimately triggering apoptosis. Thus in MMR deficient cells, cell death is not as efficient, promoting tolerance to platinum agents [71].

MMR-deficient cells are also more tolerant to 6-thioguanine treatment, used to treat leukaemias, than MMR-proficient cells. The anti-metabolite 6-thioguanine is incorporated into DNA, where it can be methylated by *S*-adenosylmethionine to 6-methylthioguanine (Me6-thioguanine), which has similar miscoding properties as methylguanine [68].

Nevertheless, although many preclinical studies suggest MMR-deficient cells are resistant to alkylating agents, few clinical studies have been published regarding MMR deficiency and response to alkylating agents. On the contrary, for example, Maxwell *et al.*, [72] found that MMR deficiency does not seem to be responsible for mediating TMZ resistance in adult malignant glioma. Coupled with the lack of substantial data linking polymorphisms within the MMR genes and resistance to chemotherapy or radiotherapy, published work suggests that the MMR pathway has low priority in the quest for new cancer therapies. However, ongoing research on the role of microRNAs and cancer drug resistance could increase interest in this pathway. Published work has suggested that for example miR-21 targets *MSH2* and consequently induces resistance to 5-Fluorouracil (5-FU) in colorectal cancer [73] (see the section of microRNAs and drug resistance).

5. Targeting BER in cancer drug resistance

BER is the main pathway for removing small, non-helix-distorting base lesions from the genome. Thus, BER targets predominantly base lesions that arise due to oxidative, alkylation, deamination, and depurination/depyrimidination damage. Some examples of chemotherapeutic agents that generate lesions that are targeted by BER include TMZ, melphalan, dacarbazine/procarbazine, and streptozotocin [33]. Some chemotherapeutic agents also generate ROS as a "by-product" such as platinum-based drugs (*i.e.* oxaliplatin and cisplatin), anthracyclines, (*i.e.* epirubicin, daunorubicin, doxorubicin) and paclitaxel [31, 33]. ROS induce DNA lesions that are also repaired by the BER pathway. Additionally, IR produces a number of DNA lesions that are repaired by the BER pathway. Endogenous production of ROS also gives rise to several lesions, which are variable in number and consequence. For instance the highly mutagenic 8-hydroxyguanine (8-oxoG) is formed in large quantities as a consequence of the high oxidation potential of this base, and has a miscoding effect, due to DNA polymerase activity which inserts adenine opposite to 8-oxoG, resulting in G:C to A:T transition mutations.

The BER pathway is initiated by one of many DNA glycosylases, which recognize and catalyze the removal of different damaged bases. After recognition of the damaged base by the appropriate DNA glycosylase, it catalyzes the cleavage of an *N*-glycosidic bond, thus removing the damaged base and creating an apurinic or apyrimidinic site (AP site). The DNA backbone is cleaved by either a DNA AP endonuclease or a DNA AP lyase, activity present in some glycosylases. This creates a single-stranded DNA nick 5′ to the AP site. The newly created nick is processed by the AP endonuclease, creating a single-nucleotide gap in the DNA. At this point BER can proceed through a short-patch BER, where polymerase β (pol β) introduces a single nucleotide past the abasic site and Ligase IIIα seals the DNA nick, or through a long-patch BER, where Polymerase δ/ε introduces two to eight nucleotides past the abasic site. The resulting overhang DNA is excised by FEN1 endonuclease and the nick sealed by DNA ligase I [74]. In addition to these enzymes, a number of accessory proteins are involved in BER, including the X-ray cross-complementation group 1 protein (XRCC1), PARP1, the proliferating cell nuclear antigen (PCNA), and the heterotrimer termed 9-1-1, which function in scaffolds for the core BER enzymes [75].

Preclinical evidences have implied the BER pathway in the repair of DNA lesions induced by antimetabolites, monofunctional alkylating drugs, radiotherapy and radiomimetic agents. Moreover, BER modulation may also sensitize cancer cells to the effect of chemotherapeutic drugs that are able to generate ROS [31, 33]. Therefore, targeting BER with inhibitors

http://dx.doi.org/10.5772/53952

of the multifunctional AP Endonuclease 1 and DNA pol β is an attractive field to the development of novel therapeutic compounds.

Some studies have found deregulation of BER genes in tumours. For example pol β has been shown to be overexpressed in a variety of tumour cells [76]. N-methylpurine DNA glycosylase (MPG) overexpression, together with inhibition of BER, sensitizes glioma cells to the alkylating agent TMZ in a DNA pol β - dependent manner, suggesting that the expression level of both MPG and pol β might be used to predict the effectiveness of BER inhibition and PARP-mediated potentiation of TMZ in cancer treatment [77]. We recently observed an increase in expression of the BER genes *MDB4* and *NTHL1* in Imatinib resistant K562 leukaemia cells, and knockdown of their expression in resistant cells using siRNA decreased cell survival after treatment with doxorubicin [78]. Nevertheless, the involvement of deregulated BER components in chemotherapy resistance is not completely evident at present, except for PARP, and the AP endonucleases. The following text shall describe ongoing research targeting these components of the BER pathway.

The major AP endonuclease in mammalian cells is apurinic/apyrimidinic endonuclease 1/ redox-factor-1 (APE1/Ref-1, also called APEX1), and has been found to be elevated in a number of cancers such as ovarian [79], prostate [80], osteosarcoma [81] and testicular cancer [82]. Over-expression of APE1 *in vitro* led to increased protection against bleomycin [82]. Thus elevated levels of APE1 in cancer cells have been postulated to be a reason for chemotherapeutic resistance [81, 83, 84]. Inhibition of APE1 has been shown to increase cell killing and apoptosis and also to sensitize cancer cells to chemotherapeutic agents, and thus APE1 is considered as a molecular target in therapeutics [85, 86].

APE1 endonuclease activity is indirectly inhibited by blocked AP sites that result from the binding of the small molecule methoxyamine (MX) to the DNA. With the APE1's substrate unavailable, BER cannot proceed and the cytotoxic abasic sites accumulate in the cell, eventually leading to cell death. The promising results from *in vitro* and *in vivo* experiments showing MX sensitization to the cytotoxic effect of TMZ [87-90], carmustine [91], pemetrexed [92] and 5-iodo-2'-deoxyuridine (IdUrd) as well as a potentiation of IdUrd-mediated radiosensitization [93, 94], in multiple solid tumours models, provided the proof-of-concept to conduct clinical trials with MX as adjuvant therapy of anticancer agents. A Phase I clinical trial of pemetrexed and oral methoxyamine hydrochloride (TRC102) in patients with advanced refractory cancer is already completed [95]. According to the authors, this drug is well tolerated after daily oral administration and potentiates the activity of chemotherapy. Safety, pharmacokinetic and pharmacodynamic profile of MX was also evaluated in combination with TMZ in a Phase I clinical trial for patients with advanced solid tumours [96]. Currently, two clinical trials (Phase I) are recruiting patients to study the side effects and the best dose of MX to be administered in combination with TMZ and fludarabine phosphate in patients with advanced solid tumours and relapsed or refractory hematologic malignancies, respectively.

In view of the emerging roles of APE1, many efforts have been made to develop small molecule inhibitors that can be translated to the clinic. *In silico* based approaches with design of pharmacophore models [97, 98] and high-throughput screening of several commercially available libraries of compounds have been performed to identify a pharmacologically active inhibitor for APE1 [86, 99-102]. Lucanthone acts as a direct inhibitor of APE1 but also interacts with other cellular targets and the associated toxicity hinders their therapeutic use [103, 104]. CRT0044876 was identified by a fluorescence-based high-throughput assay and showed promising results in *in vitro* studies [105]. However, some authors were not able to reproduce the reported effects of this compound [85].

Hypersensitivity of DNA pol β-null cells to methyl methanesulfonate (MMS), a DNA-methylating agent, displayed another potential target in BER [106]. Several small-molecule inhibitors of DNA pol β have been identified and many of these compounds are natural products, such as koetjapic acid (KJA), a triterpenoid. Pamoic acid was one of the first synthetic small molecule inhibitors of DNA pol β to be characterized and is more active than the former compound [107]. Nevertheless, the actually known inhibitors of DNA pol β have low potency and specificity that make them weak candidates to drug development (for a comprehensive review see [108]). In view of the preclinical data that suggest an important role of DNA Pol β in the repair of chemotherapeutic-induced DNA damage, the design of effective DNA Pol β inhibitors is an attractive research area.

In what concerns PARP1, this enzyme is a DNA damage sensor that binds to DNA breaks to activate the repair pathways. PARP1 is not directly involved in the repair of the lesions but is essential to signal the damage and to coordinate the functions of several BER and DSB repair proteins. PARP inhibitors have been thoroughly developed and several reviews papers published under this topic. For a recent comprehensive review on PARP inhibitors see Javle *et al* [109]. PARP inhibitors were first evaluated in clinical trials as chemosensitizers. After AG014699 combination with TMZ [110], other PARP inhibitors, specifically INO-1001, ABT-888 and AZD2281 were also tested as adjuvant therapy of multiple anticancer agents such as gemcitabine, carboplatin, TMZ or chemotherapeutic combinations (e.g. cisplatin plus gemcitabine) [111]. Currently, several PARP inhibitors are being evaluated in clinical trials, either in combination with chemotherapeutic drugs or in monotherapy [28, 109, 112-117].

Some of these chemicals showed an enhancement of the toxicity in normal tissues that required dose adjustments and optimization of the therapeutic schedule. Interestingly, preclinical and clinical data revealed that PARP inhibitors as single agents could be less toxic to the normal cells and are more effective in killing *BRCA1*- and *BRCA2*-mutated cancer cells since these cells are defective in HR, the backup pathway responsible for the repair of DSBs generated after PARP chemical inhibition. Similarly, mutations in other proteins related to the DNA damage response, such as ATM and PTEN have also been associated to defects in DSB repair and may be involved in an increased sensitivity to PARP inhibitors [118-120]. These findings led to a novel potential therapeutic indication of the DNA repair inhibitors as single agents in cancer therapy which is currently being evaluated in clinical trials [121]. This synthetic lethal approach was also reported in an *in vitro* study with APE1 inhibitors in BRCA and ATM deficient cells [116, 122].

Recently, negative results from the first phase III clinical trial in breast cancer patients with a combination of iniparib (BSI-201) and gemcitabine/carboplatin were reported [123]. The mechanism of action of this inhibitor is not fully understood, an issue that should be further clarified. Nonetheless, promising positive outcomes have already been suggested with other PARP inhibitors [124, 125]. A further understanding of the complex PARP interactome, the discovery of PARP1 specific small molecule inhibitors and an accurate selection of the best candidates to the treatment is still needed to improve the quality of information obtained from preclinical and clinical trials and to promote the development of currently known PARP inhibitors as well to discover novel compounds.

6. Targeting NER in drug resistance

NER repairs DNA lesions which alter the helical structure of the DNA molecule and interfere with DNA replication and transcription, such as bulky adducts and cross-linking agents [2]. Briefly, NER consists of the recognition of DNA damage and demarcation of the specific area affected, followed by the formation of a complex to unwind the damaged portion and excise a 24-32 oligonucleotide section that contains the lesion. Finally, the excised nucleotides are resynthesized and ligated. Two NER sub-pathways exist with partly distinct substrate specificity: global genome nucleotide excision repair (GGR) surveys the entire genome for distorting lesions and transcription-coupled repair (TCR) focuses specifically in the transcribed strand of expressed genes, by targeting damage that blocks elongating RNA polymerases. In total more than 30 proteins participate in NER [126]. The genes involved in GGR are DNA damage recognition by XPC-HR23B complex, lesion demarcation and verification by a TFIIH complex, assembly of a pre-incision complex (RPA, XPA and XPG), DNA opening by XPB and XPD helicases, dual incision by ERCC1-XPF and XPG endonucleases, release of the excised oligomer, repair synthesis to fill in the resulting gap, and ligation by ligase I. Defects in the proteins involved in NER result in three autosomal recessive disorders XP, CS, and TTD.

The most relevant class of chemotherapeutics associated with NER is the platinum-based group of agents. Platinum-based chemotherapy has been used for the treatment of a wide variety of solid tumours including lung, head and neck, ovarian, cervical, and testicular cancer for many years [127]. These agents interact with DNA to form predominantly intra-strand cross-link DNA adducts that trigger a series of intracellular events that ultimately result in cell death. The most studied platinum based cancer therapeutics are cisplatin and the less toxic carboplatin and oxaliplatin, but there has been a resurgence in the development of platinum based drugs, and more platinum based chemotherapeutics are in clinical trials [128].

The basic mechanism of action of cisplatin (and carboplatin) involves covalent binding to purine DNA bases: platinum binding to the N7 position of the imidazole ring of the purine bases of DNA — guanine (G) and adenine (A) — to form either monofunctional or bifunctional adducts. In the case of cisplatin, most occur on the same DNA strand and involve bases adjacent to one another, and are therefore known as intra-strand adducts or crosslinks, namely GpG 1,2 intra-strand (60–65% of all adducts) and ApG 1,2 intra-strand (20–25%) which primarily leads to cellular apoptosis [128]. These DNA lesions are repaired by the NER pathway.

Cisplatin has been used successfully as therapy to treat metastatic testicular cancer with >90 % cure rate. The high sensitivity of testicular tumour cells is attributed to reduced DNA-repair capacity in response to platinum–DNA adducts [129]. Extracts from testicular cancer cells had low constitutive NER capacity and, in particular, low levels of the protein XPA [130]. Further studies have shown low levels of XPA and other NER proteins (XPF and ERCC1), in testicular cancers. This suggested that reducing NER capacity in a cancer holds the potential to sensitize the cancer to cisplatin. Parallel studies revealed that increased DNA repair capacity was a common function in cancers that were inherently resistant to cisplatin or that acquired resistance following treatment [130].

Clinical studies in ovarian cancer patients have correlated increased excision repair cross-complementation group 1 – (*ERCC1)* mRNA levels with clinical resistance to platinum based chemotherapy [131, 132]. In metastatic colorectal cancer patients, higher *ERCC1* expression levels were considered as predictive for lower survival rates when treated with oxaliplatin in combination with 5-fluorouracil, suggesting that enhanced DNA repair decreases the efficacy of platinum-based treatment [133]. In another study a subgroup of 761 patients with metastatic lung cancer treated with a platinum based compound were retrospectively evaluated by immunohistochemical analysis of ERCC1. This study showed a statistically significant survival benefit in patients with low levels of ERCC1 who had received platinum based chemotherapy, compared to patients with low levels of ERCC1 who did not receive chemotherapy and patients with high levels of ERCC1 who received cisplatin chemotherapy [134]. Also, low *ERCC1* expression correlated with prolonged survival after cisplatin plus gemcitabine chemotherapy in non-small cell lung cancer (NSCLC) [135].

Hence, it is hypothesized that high expression of the *ERCC1* gene might be a positive prognostic factor, and could predict decreased sensitivity to platinum-based chemotherapy. Expression of *ERCC1* has been used to stratify patients treated with platinum based chemotherapeutics with some success, and also to predict improved survival in platinum treated patients [136]. Nonetheless, results from the published data are inconsistent. To derive a more precise estimation of the relationship between *ERCC1* and the prognosis and predictive response to chemotherapy of NSCLC, a meta-analysis was performed and results indicated that high *ERCC1* expression might indeed be a favourable prognostic and a drug resistance predictive factor for NSCLC [137].

Other studies with different tumour/chemotherapy associations have shown that *ERCC1* mRNA expression in tumours may be a predictive marker of survival for Irinotecan-resistant metastatic colorectal cancer receiving 5-FU and Oxaliplatin combination chemotherapy [133]. In this study patients whose tumours had low *ERCC1* mRNA expression had a significantly longer median survival than those with high *ERCC1* expression.

Other genes involved in NER have been shown to influence drug resistance. For example, increased expression of excision repair cross-complementation group 4 (*ERCC4* or *XPF*) was observed in hydroxycamptothecin (HCPT) treated bladder cancer tissue compared to untreated samples. Complementary *in vitro* studies showed that enhanced *ERCC4* expression decreased the sensitivity of bladder T24 cells and 5637 cells to HCPT, whereas after gene silencing of *ERCC4* the chemotherapeutic resistance of bladder cancer cells to HCPT was significantly decreased [138].

Since the NER pathway is crucial for the repair of bulky adducts and cross-linking agents in normal cells, the development and application of NER inhibitors in clinical settings is scarce, although preclinical data show that the manipulation of this pathway could be a relevant strategy in cancer chemotherapy. For example, preclinical studies have demonstrated that the chemotherapeutic action of the platinum agent oxaliplatin is improved when combined with cetuximab, a chimeric IgG1 monoclonal antibody targeting the epidermal growth factor receptor. This antibody has been shown to reduce the expression of *ERCC4* and *ERCC1*. A concomitant increase in the accumulation of platinum and apurinic/apyrimidinic sites on DNA during oxaliplatin treatment was observed, thus leading to an increase in apoptosis [139, 140]. These interesting results are suggestive that targeting other pathways that regulate expression of DNA repair genes could be a promising strategy.

7. HR and drug resistance

HR repairs DSBs, which occur through exposure to various chemotherapeutic agents, including IR, topoisomerase inhibitors and DNA crosslinking agents (e.g. mitomycin, camptothecins, etoposide, doxorubicin, daunorubicin and bleomycin). HR is also recruited to restart stalled replication forks and to repair ICL, the repair of which also involves the FA protein complex. HR ensures the accurate repair of DSBs by using a homologous undamaged DNA strand from an intact sister chromatid as a template for DNA polymerase to extend past the break, and is thus restricted to late S and G2 of the cell cycle. Components of HR include the RAD group of proteins (including RAD50, RAD51, RAD52, and RAD54), RPA, XRCC2, XRCC3, and the BRCA proteins. Briefly, HR occurs through pre-synapsis, preparation of a recombination proficient DNA end; synapsis, formation of a joint molecule between the recombination proficient DNA end and a double-stranded homologous template DNA; post-synapsis and resolution, repair of DNA strands and separation of the recombined DNA molecules [19]. DSBs can also be repaired by NHEJ that do not utilize significant homology at the broken ends. In NHEJ, DSBs are recognized by the Ku protein that then binds and activates the protein kinase DNA-PKcs, leading to recruitment and activation of end-processing enzymes, polymerases and DNA ligase IV. Whereas HR is restricted to late S and G2, NHEJ functions in all phases of the cell cycle and ligates broken DNA ends without the need of an undamaged template.

Following DNA lesions initial checkpoint signalling is performed by the kinases ATR and ATM, two phosphatidylinositol 3-kinase family members. Activation of these kinases leads to activation of the effector kinases, checkpoint kinases 1 and 2 (Chk1 and Chk2; serine/threonine kinases). The activated effector kinases are then able to transiently delay cell cycle progression through the G1, S, or the G2 phases so that DNA can be efficiently repaired. The

ATM/Chk2 pathway predominantly regulates the G1 checkpoint and the ATR/Chk1 pathway the S and G2 checkpoints. However, there is cross-talk between the pathways implying a role for both ATR and ATM pathways in all cell cycle checkpoints. In addition to directly regulating the cell cycle, the pathways also affect DNA repair, transcription, chromatin regulation, and cell death. Many details of these pathways are not fully known.

One consequence of DSBs is the localized alteration of chromatin adjacent to DSBs in order to facilitate recruitment of repair proteins. For examples, ATM not only phosphorylates DNA repair proteins recruited to DNA ends but also the histone variant H2AX in nucleosomes adjacent to DSBs, which is also phosphorylated by DNA-dependent protein kinase (DNA-PK), another protein kinase activated by DSBs. Phosphorylated H2AX (known as γ-H2AX) around DSBs facilitates the recruitment of a number of DNA repair proteins and chromatin modulating factors. The presence of large patches of γ-H2AX around a DSB has made its detection by fluorescent tagged antibodies a biomarker for DSBs [141, 142].

There is accumulating evidence for the existence of HR defects not only in familial cancers but also in sporadic cancers. Mutations or epigenetic alterations have been observed in several genes known to be involved in HR regulation and repair, such as *BRCA1* and *BRCA2*. Functional analysis of human cancer tissues and cancer cell lines has revealed HR deficiency, chromatid-type chromosomal aberrations, severe ICL hypersensitivity, and impaired formation of damage-induced RAD51 foci. For example, although genetic mutations in *BRCA1* or *BRCA2* are only rarely found in sporadic tumors, in contrast to familial breast and ovarian cancers, epigenetic gene inactivation of the *BRCA1* promoter is a fairly common event in sporadic breast cancers, with aberrant methylation being detected in 11 to 14% of cases [143]. Non-triple-negative sporadic breast cancers may also harbor HR defects. It has been suggested that ~20% of these cancers are defective in HR as measured by an impaired ability to mount RAD51 foci in response to chemotherapy [144]. There is emerging evidence that approximately up to one fifth of non-familial breast cancers harbour HR defects that may be useful targets for therapy.

The BRCA1 and BRCA2 proteins are involved in HR, in association with FA proteins, forming a complex DNA damage response network [145]. *BRCA1* expression levels have been demonstrated to be a biomarker of survival following cisplatin-based chemotherapy for NSCLC and ovarian cancer, suggesting that this gene could be involved in response to platinum therapy [146, 147]. *In vitro* studies indicate that loss of *BRCA1* or *BRCA2* increases sensitivity to agents that cause DSBs such as bleomycin and/or ICLs including platinum agents. Conversely, loss of *BRCA1* or *BRCA2* may increase resistance to microtubule interfering agents such as taxanes and vincristine [148, 149]. In contrast, *BRCA1* may increase sensitivity to spindle poisons by activating the mitotic spindle checkpoint and signalling through a proapoptotic pathway. This dual role of increasing apoptosis and therefore sensitivity to spindle poisons and also promoting DNA repair and cell survival after treatment with DNA-damaging drugs may influence the response of breast and ovarian cancer cells to treatment [150]. Chemotherapy in breast and ovarian cancers is attained by treatment with platinum based compounds and anthracyclines and also taxanes, all of which induce both

SSBs and DSBs. Efforts are underway to use *BCRA1* as a predictive marker for chemotherapy customization and response [151].

Regarding other types of cancer, *BRCA1* promoter hypermethylation is also found in approximately 5-30% of sporadic ovarian cancers. Also, mutations in *BRCA1* and *BRCA2* have recently been found in up to 20% of unselected ovarian cancers [152]. Thus, these HR deficient cancers are viable targets for synthetic lethality approaches with PARP inhibitors. Defects in the FA/BRCA pathway as well as ATM defects have been described in a variety of other malignancies, such as prostatic adenocarcinoma, colorectal cancer, leukaemia, lymphoma, and medulloblastoma [153, 154]. However, it remains to be seen whether these defects can be targeted effectively in the clinic.

Single-agent chemotherapy with a nitrogen mustard, usually Chlorambucil, is the standard initial therapy for Chronic lymphocytic leukaemia (CLL) and at least 60–80% of patients respond but eventually all patients become resistant to these agents. XRCC3 protein levels and DNA-damage induced RAD51 foci correlates with chlorambucil drug resistance in lymphocytes from CLL patients and with melphalan and cisplatin resistance in epithelial tumor cell lines, indicating that increased HR can be involved in drug resistance to these agents [155].

Another component of the HR pathway, *RAD51,* has been found to be increased in expression in a wide range of human tumors, most likely contributing to drug resistance of these tumors. Over-expression of *RAD51* in different cell types leads to increased homologous recombination and increased resistance to DNA damaging agents to disruption of the cell cycle and apoptotic cell death. *RAD51* expression is increased in p53-negative cells, and since *TP53* is often mutated in tumor cells, there is a tendency for *RAD51* to be overexpressed in tumor cells, leading to increased resistance to DNA damage and drugs used in chemotherapies [156].

Chronic myeloid leukaemia (CML) cell lines expressing the fusion protein BCR-ABL1 utilize an alternative non-homologous end-joining pathway (ALT NHEJ) to repair DSBs. The expression levels of PARP1 and DNA ligase IIIα served as biomarkers to identify a subgroup of CML patients who may be candidates for therapies that target the ALT NHEJ pathway when treatment with TKIs has failed [157]. Tamoxifen- and aromatase-resistant derivatives of MCF7 cells and Estrogen Receptor$^-$/Progesterone Receptor$^-$ (ER$^-$/PR$^-$) cells have higher steady-state levels of DNA ligase IIIα and increased levels of PARP1, another ALT NHEJ component. Notably, therapy-resistant derivatives of MCF7 cells and ER$^-$/PR$^-$ cells exhibited significantly increased sensitivity to a combination of PARP and DNA ligase III inhibitors that increased the number of DSBs. Thus, ALT NHEJ may be a novel therapeutic target in breast cancers that are resistant to frontline therapies and changes in NHEJ protein levels may serve as biomarkers to identify tumors that are candidates for this therapeutic approach [158].

Another interesting approach in this field is to target components of the DNA damage response, namely DNA damage signalling and cell-cycle checkpoints [34]. The members of the phosphatidylinositol (PI) 3-kinase-like (PIKK) family perform crucial roles in the activation of DSB repair pathways, namely in HR and NHEJ. ATM, a PIKK family member, is a DSB signalling protein mainly implicated in the phosphorylation of effector proteins from HR. ATM has been also involved in the regulation of NHEJ. KU55933, 2-morpholin-4-yl-6-thianthren-1-yl-pyran-4-one is a specific and potent small-molecule inhibitor of ATM identified by screening of a combinatorial library. Preclinical studies have shown an increase in the cytotoxicity of multiple chemotherapeutic drugs as doxorubicin, etoposide, camptothecin and ionizing radiation [159, 160] while the UV-induced cellular effects were not modified. More recently, KU60019, an improved analogue of KU55933, was developed. Besides its radiosensitizing properties, *in vitro* studies revealed that KU60019 may also impair the migration and invasion of tumor cells by inhibiting ATM-mediated AKT phosphorylation [161].

DNA-PK is also a target to the development of chemo- and radiosensitizers [162]. In fact, the identification of specific small molecule modulators of DNA-PK [163-165], namely NU7441 and NU7026, was shown to potentiate the effects of ionizing radiation as well as chemotherapeutic agents in human tumor cell lines and in *in vivo* xenograft models.

Another example is the development of AZD7762, which potently inhibits Chk1 and Chk2, abrogates DNA damage-induced S and G2 checkpoints, enhances the efficacy of gemcitabine and topotecan, and modulates downstream checkpoint pathway proteins [166]. This agent has been evaluated in clinical trials, however due to an inadequate response the drug has been discontinued in 2011 (http://www.astrazenecaclinicaltrials.com).

8. MicroRNAs and chemotherapy resistance

MicroRNAs (miRs) are small non-coding RNAs (19 to 25 nucleotides) that regulate gene expression by binding to 3′ untranslated region (UTR) of several mRNAs, thus blocking translation. Recently, it was also shown that miRs can act by binding to open reading frames or 5′UTR of mRNAs, as revised by Iorio and Croce [167]. Due to small size and incomplete complementarity to mRNA, one miR can have a widespread effect on the transcriptome of a cell, acting as a hallmark of several diseases, including cancer. Numerous studies have been performed regarding biogenesis and function of miRs, being revised elsewhere [168-170]. *In vitro* and *in vivo* studies have suggested that miRNAs might be useful as diagnostic and prognostic markers, and recent data suggest that miRNA profiling can be used for tumor typing.

Although it is well established that miRs have an important role in cancer, the complexity of their action remains to be understood and questions regarding their use as cancer therapy need further investigation. The strong pleiotropy of miRs in deregulating normal cellular homeostasis due to misexpression, has led investigators to believe that they are valuable targets for cancer therapy and consequently for drug resistance. Two major approaches for using miRs as therapeutics can be described. First, miRs can be used as single molecules or combined in order to target one or multiple transcripts. In this approach, a miR or a set of miRs are antagonized or mimicked to alter miR levels and consequently change the protein outcome in a cancer cell. Second, miRs can act as modulators of cell sensitivity for cancer therapy [167, 171]. This second approach will be our focus.

Many studies regarding miRs expression patterns in cancer cells have been performed. These studies not only allow investigators to determine novel biomarkers for a better and easily prognostication of several types of cancer but also the functional role of the same miRs. These can give us the knowledge if the loss or gain of miR function interferes with the original balance of protein levels which may be important, but not only, in drug response and consequently lead to drug resistance. Since miRs expression seems to be tissue, grade and stage specific, the ectopic expression or repression of miRs in conjugation with cancer therapy seems promising. For that reason, recent studies that evaluate miR expression profiles of sensitive and resistant cell lines have been made in order to find the key miR signatures related to drug response, which not only promote further analysis of the mechanisms of cancer drug resistance, but also allow the discovery of new drug targets and individualized medicine.

Although the study of the therapeutic potential of miRs is still recent, several studies have been published and compiled. For example, Tian *et al.* [172] and Kutanzi *et al.* [173], published compilations of several studies reporting influence of miRs in mechanisms of drug resistance and how they can modulate drug response in breast cancer.

With regard to miRs and modulation of drug resistance through regulation of DNA damage and repair genes, studies are scarce. It is known that miRs have an important role in DNA damage response, which includes DNA repair [174, 175]. One example how miRs can influence drug resistance through DNA repair is demonstrated by Valerie et al. [73]. The authors showed that miR-21 targets *MSH2* and consequently induces resistance to 5-FU in colorectal cancer. Since miR-21 has a pleiotropic effect, it is possible that it could regulate other genes associated with drug resistance. However, the impact of *MSH2* seems to be of extreme importance on acquired 5-FU resistance since when knocked out cells for *MSH2* are transfected with miR-21, cell-cycle arrest or apoptosis is not altered. These results show that the inhibition of miR-21 action might represent an important treatment to overcome 5-FU resistance. A correlation between miR-21 and *MSH2* in breast cancer was also found [176]. It is recognized that TGF-β is a promoter of miR-21 processing through the interaction with the SMAD and DROSHA complex. On the other hand, *MSH2* is a proven target of miR-21. Thus, TGF-β inhibits *MSH2* gene expression and consequently increases drug resistance. Indeed, to find out if TGF-β contributes to drug resistance through *MSH2*, the authors tested the response of breast cancer MDA-MB-231 cell line to cisplatin, methyl methanesulfonate (MMS) and doxorubicin in the presence and absence of TGF-β. Exposure to TGF-β for 24 h increased cell viability upon treatment with these DNA damaging agents and knock down of *MSH2* induced resistance to both cisplatin and doxorubicin. In contrast, transfection of the anti-miR-21 enhanced the effect of cisplatin in MDA-MB-231 cells.

Another example of miR influence in DNA repair and consequent drug response is miR-182 that targets *BRCA1*. Moskwa and colleagues showed that ectopic expression of miR-182 represses BRCA1 protein expression and sensitizes breast cancer cells to PARP inhibitors [177]. However, PARP inhibitors are mostly used in patients with BRCA1 inherited mutations. Therefore, the question if PARP inhibitors are useful therapeutic drugs in sporadic breast cancer rises. Theoretically, if administrated with BRCA1 repressors such as miR-182, PARP inhibitors can have the same effect as in inherited breast cancer. Further studies need to be done in order to clarify this issue.

As described previously, MGMT has DNA repair activity insofar as it can remove mutagenic O^6-alkylguanine induced by alkylating agents. Although TMZ has been widely used in glioblastoma multiforme (GBM), many patients become or are resistant to this chemotherapy agent, since MGMT can repair the DNA damage induced by TMZ. Epigenetic regulation mechanisms, such as methylation of the *MGMT* gene promoter can sensitize cancer cells to alkylating chemotherapeutic drugs. Glioblastoma patients with positive methylation status of *MGMT* gene promoter have been reported to present a better response to TMZ treatment [44], but these results have not been confirmed by other studies, and therefore results are ambiguous [178]. Indeed, some patients with unmethylated status of *MGMT* promoter gene also have good response to TMZ, which points out to other regulatory mechanisms of *MGMT* expression [179]. Thus, miRs appear as good alternative regulation candidates of *MGMT* expression levels. Recent evidence also suggests that the miR-181 family might be associated to drug response [180]. The authors found that glioblastoma patients with low expression of miR-181b and miR-181c have a better response to TMZ. On the contrary, miR-181d seems to post-transcriptionally regulate *MGMT* since both directly interact and inversely correlate in relation to expression levels [181]. This fact is important because it could be a predictive biomarker for chemotherapy response in GBM. Lakomy and collaborators found that high expression of miR-195 and miR-196b is significantly associated with longer survival of GBM patients and miR-21 and miR-181c with high risk GBM patients [182]. However none of these miRs were associated with *MGMT* gene promoter status.

Altogether the potential for use of miRs in cancer therapy is high, so are the challenges, since each miR can target up to hundreds of mRNA targets. The rapid elucidation of the role they play in cancer suggest that translation of this knowledge will rapidly reach the clinic.

9. Phytochemicals as alternative therapies against drug resistance

As discussed previously, frequently novel therapeutics that show promising results in preclinical assays reveal unacceptable toxicity in clinical trials. Since cancer cells frequently present deregulation of multiple cellular pathways, targeting multiple pathways seems more promising than using single agents that target single pathways. In recent years natural dietary compounds such as curcumin, resveratrol and soy isoflavones such as genistein, have received attention due to the fact that they frequently target multiple cell signalling pathways, including the cell cycle, apoptosis, proliferation, survival, invasion, angiogenesis, metastasis and inflammation. Thus their use in chemoprevention has gained attention [183, 184]. Additionally, since most of the cancer drugs developed have been deliberately directed toward specific molecular targets that are involved in one way or another in enabling particular cellular functions, in response to monotherapy cancer cells may reduce their dependence on a particular proficiency (e.g. a single repair pathway), becoming more dependent on another, thus contributing to acquire drug resistance. Thus, as an alternative approach, selective co-targeting of multiple core and emerging hallmark proficiencies in mechanism-guided combinations could result in more effective and durable therapies for human cancer [185]. Phytochemicals can be highly pleiotropic, modulating numerous targets, including the activation of transcription factors, receptors, kinases, cytokines, enzymes, and growth factors [186]. Therefore current efforts are highly engaged in discovering natural plant-based chemicals that could assist in the fight against drug resistance.

For example soy isoflavones inhibited APE1 expression in prostate cancer cells in a time- and dose-dependent manner, whereas IR up-regulated expression of this BER gene, in response to DNA damage [187-190]. Pretreatment of cancer cells with soy isoflavones inhibited the increase in expression of APE1, and enhanced the efficacy of chemotherapy and radiation therapy of multiple cancers models *in vitro* and *in vivo*, possibly through down-regulation of this DNA repair gene [188]. Another phytochemical, resveratrol, was also shown to inhibit APE1 endonuclease activity and render melanoma cells more sensitive to treatment with the alkylating agent dacarbazine [191]. Thus both resveratrol and isoflavones such as genistein can have therapeutic potential as an APE inhibitor. A series of analogs of resveratrol have been generated in recent years, which exhibit increased potency and/or a range of selective activities compared to the parental compound resveratrol, and possibly improved pharmacokinetic properties [192]. A clinical trial of resveratrol in colon cancer has recently been completed (http://www.clinicaltrials.gov).

Resveratrol can also increase *BRCA1* and *BRCA2* expression, although no effect is seen at the protein level [193]. An increase in BRAC1 expression can lead to increased arrest of cells in the G2 phase, thus making them much more sensitive to conventional therapy. One common chemotherapeutic drug is doxorubicin, which predominantly induces DNA damage in G2 phase cells [194]. Resveratrol, curcumin and the naturally occurring flavolignan deoxypodophyllotoxin [195] can induce G2/M cell cycle arrest, and alter the expression of cell cycle regulatory proteins, thus allowing doxorubicin to induce lesions and as a consequence enhance the apoptotic effect [186, 196, 197]. Le Corre *et al.*, also demonstrated that resveratrol has an effect on the expression of genes implicated in the regulation of BRCA1 protein functions and in multiple nuclear processes modulated by BRCA1 in human breast cancer and fibrocystic breast cells [198]. One of the mechanisms by which resveratrol can enhance *BRAC1* expression is by association with BRCA1, repressing the aromatic hydrocarbon receptor (AhR). AhR binds many natural dietary bioactive compounds therefore combination diets with AhR antagonists may offer the advantage of higher cancer prevention efficacies [199]. In HR-deficient tumours, patients with heterozygous mutations in the HR genes *BRCA1* and *BRCA2* develop breast and ovarian tumours with functional loss of HR activity, and deficiency in this pathway may dictate the sensitivity of tumours to certain DNA-damaging agents and this may be another possible approach to test natural compounds to overcome resistance, and once more enhance combinatory strategies to optimize treatment outcome [32].

Recently an extract of neem leaves was characterized and a significant up-regulation of genes associated with metabolism, inflammation and angiogenesis, such as *HMOX1* and

AKR was observed. However genes associated with cell cycle, DNA replication, recombination, and repair functions were down-regulated [200]. One study analysed 531 compounds derived from plants and found no correlation with genes involved in NER (*ERCC1, XPA, XPC, DDB2, ERCC4, ERCC5*) or BER (*MPG, APE1, OGG1, XRCC1, LIG3, POLB*). It is possible that natural compounds may target different molecular pathways from those of standard anti-tumor drugs, hence if DNA repair is involved in the development of resistance to established anticancer drugs, natural compounds may be attractive sources of novel drugs suitable to treat drug resistant tumours, with the advantage of having reduced side effects [201].

Likewise, most plant derivatives can act as antioxidants and some of them can increase human *MGMT* expression (e.g. curcumin, silymarin, sulforaphane and resveratrol) beyond its steady-state levels, having a role in cancer chemoprevention [202]. Additionally, both *BRCA1* and *MGMT* genes are susceptible to hypermethylation, and green tea polyphenols and bioflavonoids have been shown to reverse the effects of DNA hypermethylation [203].These results suggest that some dietary compounds may have a potential demethylating effect, and could be promising adjuvants to chemotherapy in drug resistant settings.

Another issue in cancer chemotherapy is the use of monotherapy *vs* combined therapy, and several studies have been performed regarding possible combinatory chemotherapy with natural compounds (less aggressive than the majority of chemotherapeutic drugs), albeit in preclinical settings, *e.g.* silibinin extract [204], ixabepilone [205] and curcumin [206]. Some of these agents are being evaluated in clinical trials. Silibinin strongly synergized the growth-inhibitory effect of doxorubicin in prostate carcinoma cells, which was associated with a strong G2-M arrest followed by apoptosis [204]. Ixabepilone, an analogue of the natural product epothilone B, is already indicated for the treatment of locally advanced or metastatic breast cancer in the US. In a phase III trial in women with locally advanced or metastatic breast cancer that were pretreated with, or resistant to, anthracyclines (e.g. doxorubicin) and resistant to taxanes, progression-free survival was significantly longer in ixabepilone plus capecitabine recipients compared with recipients of capecitabine monotherapy [205]. Combination therapy using curcumin with gemcitabine-based chemotherapy, in a phase I/II study, in patients with pancreatic cancer warrants further investigation into its efficacy [206].

Finally, an interesting recent development concerns the observation that miRs could be regulated by natural agents, leading to the inhibition of cancer cell growth, epithelial to mesenchymal transition (EMT), drug resistance, and metastasis [207]. For most epithelial tumors, progression toward malignancy is accompanied by a loss of epithelial differentiation and a shift toward mesenchymal phenotype [185]. During the acquisition of EMT characteristics, cancer cells lose the expression of proteins that promote cell-cell contact, such as E-cadherin and γ-catenin, and gain the expression of mesenchymal markers, such as vimentin, fibronectin, and N-cadherin, leading to enhanced cancer cell migration and invasion. It has been shown that down-regulation or the loss in the expression of the miR-200 family is associated with EMT. Gemcitabine-resistant pancreatic cells having EMT characteristics showed low expression of the miR-200 family and miR-200 is lost in invasive breast cancer cell lines with mesenchymal phenotype. Hence the interesting observation that isoflavone could induce miR-200 expression in gemcitabine-resistant pancreatic cells, resulting in altered cellular morphology from mesenchymal-to-epithelial appearance and induced E-cadherin distribution that is more similar to epithelial-like cells. Likewise, let-7 has been found to regulate cell proliferation and differentiation, and inhibit the expression of multiple oncogenes, including ras and myc, and again it was observed that isoflavone could significantly up-regulate the expression of let-7 family, suggesting that this phytochemical could reverse EMT characteristics in part due to the up-regulation of let-7 [207]. Other reports have shown that curcumin, isoflavone, indole-3-carbinol (I3C), 3,3′-diindolylmethane (DIM), (−)-epigallocatechin-3-gallate (EGCG) or resveratrol, can alter miRNA expression profiles, leading to the inhibition of cancer growth, induction of apoptosis, reversal of EMT phenotype, and increasing drug sensitivity [208].

It remains to be seen if phytochemicals can affect miRs that regulate DNA repair pathways, but since any given miR can target several transcripts, this regulation is highly likely. Overall, natural compounds, may have an important role in chemoprevention and in combined therapy, and may prevent resistance to chemotherapy [188, 189, 208-210].

10. Conclusion and future directions

As discussed in this chapter, the ultimate target of chemotherapy and radiotherapy is the cancer cell, and use of DNA damaging agents is justifiable since most of these cells are highly cycling cells. The targeting of DNA repair pathways is but one of the many strategies developed in the fight against cancer. Cancer cells frequently possess altered DNA repair capacities, and this can be put to use in the clinic. Thus the quest for specific therapies that target DNA repair has produced many potentially useful agents (Table 1). Using such agents can theoretically increase the efficacy of existing chemotherapy and/or radiotherapy. Nevertheless, the same difficulties encountered by all other alternative strategies are also arising when we disrupt DNA repair processes.

The success of these agents ultimately will depend on our basic knowledge of the various DNA repair processes present in a given cell type or tissue. Not all DNA repair pathways are present in all tissues, as evidenced by the fact that mutations in specific pathways give rise preferentially to certain tumour types and not others. Secondly, the success will also depend on the specific genomic and genetic landscape of each tumour, implying that different combinations of inhibitors and chemical agents shall have to be tailored to each tumour. We are still far from achieving this goal, but great strides have been taken in the past years. Thirdly, we shall have to redirect the strategy to discover a "cure for cancer" and instead follow strategies that allow us to accompany the inevitable and inexorable evolution of the cancer cell and consistently find and implement more and more targeted therapies, even if these strategies lead us to return to abandoned therapies. The resurgence of drug holidays, in which a therapy is abandoned temporarily to be taken up after a certain period, not unlike what can be adopted with antibiotics, is one such strategy. In this case the absence of a selective pressure imposed by a specific agent may lead cancer cells to lose resistance to this agent, making them again vulnerable to the same agent. This strategy has been followed in certain cancers and could be adapted in others, with the advantage of offering reduced time on chemotherapy, reduced cumulative toxic effects, and improved quality of life [211, 212].

Target	Drug	Condition or tumor	Combination therapy agent(s)	Phase of clinical trial planned, ongoing or recently completed*	Reference
MGMT	O^6-Benzylguanine	Multiple Myeloma and Plasma Cell Neoplasm Glioblastoma, Gliosarcoma Melanoma Colorectal Cancer	Carmustine Temodar Carmustine Carmustine	Phase II completed Phase II completed Phase II completed Phase II completed	www.cancer.gov
PARP1	AZD-2281/ KU59436 (Olaparib)	Triple Negative Breast Cancer Triple Negative Metastatic Breast Cancer Known BRCA Ovarian Cancer or Known BRCA/ Triple Neg. Breast Cancer	Cisplatin Paclitaxel	Phase I/II active Phase I/II completed	www.astrazeneca.com
	AG014699/ PF-01367338 (Rucaparib)	Solid tumors Melanoma	Temozolomide Various agents	Phase I completed Phase II ongoing	www.pfizer.com
	INO-1001	Melanoma	Temozolomide	Phase I terminated	www.inotekcorp.com
	BSI-201/ (Iniparib)	Uterine Carcinosarcoma	Carboplatin, Paclitaxel,	Phase II active	www.biparsciences.com www.sanofi.com
		Breast Cancer	Gemcitabine/ Carboplatin	Phase II completed Phase III active	
	ABT-888/ (Veliparib)	Breast cancer	Carboplatin Temozolomide	Phase II active	www.abbott.com
		Prostate Cancer	Temozolomide	Phase I active	
		Melanoma	Temozolomide	Phase II active	
		Various cancers	Various agents	Phase I/II active	
	MK4827	Solid BRCA Ovarian	Single agent Various agents	Phase I ongoing	www.merck.com
	CEP-9722	Solid tumours	TMZ Various agents	Phase I	www.cephalon.com www.tevapharm.com
	GPI 1016/ E7016	Solid tumours	TMZ Various agents	Phase I	www.eisai.com
	LT673	Hematological cancers Solid tumours	Various agents	Phase I ongoing	www.bmrn.com
	NMS-P118			Preclinical; highly selective against PARP-5 (tankyrase)	www.nervianoms.com
BER	Methoxyamine/ TRC-102	Advanced refractory solid cancers Hematological cancers	Pemetrexed TMZ Fludarabine	Phase I active Phase I ongoing	www.traconpharma.co m
ATM Kinase	KU55933			Preclinical	www.astrazeneca.com
CHK1	AZD7762				www.astrazeneca.com
	PF-00477736				www.pfizer.com
	XL844				www.exelixis.com
FA	Curcumin	Gastrointestinal cancers		Phase II	

Target	Drug	Condition or tumor	Combination therapy agent(s)	Phase of clinical trial planned, ongoing or recently completed*	Reference
Pathway					
c-ABL	Imatinib	Various solid tumours		Phase III	www.novartis.com
EGFR	Erlotinib	NSCLC	Monotherapy or combination	Phase II/III	www.gene.com
	Gefinitib				www.astrazeneca.com

* As of 10 September 2012, http://clinicaltrials.gov

Table 1. Targeted therapeutics in development, in clinical use or in clinical trials*.

This leads to the final and perhaps most challenging problem in the development of agents that modulate DNA repair, which is toxicity to normal cells, in particular to the hematopoietic system and the gastrointestinal epithelia. Various strategies are being followed to minimize toxicity, which include the intermittent administration during therapy, mentioned above, alternating with other therapies, using highly localized radiotherapy together with inhibitors to minimize collateral damage, and using inhibitors as single agents [213, 214]. Altogether, the combined use of the various weapons at our disposal in a coordinated, comprehensive fashion could effectively lead to improved patient treatment.

Acknowledgements

This work was supported by grants PTDC/SAUGMG/71720/2006 from Fundação de Ciência e Tecnologia (FCT), and PEst-OE/SAU/UI0009/2011-12 from FCT. M.G. was supported by CIENCIA 2008 (FCT). CIGMH is supported by FCT. B.G. (SFRH/BD/64131/2009), P.G. (SFRH/BD/70293/2010) and C.M. (SFRH/BD/ 81097/2011) are supported by Ph.D. grants from FCT.

Author details

António S. Rodrigues[1*], Bruno Costa Gomes[1], Célia Martins[1], Marta Gromicho[1], Nuno G. Oliveira[2], Patrícia S. Guerreiro[2] and José Rueff[1]

*Address all correspondence to: sebastiao.rodrigues@fcm.unl.pt

1 CIGMH – Department of Genetics, Faculty of Medical Sciences, Universidade Nova de Lisboa, Lisboa, Portugal

2 Research Institute for Medicines and Pharmaceutical Sciences (iMed.UL), UL, Faculty of Pharmacy, Universidade de Lisboa, Lisboa, Portugal

References

[1] Friedberg EC. DNA Repair And Mutagenesis: ASM Press; 2006.

[2] Hoeijmakers J. Genome maintenance mechanisms for preventing cancer. Nature. 2001;411:366 - 74.

[3] Harper JW, Elledge SJ. The DNA Damage Response: Ten Years After. Molecular cell. 2007;28(5):739-45.

[4] Lin Z, Nei M, Ma H. The origins and early evolution of DNA mismatch repair genes —multiple horizontal gene transfers and co-evolution. Nucleic Acids Research. 2007;35(22):7591-603.

[5] Lehmann A, McGibbon D, Stefanini M. Xeroderma pigmentosum. Orphanet Journal of Rare Diseases. 2011;6(1):70.

[6] Paradiso A, Formenti S. Hereditary breast cancer: clinical features and risk reduction strategies. Annals of Oncology. 2011;22(suppl 1):i31-i6.

[7] Hoeijmakers JHJ. DNA Damage, Aging, and Cancer. New England Journal of Medicine. 2009;361(15):1475-85.

[8] Lengauer C, Kinzler KW, Vogelstein B. Genetic instabilities in human cancers. Nature. 1998;396(6712):643-9.

[9] Loeb LA. A Mutator Phenotype in Cancer. Cancer Research. 2001;61(8):3230-9.

[10] Lagerwerf S, Vrouwe MG, Overmeer RM, Fousteri MI, Mullenders LHF. DNA damage response and transcription. DNA Repair. 2011;10(7):743-50.

[11] Rodrigues AS, Dinis, J., Gromicho, M., Martins, M., Laires, A. and Rueff, J.. Genomics and Cancer Drug Resistance. Current Pharmaceutical Biotechnology. 2012;13(5): 651-73.

[12] Gillet J-P, Gottesman MM. Mechanisms of Multidrug Resistance in Cancer Multi-Drug Resistance in Cancer. In: Zhou J, editor.: Humana Press; 2010. p. 47-76.

[13] O'Connor MJ, Martin NMB, Smith GCM. Targeted cancer therapies based on the inhibition of DNA strand break repair. Oncogene. 2007;26(56):7816-24.

[14] Al-Ejeh F, Kumar R, Wiegmans A, Lakhani SR, Brown MP, Khanna KK. Harnessing the complexity of DNA-damage response pathways to improve cancer treatment outcomes. Oncogene. 2010;29(46):6085-98.

[15] Hurley LH. DNA and its associated processes as targets for cancer therapy. Nat Rev Cancer. 2002;2(3):188-200.

[16] Kokkinakis DM, Ahmed MM, Delgado R, Fruitwala MM, Mohiuddin M, Albores-Saavedra J. Role of O6-Methylguanine-DNA Methyltransferase in the Resistance of Pancreatic Tumors to DNA Alkylating Agents. Cancer Research. 1997;57(23):5360-8.

[17] Sancar A, Lindsey-Boltz LA, Ünsal-Kaçmaz K, Linn S. Molecular Mechanisms of Mammalian DNA repair and the DNA Damage Checkpoints. Annual Review of Biochemistry. 2004;73(1):39-85.

[18] Lieberman HB. DNA Damage Repair and Response Proteins as Targets for Cancer Therapy. Current Medicinal Chemistry. 2008;15(4):360-7.

[19] Jackson SP, Bartek J. The DNA-damage response in human biology and disease. Nature. 2009;461(7267):1071-8.

[20] Schofield M, Hsieh P. DNA mismatch repair: molecular mechanisms and biological function. Annu Rev Microbiol. 2003;57:579 - 608.

[21] Peltomäki P. Role of DNA Mismatch Repair Defects in the Pathogenesis of Human Cancer. Journal of Clinical Oncology. 2003;21(6):1174-9.

[22] Nguewa PA, Fuertes MA, Valladares B, Alonso C, Pérez JM. Poly(ADP-Ribose) Polymerases: Homology, Structural Domains and Functions. Novel Therapeutical Applications. Progress in Biophysics and Molecular Biology. 2005;88(1):143-72.

[23] Kass EM, Jasin M. Collaboration and competition between DNA double-strand break repair pathways. FEBS Letters. 2010;584(17):3703-8.

[24] Li SX, Sjolund A, Harris L, Sweasy JB. DNA repair and personalized breast cancer therapy. Environmental and Molecular Mutagenesis. 2010;51(8-9):897-908.

[25] Helleday T. Homologous recombination in cancer development, treatment and development of drug resistance. Carcinogenesis. 2010;31(6):955-60.

[26] Bryant HE, Schultz N, Thomas HD, Parker KM, Flower D, Lopez E, et al. Specific killing of BRCA2-deficient tumours with inhibitors of poly(ADP-ribose) polymerase. Nature. 2005;434(7035):913-7.

[27] Farmer H, McCabe N, Lord CJ, Tutt ANJ, Johnson DA, Richardson TB, et al. Targeting the DNA repair defect in BRCA mutant cells as a therapeutic strategy. Nature. 2005;434(7035):917-21.

[28] Chiarugi A. A snapshot of chemoresistance to PARP inhibitors. Trends in Pharmacological Sciences. 2012;33(1):42-8.

[29] Davar D, Beumer JH, Hamieh L, Tawbi H. Role of PARP Inhibitors in Cancer Biology and Therapy. Curr Med Chem. 2012;19(23):3907-21. Epub 2012/07/14.

[30] Fong PC, Boss DS, Yap TA, Tutt A, Wu P, Mergui-Roelvink M, et al. Inhibition of Poly(ADP-Ribose) Polymerase in Tumors from BRCA Mutation Carriers. New England Journal of Medicine. 2009;361(2):123-34.

[31] Kelley MR, Fishel ML. DNA repair proteins as molecular targets for cancer therapeutics. Anti-Cancer Agents in Medicinal Chemistry. 2008;8(4):417-25.

[32] Evers B, Helleday T, Jonkers J. Targeting homologous recombination repair defects in cancer. Trends in Pharmacological Sciences. 2010;31(8):372-80.

[33] Helleday T, Petermann E, Lundin C, Hodgson B, Sharma RA. DNA repair pathways as targets for cancer therapy. Nature Reviews Cancer. 2008;8(3):193-204.

[34] Bouwman P, Jonkers J. The effects of deregulated DNA damage signalling on cancer chemotherapy response and resistance. Nat Rev Cancer. 2012;12(9):587-98.

[35] Longley DB, Johnston PG. Molecular mechanisms of drug resistance. The Journal of Pathology. 2005;205(2):275-92.

[36] Stratton MR, Campbell PJ, Futreal PA. The cancer genome. Nature. 2009;458(7239): 719-24.

[37] Drabløs F, Feyzi E, Aas PA, Vaagbø CB, Kavli B, Bratlie MS, et al. Alkylation damage in DNA and RNA—repair mechanisms and medical significance. DNA Repair. 2004;3(11):1389-407.

[38] Kaina B, Christmann M, Naumann S, Roos WP. MGMT: Key node in the battle against genotoxicity, carcinogenicity and apoptosis induced by alkylating agents. DNA Repair. 2007;6(8):1079-99.

[39] Jacinto FV, Esteller M. MGMT hypermethylation: A prognostic foe, a predictive friend. DNA Repair. 2007;6(8):1155-60.

[40] Margison GP, Santibáñez Koref MF, Povey AC. Mechanisms of carcinogenicity/ chemotherapy by O6-methylguanine. Mutagenesis. 2002;17(6):483-7.

[41] Zaidi NH, Liu L, Gerson SL. Quantitative immunohistochemical estimates of O6-alkylguanine-DNA alkyltransferase expression in normal and malignant human colon. Clinical Cancer Research. 1996;2(3):577-84.

[42] Lee SM, Rafferty JA, Elder RH, Fan CY, Bromley M, Harris M, et al. Immunohistological examination of the inter- and intracellular distribution of O6-alkylguanine DNA-alkyltransferase in human liver and melanoma. Br J Cancer. 1992;66(2):355-60.

[43] Augustine CK, Yoo JS, Potti A, Yoshimoto Y, Zipfel PA, Friedman HS, et al. Genomic and Molecular Profiling Predicts Response to Temozolomide in Melanoma. Clinical Cancer Research. 2009;15(2):502-10.

[44] Hegi ME, Liu L, Herman JG, Stupp R, Wick W, Weller M, et al. Correlation of O6-Methylguanine Methyltransferase (MGMT) Promoter Methylation With Clinical Outcomes in Glioblastoma and Clinical Strategies to Modulate MGMT Activity. Journal of Clinical Oncology. 2008;26(25):4189-99.

[45] Hegi ME, Diserens A-C, Gorlia T, Hamou M-F, de Tribolet N, Weller M, et al. MGMT Gene Silencing and Benefit from Temozolomide in Glioblastoma. New England Journal of Medicine. 2005;352(10):997-1003.

[46] Hegi ME, Diserens A-C, Godard S, Dietrich P-Y, Regli L, Ostermann S, et al. Clinical Trial Substantiates the Predictive Value of O-6-Methylguanine-DNA Methyltransferase Promoter Methylation in Glioblastoma Patients Treated with Temozolomide. Clinical Cancer Research. 2004;10(6):1871-4.

[47] Hegi ME, Sciuscio D, Murat A, Levivier M, Stupp R. Epigenetic Deregulation of DNA Repair and Its Potential for Therapy. Clinical Cancer Research. 2009;15(16): 5026-31.

[48] Suzuki T, Nakada M, Yoshida Y, Nambu E, Furuyama N, Kita D, et al. The Correlation between Promoter Methylation Status and the Expression Level of O6-Methylguanine-DNA Methyltransferase in Recurrent Glioma. Japanese Journal of Clinical Oncology. 2011;41(2):190-6.

[49] Esteller M, Hamilton SR, Burger PC, Baylin SB, Herman JG. Inactivation of the DNA repair gene O6-methylguanine-DNA methyltransferase by promoter hypermethylation is a common event in primary human neoplasia. Cancer Res. 1999;59(4):793-7. Epub 1999/02/24.

[50] Nakada M, Furuta T, Hayashi Y, Minamoto T, Hamada J-i. The strategy for enhancing temozolomide against malignant glioma. Frontiers in Oncology. 2012;2.

[51] Quinn JA, Desjardins A, Weingart J, Brem H, Dolan ME, Delaney SM, et al. Phase I Trial of Temozolomide Plus O6-Benzylguanine for Patients With Recurrent or Progressive Malignant Glioma. Journal of Clinical Oncology. 2005;23(28):7178-87.

[52] Maki Y, Murakami J, Asaumi J-i, Tsujigiwa H, Nagatsuka H, Kokeguchi S, et al. Role of O6-methylguanine–DNA methyltransferase and effect of O6-benzylguanine on the anti-tumor activity of cis-diaminedichloroplatinum(II) in oral cancer cell lines. Oral oncology. 2005;41(10):984-93.

[53] Batts E, Maisel C, Kane D, Liu L, Fu P, O'Brien T, et al. O^6-benzylguanine and BCNU in multiple myeloma: a phase II trial. Cancer Chemotherapy and Pharmacology. 2007;60(3):415-21.

[54] Ranson M, Hersey P, Thompson D, Beith J, McArthur GA, Haydon A, et al. Randomized Trial of the Combination of Lomeguatrib and Temozolomide Compared With Temozolomide Alone in Chemotherapy Naive Patients With Metastatic Cutaneous Melanoma. Journal of Clinical Oncology. 2007;25(18):2540-5.

[55] Khan OA, Ranson M, Michael M, Olver I, Levitt NC, Mortimer P, et al. A phase II trial of lomeguatrib and temozolomide in metastatic colorectal cancer. Br J Cancer. 2008;98(10):1614-8.

[56] Tawbi HA, Villaruz L, Tarhini A, Moschos S, Sulecki M, Viverette F, et al. Inhibition of DNA repair with MGMT pseudosubstrates: phase I study of lomeguatrib in combination with dacarbazine in patients with advanced melanoma and other solid tumours. Br J Cancer. 2011;105(6):773-7.

[57] Ranson M, Middleton MR, Bridgewater J, Lee SM, Dawson M, Jowle D, et al. Lomeguatrib, a potent inhibitor of O6-alkylguanine-DNA-alkyltransferase: phase I safety, pharmacodynamic, and pharmacokinetic trial and evaluation in combination with temozolomide in patients with advanced solid tumors. Clin Cancer Res. 2006;12(5): 1577-84. Epub 2006/03/15.

[58] Caporaso P, Turriziani M, Venditti A, Marchesi F, Buccisano F, Tirindelli MC, et al. Novel role of triazenes in haematological malignancies: Pilot study of Temozolomide, Lomeguatrib and IL-2 in the chemo-immunotherapy of acute leukaemia. DNA Repair. 2007;6(8):1179-86.

[59] Sabharwal A, Corrie PG, Midgley RS, Palmer C, Brady J, Mortimer P, et al. A phase I trial of lomeguatrib and irinotecan in metastatic colorectal cancer. Cancer Chemother Pharmacol. 2010;66(5):829-35. Epub 2009/12/30.

[60] Kaina B, Margison GP, Christmann M. Targeting O(6)-methylguanine-DNA methyltransferase with specific inhibitors as a strategy in cancer therapy. Cell Mol Life Sci. 2010;67(21):3663-81. Epub 2010/08/19.

[61] Koch D, Hundsberger T, Boor S, Kaina B. Local intracerebral administration of O^6-benzylguanine combined with systemic chemotherapy with temozolomide of a patient suffering from a recurrent glioblastoma. Journal of Neuro-Oncology. 2007;82(1): 85-9.

[62] Jiricny J. The multifaceted mismatch-repair system. Nat Rev Mol Cell Biol. 2006;7:335 - 46.

[63] Li G. Mechanisms and functions of DNA mismatch repair. Cell Res. 2008;18:85 - 98.

[64] Aaltonen L, Peltomaki P, Leach F, Sistonen P, Pylkkanen L, Mecklin J, et al. Clues to the pathogenesis of familial colorectal cancer. Science. 1993;260(5109):812-6.

[65] Boland CR, Thibodeau SN, Hamilton SR, Sidransky D, Eshleman JR, Burt RW, et al. A National Cancer Institute Workshop on Microsatellite Instability for Cancer Detection and Familial Predisposition: Development of International Criteria for the Determination of Microsatellite Instability in Colorectal Cancer. Cancer Research. 1998;58(22):5248-57.

[66] Aebi S, Kurdi-Haidar B, Gordon R, Cenni B, Zheng H, Fink D, et al. Loss of DNA Mismatch Repair in Acquired Resistance to Cisplatin. Cancer Research. 1996;56(13): 3087-90.

[67] Hawn MT, Umar A, Carethers JM, Marra G, Kunkel TA, Boland CR, et al. Evidence for a Connection between the Mismatch Repair System and the G2 Cell Cycle Checkpoint. Cancer Research. 1995;55(17):3721-5.

[68] Lage H, Dietel M. Involvement of the DNA mismatch repair system in antineoplastic drug resistance. Journal of cancer research and clinical oncology. 1999;125(3):156-65.

[69] Diouf B, Cheng Q, Krynetskaia NF, Yang W, Cheok M, Pei D, et al. Somatic deletions of genes regulating MSH2 protein stability cause DNA mismatch repair deficiency and drug resistance in human leukemia cells. Nat Med. 2011;17(10):1298-303.

[70] Kaplan E, Gunduz U. Expression analysis of TOP2A, MSH2 and MLH1 genes in MCF7 cells at different levels of etoposide resistance. Biomed Pharmacother. 2012;66(1):29-35. Epub 2012/01/31.

[71] Povey AC, Badawi AF, Cooper DP, Hall CN, Harrison KL, Jackson PE, et al. DNA Alkylation and Repair in the Large Bowel: Animal and Human Studies. The Journal of Nutrition. 2002;132(11):3518S-21S.

[72] Maxwell JA, Johnson SP, McLendon RE, Lister DW, Horne KS, Rasheed A, et al. Mismatch Repair Deficiency Does Not Mediate Clinical Resistance to Temozolomide in Malignant Glioma. Clinical Cancer Research. 2008;14(15):4859-68.

[73] Valeri N, Gasparini P, Braconi C, Paone A, Lovat F, Fabbri M, et al. MicroRNA-21 induces resistance to 5-fluorouracil by down-regulating human DNA MutS homolog 2 (hMSH2). Proceedings of the National Academy of Sciences. 2010;107(49): 21098-103.

[74] Robertson A, Klungland A, Rognes T, Leiros I. DNA Repair in Mammalian Cells. Cellular and Molecular Life Sciences. 2009;66(6):981-93.

[75] Wallace SS, Murphy DL, Sweasy JB. Base excision repair and cancer. Cancer Letters. 2012(0).

[76] Srivastava DK, Husain I, Arteaga CL, Wilson SH. DNA polymerase β expression differences in selected human tumors and cell lines. Carcinogenesis. 1999;20(6):1049-54.

[77] Tang J-b, Svilar D, Trivedi RN, Wang X-h, Goellner EM, Moore B, et al. N-methylpurine DNA glycosylase and DNA polymerase β modulate BER inhibitor potentiation of glioma cells to temozolomide. Neuro-Oncology. 2011;13(5):471-86.

[78] Dinis J, Silva V, Gromicho M, Martins C, Laires A, Tavares P, et al. DNA damage response in imatinib resistant chronic myeloid leukemia K562 cells. Leuk Lymphoma. 2012;53(10):2004-14. Epub 2012/04/06.

[79] Moore DH, Michael H, Tritt R, Parsons SH, Kelley MR. Alterations in the Expression of the DNA Repair/Redox Enzyme APE/ref-1 in Epithelial Ovarian Cancers. Clinical Cancer Research. 2000;6(2):602-9.

[80] Kelley MR, Cheng L, Foster R, Tritt R, Jiang J, Broshears J, et al. Elevated and Altered Expression of the Multifunctional DNA Base Excision Repair and Redox Enzyme Ape1/ref-1 in Prostate Cancer. Clinical Cancer Research. 2001;7(4):824-30.

[81] Wang D, Luo M, Kelley MR. Human apurinic endonuclease 1 (APE1) expression and prognostic significance in osteosarcoma: enhanced sensitivity of osteosarcoma to DNA damaging agents using silencing RNA APE1 expression inhibition. Mol Cancer Ther. 2004;3(6):679-86. Epub 2004/06/24.

[82] Robertson KA, Bullock HA, Xu Y, Tritt R, Zimmerman E, Ulbright TM, et al. Altered Expression of Ape1/ref-1 in Germ Cell Tumors and Overexpression in NT2 Cells Confers Resistance to Bleomycin and Radiation. Cancer Research. 2001;61(5):2220-5.

[83] Bobola MS, Finn LS, Ellenbogen RG, Geyer JR, Berger MS, Braga JM, et al. Apurinic/Apyrimidinic Endonuclease Activity Is Associated with Response to Radiation and

Chemotherapy in Medulloblastoma and Primitive Neuroectodermal Tumors. Clinical Cancer Research. 2005;11(20):7405-14.

[84] Silber JR, Bobola MS, Blank A, Schoeler KD, Haroldson PD, Huynh MB, et al. The Apurinic/Apyrimidinic Endonuclease Activity of Ape1/Ref-1 Contributes to Human Glioma Cell Resistance to Alkylating Agents and Is Elevated by Oxidative Stress. Clinical Cancer Research. 2002;8(9):3008-18.

[85] Bapat A, Fishel ML, Kelley MR. Going ape as an approach to cancer therapeutics. Antioxidants & redox signaling. 2009;11(3):651-68. Epub 2008/08/22.

[86] Bapat A, Glass LS, Luo M, Fishel ML, Long EC, Georgiadis MM, et al. Novel small-molecule inhibitor of apurinic/apyrimidinic endonuclease 1 blocks proliferation and reduces viability of glioblastoma cells. J Pharmacol Exp Ther. 2010;334(3):988-98. Epub 2010/05/28.

[87] Taverna P, Liu L, Hwang HS, Hanson AJ, Kinsella TJ, Gerson SL. Methoxyamine potentiates DNA single strand breaks and double strand breaks induced by temozolomide in colon cancer cells. Mutat Res. 2001;485(4):269-81. Epub 2001/10/05.

[88] Rinne M, Caldwell D, Kelley MR. Transient adenoviral N-methylpurine DNA glycosylase overexpression imparts chemotherapeutic sensitivity to human breast cancer cells. Mol Cancer Ther. 2004;3(8):955-67. Epub 2004/08/10.

[89] Yan L, Bulgar A, Miao Y, Mahajan V, Donze JR, Gerson SL, et al. Combined treatment with temozolomide and methoxyamine: blocking apurininc/pyrimidinic site repair coupled with targeting topoisomerase IIalpha. Clin Cancer Res. 2007;13(5): 1532-9. Epub 2007/03/03.

[90] Fishel ML, He Y, Smith ML, Kelley MR. Manipulation of base excision repair to sensitize ovarian cancer cells to alkylating agent temozolomide. Clin Cancer Res. 2007;13(1):260-7. Epub 2007/01/04.

[91] Liu L, Yan L, Donze JR, Gerson SL. Blockage of abasic site repair enhances antitumor efficacy of 1,3-bis-(2-chloroethyl)-1-nitrosourea in colon tumor xenografts. Mol Cancer Ther. 2003;2(10):1061-6. Epub 2003/10/28.

[92] Bulgar AD, Weeks LD, Miao Y, Yang S, Xu Y, Guo C, et al. Removal of uracil by uracil DNA glycosylase limits pemetrexed cytotoxicity: overriding the limit with methoxyamine to inhibit base excision repair. Cell Death Dis. 2012;3:e252. Epub 2012/01/13.

[93] Taverna P, Hwang HS, Schupp JE, Radivoyevitch T, Session NN, Reddy G, et al. Inhibition of base excision repair potentiates iododeoxyuridine-induced cytotoxicity and radiosensitization. Cancer Research. 2003;63(4):838-46.

[94] Yan T, Seo Y, Schupp JE, Zeng XH, Desai AB, Kinsella TJ. Methoxyamine potentiates iododeoxyuridine-induced radiosensitization by altering cell cycle kinetics and enhancing senescence. Molecular Cancer Therapeutics. 2006;5(4):893-902.

[95] Weiss G, Gordon M, Rosen L, Savvides P, Adams B, Alvarez D, et al. Final results from a phase I study of oral TRC102 (methoxyamine HCl), an inhibitor of base-excision repair, to potentiate the activity of pemetrexed in patients with refractory cancer. [abstract]. J Clin Oncol. 2010;28(15s):abstract 2576.

[96] Sawides P, Xu Y, Liu L, Bokar J, Silverman P, Dowlati A, et al. Pharmacokinetic profile of the base-excision repair inhibitor methoxyamine-HCl (TRC102; MX) given as an one-hour intravenous infusion with temozolomide (TMZ) in the first-in-human phase I clinical trial. [abstract]. J Clin Oncol 2010;28(15s):abstract e13662.

[97] Mohammed MZ, Vyjayanti VN, Laughton CA, Dekker LV, Fischer PM, Wilson DM, 3rd, et al. Development and evaluation of human AP endonuclease inhibitors in melanoma and glioma cell lines. Br J Cancer. 2011;104(4):653-63. Epub 2011/01/27.

[98] Zawahir Z, Dayam R, Deng J, Pereira C, Neamati N. Pharmacophore guided discovery of small-molecule human apurinic/apyrimidinic endonuclease 1 inhibitors. J Med Chem. 2009;52(1):20-32. Epub 2008/12/17.

[99] Simeonov A, Kulkarni A, Dorjsuren D, Jadhav A, Shen M, McNeill DR, et al. Identification and characterization of inhibitors of human apurinic/apyrimidinic endonuclease APE1. PLoS One. 2009;4(6):e5740. Epub 2009/06/02.

[100] Seiple LA, Cardellina JH, 2nd, Akee R, Stivers JT. Potent inhibition of human apurinic/apyrimidinic endonuclease 1 by arylstibonic acids. Mol Pharmacol. 2008;73(3): 669-77. Epub 2007/11/29.

[101] Rai G, Vyjayanti VN, Dorjsuren D, Simeonov A, Jadhav A, Wilson DM, et al. Synthesis, Biological Evaluation, and Structure-Activity Relationships of a Novel Class of Apurinic/Apyrimidinic Endonuclease 1 Inhibitors. Journal of Medicinal Chemistry. 2012;55(7):3101-12.

[102] Srinivasan A, Wang L, Cline C, Xie Z, Sobol RW, Xie X, et al. Identification and Characterization of Human Apurinic/Apyrimidinic Endonuclease-1 Inhibitors. Biochemistry. 2012;[Epub ahead of print].

[103] Luo M, Kelley MR. Inhibition of the human apurinic/apyrimidinic endonuclease (APE1) repair activity and sensitization of breast cancer cells to DNA alkylating agents with lucanthone. Anticancer Res. 2004;24(4):2127-34. Epub 2004/08/28.

[104] Naidu MD, Agarwal R, Pena LA, Cunha L, Mezei M, Shen M, et al. Lucanthone and its derivative hycanthone inhibit apurinic endonuclease-1 (APE1) by direct protein binding. PLoS One. 2011;6(9):e23679. Epub 2011/09/22.

[105] Madhusudan S, Smart F, Shrimpton P, Parsons JL, Gardiner L, Houlbrook S, et al. Isolation of a small molecule inhibitor of DNA base excision repair. Nucleic Acids Res. 2005;33(15):4711-24. Epub 2005/08/23.

[106] Horton JK, Joyce-Gray DF, Pachkowski BF, Swenberg JA, Wilson SH. Hypersensitivity of DNA polymerase beta null mouse fibroblasts reflects accumulation of cytotoxic

repair intermediates from site-specific alkyl DNA lesions. DNA Repair. 2003;2(1): 27-48.

[107] Hu HY, Horton JK, Gryk MR, Prasad R, Naron JM, Sun DA, et al. Identification of small molecule synthetic inhibitors of DNA polymerase beta by NMR chemical shift mapping. J Biol Chem. 2004;279(38):39736-44. Epub 2004/07/20.

[108] Barakat K, Gajewski M, Tuszynski JA. DNA Repair Inhibitors: The Next Major Step to Improve Cancer Therapy. Curr Top Med Chem. 2012;12(12):1376-90.

[109] Javle M, Curtin NJ. The role of PARP in DNA repair and its therapeutic exploitation. Brit J Cancer. 2011;105(8):1114-22.

[110] Plummer R, Jones C, Middleton M, Wilson R, Evans J, Olsen A, et al. Phase I Study of the Poly (ADP-Ribose) Polymerase Inhibitor, AG014699, in Combination with Temozolomide in Patients with Advanced Solid Tumors. Clin Cancer Res. 2008;14(23): 7917-23.

[111] Underhill C, Toulmonde M, Bonnefoi H. A review of PARP inhibitors: from bench to bedside. Annals of Oncology. 2011;22(2):268-79.

[112] Ashworth A. A Synthetic Lethal Therapeutic Approach: Poly(ADP) Ribose Polymerase Inhibitors for the Treatment of Cancers Deficient in DNA Double-Strand Break Repair. Journal of Clinical Oncology. 2008;26(22):3785-90.

[113] de Bono JS, Ashworth A. Translating cancer research into targeted therapeutics. Nature. 2010;467(7315):543-9.

[114] Rouleau M, Patel A, Hendzel MJ, Kaufmann SH, Poirier GG. PARP inhibition: PARP1 and beyond. Nat Rev Cancer. 2010;10(4):293-301.

[115] Calvert H, Azzariti A. The clinical development of inhibitors of poly(ADP-ribose) polymerase. Annals of Oncology. 2011;22(suppl 1):i53-i9.

[116] Yap TA, Sandhu SK, Carden CP, de Bono JS. Poly(ADP-Ribose) polymerase (PARP) inhibitors: Exploiting a synthetic lethal strategy in the clinic. CA: A Cancer Journal for Clinicians. 2011;61(1):31-49.

[117] Kummar S, Chen A, Parchment R, Kinders R, Ji J, Tomaszewski J, et al. Advances in using PARP inhibitors to treat cancer. BMC medicine. 2012;10(1):25.

[118] Bryant HE, Helleday T. Inhibition of poly (ADP-ribose) polymerase activates ATM which is required for subsequent homologous recombination repair. Nucleic Acids Res. 2006;34(6):1685-91. Epub 2006/03/25.

[119] Mendes-Pereira AM, Martin SA, Brough R, McCarthy A, Taylor JR, Kim JS, et al. Synthetic lethal targeting of PTEN mutant cells with PARP inhibitors. EMBO Mol Med. 2009;1(6-7):315-22. Epub 2010/01/06.

[120] Leung M, Rosen D, Fields S, Cesano A, Budman DR. Poly(ADP-ribose) polymerase-1 inhibition: preclinical and clinical development of synthetic lethality. Mol Med. 2011;17(7-8):854-62. Epub 2011/03/23.

[121] Tutt A, Robson M, Garber JE, Domchek SM, Audeh MW, Weitzel JN, et al. Oral poly(ADP-ribose) polymerase inhibitor olaparib in patients with BRCA1 or BRCA2 mutations and advanced breast cancer: a proof-of-concept trial. Lancet. 2010;376(9737):235-44. Epub 2010/07/09.

[122] Sultana R, McNeill DR, Abbotts R, Mohammed MZ, Zdzienicka MZ, Qutob H, et al. Synthetic lethal targeting of DNA double-strand break repair deficient cells by human apurinic/apyrimidinic endonuclease inhibitors. Int J Cancer. 2012. Epub 2012/03/02.

[123] Guha M. PARP inhibitors stumble in breast cancer. Nat Biotechnol. 2011;29(5):373-4.

[124] Dent R, Lindeman G, Clemons M, Wildiers H, Chan A, McCarthy N, et al. Safety and efficacy of the oral PARP inhibitor olaparib (AZD2281) in combination with paclitaxel for the first- or second-line treatment of patients with metastatic triple-negative breast cancer: Results from the safety cohort of a phase I/II multicenter trial [abstract]. J Clin Oncol 2010;28(15s):abstr 1018.

[125] Gelmon KA, Tischkowitz M, Mackay H, Swenerton K, Robidoux A, Tonkin K, et al. Olaparib in patients with recurrent high-grade serous or poorly differentiated ovarian carcinoma or triple-negative breast cancer: a phase 2, multicentre, open-label, non-randomised study. The Lancet Oncology. 2011;12(9):852-61.

[126] Wood RD, Mitchell M, Lindahl T. Human DNA repair genes, 2005. Mutation Research/Fundamental and Molecular Mechanisms of Mutagenesis. 2005;577(1–2): 275-83.

[127] Rabik CA, Dolan ME. Molecular mechanisms of resistance and toxicity associated with platinating agents. Cancer Treatment Reviews. 2007;33(1):9-23.

[128] Kelland L. The resurgence of platinum-based cancer chemotherapy. Nat Rev Cancer. 2007;7(8):573-84.

[129] Köberle B, Grimaldi KA, Sunters A, Hartley JA, Kelland LR, Masters JRW. DNA Repair capacity and cisplatin sensitivity of human testis tumour cells. International Journal of Cancer. 1997;70(5):551-5.

[130] Masters JRW, Koberle B. Curing metastatic cancer: lessons from testicular germ-cell tumours. Nat Rev Cancer. 2003;3(7):517-25.

[131] Dabholkar M, Bostick-Bruton F, Weber C, Bohr VA, Egwuagu C, Reed E. ERCC1 and ERCC2 Expression in Malignant Tissues From Ovarian Cancer Patients. Journal of the National Cancer Institute. 1992;84(19):1512-7.

[132] Reed E. ERCC1 and Clinical Resistance to Platinum-Based Therapy. Clinical Cancer Research. 2005;11(17):6100-2.

[133] Shirota Y, Stoehlmacher J, Brabender J, Xiong Y-P, Uetake H, Danenberg KD, et al. ERCC1 and Thymidylate Synthase mRNA Levels Predict Survival for Colorectal Cancer Patients Receiving Combination Oxaliplatin and Fluorouracil Chemotherapy. Journal of Clinical Oncology. 2001;19(23):4298-304.

[134] Olaussen KA, Dunant A, Fouret P, Brambilla E, André F, Haddad V, et al. DNA Repair by ERCC1 in Non–Small-Cell Lung Cancer and Cisplatin-Based Adjuvant Chemotherapy. New England Journal of Medicine. 2006;355(10):983-91.

[135] Lord RVN, Brabender J, Gandara D, Alberola V, Camps C, Domine M, et al. Low ERCC1 Expression Correlates with Prolonged Survival after Cisplatin plus Gemcitabine Chemotherapy in Non-Small Cell Lung Cancer. Clinical Cancer Research. 2002;8(7):2286-91.

[136] Weberpals J, Garbuio K, O'Brien A, Clark-Knowles K, Doucette S, Antoniouk O, et al. The DNA repair proteins BRCA1 and ERCC1 as predictive markers in sporadic ovarian cancer. International Journal of Cancer. 2009;124(4):806-15.

[137] Jiang J, Liang X, Zhou X, Huang R, Chu Z, Zhan Q. ERCC1 expression as a prognostic and predictive factor in patients with non-small cell lung cancer: a meta-analysis. Molecular Biology Reports. 2012;39(6):6933-42.

[138] Li J, Zhang J, Liu Y, Ye G. Increased expression of DNA repair gene XPF enhances resistance to hydroxycamptothecin in bladder cancer. Medical science monitor : international medical journal of experimental and clinical research. 2012;18(4):BR156-62. Epub 2012/03/31.

[139] Prewett M, Deevi DS, Bassi R, Fan F, Ellis LM, Hicklin DJ, et al. Tumors Established with Cell Lines Selected for Oxaliplatin Resistance Respond to Oxaliplatin if Combined with Cetuximab. Clinical Cancer Research. 2007;13(24):7432-40.

[140] Balin-Gauthier D, Delord JP, Pillaire MJ, Rochaix P, Hoffman JS, Bugat R, et al. Cetuximab potentiates oxaliplatin cytotoxic effect through a defect in NER and DNA replication initiation. Br J Cancer. 2008;98(1):120-8.

[141] Rogakou EP, Pilch DR, Orr AH, Ivanova VS, Bonner WM. DNA Double-stranded Breaks Induce Histone H2AX Phosphorylation on Serine 139. Journal of Biological Chemistry. 1998;273(10):5858-68.

[142] Paull TT, Rogakou EP, Yamazaki V, Kirchgessner CU, Gellert M, Bonner WM. A critical role for histone H2AX in recruitment of repair factors to nuclear foci after DNA damage. Current biology : CB. 2000;10(15):886-95.

[143] Esteller M, Silva JM, Dominguez G, Bonilla F, Matias-Guiu X, Lerma E, et al. Promoter Hypermethylation and BRCA1 Inactivation in Sporadic Breast and Ovarian Tumors. Journal of the National Cancer Institute. 2000;92(7):564-9.

[144] Graeser M, McCarthy A, Lord CJ, Savage K, Hills M, Salter J, et al. A Marker of Homologous Recombination Predicts Pathologic Complete Response to Neoadjuvant

Chemotherapy in Primary Breast Cancer. Clinical Cancer Research. 2010;16(24): 6159-68.

[145] Wang W. Emergence of a DNA-damage response network consisting of Fanconi anaemia and BRCA proteins. Nat Rev Genet. 2007;8(10):735-48.

[146] Taron M, Rosell R, Felip E, Mendez P, Souglakos J, Ronco MS, et al. BRCA1 mRNA expression levels as an indicator of chemoresistance in lung cancer. Human Molecular Genetics. 2004;13(20):2443-9.

[147] Quinn JE, Carser JE, James CR, Kennedy RD, Harkin DP. BRCA1 and implications for response to chemotherapy in ovarian cancer. Gynecologic Oncology. 2009;113(1): 134-42.

[148] Quinn JE, Kennedy RD, Mullan PB, Gilmore PM, Carty M, Johnston PG, et al. BRCA1 Functions as a Differential Modulator of Chemotherapy-induced Apoptosis. Cancer Research. 2003;63(19):6221-8.

[149] Husain A, He G, Venkatraman ES, Spriggs DR. BRCA1 Up-Regulation Is Associated with Repair-mediated Resistance to cis-Diamminedichloroplatinum(II). Cancer Research. 1998;58(6):1120-3.

[150] Kennedy RD, Quinn JE, Mullan PB, Johnston PG, Harkin DP. The Role of BRCA1 in the Cellular Response to Chemotherapy. Journal of the National Cancer Institute. 2004;96(22):1659-68.

[151] Margeli M, Cirauqui B, Castella E, Tapia G, Costa C, Gimenez-Capitan A, et al. The Prognostic Value of BRCA1 mRNA Expression Levels Following Neoadjuvant Chemotherapy in Breast Cancer. PLoS ONE. 2010;5(3):e9499.

[152] Hennessy BTJ, Timms KM, Carey MS, Gutin A, Meyer LA, Flake DD, et al. Somatic Mutations in BRCA1 and BRCA2 Could Expand the Number of Patients That Benefit From Poly (ADP Ribose) Polymerase Inhibitors in Ovarian Cancer. Journal of Clinical Oncology. 2010;28(22):3570-6.

[153] Weston VJ, Oldreive CE, Skowronska A, Oscier DG, Pratt G, Dyer MJS, et al. The PARP inhibitor olaparib induces significant killing of ATM-deficient lymphoid tumor cells in vitro and in vivo. Blood. 2010;116(22):4578-87.

[154] Offit K, Levran O, Mullaney B, Mah K, Nafa K, Batish SD, et al. Shared Genetic Susceptibility to Breast Cancer, Brain Tumors, and Fanconi Anemia. Journal of the National Cancer Institute. 2003;95(20):1548-51.

[155] Panasci L, Paiement J-P, Christodoulopoulos G, Belenkov A, Malapetsa A, Aloyz R. Chlorambucil Drug Resistance in Chronic Lymphocytic Leukemia. Clinical Cancer Research. 2001;7(3):454-61.

[156] Klein HL. The consequences of Rad51 overexpression for normal and tumor cells. DNA Repair. 2008;7(5):686-93.

[157] Tobin LA, Robert C, Rapoport AP, Gojo I, Baer MR, Tomkinson AE, et al. Targeting abnormal DNA double-strand break repair in tyrosine kinase inhibitor-resistant chronic myeloid leukemias. Oncogene. 2012. Epub 2012/05/30.

[158] Tobin LA, Robert C, Nagaria P, Chumsri S, Twaddell W, Ioffe OB, et al. Targeting abnormal DNA repair in therapy-resistant breast cancers. Molecular cancer research : MCR. 2012;10(1):96-107. Epub 2011/11/25.

[159] Hickson I, Zhao Y, Richardson CJ, Green SJ, Martin NMB, Orr AI, et al. Identification and Characterization of a Novel and Specific Inhibitor of the Ataxia-Telangiectasia Mutated Kinase ATM. Cancer Research. 2004;64(24):9152-9.

[160] Cowell IG, Durkacz BW, Tilby MJ. Sensitization of breast carcinoma cells to ionizing radiation by small molecule inhibitors of DNA-dependent protein kinase and ataxia telangiectsia mutated. Biochemical Pharmacology. 2005;71(1–2):13-20.

[161] Golding SE, Rosenberg E, Valerie N, Hussaini I, Frigerio M, Cockcroft XF, et al. Improved ATM kinase inhibitor KU-60019 radiosensitizes glioma cells, compromises insulin, AKT and ERK prosurvival signaling, and inhibits migration and invasion. Molecular Cancer Therapeutics. 2009;8(10):2894-902.

[162] Shinohara ET, Geng L, Tan J, Chen H, Shir Y, Edwards E, et al. DNA-Dependent Protein Kinase Is a Molecular Target for the Development of Noncytotoxic Radiation–Sensitizing Drugs. Cancer Research. 2005;65(12):4987-92.

[163] Leahy JJJ, Golding BT, Griffin RJ, Hardcastle IR, Richardson C, Rigoreau L, et al. Identification of a highly potent and selective DNA-dependent protein kinase (DNA-PK) inhibitor (NU7441) by screening of chromenone libraries. Bioorganic & Medicinal Chemistry Letters. 2004;14(24):6083-7.

[164] Collis SJ, DeWeese TL, Jeggo PA, Parker AR. The life and death of DNA-PK. Oncogene. 2004;24(6):949-61.

[165] Hardcastle IR, Cockcroft X, Curtin NJ, El-Murr MD, Leahy JJJ, Stockley M, et al. Discovery of Potent Chromen-4-one Inhibitors of the DNA-Dependent Protein Kinase (DNA-PK) Using a Small-Molecule Library Approach. Journal of Medicinal Chemistry. 2005;48(24):7829-46.

[166] Zabludoff SD, Deng C, Grondine MR, Sheehy AM, Ashwell S, Caleb BL, et al. AZD7762, a novel checkpoint kinase inhibitor, drives checkpoint abrogation and potentiates DNA-targeted therapies. Molecular Cancer Therapeutics. 2008;7(9):2955-66.

[167] Iorio MV, Croce CM. MicroRNA dysregulation in cancer: diagnostics, monitoring and therapeutics. A comprehensive review. EMBO Molecular Medicine. 2012;4(3): 143-59.

[168] Bartel D. MicroRNAs: genomics, biogenesis, mechanism, and function. Cell. 2004;116(2):281 - 97.

[169] Bartel D. MicroRNAs: target recognition and regulatory functions. Cell. 2009;136:215 - 33.

[170] Garzon R, Calin GA, Croce CM. MicroRNAs in Cancer. Annual Review of Medicine. 2009;60(1):167-79.

[171] Di Leva G, Briskin D, Croce CM. MicroRNA in cancer: New hopes for antineoplastic chemotherapy. Upsala Journal of Medical Sciences. 2012;117(2):202-16.

[172] Tian W, Chen J, He H, Deng Y. MicroRNAs and drug resistance of breast cancer: basic evidence and clinical applications. Clinical and Translational Oncology. 2012:1-8.

[173] Kutanzi KR, Yurchenko OV, Beland FA, Checkhun VF, Pogribny IP. MicroRNA-mediated drug resistance in breast cancer. Clin Epigenetics. 2011;2(2):171-85. Epub 2011/09/29.

[174] Hu H, Gatti RA. MicroRNAs: new players in the DNA damage response. Journal of Molecular Cell Biology. 2010.

[175] Wouters MD, van Gent DC, Hoeijmakers JHJ, Pothof J. MicroRNAs, the DNA damage response and cancer. Mutation Research/Fundamental and Molecular Mechanisms of Mutagenesis. 2011;717(1–2):54-66.

[176] Yu Y, Wang Y, Ren X, Tsuyada A, Li A, Liu LJ, et al. Context-Dependent Bidirectional Regulation of the MutS Homolog 2 by Transforming Growth Factor β Contributes to Chemoresistance in Breast Cancer Cells. Molecular Cancer Research. 2010;8(12): 1633-42.

[177] Moskwa P, Buffa FM, Pan Y, Panchakshari R, Gottipati P, Muschel RJ, et al. miR-182-Mediated Downregulation of BRCA1 Impacts DNA Repair and Sensitivity to PARP Inhibitors. Molecular cell. 2011;41(2):210-20.

[178] Sadones J, Michotte A, Veld P, Chaskis C, Sciot R, Menten J, et al. MGMT promoter hypermethylation correlates with a survival benefit from temozolomide in patients with recurrent anaplastic astrocytoma but not glioblastoma. European Journal of Cancer. 2009;45(1):146-53.

[179] Stupp R, Hegi ME, Mason WP, van den Bent MJ, Taphoorn MJB, Janzer RC, et al. Effects of radiotherapy with concomitant and adjuvant temozolomide versus radiotherapy alone on survival in glioblastoma in a randomised phase III study: 5-year analysis of the EORTC-NCIC trial. The Lancet Oncology. 2009;10(5):459-66.

[180] Slaby O, Lakomy R, Fadrus P, Hrstka R, Kren L, Lzicarova E, et al. MicroRNA-181 family predicts response to concomitant chemoradiotherapy with temozolomide in glioblastoma patients. Neoplasma. 2010;57(3):264-9. Epub 2010/04/01.

[181] Zhang W, Zhang J, Hoadley K, Kushwaha D, Ramakrishnan V, Li S, et al. miR-181d: a predictive glioblastoma biomarker that downregulates MGMT expression. Neuro-Oncology. 2012;14(6):712-9.

[182] Lakomy R, Sana J, Hankeova S, Fadrus P, Kren L, Lzicarova E, et al. MiR-195, miR-196b, miR-181c, miR-21 expression levels and O-6-methylguanine-DNA methyltransferase methylation status are associated with clinical outcome in glioblastoma patients. Cancer Science. 2011;102(12):2186-90.

[183] Surh Y-J. Cancer chemoprevention with dietary phytochemicals. Nat Rev Cancer. 2003;3(10):768-80.

[184] Khan N, Afaq F, Mukhtar H. Apoptosis by dietary factors: the suicide solution for delaying cancer growth. Carcinogenesis. 2006;28(2):233-9.

[185] Hanahan D, Weinberg Robert A. Hallmarks of Cancer: The Next Generation. Cell. 2011;144(5):646-74.

[186] Anand P, Sundaram C, Jhurani S, Kunnumakkara AB, Aggarwal BB. Curcumin and cancer: An "old-age" disease with an "age-old" solution. Cancer Letters. 2008;267(1): 133-64.

[187] Raffoul JJ, Banerjee S, Che M, Knoll ZE, Doerge DR, Abrams J, et al. Soy isoflavones enhance radiotherapy in a metastatic prostate cancer model. Int J Cancer. 2007;120(11):2491-8. Epub 2007/02/17.

[188] Raffoul JJ, Banerjee S, Singh-Gupta V, Knoll ZE, Fite A, Zhang H, et al. Down-regulation of Apurinic/Apyrimidinic Endonuclease 1/Redox Factor-1 Expression by Soy Isoflavones Enhances Prostate Cancer Radiotherapy In vitro and In vivo. Cancer Research. 2007;67(5):2141-9.

[189] Raffoul JJ, Heydari AR, Hillman GG. DNA Repair and Cancer Therapy: Targeting APE1/Ref-1 Using Dietary Agents. Journal of oncology. 2012;2012:11.

[190] Raffoul JJ, Sarkar FH, Hillman GG. Radiosensitization of prostate cancer by soy isoflavones. Curr Cancer Drug Targets. 2007;7(8):759-65. Epub 2008/01/29.

[191] Yang S, Irani K, Heffron SE, Jurnak F, Meyskens FL. Alterations in the expression of the apurinic/apyrimidinic endonuclease-1/redox factor-1 (APE/Ref-1) in human melanoma and identification of the therapeutic potential of resveratrol as an APE/Ref-1 inhibitor. Molecular Cancer Therapeutics. 2005;4(12):1923-35.

[192] Fulda S. Resveratrol and derivatives for the prevention and treatment of cancer. Drug Discovery Today. 2010;15(17–18):757-65.

[193] Fustier P, Le Corre L, Chalabi N, Vissac-Sabatier C, Communal Y, Bignon YJ, et al. Resveratrol increases BRCA1 and BRCA2 mRNA expression in breast tumour cell lines. Br J Cancer. 2003;89(1):168-72.

[194] Potter AJ, Gollahon KA, Palanca BJA, Harbert MJ, Choi YM, Moskovitz AH, et al. Flow cytometric analysis of the cell cycle phase specificity of DNA damage induced by radiation, hydrogen peroxide and doxorubicin. Carcinogenesis. 2002;23(3): 389-401.

[195] Shin SY, Yong Y, Kim CG, Lee YH, Lim Y. Deoxypodophyllotoxin induces G2/M cell cycle arrest and apoptosis in HeLa cells. Cancer Letters. 2010;287(2):231-9.

[196] Park C, Kim GY, Kim GD, Choi BT, Park YM, Choi YH. Induction of G2/M arrest and inhibition of cyclooxygenase-2 activity by curcumin in human bladder cancer T24 cells. Oncol Rep. 2006;15(5):1225-31. Epub 2006/04/06.

[197] Sa G, Das T. Anti cancer effects of curcumin: cycle of life and death. Cell Division. 2008;3(1):14.

[198] Le Corre L, Fustier P, Chalabi N, Bignon Y-J, Bernard-Gallon D. Effects of resveratrol on the expression of a panel of genes interacting with the BRCA1 oncosuppressor in human breast cell lines. Clinica Chimica Acta. 2004;344(1–2):115-21.

[199] Papoutsis AJ, Lamore SD, Wondrak GT, Selmin OI, Romagnolo DF. Resveratrol Prevents Epigenetic Silencing of BRCA-1 by the Aromatic Hydrocarbon Receptor in Human Breast Cancer Cells. The Journal of Nutrition. 2010;140(9):1607-14.

[200] Mahapatra S, Karnes R, Holmes M, Young C, Cheville J, Kohli M, et al. Novel Molecular Targets of <i>Azadirachta indica Associated with Inhibition of Tumor Growth in Prostate Cancer. The AAPS Journal. 2011;13(3):365-77.

[201] Konkimalla VSB, Wang G, Kaina B, Efferth T. Microarray-based Expression of DNA Repair Genes Does not Correlate with Growth Inhibition of Cancer Cells by Natural Products Derived from Traditional Chinese Medicine. Cancer Genomics - Proteomics. 2008;5(2):79-83.

[202] Niture SK, Velu CS, Smith QR, Bhat GJ, Srivenugopal KS. Increased expression of the MGMT repair protein mediated by cysteine prodrugs and chemopreventative natural products in human lymphocytes and tumor cell lines. Carcinogenesis. 2006;28(2): 378-89.

[203] Aggarwal BB, Shishodia S. Molecular targets of dietary agents for prevention and therapy of cancer. Biochemical Pharmacology. 2006;71(10):1397-421.

[204] Tyagi AK, Singh RP, Agarwal C, Chan DCF, Agarwal R. Silibinin Strongly Synergizes Human Prostate Carcinoma DU145 Cells to Doxorubicin-induced Growth Inhibition, G2-M Arrest, and Apoptosis. Clinical Cancer Research. 2002;8(11):3512-9.

[205] Moen MD. Ixabepilone: In Locally Advanced or Metastatic Breast Cancer. Drugs. 2009;69(11):1471-81 10.2165/00003495-200969110-00006.

[206] Kanai M, Yoshimura K, Asada M, Imaizumi A, Suzuki C, Matsumoto S, et al. A phase I/II study of gemcitabine-based chemotherapy plus curcumin for patients with gemcitabine-resistant pancreatic cancer. Cancer Chemotherapy and Pharmacology. 2011;68(1):157-64.

[207] Li Y, VandenBoom TG, Kong D, Wang Z, Ali S, Philip PA, et al. Up-regulation of miR-200 and let-7 by Natural Agents Leads to the Reversal of Epithelial-to-Mesen-

chymal Transition in Gemcitabine-Resistant Pancreatic Cancer Cells. Cancer Research. 2009;69(16):6704-12.

[208] Li Y, Kong D, Wang Z, Sarkar F. Regulation of microRNAs by Natural Agents: An Emerging Field in Chemoprevention and Chemotherapy Research. Pharmaceutical research. 2010;27(6):1027-41.

[209] Sarkar FH, Li Y. Harnessing the fruits of nature for the development of multi-targeted cancer therapeutics. Cancer Treatment Reviews. 2009;35(7):597-607.

[210] Sarkar FH, Li Y, Wang Z, Kong D, Ali S. Implication of microRNAs in drug resistance for designing novel cancer therapy. Drug resistance updates : reviews and commentaries in antimicrobial and anticancer chemotherapy. 2010;13(3):57-66.

[211] Adams RA, Meade AM, Seymour MT, Wilson RH, Madi A, Fisher D, et al. Intermittent versus continuous oxaliplatin and fluoropyrimidine combination chemotherapy for first-line treatment of advanced colorectal cancer: results of the randomised phase 3 MRC COIN trial. The Lancet Oncology. 2011;12(7):642-53.

[212] Becker A, Crombag L, Heideman DAM, Thunnissen FB, van Wijk AW, Postmus PE, et al. Retreatment with erlotinib: Regain of TKI sensitivity following a drug holiday for patients with NSCLC who initially responded to EGFR-TKI treatment. European journal of cancer (Oxford, England : 1990). 2011;47(17):2603-6.

[213] Kelley MR. Chapter 14 - Future Directions with DNA Repair Inhibitors: A Roadmap for Disruptive Approaches to Cancer Therapy. In: Mark RK, editor. DNA Repair in Cancer Therapy. San Diego: Academic Press; 2012. p. 301-10.

[214] Kelley MR. DNA repair inhibitors: where do we go from here? DNA Repair (Amst). 2011;10(11):1183-5. Epub 2011/10/04.

Chapter 19

DNA Base Excision Repair: Evolving Biomarkers for Personalized Therapies in Cancer

Vivek Mohan and Srinivasan Madhusudan

Additional information is available at the end of the chapter

http://dx.doi.org/10.5772/54607

1. Introduction

DNA repair is critical for maintaining genomic integrity. The DNA damage such as those induced by endogenous processes (methylation, hydroxylation, oxidation by free radicals) or by exogenous agents such as ionizing radiation, environmental toxins, and chemotherapy is processed through the DNA repair machinery in cells. At least six distinct DNA repair pathways have been described. A detailed discussion of individual pathways is beyond the scope of this chapter as several recent excellent reviews on DNA repair are available [1-6]. Briefly, direct repair is involved in the repair of alkylated bases (such as O^6 methyl guanine) by MGMT (O^6 methyl guanine DNA methyl transferases [7-10]. DNA mismatch repair (MMR) corrects base-base mismatches and insertion-deletion loops (IDLs) erroneously generated during DNA replication and by exogenous DNA damage [11-13]. Bulky DNA adducts are processed through the nucleotide excision repair pathway (NER) [14-16]. DNA double strand breaks are repaired through the homologous recombination pathway (predominantly during S-phase of cell cycle) [17-19] or the non-homologous end joining pathway (NHEJ), that operates outside the S-phase of the cell cycle [20-22]. DNA base damage is processed by the base excision repair (BER) machinery. In the current chapter we focus on BER. Evolving preclinical and clinical data suggests that BER factors are likely to be important prognostic, predictive and therapeutic targets in cancer.

2. Base excision repair pathway (BER)

Exogenous as well as endogenously derived reactive metabolites cause DNA damage such as base oxidation, deamination and alkylation. If the damaged bases are left unrepaired, then during replication or transcription misincorporation of erroneous complementary bases usher mutagenesis. For example, reactive oxygen species (ROS) generated during cellular respiration, phagocytosis, inflammation and in tumour hypoxia milieu can lead to base oxidation and generation of oxidised bases such as 8-hydroxyguanine (8-oxoG) [23]. DNA polymerase inserts adenine opposite to 8-oxoG, resulting in GC to AT transversion mutations after replication. Similarly, pyrimidine oxidation leads to the formation of 5-hydroxycytosine (5-OHC) which leads to the insertion of a thymine creating a potential mutagenic lesion [24]. Purine deamination products such as hypoxanthine and xanthine generated from adenine and guanine respectively are highly mutagenic. Hypoxanthine in DNA can cause AT to GC mutations, whereas xanthine generate GC to AT mutations [25]. Deamination of cytosine generates uracil which can occur in DNA at a frequency of upto 100–500 per cell per day. Uracil misincorporation can induce CG to TA transition mutations [26]. Although endogenous *S*-adenosyl methionine (SAM) participates in targeted enzymatic DNA base methylation, non-enzymatic methylation of ring nitrogen of purine base adenine can be cytotoxic[26]. Exogeneous agents that cause base alkylation are common chemotherapeutic agents and include mono functional alkylating agents [27] (e.g. temozolomide, nitrosurea compounds, alkylsulfonates) and bifunctional alkylating agents (e.g. cisplatin, mitomycin C, nitrogen mustards). DNA bases damaged by oxidation, deamination and alkylation produce a non-helix distorting, non-bulky base lesion. Such lesions are the prime repair target of BER [6, 28-30].

BER is a complex process and utilizes a number of enzymes and accessory scaffold proteins (Figure 1). DNA glycosylases, AP endonuclease (APE-1) also called REF-1(Redox Effector Factor-1), DNA Polymerases, flap endonuclease (FEN-1), poly (ADP-ribose) polymerase 1(PARP-1) and DNA ligases are the key enzymes involved in BER. The core enzymes depend on accessory proteins such as X-ray cross complementation group 1 protein (XRCC1), proliferating cell nuclear antigen (PCNA), and protein 9-1-1 for coordinated action. DNA glycosylases initiate BER by excising the damaged base from DNA and generating an abasic site. APE1 hydrolyzes the phosphate bond 5′ to the AP site leaving a 3′-OH group and a 5′-dRP flanking the nucleotide gap. Polymerase β (pol β) excises the 5′-dRP moiety generating a 5′-P. Members of the poly (ADP-ribose) polymerase (PARP) family of proteins get activated by single strand DNA breaks induced by APE1 and catalyze the addition of poly (ADP-ribose) polymers to target proteins, affecting protein-protein interactions. PARP may also be involved in the coordination of BER. At this point, BER can proceed through the short-patch (SP-BER) where pol β introduces a single nucleotide with the help of XRCC1. Ligase-IIIα subsequently seals the DNA nick establishing the phosphodiester DNA backbone. The long patch (LP-BER) processes those lesions that cannot be handled by the short patch such as oxidised AP sites. PCNA mediated Polymerase δ/ε introduces two to eight nucleotides past the abasic site. The resulting overhang DNA is excised by FEN1 endonuclease and the nick is then sealed by DNA ligase I.[28-32]

2.1. BER factors are promising biomarkers in cancer

Prognostic factors are defined as patient and/or cancer characteristics that help to estimate patient survival independent of treatment. Conventionally these include patient age, fitness to withstand treatment toxicity (usually measured as performance status), tumour stage, histological grade, neuro-lymphovascular invasion by cancer cells, presence or absence of certain signal protein expression (for example Her-2 in breast cancer is a poor prognostic marker). Predictive factors are those factors that help estimate the probability of a patient responding to a specific treatment. For example BRAF V 600 gene mutation in patients with metastatic melanoma predicts the response to treatment with Vemurafenib [33].

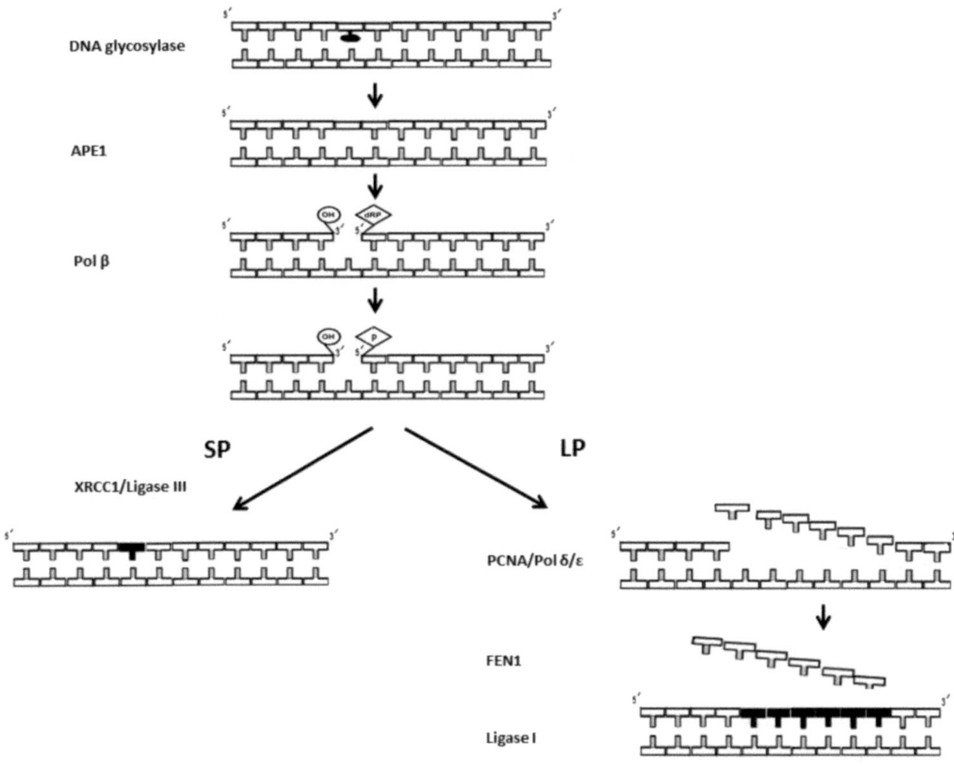

Figure 1. DNA glycosylase initiates BER by excising the damaged base from DNA and generating an abasic site. APE 1 nicks the phosphodiester bond and hydrolyzes the phosphate bond 5′ to the AP site leaving a 3′-OH group and a 5′-dRP flanking the nucleotide gap. Pol β excises the 5′-dRP moiety generating a 5′-P. The short-patch (SP-BER) where pol β introduces a single nucleotide with the help of XRCC1. Ligase-IIIα subsequently seals the DNA nick establishing the phosphodiester DNA backbone. The long patch (LP-BER) processes those lesions that cannot be handled by the short patch such as oxidised AP sites. PCNA mediated Polymerase δ/ε introduces two to eight nucleotides past the abasic site. The resulting overhang DNA is excised by FEN1 endonuclease and the nick is then sealed by DNA ligase I.

Chemotherapeutic agents and ionizing radiation achieve cellular cytotoxicity by inducing DNA base damages [34]. However proficient BER in cancer cells results in therapeutic resistance and adversely impact patient outcomes. BER factors, therefore, are emerging as important prognostic factors as well as predictors of response to cytotoxic therapy in patients. For example, Temozolomide is an effective treatment for patients with high grade brain tumours. It induces *O*6-meG, N3-meA and N7-meG base alkylation lesions which are processed by BER. [35]. Similarly, Melphalan which is used in the treatment of multiple myeloma induces N3-meA lesions that is processed through BER [36]. Thiotepa is used with or without total body irradiation as a conditioning treatment prior to allogeneic or autologous haematopoietic progenitor cell transplantation in haematological diseases in adult and paediatric patients. Thiotepa produces formamidopyrimidine, 7-Methyl-formamidopyrimidine base lesions [37] which is repaired by BER. Dacarbazine is used in the treatment of patients with advanced malignant melanoma and Procarbazine is used in the treatment of Hodgkin's disease. They both produce O6-meG, N7-meG alkylation lesions which are targets of BER [38]. Streptozotocin generates O6-meG, N3-meA, N7-meG metabolites and is used in the treatment of neuroendocrine tumours of the gastro-intestinal (GI) tract.[39]. Platinating agents usually cause DNA inter-strand lesions which are repaired via NER, MMR and HR pathways (see table 1). Cisplatin is used in the treatment of advanced and metastatic non-small cell lung cancer (NSCLC), small cell carcinoma (SCLC), head and neck squamous cell carcinoma (HNSCC), germ cell tumour (GCT), gastric, pancreatic, bladder and cervical cancer. In addition to the DNA inter-strand lesions it also generates reactive oxygen species (ROS) that results in oxidative base damages. ROS derived base damages are also seen in patients with colorectal cancer (CRC) treated with Oxaliplatin. ROS induced base damages are also seen with anthracyclines (epirubicin and doxorubicin), used in the treatment of breast, gastric, ovarian, sarcoma and in haematological malignancy. The antimetabolite gemcitabine used in the treatment of NSCLC, pancreatico-biliary, bladder, breast and ovarian cancer also causes DNA base damage. Given the essential role of BER in cytotoxic therapy induced base damage, it is perhaps not surprising to note that several components of BER are promising prognostic and predictive factors. The following section will review individual markers and their relevance to cancer therapy.

2.2 APE1

Human apurinic / apyrimidinic endonuclease 1 (APE1) is a major endonuclease accounting for > 95% of the cellular AP endonuclease activity in most of the human cell lines [40]. It is also involved in redox regulation of transcription factors [41-43]. APE1 may be expressed in the cytoplasm and/ or in the nucleus of cancer cells. Although the precise sub-cellular localization and regulation is not clearly known, altered localization may have prognostic or predictive significance in patients. Table 2 summarizes the current knowledge regarding the association between APE1 and its role as a biomarker. We recently demonstrated that APE1 is over expressed in Ovarian, Gastro-oesophageal and pancreatico-biliary cancers [44]. In ovarian cancers, nuclear APE1 expression was seen in 71.9% of tumours and correlated with tumour type (P 0.006), optimal debulking (P 0.009), and overall survival (P 0.05). In gastro-oesophageal cancers previously exposed to neoadjuvant chemotherapy, 34.8% of tumours were positive in the nucleus and this correlated with shorter overall survival (P 0.005), whereas cytoplasmic localisation correlated with tumour de-differentiation (P 0.034). In pancreatico-biliary cancer, nuclear staining was seen in 44% of tumours. Absence of cytoplasmic staining was associated with perineural invasion (P 0.007), vascular invasion (P 0.05), and poorly differentiated tumours (P 0.068). [45]. In another study, a cohort of ninety one NSCLC patients treated with radical resection, tumour samples were analyzed for expression of APE1 protein. In patients with adenocarcinoma, cytoplasmic expression of APE1 was significantly associated with poor survival rate in univariate (P 0.01) and multivariate (P 0.07) analyses. In addition, a cytoplasmic expression was also predictive of worse prognosis (log-rank test, P 0.02) in NSCLC patients with lymph node involvement, regardless of the histology [46]. In another study, high nuclear and cytoplasmic APE1 expression was demonstrated in prostate cancer biopsy samples [47].

	DNA damaging agents	**DNA Lesions**	**DNA repair pathways [104, 105]**
1	Mono-functional alkylators: temozolomide, nitrosurea, alkylsulfonates	Small alkyl base adducts	Direct reversal
		Non-bulky alkyl adducts, base oxidation, deamination, AP sites	BER
		Bulky alkyl adducts, helix distorting lesions	NER
		Mismatched base pairs, insertion deletion loops	MMR
		DS DNA break	HR
2	Bi-functional alkylators: cisplatin, mitomycin C, nitrogen mustards, psoralen	DNA cross-links	NER
		DS DNA break	HR
		Bulky adducts	NER, MMR
		Replication fork arrest	BER
3	Anti-metabolites: 5-Fluorouracil (5FU) Thiopurines Folate analogues	Base damages, replication fork arrest	BER
4	Topoisomerase inhibitors: Etoposide	Double-strand breaks Single-strand breaks Replication lesions	HR, NHEJ
5	Replication inhibitors: Hydroxyrea	Double-strand breaks, Replication lesions	HR, NHEJ
6	Ionising Radiation and Radiomimetics: Bleomycin	Single-strand breaks Double-strand breaks Base damage	NHEJ, HR,BER

Abbreviations: BER : base excision repair pathway, NER: Nucleotide excision repair pathway, MMR: mis match repair pathway, HR: homologous repair pathway, NHEJ: non homologous end joining repair pathway.

Table 1. Cytotoxic agents and DNA Repair pathways

	BER factor	Key findings	Year of publication	Ref
1	APE1	Profound deregulation of APE1 acetylation status in triple negative breast cancer	2012	[52]
2	APE1	Ape1 expression elevated by p53 aberration may be used to predict poor survival and relapse in patients with NSCLC.	2012	[53]
3	APE1, XRCC1,HOGG1	APE1 genetic variants may be associated with endometrial cancer in Turkish women.	2012	[54]
4	APE1	APE1 T1349G polymorphism may be a marker for the development of gastric cancer in the Chinese population	2012	[55]
5	APE1, XRCC1	APE1 allele and the 399Gln XRCC1 allele apparently increased the risk of colon cancer	2012	[57]
6	APE1	APE1-656 T "/> G polymorphism has a possible protective effect on cancer risk particularly among Asian populations	2011	[106]
7	APE1, XRCC, OOG1	Polymorphisms within BER genes may contribute to the tumorigenesis of lung cancer.	2011	[59]
8	APE1	Loss of APE1 expression causes cell growth arrest, mitochondrial impairment and apoptosis	2011	[107]
9	APE1	Genetic variant rs1760944 in APE1 was associated with gastric cancer survival in a Chinese population.	2011	[56]
10	APE1, OGG1, XRCC1	APE1 Asp148Glu and hOGG1 Ser326Cys polymorphisms might be associated with increasing risk of CRC in a Turkish population.	2011	[58]
11	APE1	Polymorphisms of APE1 may confer susceptibility to RCC.	2011	[60]
12	APE1	Cytoplasmic localization of APE1 is associated with tumor progression and might be a valuable prognostic marker for EOC	2011	[51]
13	APE1	Genetic variant in the APE1 promoter may modulate risk of glioblastoma.	2011	[61]
14	APE1	Changes in the expression of APE1 might contribute to lip carcinogenesis.	2011	[108]
15	APE1	APE1 inhibitors potentiated the cytotoxicity of alkylating agents in melanoma and glioma cell lines	2011	[109]
16	APE1	Ape1 promotes radiation resistance in pediatric ependymomas	2011	[110]
17	APE1	The APE1 expression had significant correlation with osteosarcoma local recurrence and/or metastasis.	2010	[111]
18	APE1	APE1 may be a potential therapeutic target of MM.	2010	[112]
19	APE1	APE1 is a potential drug target in ovarian, gastro-oesophageal, and pancreatico-biliary cancers.	2010	[44]

	BER factor	Key findings	Year of publication	Ref
20	APE1	Nuclear expression of APE1 in gastro-oesophageal cancer patients treated with neo-adjuvant chemotherapy is associated with poor prognosis.	2010	[45]
21	APE1	Polymorphism in APE1 gene may affect response to palliative chemotherapy in NSCLC.	2009	[113]
22	APE1	Altered APE1 expression found in platinum resistant ovarian cancer patients	2009	[114]
23	APE1	APE1 is up-regulated in the NSCLC	2008	[115]
24	APE1	APE1 activity promotes resistance to radiation plus chemotherapy in Medulloblastomas and primitive neuroectodermaltumours	2005	[116]
25	APE1, XRCC1	High APE1 and XRCC1 protein expression levels predict better cancer-specific survival following radical radiotherapy in bladder cancer.	2005	[77]
26	APE1	APE1 over expression corresponds to poor prognosis in osteosarcoma	2004	[117]
27	APE1	APE 1 activity mediates resistance to alkylating agents and radiation and may be a useful predictor of progression after adjuvant therapy in a subset of gliomas.	2004	[118]
28	APE1	Cytoplasmic localization of APE1 seems to confer a poor survival outcome in patients with lung adenocarcinoma. Cytoplasmic expression of APE1 is a poor prognostic marker in node positive NSCLC regardless of the Histology.	2002	[46]
29	APE1	Increased expression of APE1 is seen in GCT and may be responsible for resistance to treatment with chemotherapy and IR	2001	[119]
30	APE1	APE1 nuclear expression in HNSCC is directly related to resistance to chemoradiotherapy and poor survival	2001	[120]
31	APE1	Increased APE1 cytoplasmic staining in prostate carcinoma as compared to BPH	2001	[47]
32	APE1	APE1 expression in carcinompa of the cervix is a marker of radio-resistance	1998	[121]

Abbreviations: NSCLC: non small cell lung cancer, CRC: colorectal cancer, RCC: renal cell carcinoma, EOC: epithelial ovarian carcinoma, GCT: germ cell tumour, HNSCC: Head and neck Squamous cell carcinoma, BPH: benign prostatic hypertrophy.

Table 2. APE1

The commonly reported APE1 polymorphisms include Asp148Glu, Leu104Arg, Glu126Asp, Arg237Ala, Asp283Gly, Gln51His, Ile64Val, Gly306Glu and Thr141Gly [48-50]. In a cohort of epithelial ovarian cancer patients, cytoplasmic APE1 positivity was significantly associated with higher grade of tumour ($P = 0.002$), advanced stage (III + IV) compared to early stage (I + II) patients (40.7% vs. 11.8%; $P = 0.002$) and a lower survival rate compared to patients with cytoplasmic negative localization ($P < 0.05$) of APE1 [51]. Profound deregulation of APE1 acetylation status in triple negative breast cancer patients has recently been demonstrated. This may be a potential biomarker for breast cancer aggressiveness [52]. In another study, one hundred and twenty five lung tumour samples were analysed for APE1 protein and mRNA expression by immunohistochemistry and real-time RT-PCR respectively. Cytoplasmic APE1 overexpression and p53 aberration was shown to be a potential predictor of poor survival and relapse in patients with NSCLC[53]. In a case control study of one hundred and four endometrial cancer patients with aged matched normal controls, APE1 Asp148Glu genotypes were determined by PCR-RFLP assays. Frequencies of Glu+ and Asp/Glu genotypes of APE1 were found to be more prevalent in patients than controls. This may represent a future diagnostic biomarker in endometrial cancer [54]. In a study involving three hundred and thirty eight newly diagnosed gastric cancer patients and matched control, APE1 genotype T1349G polymorphism was assessed. Compared with the APE1 TT genotype, individuals with the variant TG/GG genotypes had a significantly increased risk of gastric cancer (OR 1.69, 95% CI 1.19-2.40). Further analyses revealed that the variant genotypes were associated with an increased risk for diffuse-type, low depth of tumour infiltration (T1 and T2), and lymph node metastatic gastric cancer. The APE1 T1349G polymorphism may be a biomarker for the development of aggressive gastric cancer [55]. Another cohort of nine hundred and twenty five gastric cancer patients was evaluated for the genetic variant rs1760944 in APE1. Survival analyses showed a statistically significant (P 0.025, log-rank test) differences in median survival time between gastric cancer patients with APE1 rs1760944 TT (55 months) versus those with GT/GG (78 months). These studies suggest that APE1 polymorphism is a potential biomarker in patients with Gastric cancer [56]. In another study, significant differences in the distribution of APE1 genotype were found between colon cancer patients and healthy individuals. The 148Asp APE1 allele apparently increased the risk of colon cancer (OR 1.9-2.3), suggesting it to be a biomarker in colorectal cancer (CRC) [57]. Polymorphisms of APE1 Asp148Glu (rs3136820) were determined by polymerase chain reaction (PCR) and restriction fragment length polymorphism (RFLP) methods in blood samples of seventy nine CRC patients at their initial staging and two hundred and forty seven healthy controls. Frequency of Glu allele of APE1 Asp148Glu was higher in CRC patients than in controls (P 0.006, OR 3.43; 95% CI 1.76-6.70)[58]. In a hospital-based case-control study of four hundred and fifty five lung cancer patients and four hundred and forty three controls, the single nucleotide polymorphisms (SNPs) of APE1 (Asp148Glu and -141T/G) were genotyped and analyzed. In a multivariate logistic regression model, individuals homozygous for the variants APE1 -141GG showed a protective effect for lung cancer (OR 0.62; 95% CI 0.42-0.91; p 0.02). This study indirectly suggests that polymorphism in APE1 genes may be a biomarker and contribute in the pathogenesis of lung cancer [59]. In a case-control study of six hundred and twelve renal cell carcinoma (RCC) patients and six hundred and thirty two age and sex matched healthy controls, APE1 polymorphisms (-656 T>G, rs1760944 and 1349 T>G, rs1130409) were assessed. Compared with 1349 TT/TG genotypes, the variant genotype 1349 GG had a significantly increased risk of RCC (adjusted odds ratio 1.47; 95% CI 1.10-1.95), suggesting a role for APE1 polymorphism as a biomarker in RCC [60]. In a case-control study of seven hundred and sixty six glioma patients and eight hundred and twenty four cancer-free controls APE1/Ref-1 promoter -141T/G variant (rs1760944) was evaluated. Allele G was associated with significant decreased glioblastoma risk (OR 0.80; 95% CI 0.65-0.98; P 0.032) [61].In conclusion emerging studies of APE1 in tumours suggest that APE1 is a promising biomarker in cancer. However, large prospective studies are required to confirm these observations.

2.3. XRCC1

X-ray repair cross-complementing group 1 (XRCC1) is a scaffolding protein and coordinates BER [62]. Cells deficient in XRCC1 are hypersensitive to DNA damaging agents such as ionizing radiation and alkylating agents. Pre-clinically XRCC1 deficiency can induce mutagenesis [63]. Embryonic knock out of XRCC1 is lethal. The most extensively studied polymorphisms of XRCC1 are Arg194Trp, Arg280His, Arg399Gln, Arg399Gln, Pro161Leu and Tyr576S. Ensembl data base records ten somatic mutations and six genetic variations of human XRCC1gene. Table 3 summarizes the current knowledge regarding the association between APE1 and its role as a biomarker. XRCC1 SNPs rs1799782 and rs25487 were investigated using the TaqMan assay in one hundred and eighty five pancreatic cancer cases and one thousand four hundred and sixty five controls. The minor allele, rs25487 was significantly associated with pancreatic cancer risk in the per-allele model (OR 1.29; CI 1.01-1.65; P 0.043). Haplotype analysis of XRCC1 also showed a statistically significant association with pancreatic cancer risk [64]. Endometrial biopsy samples in a case control study assessed the polymorphisms Arg399Gln. Gln/Gln genotype of XRCC1was more prevalent in patients than in controls suggesting XRCC1 polymorphisms as a biomarker in endometrial cancer [54]. In a case control study, polymorphisms of XRCC1 Arg399Gln allele increased the risk of colon cancer (OR 1.5-2.1)[57]. In a cohort of ninety nine advanced colorectal cancer patients treated with oxaliplatin based chemotherapy, polymorphisms of XRCC1 Arg399Gln (G-->A) genotypes were detected by TaqMan-MGB probe allelic discrimination method. Cox proportional hazards model, adjusted for stage, performance status, and chemotherapy regimen, showed that XRCC1 G/G genotype increased the OR significantly (OR 3.555; 95 % CI, 2.119 - 5.963; $P < 0.01$). The result suggests that XRCC1 Arg399Gln polymorphism is associated with response to chemotherapy and time to progression in advanced colorectal cancer patients. This study pointed XRCC1 polymorphism as a predictive biomarker in advanced CRC patients treated with oxaliplatin based chemotherapy [65].

	BER factor	Key findings	Year of publication	Ref
1	XRCC1	XRCC1 polymorphisms affect pancreatic cancer risk in Japanese.	2012	[64]
2	XRCC1	Elevated cancer risk associated with XRCC1 polymorphism.	2012	[66]
3	XRCC1	XRCC1 polymorphism might influence the risk of developing glioma	2012	[68]
4	XRCC1, XRCC3	Polymorphisms in DNA repair genes have roles in the susceptibility and survival of ovarian cancer patients.	2012	[69]
5	XRCC1	XRCC1 polymorphism is associated with significantly increased risk of gastric cancer	2012	[70]
6	XRCC1	High XRCC1 and low ATM were independently associated with poor survival in gastric cancer	2012	[76]
7	XRCC1	XRCC1 polymorphisms affect pancreatic cancer risk in Japanese.	2012	[64]
8	XRCC1	Genetic variations in XRCC1 exhibit variation in the sensitivity to platinum based chemotherapy in NSCLC	2012	[71]
9	XRCC1	Polymorphisms of XRCC1 gene might have contributed to individual susceptibility to lung cancer.	2012	[72]
10	XRCC1	Arg194Trp polymorphism could be associated with nonmelanoma skincancer and extramammary Paget's disease risk in a Japanese population.	2012	[Chiyomaru, 2012 #1047] [122]
11	XRCC1	Polymorphism of XRCC1 Arg399Gln may be a candidate for contributing to the difference in the OS of gemcitabine/platinum-treated advanced NSCLC patients.	2012	[73]
12	XRCC1	XRCC1 Arg399Gln polymorphisms is associated with a response to oxaliplantin-based chemotherapy and time to progression in advanced colorectal cancer in Chinese population.	2012	[65]

	BER factor	Key findings	Year of publication	Ref
13	XRCC1	The 751 Lys/Gln polymorphism of the ERCC2 gene may be linked to endometrial cancer	2012	[Sobczuk, 2012 #1050][123]
14	XRCC1, XRCC3	XRCC1 and XRCC3 gene polymorphisms for risk of colorectal cancer in the Chinese population.	2012	[124]
15	XRCC1	XRCC1 399Gln is an independent unfavourable prognostic factor in unresected NSCLC treated with radiotherapy and chemoradiotherapy	2012	[125]
16	XRCC1	XRCC1-Arg399Cln polymorphism is associated with susceptibility to HCC, and XRCC1 Gln allele genotype showed significant prognostic associations.	2012	[126]
17	XRCC1	XRCC1 -77T"/>C polymorphism is associated with cancer risk, and individuals with XRCC1-77C variant have a significantly higher cancer risk, particularly in the Asian population	2012	[67]
18	XRCC1	XRCC1 protein expressions in tumor is novel candidate prognostic markers and predictive factor for benefit from adjuvant platinum-based chemotherapy in resectable gastric carcinoma.	2012	[75]
19	XRCC1	Genetic polymorphisms in XRCC1 gene might be associated with overall survival and response to platinum-based chemotherapy in lung cancer patients.	2012	[127]
20	XRCC1	XRCC1 T-77C and eNOS G874T may confer an increased risk of acute skin reactions to radiotherapy in breast cancer patients	2012	[128]
21	XRCC1	XRCC1 399Gln/Gln genotype have an increased risk of colorectal cancer	2012	[129]
22	XRCC1	XRCC1 Arg399Gln allele is a risk factor for the development breast cancer, especially among Asian and African populations.	2011	[130]
23	XRCC1	genetic polymorphisms in XRCC1 may affect survival post radiotherapy for localized prostate cancer.	2010	[131]
24	XRCC1	Combined polymorphisms of ERCC1 and XRCC1 may predict OS and response to palliative chemotherapy with FOLFOX / XELOX in metastatic CRC patients	2010	[132]

	BER factor	Key findings	Year of publication	Ref
25	XRCC1	XRCC1 194 CT genotype associated with inferior overall survival in advanced gastric cancer patients treated with Cisplatin-Taxane combined chemotherapy.	2010	[133]
26	XRCC1	XRCC1 codon 194 and codon 399 polymorphisms may predict the sensitivity of advanced NSCLC to palliative chemotherapy treatment with vinorelbine and Cisplatin.	2009	[134]
27	XRCC1	XRCC 1 polymorphism may predict higher response rate to palliative Cisplatin based chemotherapy in NSCLC patients	2009	[135]
28	XRCC1	XRCC1 polymorphism in clinical stage III may be a prognostic survival marker in HNSCC.	2009	[136]
29	XRCC1	SNP of XRCC1 gene at codon 399 influences the response to platinum based neo-adjuvant chemotherapy treatment in patients with cervical cancer.	2009	[137]
30	XRCC1, APE1	Polymorphism in APE1 and XRCC1 may represent prognostic factors in metastatic melanoma.	2009	[138]
31	XRCC1	A rarely occurring XRCC1 variant may predict response to Neoadjuvant chemo-radiotherapy for the treatment of oesophageal cancer.	2009	[139]
32	XRCC1	XRCC1 variant alleles may be associated with shorter overall survival in lung cancer patients	2008	[140]
33	XRCC1	Genotypes of XRCC1 Arginine194Tryptophan and GGH-401Cytosine/Thymine associated with the response to platinum based neo-adjuvant chemotherapy treatment in patients with cervical cancer	2008	[141]
34	XRCC1	XRCC1 variant may predict the risk of recurrence of bladder TCC post BCG treatment.	2008	[142]
35	XRCC1	XRCC1 gene polymorphism may predict survival in good PS advanced Gastric cancer patients treated with Oxalipaltin based palliative chemotherapy.	2007	[143]
36	XRCC1	Polymorphism in XRCC1 gene is a potential prognostic and predictive marker in breast cancer patients treated with adjuvant CMF chemotherapy	2007	[144]

	BER factor	Key findings	Year of publication	Ref
37	XRCC1	XRCC1 polymorphism may predict survival advantage for SCLC and NSCLC patients after platinum based treatment	2007	[145]
38	XRCC1	XRCC1 polymorphism may predict response to palliative FOLFOX and can also be a prognostic survival factor in metastatic colorectal cancer.	2006	[146]
39	XRCC1	Variant alleles of XRCC1 associated with the absence of pathologic complete response and poor survival in oesophageal cancer	2006	[147]
40	XRCC1	XRCC1 polpmorphism may represent a prognostic factor in advanced NSCLC patients treated with palliative Cisplatin and Gemcitabine.	2006	[148]
41	OGG1, LIG3, APE1, POLB, XRCC1, PCNA	XRCC1 polymorphism may be a prognostic factor in patients with CRC	2006	[95]
42	XRCC1	XRCC1-01may predict survival outcome in patients with MBC treated with high dose chemotherapy.	2006	[74]
43	XRCC1	Combined XPD and XRCC1 genotypes might be prognostic factors in muscle-invasive bladder cancer patients treated with CRT.	2006	[149]
44	XRCC1	Polymorphism of XRCC1 R399Q is associated with response to platinum-based NAC in bulky cervical cancer	2006	[150]
45	XRCC1	Polymorphisms in the XRCC1 gene may impact the response rate to platinum based palliative chemotherapy in NSCLC patients.	2004	[151]
46	XRCC1	Polymorphism of XRCC1 gene may be associated with resistance to oxaliplatin/5-FU chemotherapy in advanced colorectal cancer.	2001	[152]

Abbreviations:ATM: ataxia telangiectasia mutated protein, FOLFOX: oxaliplatin and 5FU based chemotherapy, XELOX: oxliplatin and Capecitabine based chemotherapy, TCC: transitional cell carcinoma, BCG: Bacillus Calmette–Guérin, CRT: chemoradiotherapy, MBC: metastatic breast cancer.

Table 3. XRCC1

Meta-analysis of fifty three case-control studies with twenty one thousand three hundred and forty nine cases and twenty three thousand six hundred forty nine controls for XRCC1 Arg280His polymorphism and its cancer risk were estimated using fixed or random effect models. Minor variant His allele and Arg-His/His-His genotypes showed a statistical association with the risk of cancer (OR 1.16; 95% CI 1.08-1.25) [66]. Meta-analysis of thirteen studies involving a total of eleven thousand six hundred and seventy eight individuals showed that there was significant association between the C variant of XRCC1-77T>C polymorphism and cancer risk in all four genetic comparison models (OR C vs. T 1.19; 95% CI 1.07-1.31; P 0.001; OR homozygote model 1.28; 95% CI 1.07-1.52; P 0.007; OR recessive genetic model 1.22; 95% CI 1.04-1.44; P 0.015; OR dominant model 1.21; 95% CI 1.07-1.35, P 0.001). XRCC1 -77T>C polymorphism is associated with cancer risk, and individuals with XRCC1 -77C variant have a significantly higher cancer risk, particularly in the Asian population [67]. Using a PCR-RFLP method, XRCC1 Arg194Trp, Arg280His and Arg399Gln were genotyped in six hundred and twenty four glioma patients and five hundred and eighty healthy controls. Significant differences in the distribution of the Arg399Gln allele were detected between glioma patients and healthy controls by a logistic regression analysis (OR 1.35; 95% CI 1.17-1.68; P 0.001). Arg399Gln variant (allele A) carriers had an increased glioma risk compared to the wild-type (allele G) homozygous carriers (OR 1.40, 95%CI 1.12-1.76, P 0.003)[68]. In a prospective follow-up study, a cohort of three hundred and ten ovarian cancer patients treated with platinum-based chemotherapy between January 2005 to January 2007 were followed up to 2010. Genotyping of XRCC1 and XRCC3 polymorphisms was conducted by TaqMan Gene Expression assays. Lower survival rate in XRCC1 399 Arg/Arg genotype than in Gln/ Gln, with a significant increased risk of death (HR 1.69; 95% CI 1.07-2.78) were observed. However no significant association between XRCC1 Arg194Trp and XRCC1 Arg280His gene polymorphisms and ovarian cancer death was observed. [69]. A multicenter 1:1 matched case- control study of three hundred and seven pairs of gastric cancers patients and controls between October 2010 and August 2011 was undertaken. XRCC1 Arg194Trp and ADPRT Val762Ala were sequenced. Demographic data collected using a self-designed questionnaire. Individuals carrying XRCC1 Trp/Trp or Arg/Trp variant genotype had a significantly increased risk of gastric cancer (OR 1.718; 95% CI, 1.190-2.479). [70]. In a cohort of advanced NSCLC patients treated with platinum based chemotherapy, XRCC1 polymorphism was evaluated. XRCC1 Arg194Arg, FAS-1377GG, and FASL-844T allele displayed no response to platinum, whereas patients with XRCC1 194Trp allele and XPC PAT +/+ had 68.8% response rate to platinum. In Logistic Regression analysis, a significant gene-dosage effect was detected along with the increasing number of favourable genotypes of these four polymorphisms (P 0.00002). Multi-loci analysis showed the importance of genetic variations involved in BER repair and apoptotic pathways in sensitivity of platinum-based chemotherapy in NSCLC [71]. In a meta-analysis of forty four published case-control studies demonstrated that codon 194, codon 399 and -77 T > C polymorphisms of XRCC1 gene might have contributed to individual susceptibility to lung cancer [72]. In a another study, sixty two advanced NSCLC patients in a training set and forty five patients in a validation set treated with gemcitabine/platinum were genotyped for XRCC1 polymorphism. Wild-type genotype of XRCC1 Arg399Gln (G/G) was associated with decreased median overall survival than those carrying variant genotypes (G/A+A/A). In addition, there was a statistically significant longer median OS in patients carrying wild-type ERCC2 Asp312Asn genotype (G/G) (51 months, 95% CI, 19-82 months versus 10 months, log-rank test, P < 0.001) than those carrying heterozygous variant genotypes (G/A). This points out the predictive biomarker status of XRCC1 in platinum treated NSCLC patients[73]. XRCC1 polymorphism is a potential predictive marker of platinum based treatment response in non-small cell lung carcinoma, colorectal carcinoma, advanced gastric, advanced cervical, advanced operable oesophageal cancer. It may also predict response to adjuvant CMF chemotherapy and high dose chemotherapy in breast cancer [74].

In a training and validating cohort of Gastric cancer patients, XRCC1 protein levels were significantly downregulated in gastric cancers compared to adjacent non-cancerous tissues. Low tumour XRCC1 expression significantly correlated with shorter overall survival as well as with clinic-pathologic characteristics in patients without adjuvant treatment. Multivariate regression analysis showed that low XRCC1 expressions, separately and together, were independent negative markers of OS. Adjuvant fluorouracil-leucovorin-oxaliplatin (FLO) significantly improved OS compared with surgery alone (log-rank test, P 0.01). However, this effect was evident only in the XRCC1 low expression group (HR 0.44, 95% CI 0.26-0.75; P 0.002); Adjuvant fluorouracil-leucovorin-platinum (FLP) did not improve OS, except in the patients with low XRCC1 expressions (P 0.024). XRCC1 protein expressions in tumour are novel candidate prognostic markers and predictive factors for benefit from adjuvant platinum-based chemotherapy (FLO or FLP) in patients with resectable gastric carcinoma [75]. SMUG1, FEN1, XRCC1 and ATM are involved in ROS induced oxidative DNA damage repair in gastric cancer patients. High expression of SMUG1, FEN1 and XRCC1 correlated to high T-stage (T3/T4) (P 0.001, 0.005 & 0.02 respectively). High expression of XRCC1 and FEN1 also correlated to lymph node positive disease (P 0.009 and 0.02 respectively). High expression of XRCC1, FEN1 & SMUG1 correlated with poor disease specific survival (P 0.001, 0.006 and 0.05 respectively) and poor disease free survival (P 0.001, 0.001 & 0.02 respectively) [76]. Muscle-invasive transitional cell carcinoma tumour samples from ninety patients treated with radical radiotherapy was evaluated for XRCC1 protein expression. Nuclear staining of XRCC1 was 96.5% (range, 0.6-99.6%). High expression levels of XRCC1 (> or = 95% positivity) were associated with improved patient cancer-specific survival (log-rank, P 0.006) [77].

XRCC1 has shown to be a promising prognostic biomarker in a majority of cancer groups including HNSCC, breast, ovarian, endometrial, cervical, lung, gastric, oesophageal, pancreatic, glial, colorectal, hepatocellular, bladder transitional cell carcinoma, metastatic melanoma and non melanomatous skin cancer.

2.4. FEN1

FEN1 is a structure-specific 5′ endo/exonuclease with a range of functions during DNA repair and replication. It is a BER long patch protein. FEN1 also has a role in the processing of the okazaki lagging DNA strand synthesis. As an endonuclease, FEN1 recognizes double-stranded DNA with a 5′-unannealed flap and makes an endonucleolytic cleavage at the base of the flap. As a 5′ exonuclease, it degrades nucleotides from a nick or a gap. It may also be involved in maintaining stability of telomeres, inhibiting repeat sequence expansion and involved in creation of double-stranded DNA breaks when mammalian cells are subjected to X-ray irradiation[78]. Human flap endonuclease 1 gene has been shown to have 4 somatic mutations, one polymorphism, and two transcripts in the Ensembl data base. In the following section we will review the potential of FEN1 as a prognostic, predictive biomarker and its feasibility as a drug target in cancer treatment (See Table 4).

	BER factor	Key findings	Year of publication	Ref
1	FEN1	Polymorphisms in FEN1 confer susceptibility to gastrointestinal cancers	2012	[79]
2	FEN1	High expression of XRCC1, FEN1 & SMUG1 correlated with poor disease free survival	2012	[76]
3	FEN1	FEN1 protein expression was also associated with poor prognosis in prostatectomy-treated patients. Knock-down of FEN1 with small interfering RNA inhibited the growth of LNCaP cells.	2012	[83]
4	FEN1	Genetic polymorphisms in FEN1 confer susceptibility to lung cancer.	2009	[153]
5	FEN1	FEN1 overexpression is common in testis, lung and brain tumors. Down-regulation of FEN1 by siRNA increased sensitivity to methylating agents (temozolomide, MMS) and cisplatin in LN308 glioma cells	2009	[81]
6	FEN1	RAD54B-deficient human colorectal cancer cells are sensitive to SL killing by reduced FEN1 expression	2009	[85]
7	FEN1	FEN1 is significantly up-regulated in multiple cancers. The overexpression and promoter hypomethylation of FEN1 may serve as biomarkers for monitoring the progression of cancers	2008	[82]
8	FEN1	FEN-1 is overexpressed in prostate cancer and is associated with higher Gleason score.	2006	[84]

Abbreviations: SMUG1: Single-strand selective monofunctional uracil-DNA glycosylase

Table 4. FEN1

Human germ line variants (-69G >A and 4150G > T) in the FEN1 gene have been associated with DNA damage in coke oven workers and lung cancer risk in general populations. This was studied in one thousand eight hundred and fifty gastrointestinal cancer (hepatocellular carcinoma, esophageal cancer, gastric cancer and colorectal cancer) patients and two thousand two hundred and twenty two healthy controls. It was found that the FEN1 -69GG genotypes were significantly correlated to increased risk for developing gastrointestinal cancer compared with the -69AA genotype highlighting FEN1 as an important gene in human gastrointestinal oncogenesis and a potential biomarker [79]. We recently investigated this relationship in a cohort of gastric cancer patients and found high expression of FEN1 correlated to lymph node positive disease with poor disease specific survival and poor disease free survival [76]. In pro-myelocytic leukemia cell line HL-60, gene expression of FEN-1 has been shown to be higher in cells during mitotic phase as compared to cells in the resting phase. FEN1 expression markedly decreases when these cells reach maturity upon induction of terminal differentiation [80]. This study pointed out the relationship between increased FEN1 expression and proliferating cancer cells. Subsequent studies showed increased FEN 1 expression in testis, lung and brain cancer specimens as studied by Western blot analysis and compared with the normal tissue from the same patient. FEN1 over expression was observed in nineteen samples from testicular tumours (mostly seminomas), four samples from NSCLC, nine samples from glioblastoma multiforme and in five samples from astrocytomas. Down regulation of FEN1 expression in LN308 glioblastoma cell line by siRNA resulted in hypersensitivity to cisplatin, temozolomide, nimustine and methyl methanesulfonate (MMS)[81]. Statistically significant increased amount of FEN1 expression has been demonstrated in breast tumor tissue (~2.4 fold, $P< 0.0001$, $n = 50$), uterine tumor tissue (~2.3 fold, $P = 0.0006$, $n = 42$), colon tumor tissue (~1.5 fold, $P < 0.0001$, $n = 35$), stomach tumor tissue (~1.5 fold, $P= 0.0005$, $n = 28$), lung tumor tissue (~1.9 fold, $P = 0.0066$, $n=21$) and kidney tumor tissue (~2.3 fold, $P = 0.0063$, $n = 20$), compared to matched normal tissues[82]. FEN1 also found to be increased in castration refractory prostate cancer (CRPC) cells. The knock-down of FEN1 with si RNA inhibited the growth of these LNCaP cells [83] pointing it as a potential drug target in prostate cancer. In primary prostate cancer from two hundred and forty six patients who had had a radical prostatectomy, FEN-1 nuclear expression correlated with Gleason score. These results suggest that FEN-1 might be a potential marker for selecting patients at high risk and therapy [84]. Interestingly, synthetic lethality (SL) has been observed in RAD54B-deficient human colorectal cancer cell line by iatrogenic reduction of FEN1 expression thus demonstrating it to be a potential novel therapeutic biological target [85].

2.5. Polymerase beta, PCNA

Polymerase beta (pol β) is essential for short patch BER. It is present in all tissues at a lower level [86] and has no cell-cycle dependence. Majority of BER proceeds through the short-patch whereby a single nucleotide is removed and replaced. Unlike other DNA polymerases, pol β has no proof reading capability[87] hence its over expression has the potential for mutagenesis[88, 89]. Proliferating cell nuclear antigen(PCNA) is an accessory protein required for replication by DNA polymerase δ, and as a consequence, PCNA is required during the long patch BER [90]. Lesions left unrepaired by the short patch BER is facilitated by PCNA to switch to the long patch BER. PCNA then helps polymerase δ to excise and replace 2-8 nucleotide patch in the long path of BER. Table 5 summarizes recent insight into the prognostic and predictive significance of pol β and PCNA.

Twenty somatic pol β mutations in prostate tumors are already known. The somatic missense pol β mutations (p.K27N, p.E123K, p.E232K, p.P242R, p.E216K, p.M236L, and the triple mutant p.P261L/T292A/I298T) were assessed *in vitro* for the biochemical properties of the polymerase. Experiments suggest that interfering with normal polymerase beta function may be a frequent mechanism of prostate tumour progression [91].Three non-synonymous single nucleotide substitutions, Gln8Arg, Arg137Gln and Pro242Arg have been identified as polymorphisms in DNA Pol β. The Arg137Gln variant demonstrates significantly reduced polymerase activity and impaired interaction with PCNA, and reduced BER efficiency when assayed in a reconstitution assay or with cellular extracts. Other polymorphisms within DNA Pol β include *A165G* and *T2133C*, which were associated with overall survival in a study of patients with pancreatic cancer [92, 93]. One hundred and fifty two ovarian cancer samples subjected to RT-PCR and sequencing, a variant of polymerase beta (deletion of exon 4-6 and 11-13, comprising of amino acid 63-123, and 208- 304) was detected in heterozygous condition. Statistical analysis showed this variant to be associated with risk of stage IV, endometrioid type ovarian carcinoma[94]. In a case-control study (three hundred and seventy seven cases along with three hundred and twenty nine controls) designed to assess gene-environment interactions, samples were genotyped by use of an oligonucleotide microarray and the arrayed primer extension technique. Twenty-eight single nucleotide polymorphisms in 15 DNA repair genes including pol β P242R were evaluated. It was demonstrated that pol β polymorphism is associated with a decreased risk of colorectal cancer [95]. Pol β over expression reduces the efficacy of anticancer drug therapies including ionizing radiation, bleomycin, monofunctional alkylating agents and cisplatin. Small-scale studies in different cancers showed that pol β is mutated in approximately 30% of tumours. These mutations further lower pol β fidelity in DNA synthesis exposing the genome to serious mutations. These findings suggested pol β to be a promising therapeutic target in cancer treatment [96].

	BER factor	**Key findings**	**Year of publication**	**Ref**
1	Pol beta	variant form of Pol β cDNA is associated with edometrioid type, stage IV ovarian carcinoma	2012	[94]
2	Pol beta	A proportion of prostate cancer patients express functionally important somatic mutations of pol β.	2011	[91]
3	Pol Beta	Over expression of pol β reduces the efficacy of anticancer drug therapies including, Cisplatin, bleomycin, monofunctional alkylating agents and ionizing radiation.	2011	[96]
4	Pol beta, PCNA	More than 30% of human tumors characterized to date express DNA pol β variants, a polymorphism encoding an arginine to glutamine substitution, R137Q, has lower polymerase activity	2009	[92]
4	Pol beta, PCNA	Pancreatic cancer patients carrying at least 1 of the 2 homozygous variant pol β GG or CC genotypes have a significantly better overall survival	2007	[93]
5	OGG1, LIG3, APE1, POLB, XRCC1, PCNA	pol β P242R was also associated with decreased risk of colorectal cancer	2006	[95]

Table 5. Other BER factors

http://dx.doi.org/10.5772/54607

3. Summary and the future developments

Numerous DNA base excision repair proteins are currently under development as potential biomarkers and therapeutic targets. Studies presented above provide compelling evidence that BER factors are promising prognostic and predictive biomarkers in cancer. More recent evidence also suggests that BER is an attractive target for drug discovery. APE1 inhibitors, for example, are currently in development and may have therapeutic application in the near future. [34, 97, 98]. Moreover, DNA polymerase beta inhibitor is also currently under developmental stage and early reports reveal the ability of DNA pol β inhibitors to potentiate the cytotoxicity of alkylating agents [99]. In contrast, several other studies demonstrate that pol β-null cells, although sensitive to temozolomide, are not sensitive to other chemotherapeutic agents such as melphalan, mitozolomide, BCNU, and IR [34, 100, 101]. Therefore further research is warranted to confirm pol β as a drug target in cancer.The principles of synthetic lethality has been transferred from the bench to the bedside with PARP-1 inhibitors in BRCA-deficient (HR-defective) cancer cells [102, 103]. Recent evidence suggests that other factors in BER are also important synthetic lethality targets for personalized cancer therapy.

Author details

Vivek Mohan and Srinivasan Madhusudan*

*Address all correspondence to: srinivasan.madhusudan@nottingham.ac.uk

Translational DNA Repair Group, Academic Unit of Oncology, School of Molecular Medical Sciences, University of Nottingham, Nottingham University Hospitals, Nottingham NG 1PB, UK

References

[1] Friedberg, E. C. A brief history of the DNA repair field. Cell Res, (2008). , 3-7.

[2] Hoeijmakers, J. H. DNA damage, aging, and cancer. N Engl J Med, (2009). , 1475-1485.

[3] Hanawalt, P. C. Subpathways of nucleotide excision repair and their regulation. Oncogene, (2002). , 8949-8956.

[4] Fleck, O, & Nielsen, O. DNA repair. J Cell Sci, (2004). Pt 4): , 515-517.

[5] Essers, J, et al. Homologous and non-homologous recombination differentially affect DNA damage repair in mice. EMBO J, (2000). , 1703-1710.

[6] Kelley, M. R. DNA repair in cancer therapy : molecular targets and clinical applications. 1st ed. (2012). London ; Waltham, MA: Elsevier/Academic Press. xiii, 316 p.

[7] Kokkinakis, D. M, et al. Role of O6-methylguanine-DNA methyltransferase in the resistance of pancreatic tumors to DNA alkylating agents. Cancer Res, (1997). , 5360-5368.

[8] Milsom, M. D, & Williams, D. A. Live and let die: in vivo selection of gene-modified hematopoietic stem cells via MGMT-mediated chemoprotection. DNA Repair (Amst), (2007). , 1210-1221.

[9] Cai, S, et al. Mitochondrial targeting of human O6-methylguanine DNA methyltransferase protects against cell killing by chemotherapeutic alkylating agents. Cancer Res, (2005). , 3319-3327.

[10] Bobola, M. S, et al. O6-Methylguanine-DNA methyltransferase in pediatric primary brain tumors: relation to patient and tumor characteristics. Clin Cancer Res, (2001). , 613-619.

[11] Modrich, P, & Lahue, R. Mismatch repair in replication fidelity, genetic recombination, and cancer biology. Annu Rev Biochem, (1996). , 101-133.

[12] Brown, K. D, et al. The mismatch repair system is required for S-phase checkpoint activation. Nat Genet, (2003). , 80-84.

[13] Charara, M, et al. Microsatellite status and cell cycle associated markers in rectal cancer patients undergoing a combined regimen of 5-FU and CPT-11 chemotherapy and radiotherapy. Anticancer Res, (2004). B): , 3161-3167.

[14] Dip, R, Camenisch, U, & Naegeli, H. Mechanisms of DNA damage recognition and strand discrimination in human nucleotide excision repair. DNA Repair (Amst), (2004). , 1409-1423.

[15] Nouspikel, T. Nucleotide excision repair and neurological diseases. DNA Repair (Amst), (2008). , 1155-1167.

[16] Koberle, B, Roginskaya, V, & Wood, R. D. XPA protein as a limiting factor for nucleotide excision repair and UV sensitivity in human cells. DNA Repair (Amst), (2006). , 641-648.

[17] San FilippoJ., P. Sung, and H. Klein, Mechanism of eukaryotic homologous recombination. Annu Rev Biochem, (2008). , 229-257.

[18] Zou, L. DNA repair: A protein giant in its entirety. Nature, (2010). , 667-668.

[19] Heyer, W. D, et al. Rad54: the Swiss Army knife of homologous recombination? Nucleic Acids Res, (2006). , 4115-4125.

[20] Hartlerode, A. J, & Scully, R. Mechanisms of double-strand break repair in somatic mammalian cells. Biochem J, (2009). , 157-168.

[21] Lieber, M. R, et al. Nonhomologous DNA end joining (NHEJ) and chromosomal translocations in humans. Subcell Biochem, (2010). , 279-296.

[22] Adachi, N, et al. Hypersensitivity of nonhomologous DNA end-joining mutants to VP-16 and ICRF-193: implications for the repair of topoisomerase II-mediated DNA damage. J Biol Chem, (2003). , 35897-35902.

[23] Kasai, H, et al. Hydroxyguanine, a DNA adduct formed by oxygen radicals: its implication on oxygen radical-involved mutagenesis/carcinogenesis. J Toxicol Sci, (1991). Suppl 1: , 95-105.

[24] Lindahl, T. Instability and decay of the primary structure of DNA. Nature, (1993). , 709-715.

[25] Kow, Y. W. Repair of deaminated bases in DNA. Free Radic Biol Med, (2002). , 886-893.

[26] Huffman, J. L, Sundheim, O, & Tainer, J. A. DNA base damage recognition and removal: new twists and grooves. Mutat Res, (2005). , 55-76.

[27] Beranek, D. T. Distribution of methyl and ethyl adducts following alkylation with monofunctional alkylating agents. Mutat Res, (1990). , 11-30.

[28] Sancar, A, et al. Molecular mechanisms of mammalian DNA repair and the DNA damage checkpoints. Annu Rev Biochem, (2004). , 39-85.

[29] Wilson, D. M, & Rd, V. A. Bohr, The mechanics of base excision repair, and its relationship to aging and disease. DNA Repair (Amst), (2007). , 544-559.

[30] Dianov, G. L, et al. Repair of abasic sites in DNA. Mutat Res, (2003). , 157-163.

[31] Almeida, K. H, & Sobol, R. W. A unified view of base excision repair: lesion-dependent protein complexes regulated by post-translational modification. DNA Repair (Amst), (2007). , 695-711.

[32] Fortini, P, & Dogliotti, E. Base damage and single-strand break repair: mechanisms and functional significance of short- and long-patch repair subpathways. DNA Repair (Amst), (2007). , 398-409.

[33] Sosman, J. A, et al. Survival in BRAF advanced melanoma treated with vemurafenib. N Engl J Med, (2012). , 600-mutant, 707-714.

[34] Kelley, M. R, & Fishel, M. L. DNA repair proteins as molecular targets for cancer therapeutics. Anticancer Agents Med Chem, (2008). , 417-425.

[35] Denny, B. J, et al. NMR and molecular modeling investigation of the mechanism of activation of the antitumor drug temozolomide and its interaction with DNA. Biochemistry, (1994). , 9045-9051.

[36] Mchugh, P. J, et al. Excision repair of nitrogen mustard-DNA adducts in Saccharomyces cerevisiae. Nucleic Acids Res, (1999). , 3259-3266.

[37] Xu, Y, et al. Protection of mammalian cells against chemotherapeutic agents thiotepa, 1,3-N,N'-bis(2-chloroethyl)-N-nitrosourea, and mafosfamide using the DNA base excision repair genes Fpg and alpha-hOgg1: implications for protective gene therapy applications. J Pharmacol Exp Ther, (2001). , 825-831.

[38] Pletsa, V, et al. DNA damage and mutagenesis induced by procarbazine in lambda lacZ transgenic mice: evidence that bone marrow mutations do not arise primarily through miscoding by O6-methylguanine. Carcinogenesis, (1997). , 2191-2196.

[39] Drablos, F, et al. Alkylation damage in DNA and RNA--repair mechanisms and medical significance. DNA Repair (Amst), (2004). , 1389-1407.

[40] Demple, B, Herman, T, & Chen, D. S. Cloning and expression of APE, the cDNA encoding the major human apurinic endonuclease: definition of a family of DNA repair enzymes. Proc Natl Acad Sci U S A, (1991). , 11450-11454.

[41] Evans, A. R, Limp-foster, M, & Kelley, M. R. Going APE over ref-1. Mutat Res, (2000). , 83-108.

[42] Mitra, S, et al. Intracellular trafficking and regulation of mammalian AP-endonuclease 1 (APE1), an essential DNA repair protein. DNA Repair (Amst), (2007). , 461-469.

[43] Tell, G, et al. The intracellular localization of APE1/Ref-1: more than a passive phenomenon? Antioxid Redox Signal, (2005). , 367-384.

[44] Al-attar, A, et al. Human apurinic/apyrimidinic endonuclease (APE1) is a prognostic factor in ovarian, gastro-oesophageal and pancreatico-biliary cancers. Br J Cancer, (2010). , 704-709.

[45] Fareed, K. R, et al. Tumour regression and ERCC1 nuclear protein expression predict clinical outcome in patients with gastro-oesophageal cancer treated with neoadjuvant chemotherapy. Br J Cancer, (2010). , 1600-1607.

[46] Puglisi, F, et al. Prognostic significance of Ape1/ref-1 subcellular localization in non-small cell lung carcinomas. Anticancer Res, (2001). A): , 4041-4049.

[47] Kelley, M. R, et al. Elevated and altered expression of the multifunctional DNA base excision repair and redox enzyme Ape1/ref-1 in prostate cancer. Clin Cancer Res, (2001). , 824-830.

[48] Hung, R. J, et al. Genetic polymorphisms in the base excision repair pathway and cancer risk: a HuGE review. Am J Epidemiol, (2005). , 925-942.

[49] Hadi, M. Z, et al. Functional characterization of Ape1 variants identified in the human population. Nucleic Acids Res, (2000). , 3871-3879.

[50] Lu, J, et al. Functional characterization of a promoter polymorphism in APE1/Ref-1 that contributes to reduced lung cancer susceptibility. FASEB J, (2009). , 3459-3469.

[51] Sheng, Q, et al. Prognostic significance of APE1 cytoplasmic localization in human epithelial ovarian cancer. Med Oncol, (2012). , 1265-1271.

[52] Poletto, M, et al. Acetylation on critical lysine residues of Apurinic/apyrimidinic endonuclease 1 (APE1) in triple negative breast cancers. Biochem Biophys Res Commun, (2012). , 34-39.

[53] Wu, H. H, et al. Cytoplasmic Ape1 Expression Elevated by Aberration May Predict Survival and Relapse in Resected Non-Small Cell Lung Cancer. Ann Surg Oncol, (2012). , 53.

[54] Cincin, Z. B, et al. DNA repair gene variants in endometrial carcinoma. Med Oncol, (2012).

[55] Gu, D, et al. The DNA repair gene APE1 T1349G polymorphism and risk of gastric cancer in a Chinese population. PLoS One, (2011). , e28971.

[56] Zhao, Q, et al. A genetic variation in APE1 is associated with gastric cancer survival in a Chinese population. Cancer Sci, (2011). , 1293-1297.

[57] Jelonek, K, et al. Association between single-nucleotide polymorphisms of selected genes involved in the response to DNA damage and risk of colon, head and neck, and breast cancers in a Polish population. J Appl Genet, (2010). , 343-352.

[58] Canbay, E, et al. Association of APE1 and hOGG1 polymorphisms with colorectal cancer risk in a Turkish population. Curr Med Res Opin, (2011). , 1295-1302.

[59] Li, Z, et al. Genetic polymorphism of DNA base-excision repair genes (APE1, OGG1 and XRCC1) and their correlation with risk of lung cancer in a Chinese population. Arch Med Res, (2011). , 226-234.

[60] Cao, Q, et al. Genetic polymorphisms in APE1 are associated with renal cell carcinoma risk in a Chinese population. Mol Carcinog, (2011). , 863-870.

[61] Zhou, K, et al. A genetic variant in the APE1/Ref-1 gene promoter-141T/G may modulate risk of glioblastoma in a Chinese Han population. BMC Cancer, (2011). , 104.

[62] Caldecott, K. W. XRCC1 and DNA strand break repair. DNA Repair (Amst), (2003). , 955-969.

[63] Thompson, L. H, & West, M. G. XRCC1 keeps DNA from getting stranded. Mutat Res, (2000). , 1-18.

[64] Nakao, M, et al. Selected Polymorphisms of Base Excision Repair Genes and Pancreatic Cancer Risk in Japanese. J Epidemiol, (2012).

[65] Lv, H, et al. Genetic Polymorphism of XRCC1 Correlated with Response to Oxaliplatin-Based Chemotherapy in Advanced Colorectal Cancer. Pathol Oncol Res, (2012).

[66] Zhang, K, et al. The XRCC1 Arg280His polymorphism contributes to cancer susceptibility: an update by meta-analysis of 53 individual studies. Gene, (2012).

[67] Wang, Y. G, Zheng, T. Y, & Xrcc, T. C polymorphism and cancer risk: a meta- analysis. Asian Pac J Cancer Prev, (2012). , 111-115.

[68] Wang, D, et al. Genetic polymorphisms in the DNA repair gene XRCC1 and susceptibility to glioma in a Han population in northeastern China: A case-control study. Gene, (2012).

[69] Cheng, C. X, et al. Predictive Value of XRCC1 and XRCC3 Gene Polymorphisms for Risk of Ovarian Cancer Death After Chemotherapy. Asian Pac J Cancer Prev, (2012). , 2541-2545.

[70] Wen, Y. Y, et al. ADPRT Val762Ala and XRCC1 Arg194Trp Polymorphisms and Risk of Gastric Cancer in Sichuan of China. Asian Pac J Cancer Prev, (2012). , 2139-2144.

[71] Liu, L, et al. Multi-loci analysis reveals the importance of genetic variations in sensitivity of platinum-based chemotherapy in non-small-cell lung cancer. Mol Carcinog, (2012).

[72] Dai, L, et al. XRCC1 gene polymorphisms and lung cancer susceptibility: a meta-analysis of 44 case-control studies. Mol Biol Rep, (2012). , 9535-9547.

[73] Liao, W. Y, et al. Genetic polymorphism of XRCC1 Arg399Gln is associated with survival in non-small-cell lung cancer patients treated with gemcitabine/platinum. Journal of thoracic oncology : official publication of the International Association for the Study of Lung Cancer, (2012). , 973-981.

[74] Bewick, M. A, Conlon, M. S, & Lafrenie, R. M. Polymorphisms in XRCC1, XRCC3, and CCND1 and survival after treatment for metastatic breast cancer. J Clin Oncol, (2006). , 5645-5651.

[75] Wang, S, et al. Prognostic and predictive role of JWA and XRCC1 expressions in gastric cancer. Clin Cancer Res, (2012). , 2987-2996.

[76] Abdel-fatah, T, et al. Are DNA repair factors promising biomarkers for personalized therapy in gastric cancer? Antioxid Redox Signal, (2012).

[77] Sak, S. C, et al. APE1 and XRCC1 protein expression levels predict cancer-specific survival following radical radiotherapy in bladder cancer. Clin Cancer Res, (2005). , 6205-6211.

[78] Liu, Y, Kao, H. I, & Bambara, R. A. Flap endonuclease 1: a central component of DNA metabolism. Annu Rev Biochem, (2004). , 589-615.

[79] Liu, L, et al. Functional FEN1 genetic variants contribute to risk of hepatocellular carcinoma, esophageal cancer, gastric cancer and colorectal cancer. Carcinogenesis, (2012). , 119-123.

[80] Kim, I. S, et al. Gene expression of flap endonuclease-1 during cell proliferation and differentiation. Biochim Biophys Acta, (2000). , 333-340.

[81] Nikolova, T, Christmann, M, & Kaina, B. FEN1 is overexpressed in testis, lung and brain tumors. Anticancer Res, (2009). , 2453-2459.

[82] Singh, P, et al. Overexpression and hypomethylation of flap endonuclease 1 gene in breast and other cancers. Mol Cancer Res, (2008). , 1710-1717.

[83] Urbanucci, A, et al. Overexpression of androgen receptor enhances the binding of the receptor to the chromatin in prostate cancer. Oncogene, (2012). , 2153-2163.

[84] Lam, J. S, et al. Flap endonuclease 1 is overexpressed in prostate cancer and is associated with a high Gleason score. BJU Int, (2006). , 445-451.

[85] Mcmanus, K. J, et al. Specific synthetic lethal killing of RAD54B-deficient human colorectal cancer cells by FEN1 silencing. Proc Natl Acad Sci U S A, (2009). , 3276-3281.

[86] Hirose, F, et al. Difference in the expression level of DNA polymerase beta among mouse tissues: high expression in the pachytene spermatocyte. Exp Cell Res, (1989). , 169-180.

[87] Zhang, Q. M, & Dianov, G. L. DNA repair fidelity of base excision repair pathways in human cell extracts. DNA Repair (Amst), (2005). , 263-270.

[88] Chan, K. K, Zhang, Q. M, & Dianov, G. L. Base excision repair fidelity in normal and cancer cells. Mutagenesis, (2006). , 173-178.

[89] Chan, K, et al. Overexpression of DNA polymerase beta results in an increased rate of frameshift mutations during base excision repair. Mutagenesis, (2007). , 183-188.

[90] Klungland, A, & Lindahl, T. Second pathway for completion of human DNA base excision-repair: reconstitution with purified proteins and requirement for DNase IV (FEN1). EMBO J, (1997). , 3341-3348.

[91] An, C. L, Chen, D, & Makridakis, N. M. Systematic biochemical analysis of somatic missense mutations in DNA polymerase beta found in prostate cancer reveal alteration of enzymatic function. Hum Mutat, (2011). , 415-423.

[92] Guo, Z, et al. Human DNA polymerase beta polymorphism, Arg137Gln, impairs its polymerase activity and interaction with PCNA and the cellular base excision repair capacity. Nucleic Acids Res, (2009). , 3431-3441.

[93] Li, D, et al. Effects of base excision repair gene polymorphisms on pancreatic cancer survival. Int J Cancer, (2007). , 1748-1754.

[94] Khanra, K, Bhattacharya, C, & Bhattacharyya, N. Association of a Newly Identified Variant of DNA Polymerase Beta (polbeta63-123, 208-304) with the Risk Factor of Ovarian Carcinoma in India. Asian Pac J Cancer Prev, (2012). , 1999-2002.

[95] Moreno, V, et al. Polymorphisms in genes of nucleotide and base excision repair: risk and prognosis of colorectal cancer. Clin Cancer Res, (2006). Pt 1): , 2101-2108.

[96] Barakat, K, & Tuszynski, J. Relaxed complex scheme suggests novel inhibitors for the lyase activity of DNA polymerase beta. J Mol Graph Model, (2011). , 702-716.

[97] Srinivasan, A, et al. Identification and characterization of human apurinic/apyrimidinic endonuclease-1 inhibitors. Biochemistry, (2012). , 6246-6259.

[98] Rai, G, et al. Synthesis, biological evaluation, and structure-activity relationships of a novel class of apurinic/apyrimidinic endonuclease 1 inhibitors. J Med Chem, (2012). , 3101-3112.

[99] Jaiswal, A. S, et al. DNA polymerase beta as a novel target for chemotherapeutic intervention of colorectal cancer. PLoS One, (2011)., e16691.

[100] Horton, J. K, et al. Hypersensitivity of DNA polymerase beta null mouse fibroblasts reflects accumulation of cytotoxic repair intermediates from site-specific alkyl DNA lesions. DNA Repair (Amst), (2003)., 27-48.

[101] Sobol, R. W, et al. Requirement of mammalian DNA polymerase-beta in base-excision repair. Nature, (1996)., 183-186.

[102] Bryant, H. E, et al. Specific killing of BRCA2-deficient tumours with inhibitors of poly(ADP-ribose) polymerase. Nature, (2005)., 913-917.

[103] Farmer, H, et al. Targeting the DNA repair defect in BRCA mutant cells as a therapeutic strategy. Nature, (2005)., 917-921.

[104] Tell, G, & Wilson, D. M. rd, Targeting DNA repair proteins for cancer treatment. Cell Mol Life Sci, (2010)., 3569-3572.

[105] Helleday, T, et al. DNA repair pathways as targets for cancer therapy. Nat Rev Cancer, (2008)., 193-204.

[106] Zhou, B, et al. The association of APE1-656T > G and 1349 T > G polymorphisms and cancer risk: a meta-analysis based on 37 case-control studies. BMC Cancer, (2011)., 521.

[107] Vascotto, C, et al. Knock-in reconstitution studies reveal an unexpected role of Cys-65 in regulating APE1/Ref-1 subcellular trafficking and function. Mol Biol Cell, (2011)., 3887-3901.

[108] Souza, L. R, et al. Immunohistochemical analysis of APE1, hMSH2 and ERCC1 proteins in actinic cheilitis and lip squamous cell carcinoma. Histopathology, (2011). p. 352-60., 53.

[109] Mohammed, M. Z, et al. Development and evaluation of human AP endonuclease inhibitors in melanoma and glioma cell lines. Br J Cancer, (2011)., 653-663.

[110] Bobola, M. S, et al. Apurinic/apyrimidinic endonuclease is inversely associated with response to radiotherapy in pediatric ependymoma. Int J Cancer, (2011)., 2370-2379.

[111] Yang, J, et al. APEX1 gene amplification and its protein overexpression in osteosarcoma: correlation with recurrence, metastasis, and survival. Technol Cancer Res Treat, (2010)., 161-169.

[112] Xie, J. Y, et al. Elevated expression of APE1/Ref-1 and its regulation on IL-6 and IL-8 in bone marrow stromal cells of multiple myeloma. Clin Lymphoma Myeloma Leuk, (2010)., 385-393.

[113] Su, D, et al. Genetic polymorphisms and treatment response in advanced non-small cell lung cancer. Lung Cancer, (2007)., 281-288.

[114] Zhang, Y, et al. Alterations in the expression of the apurinic/apyrimidinic endonuclease-1/redox factor-1 (APE1/Ref-1) in human ovarian cancer and indentification of the therapeutic potential of APE1/Ref-1 inhibitor. Int J Oncol, (2009). , 1069-1079.

[115] Yoo, D. G, et al. Alteration of APE1/ref-1 expression in non-small cell lung cancer: the implications of impaired extracellular superoxide dismutase and catalase antioxidant systems. Lung Cancer, (2008). , 277-284.

[116] Bobola, M. S, et al. Apurinic/apyrimidinic endonuclease activity is associated with response to radiation and chemotherapy in medulloblastoma and primitive neuroectodermal tumors. Clin Cancer Res, (2005). , 7405-7414.

[117] Wang, D, Luo, M, & Kelley, M. R. Human apurinic endonuclease 1 (APE1) expression and prognostic significance in osteosarcoma: enhanced sensitivity of osteosarcoma to DNA damaging agents using silencing RNA APE1 expression inhibition. Mol Cancer Ther, (2004). , 679-686.

[118] Bobola, M. S, et al. Apurinic endonuclease activity in adult gliomas and time to tumor progression after alkylating agent-based chemotherapy and after radiotherapy. Clin Cancer Res, (2004). , 7875-7883.

[119] Robertson, K. A, et al. Altered expression of Ape1/ref-1 in germ cell tumors and overexpression in NT2 cells confers resistance to bleomycin and radiation. Cancer Res, (2001). , 2220-2225.

[120] Koukourakis, M. I, et al. Nuclear expression of human apurinic/apyrimidinic endonuclease (HAP1/Ref-1) in head-and-neck cancer is associated with resistance to chemoradiotherapy and poor outcome. Int J Radiat Oncol Biol Phys, (2001). , 27-36.

[121] Herring, C. J, et al. Levels of the DNA repair enzyme human apurinic/apyrimidinic endonuclease (APE1, APEX, Ref-1) are associated with the intrinsic radiosensitivity of cervical cancers. Br J Cancer, (1998). , 1128-1133.

[122] Chiyomaru, K, Nagano, T, & Nishigori, C. XRCC1 Arg194Trp polymorphism, risk of nonmelanoma skin cancer and extramammary Paget's disease in a Japanese population. Arch Dermatol Res, (2012). , 363-370.

[123] Sobczuk, A, Poplawski, T, & Blasiak, J. Polymorphisms of DNA Repair Genes in Endometrial Cancer. Pathol Oncol Res, (2012).

[124] Zhao, Y, et al. Genetic polymorphisms of DNA repair genes XRCC1 and XRCC3 and risk of colorectal cancer in Chinese population. Asian Pac J Cancer Prev, (2012). , 665-669.

[125] Butkiewicz, D, et al. Influence of DNA repair gene polymorphisms on prognosis in inoperable non-small cell lung cancer patients treated with radiotherapy and platinum-based chemotherapy. Int J Cancer, (2012). , E1100-E1108.

[126] Li, Q. W, et al. Evaluation of DNA repair gene XRCC1 polymorphism in prediction and prognosis of hepatocellular carcinoma risk. Asian Pac J Cancer Prev, (2012). , 191-194.

[127] Cui, Z, et al. Association between polymorphisms in XRCC1 gene and clinical outcomes of patients with lung cancer: a meta-analysis. BMC Cancer, (2012). , 71.

[128] Terrazzino, S, et al. Common variants of eNOS and XRCC1 genes may predict acute skin toxicity in breast cancer patients receiving radiotherapy after breast conserving surgery. Radiother Oncol, (2012). , 199-205.

[129] Yin, G, et al. Genetic polymorphisms of XRCC1, alcohol consumption, and the risk of colorectal cancer in Japan. J Epidemiol, (2012). , 64-71.

[130] Wu, Z, et al. High risk of benzo[alpha]pyrene-induced lung cancer in E160D FEN1 mutant mice. Mutat Res, (2012). , 85-91.

[131] Gao, R, et al. Genetic polymorphisms in XRCC1 associated with radiation therapy in prostate cancer. Cancer Biol Ther, (2010). , 13-18.

[132] Liang, J, et al. The combination of ERCC1 and XRCC1 gene polymorphisms better predicts clinical outcome to oxaliplatin-based chemotherapy in metastatic colorectal cancer. Cancer Chemother Pharmacol, (2010). , 493-500.

[133] Shim, H. J, et al. BRCA1 and XRCC1 polymorphisms associated with survival in advanced gastric cancer treated with taxane and cisplatin. Cancer Sci, (2010). , 1247-1254.

[134] Hong, C. Y, et al. Correlation of the sensitivity of NP chemotherapy in non-small lung cancer with DNA repair gene XRCC1 polymorphism]. Ai Zheng, (2009). , 1291-1297.

[135] Sun, X, et al. Polymorphisms in XRCC1 and XPG and response to platinum-based chemotherapy in advanced non-small cell lung cancer patients. Lung Cancer, (2009). , 230-236.

[136] Csejtei, A, et al. Association between XRCC1 polymorphisms and head and neck cancer in a Hungarian population. Anticancer Res, (2009). , 4169-4173.

[137] Cheng, X. D, et al. The association of XRCC1 gene single nucleotide polymorphisms with response to neoadjuvant chemotherapy in locally advanced cervical carcinoma. J Exp Clin Cancer Res, (2009). , 91.

[138] Figl, A, et al. Single nucleotide polymorphisms in DNA repair genes XRCC1 and APEX1 in progression and survival of primary cutaneous melanoma patients. Mutat Res, (2009). , 78-84.

[139] Warnecke-eberz, U, et al. ERCC1 and XRCC1 gene polymorphisms predict response to neoadjuvant radiochemotherapy in esophageal cancer. J Gastrointest Surg, (2009). , 1411-1421.

[140] Sreeja, L, et al. Prognostic importance of DNA repair gene polymorphisms of XRCC1 Arg399Gln and XPD Lys751Gln in lung cancer patients from India. J Cancer Res Clin Oncol, (2008). , 645-652.

[141] Kim, K, et al. XRCC1 Arginine194Tryptophan and GGH-401Cytosine/Thymine polymorphisms are associated with response to platinum-based neoadjuvant chemotherapy in cervical cancer. Gynecol Oncol, (2008)., 509-515.

[142] Mittal, R. D, et al. XRCC1 codon 399 mutant allele: a risk factor for recurrence of urothelial bladder carcinoma in patients on BCG immunotherapy. Cancer Biol Ther, (2008)., 645-650.

[143] Liu, B, et al. Polymorphism of XRCC1 predicts overall survival of gastric cancer patients receiving oxaliplatin-based chemotherapy in Chinese population. European journal of human genetics : EJHG, (2007)., 1049-1053.

[144] Jaremko, M, et al. Polymorphism of the DNA repair enzyme XRCC1 is associated with treatment prediction in anthracycline and cyclophosphamide/methotrexate/5-fluorouracil-based chemotherapy of patients with primary invasive breast cancer. Pharmacogenet Genomics, (2007)., 529-538.

[145] Giachino, D. F, et al. Prospective assessment of XPD Lys751Gln and XRCC1 Arg399Gln single nucleotide polymorphisms in lung cancer. Clin Cancer Res, (2007)., 2876-2881.

[146] Suh, K. W, et al. Which gene is a dominant predictor of response during FOLFOX chemotherapy for the treatment of metastatic colorectal cancer, the MTHFR or XRCC1 gene? Ann Surg Oncol, (2006)., 1379-1385.

[147] Wu, X, et al. Genetic variations in radiation and chemotherapy drug action pathways predict clinical outcomes in esophageal cancer. J Clin Oncol, (2006)., 3789-3798.

[148] de las PenasR., et al., Polymorphisms in DNA repair genes modulate survival in cisplatin/gemcitabine-treated non-small-cell lung cancer patients. Ann Oncol, (2006)., 668-675.

[149] Sakano, S, et al. Single nucleotide polymorphisms in DNA repair genes might be prognostic factors in muscle-invasive bladder cancer patients treated with chemoradiotherapy. Br J Cancer, (2006)., 561-570.

[150] Chung, H. H, et al. XRCC1 R399Q polymorphism is associated with response to platinum-based neoadjuvant chemotherapy in bulky cervical cancer. Gynecol Oncol, (2006)., 1031-1037.

[151] Wang, Z. H, et al. Single nucleotide polymorphisms in XRCC1 and clinical response to platin-based chemotherapy in advanced non-small cell lung cancer]. Ai Zheng, (2004)., 865-868.

[152] Stoehlmacher, J, et al. A polymorphism of the XRCC1 gene predicts for response to platinum based treatment in advanced colorectal cancer. Anticancer Res, (2001). B):, 3075-3079.

[153] Yang, M, et al. Functional FEN1 polymorphisms are associated with DNA damage levels and lung cancer risk. Hum Mutat, (2009)., 1320-1328.

Chapter 20

Nucleotide Excision Repair Inhibitors: Still a Long Way to Go

K. Barakat and J. Tuszynski

Additional information is available at the end of the chapter

http://dx.doi.org/10.5772/46014

1. Introduction

The last few decades have witnessed a new astounding trend emerge in cancer research. The new strategy materialized as a glimmer of hope to improve current standard cancer treatments that target DNA. These DNA-damaging agents induce lesions into the genome, which are aimed at preventing cancer cells from proliferating and invading the surrounding tissue. However, as was shown by many experiments, in response to that cancer cells mobilize DNA repair pathways that tend to remove the induced damage. As a consequence, they exhibit increased resistance towards what would otherwise be an efficacious treatment [1]. These findings have validated DNA repair enzymes as new molecular targets in the context of the battle against cancer [2]. Fortunately, the proof of the concept of targeting DNA repair as a cancer-therapeutic-strategy has been provided by several convincing studies, many of which are advancing through pre-clinical and clinical trials [3]. A particular example of a novel target in such pathways is the nucleotide excision repair (NER) mechanism, which correlates with the induced resistance to platinum treatments [4].

In normal cells, NER removes a broad range of DNA lesions, protecting cell integrity [5]. In cancer cells exposed to DNA damaging agents that distort the DNA helix or form bulky injuries to the genome, NER comes into play and removes the damage, in order to prevent cancer cells from lethal consequences of this damage [5, 6]. A striking example of this mechanism is represented by the use of platinum compounds such as cisplatin, the principal component of many treatments involving solid tumors including testicular, bladder, ovarian, head and neck, cervical, lung and colorectal cancer [7]. It has been demonstrated that NER is the major DNA repair mechanism that removes cisplatin-induced DNA damage, and that resistance to platinum-based therapy correlates with high expression of ERCC1, a major enzymatic element of the NER machinery. In this context, a reasonable way to increase the efficacy of platinum-based therapy and decrease drug resistance would be to regulate NER by inhibiting the activity of ERCC1 and interacting proteins using yet to be discovered therapeutic compounds [8-11].

The protein ERCC1 forms a heterodimer with XPF. The resulting complex is an endonuclease enzyme that cleaves the 5` end of the damaged DNA strand whereas XPG cleaves it in the 3′ position [6]. ERCC1-XPF is recruited to the damage site through a direct interaction between ERCC1 and XPA, an indispensible element of the NER pathway. No cellular function beyond NER has been observed for XPA and competitive inhibition of the XPA interaction with peptide fragments is considered effective at disrupting NER. Furthermore, based on clinical data, cancer patients that have been shown to have low expression levels of either XPA or ERCC1 demonstrate a correlation with a higher sensitivity to cisplatin treatments [12, 13].

This chapter reviews the state-of-the-art efforts that have been made to date to identify inhibitors of the NER pathway. These efforts have been mainly focused on targeting either the ERCC1-XPA or the ERCC1-XPF interactions. We discuss the various methods that were used toward this aim and illustrate the mode of action of the identified inhibitors. We hope that the compiled knowledge in this chapter will help researchers and clinicians in their efforts to develop new drug candidates that can improve the efficacy of and reduce resistance against platinum treatments and other DNA damaging agents as a way to arrest tumor progression.

2. Nucleotide excision repair pathway

The nucleotide excision repair process, shown in Figure 1, occurs as a stepwise mechanism and involves more than 30 different proteins. It is a "cut-and-paste" mechanism that replaces a ~30 nucleotide DNA strand that contains the lesion with a correct base pair sequence. This pathway has been extensively studied so that all the genes that are involved in it have been cloned and expressed as recombinant proteins. The main players within NER include the seven Xeroderma Pigmentosum (XP) complementation groups, XPA to XPG proteins; the Excision Repair Cross Complementing group 1 protein (ERCC1]; the human Homolog of yeast RAD23 (hHR23B), the Replication Protein A (RPA), the subunits of Transcription Factor that possess Helicase activity (TFIIH), and the Cockayne Syndrome proteins A and B (CSA and CSB) [14]. Depending on the location of the DNA damage within the genome, one can recognize two NER sub-pathways. First is the transcription-coupled repair (TCR-NER), if the DNA damage is located within the actively transcribed genes of the genome. The second is the global genome repair (GGR-NER), if the damage is located within the whole genome. The two types are thought to be identical except for the initial damage recognition step. The two mechanisms involve five sequential steps [15] described below.

The foremost step is the detection of the damage. As mentioned above, the recognition step is the only difference between TCR and GGR. In the GGR subpathway, the XPC-hHR23B-XPE complex continuously scans the genome for bulky DNA damage until it recognizes a lesion and, consequently, initiates the rest of the NER sequence. On the other hand, a stalled RNAPII and Cockayne syndrome proteins, CSA and CSB, recognize the damage and activate the TCR-NER pathway. Once the damage is recognized the second step starts by recruiting the TFIIH complex in order to unwind the DNA helix surrounding the lesion. TFIIH is composed of two major sub-complexes. The core is formed from the association of a large number of proteins including XPB, XPD, p62, p52, p44, p34 and p8. The rest of TFIIH is the cdk-activating kinase sub-complex, which contains cdk7, cyclin H and MAT1. Interestingly, TFIIH possesses both 3′-5′ and 5′-3′ helicase activities through the two ATP-dependent helicases XPB and XPD, respectively [16]. It opens the DNA structure forming a ~30 base pair bubble around the lesion. The two proteins RPA and XPA stabilize the opened DNA structure and recruit the two endonucleases that are necessary for the subsequent incision step. The interaction of XPA with the 34-kDa subunit of RPA (RPA34) activates XPA to recruit the other components of NER.

The Damaged strand-incision is the rate-limiting step for the whole pathway. The two endonucleases XBG and XPF-ERCC1 cut the two ends of the strand that contains the damage. The correct location of XPA is crucial for the recruitment of the XPF-ERCC1 heterodimer endonuclease. XPG cuts the 3′ end of the damage, while XPF-ERCC1 cuts the 5′ end [17]. The damaged strand is then released. DNA polymerases fill the single strand gap using the complementary intact strand as a template and DNA ligase I closes the 3′ nick as a final step [15].

3. ERCC1 over-expression correlates with cisplatin resistance

ERCC1 is a 33-kDa protein that forms a tight heterodimer endonuclease complex with XPF. As described above, this endonuclease cleaves the DNA strand at the phosphodiester bonds on the 5′ side of the damage. It is important to mention that the ERCC1-XPF complex has additional functions in other DNA repair pathways including inter-strand cross-link repair, double-strand break repair, and homologous recombination. Many studies have shown considerable correlation between resistance to cisplatin and the over-expression of ERCC1 [19]. This profoundly significant conclusion has been reached from several independent clinical trial investigations on ovarian [20], colorectal [21], and non–small cell lung cancer [22]. For example, a study on ~750 patients who suffer from late stages of lung cancer revealed that patients with low levels of ERCC1 and who received platinum therapy had better survival rates than those with the same levels of the protein but did not receive the platinum treatment [23]. A more recent study on 444 patients who experienced non-small lung cancer concluded that non-platinum-containing chemotherapy is more effective than platinum-based therapy on patients with high ERCC1 levels [24]. Very recently, Stefanie and coworkers [25] performed a retrospective study investigating the correlation of ERCC1 expression with patients' survival in ovarian cancer after platinum-based treatment. Their work revealed that patients with ERCC1-negative ovarian cancer had significantly better survival rates than those with ERCC1-positive ovarian cancer. They concluded that ERCC1 protein over-expression is a marker for poor survival of high-grade ovarian cancer even in patients operated on who had residual disease. All of these investigations lead to the conclusion that ERCC1 is not only a gene that is usually activated in patients subjected to platinum-based therapy but it may also act as a predictive criterion for identifying those patients who could benefit from platinum treatments [26, 27]. This latter role of ERCC1 as a biomarker is important because it can guide clinicians in their therapeutic decision-making and select the best treatment approach for a particular group of patients.

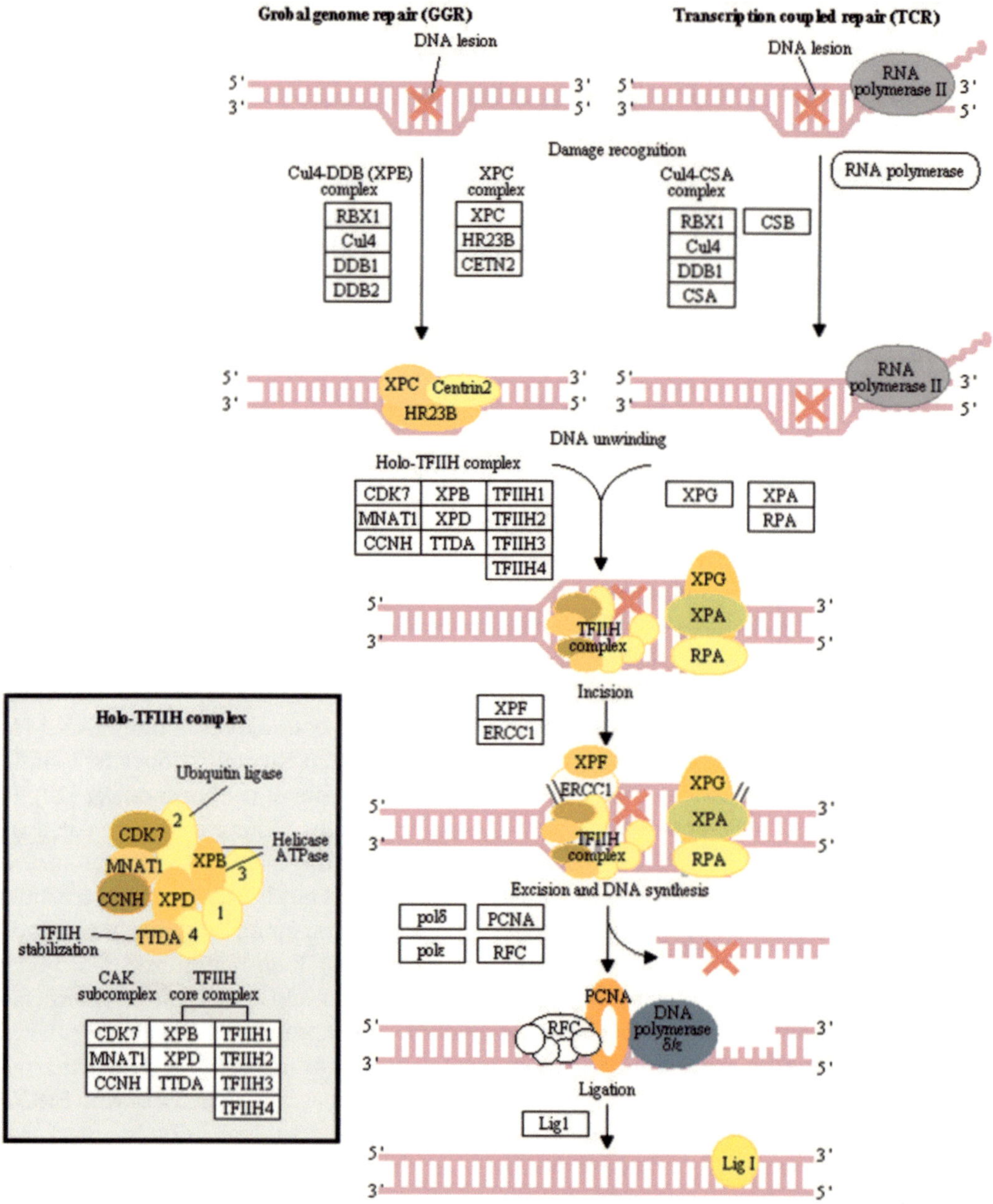

Figure 1. Steps of the nucleotide excision repair pathway. See text for details (adopted from the KEGG database [18]).

http://dx.doi.org/10.5772/46014

4. The ERCC1-XPA interaction is essential for a functional NER pathway

Regardless of the type of NER that is initiated, the XPA protein is equally essential to complete both pathways [28]. It plays a vital role in DNA lesion recognition and in the attraction of many other NER repair proteins. For example, prior to the incision step in NER, the ERCC1-XPF endonuclease is recruited to the damaged DNA site through a secondary interaction between ERCC1 and XPA [29, 30, 31]. Therefore, this protein-protein interaction is necessary for a functional NER mechanism. The NMR crystal structure was resolved by Tsodikov's group [13] and the critical residue-residue interactions were determined [4] through our binding energy predictions (see Figure 2). A 14-residue peptide from XPA that includes three essential consecutive glycines (residues 72–74) is buried within a hydrophobic cleft within the central domain of ERCC1. This peptide has two critical characteristics. First, it is necessary and sufficient for binding to ERCC1. Second, and more importantly, it can compete with the full-length XPA protein in binding to ERCC1 and disrupting NER *in vitro*.

In a recent study, Barbara et al. [32] reported mutations in the central domain of ERCC1 that had a significant impact on NER activity *in vitro* and *in vivo*. These mutations occur at the XPA binding site within ERCC1, preventing the interaction between the two proteins. Due to these mutations, the ERCC1-XPF nuclease was not recruited to the damaged DNA sites after exposing cells to ultra violet (UV) radiation. Consequently, the last incision step that is performed by ERCC1-XPF was never completed leading to a dysfunctional NER mechanism in these cells and, hence, a hypersensitivity to UV radiation. These results are consistent with previous findings on the importance of XPA in NER, where no cellular function beyond NER has been observed for XPA [12]. Interestingly, these mutations did not affect the activity of ERCC1-XPF in other DNA repair pathways leading to two distinctive conclusions. First, the XPA-ERCC1 interaction is only necessary for NER but not for other DNA repair pathways in which ERCC1-XPF is important for their activity. Second, the involvement and recruitment of ERCC1-XPF to the different DNA repair pathways is coordinated through different and not overlapping protein-protein interactions mediated by ERCC1. Based on these findings, one can selectively disrupt the activity of ERCC1-XPF within these DNA repair pathways by inhibiting its interactions with the recruitment factors to the damaged sites. These observations, coupled with the available crystal structure of this interaction make ERCC1 and XPA an extremely attractive target for computationally assisted development of small molecule inhibitors targeted for use in combination therapies involving cisplatin.

5. ERCC1 interacts massively with XPF

As shown in Figure 3, ERCC1 in engaged in a tight interaction with XPF in which almost every residue from XPF is either interacting or being affected by an interaction with ERCC1 residues. The main interaction sites are located within the C-terminal domains of the two proteins. The most tightly interacting regions in XPF include residues 828 to 835, 859 to 862, 878 to 882 and 892 to 905. These exhibit almost no flexibility in the bound structure, demonstrating a contribution to binding with ERCC1. The two proteins form the heterodimer enzyme that is responsible for the cleavage of one side of the damaged nucleotides chain.

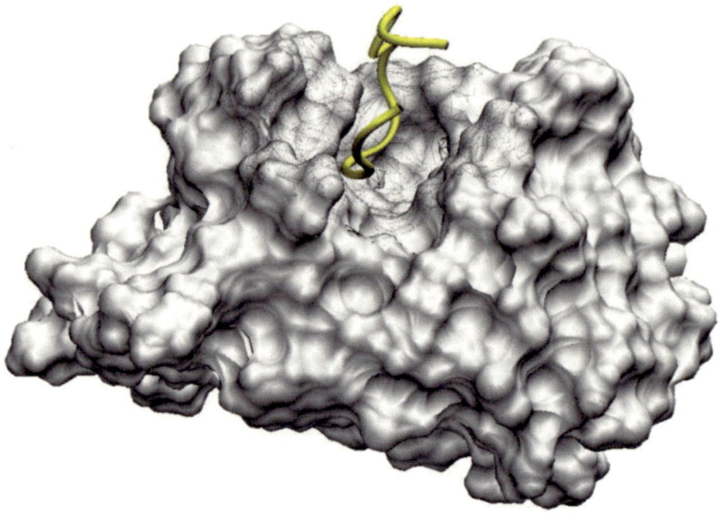

Figure 2. XPA-ERCC1 protein-protein interaction. The binding between ERCC1 (whight) and XPA (yellow) is predicted [4] to be primarily mediated by 5 residues from XPA peptide, namely; G72, G73, G74, F75 and I76. On the other hand, the contribution from the ERCC1 binding site is distributed among the following 10 residues: R106, Q107, G109, N110, P111, F140, L141, S142, Y145 and Y152.

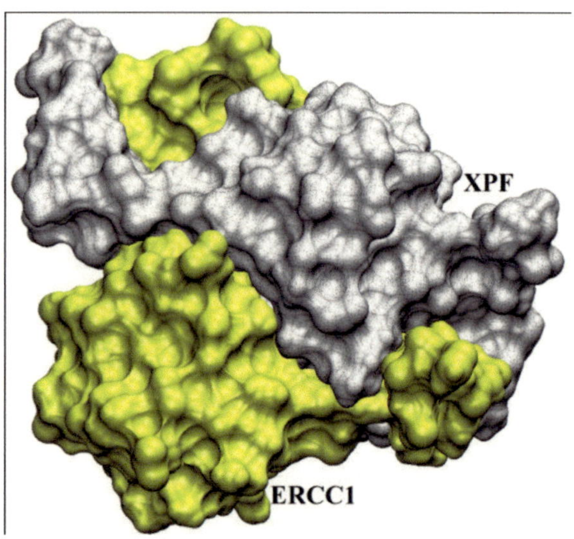

Figure 3. The ERCC1-XPF complex. The C-terminal domain of each protein interacts massively with its counterpart from the other protein forming the heterodimer endonuclease enzyme.

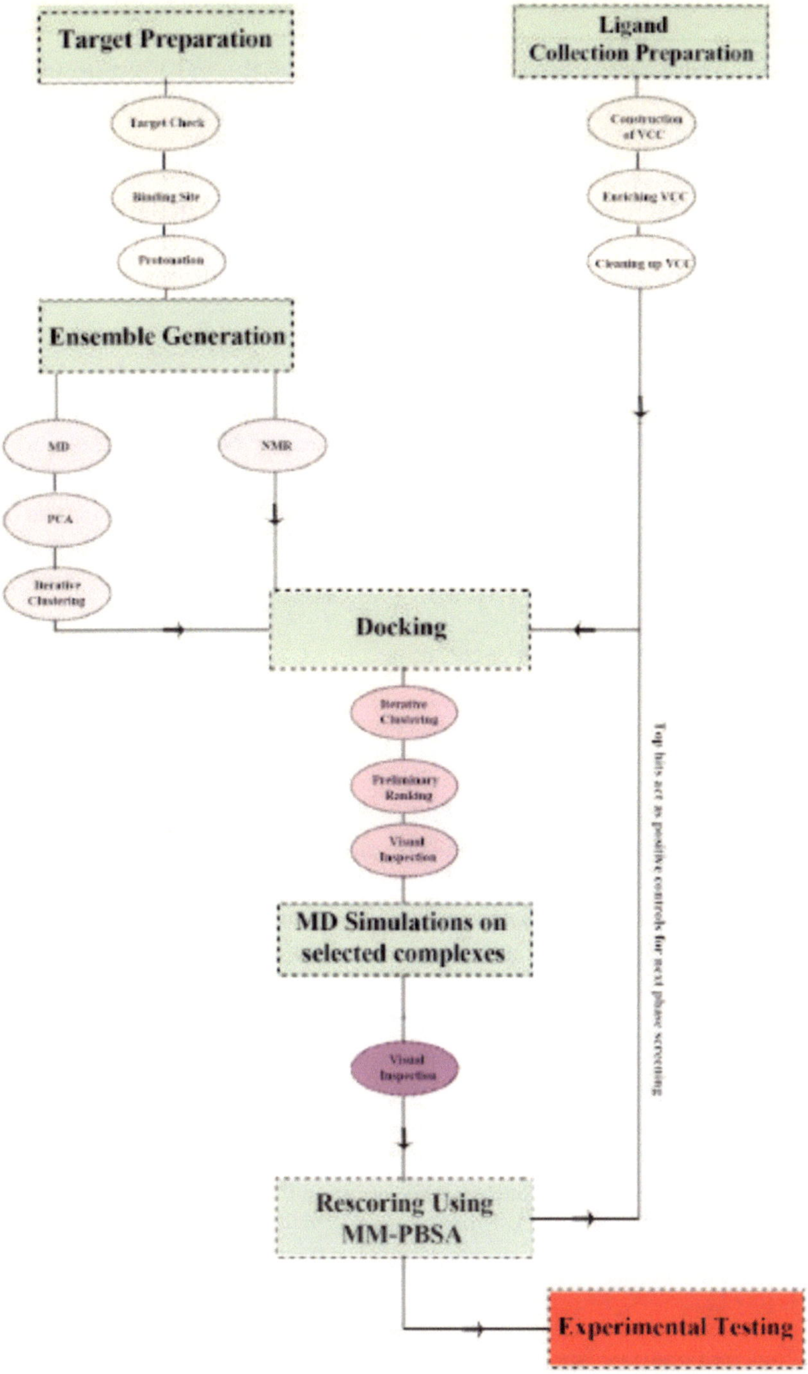

Figure 4. The implemented virtual screening protocol.

6. Earlier efforts to identify NER inhibitors

Although the NER pathway has been recognized as one of the most important factors that increase the resistance against platinum-based therapy, little work has been done so far on regulating its activity. Here, we wish to point to three major studies that identified inhibitors for the NER mechanism. First is the work done by Barret et al. [33] and their discovery of F11782. Second are the findings of Jiang and Yang [34] on the effects of the cell cycle checkpoint abrogator UCN-01 (7-hydroxystaurosporine) on NER. Finally, the work on the DNA damaging agent Et743 is a landmark result [35]. We briefly describe these outcomes below.

6.1. F11782

Using the 3D (DNA Damaged Detection) assay first proposed by Wood *et al.* [36] and later modified by Salles's team [37], Barret et al. [33] screened for NER inhibitors and identified F11782. The compound was already known as an inhibitor of both the topoisomerases II and I [38]. Moreover, F11782 did not show any activity toward other enzymes such as DNase I or T4 polynucleotide kinase, indicating that the compound targets one of the proteins that are involved in NER. Further investigations on F11782 limited its NER inhibitory activity to one of the earlier steps of the pathway, specifically either the helicase or the incision steps, with more preference given to the incision step [33].

6.2. UCN-01

Jiang and Yang [34] analyzed the effects of UCN-01, which is a well-known protein kinase C inhibitor and cell cycle checkpoint abrogator [39], on the NER pathway. These findings showed that UCN-01 inhibited the repair of cisplatin-induced DNA damage both *in vitro* and *in vivo* and indicated that UCN-01 has a dramatic inhibitory effect on the interaction of NER proteins. The drug enhanced the activity of cisplatin only in NER-proficient cells, but not in the deficient ones. However, no direct binding of UCN-01 to any of these proteins has been reported and it has been speculated that the observed inhibitory activity may result from UCN-01-mediated regulation of the signaling pathway that involves post-translational modifications of repair proteins. Although Jiang and Yang [34] attributed the loss of NER activity to an attenuation in the ERCC1-XPA protein-protein interaction, their careful and detailed binding analysis of the compound to the two proteins revealed that UCN-01 did not interact directly with either of them. However, in this work we used UCN-01 as a positive control, assuming it can bind to the XPA binding site within ERCC1, particularly because the drug can fit within the binding pocket despite its limited interactions with the protein.

6.3. Ecteinascidin 743

A final compound that has been shown [35] to interfere with NER is Ecteinascidin 743 (Et743]. At the time of writing this article, Et743 is in phase II/III clinical development and its main mode of action is as a DNA damaging agent. The drug seems to specifically obstruct the TCR-NER sub-pathway, however, it does not act as an inhibitor of any of the proteins that are involved in the NER mechanism. A model proposed by Gregory et al. [35] suggests that the DNA adducts formed by Et743 are more efficient than those of cisplatin in dealing with NER. These authors suggest that the Et743-guanine adducts trap the TCR-NER pathway at the incision or ligation steps, preventing the pathway from being completed.

7. Recent attempts to discover novel NER inhibitors

As mentioned above, most of the earlier NER inhibitors listed above were not discovered to be potent or specific NER inhibitors. In other words, they were found mainly by chance to partially inhibit the NER pathway. Given the impact of regulating the NER pathway on improving many of the chemotherapeutic drug cocktails currently in clinical use, it is very important to directly target elements of NER pathway itself. Following this path, our group has been focusing on this problem in hope of implementing a novel strategy that would reverse resistance and potentiate the efficacy of cisplatin and other similar chemotherapeutic agents. The foremost endeavor is to specifically and separately target the two protein-protein interactions described above, namely the XPA-ERCC1 [4, 40] and XPF-ERCC1 [41] interactions. These efforts have already resulted in two successful examples where inhibitors identified by us via virtual screening were able to sensitize cells to ultra violet radiation (UV) and potentiate the efficacy of cisplatin in cancer cells. Here, we briefly describe the methods used and their outcomes. The studies described below primarily utilized computational tools to develop inhibitors that disturb these interactions. This was then followed by experimental validation of the predicted effects of these inhibitors on cancer cells.

7.1. The method

In the following studies, virtual screening identified small molecules that bind to and fit within the binding site within the interacting proteins in order to disturb its binding to the other protein in the complex. The virtual screening (VS) protocol that was used is shown in Figure 4. It is an improved version of the relaxed complex scheme (RCS) technique reported by McCammon and his team [42]. In the original RCS approach, all-atom MD simulations (e.g., 2-5 ns simulation) are applied to explore the conformational space of the target, while docking is subsequently used for the fast screening of drug libraries against an ensemble of receptor conformations. This ensemble is extracted at predetermined time intervals (e.g., every 10 ps) from the simulation, resulting in hundreds of thousands of protein conformations. Each conformation is then used as a target for an independent docking experiment.

The RCS methodology has been successfully applied to a number of cases. An excellent example is that of an HIV inhibitor, raltegravir which became the first FDA approved drug targeting HIV integrase [43, 44]. Other successful examples include the identification of novel inhibitors of the acetylcholine binding protein [45], RNA-editing ligase 1 [46], the influenza protein neuraminidase [47] and *Trypanosoma brucei* uridine diphosphate galactose 4'-epimerase [48]. These applications employed alternative ways to solve two main problems with the method, namely, reducing the number of extracted target conformations and deciding on how to select the final set of hits after carrying out the screening process. For the first problem, a number of studies suggested extracting the structures at larger intervals of the MD simulation, e.g. every 5ns or so [45], condensing the structural ensemble generated from MD simulations using QR factorization [46], or clustering the MD trajectory using root-mean-square-deviation (RMSD) conformational clustering [47, 48]. On the other hand, to rank the screened compounds and suggest a final set of top hits, some studies used only docking predictions [45-47], while others suggested using a more accurate scoring method (e.g. MM/PBSA (Molecular Mechanics/ Poisson Boltzmann Surface Area)) to refine the final selected hits [42]. All of these approaches, similar to the work presented here, were aimed at keeping the balance between significantly reducing the number of target structures and retaining their capacity to describe the conformational space of the target. Figure 4 describes the approach that was used to put together and improve the RCS to target the strong protein-protein interactions described above.

Our implementation follows the same guidelines as in the RCS method. We first use MD simulations and generate large enough trajectories that can progress through the phase space of the binding site. The length of the MD simulations (usually on the order of 100 ns) is determined by applying metrics that employ principal component analysis (PCA). Once the trajectory reaches an adequate sampling of target conformations, clustering analysis extracts representative structures that describe the dominant dynamics of the binding site. The extracted structures are then used as rigid targets to screen the whole library of compounds and suggest models for the most preferred ligand-protein complexes, hence, utilizing the "conformational sampling" model. These bound structures are then solvated and used to run all-atom MD simulations to relax the two molecules and generate new trajectories that represent their "induced fit" models. The MM-PBSA method finally ranks the newly generated structures and suggests a set of top hits for experimental testing.

7.2. XPA-ERCC1 inhibitors

Our earliest challenge was to directly disturb the interaction between the ERCC1 and XPA proteins. Two subsequent screening experiments were used. The initial study screened two compound databases for inhibitors of the ERCC1-XPA interaction and constructed a pharmacophore model demonstrating the crucial features necessary for their inhibition. The databases used included the National Cancer Institute Diversity Set (NCIDS) and DrugBank compounds.

The NCIDS is a collection of approximately 2,000 compounds that are structurally representative as scaffolds of a wide range of molecules, representing almost 140,000 compounds that are available for testing at the NCI. A number of its ligands contain rare earth elements and cannot be properly parameterized for docking experiments, leaving us with 1,883 compounds that can be actually used. This work exploits a cleaned 3D version of the NCIDS formatted for use in AutoDock and it was prepared by the AutoDock Scripps team. What makes the NCIDS so valuable and extensively screened by many groups (even in HTS) is that its individual molecules have distinctive structures and are the cluster representatives of their parent families. Once screened and a number of its molecules rank high in the hit list, one can return back and screen the whole family of the representative structure, instead of screening the actual NCI set of compounds. On the other hand, the DrugBank database is not only a set of molecules representing FDA-approved drugs, but it also represents a unique bioinformatics and chem-informatics resource. It relates each drug to its target(s). It includes details about the different pathways, structural information and chemical characteristics of these targets and the way they take part in inducing a particular disease. This information is stored in a freely available website that is linked to other databases (KEGG, PubChem, ChEBI, PDB, Swiss-Prot and Gen-Bank) and a range of structure displaying applets. The DrugBank collection includes ~4,800 drug structures including >1,350 FDA-approved small molecule drugs, 123 FDA-approved biotech (protein/peptide) drugs, 71 nutraceuticals and >3,243 experimental drugs. Once a hit is identified from this library, it simply represents a drug. This means many barriers of pre-clinical and clinical tests can be readily overcome and the molecule can be tested directly for its novel biological activity. Moreover, a hit from this collection may explain a mysterious side effect that would not be discovered before its identification as a regulator for the examined target.

This initial study utilized a minimized model of the XPA binding site within ERCC1 to employ flexible residue docking as implemented in AutoDock 4.0. This was then followed by RCS docking, where MD simulations and RMSD conformational clustering were used to generate a set of forty-four representative conformations of the binding site within ERCC1. AutoDock was then used to screen against a set of seven target conformations, composed of the six most dominant cluster-representative structures along with an equilibrated folded conformation for the binding site produced by employing principal component analysis on the ERCC1 trajectory. Top hits were rescored by docking them to the whole set of cluster-representative structures and ranked by their weighted average binding energy. The non-redundant hits from these screens were then used to identify a dynamic binding-site pharmacophore that target the ERCC1-XPA interaction. The pharmacophore model was then compared to docking results for the weak inhibitor of NER, UCN-01 (7-hydroxystaurosporine). A number of selected hits from this study are shown in Figure 5.

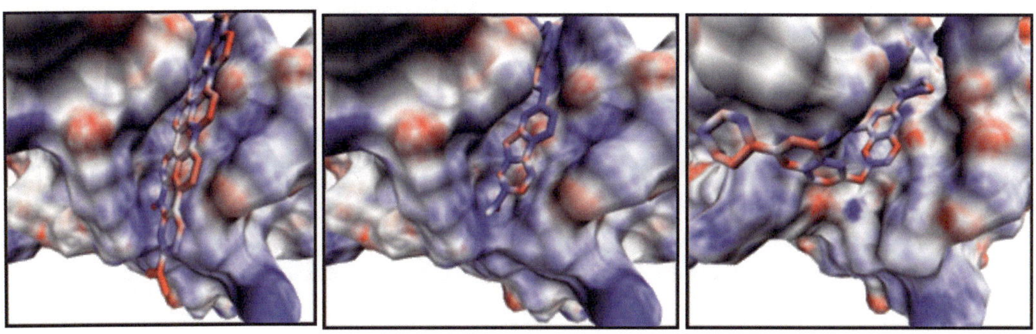

Figure 5. Three selected hits within their preferred binding site conformations. Adopted from [4].

Comparing the methodology that was used here to the workflow discussed in the above, one can make three observations. First, the virtual screening methodology depended mainly on docking scoring to rank the compounds. Second, the clustering analysis that was used to extract dominant conformations of the target was not iterative, it used a cut off RMSD value that is commonly employed in the literature. Finally, no post-docking refinements were performed on the final set of compounds. These shortcomings were properly adjusted in the subsequent study [49].

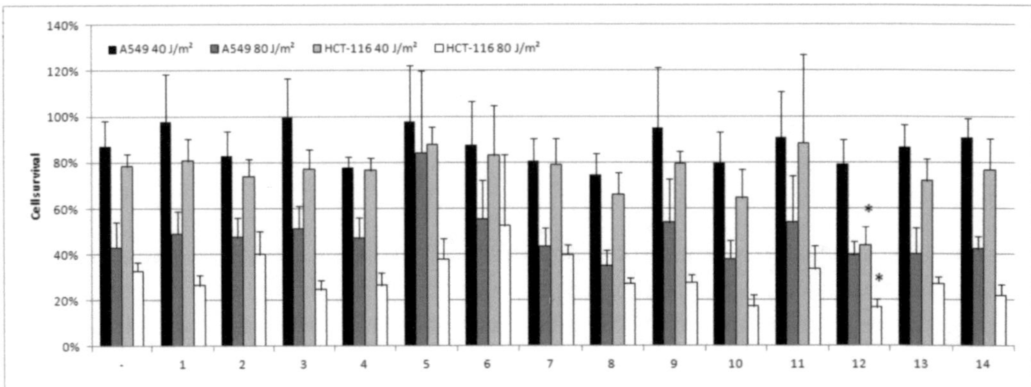

Figure 6. Sensitivity of cancer cells to UVC irradiation alone or in combination with potential inhibitors of the interaction between ERCC1 and XPA. IC50 values (J/m^2). Compound 12 showed promising effects on cancer cells and was henceforth termed NERI01.

The new study used the CN chemical library for virtual screening. The CN chemical library (~50,000 compounds) is a repository of all synthetic, natural compounds and natural extracts in the existing French public laboratories. The whole database is divided into two main categories. The first part includes information about all synthetic products, while the second contains the natural compounds and extracts. In this work, we used the whole CN database in our screening. In contrast to the previously mentioned databases, compounds in this library are represented by 2D SDF structures with no hydrogen atoms attached. This required a number of cleaning and preparation steps before using them in VS simulations.

The second ERCC1-XPA study exactly followed the screening protocol described above. The hit rate of the new study was higher than that of the one described here, indicating the importance of utilizing more accurate scoring, performing iterative clustering and refining the docked structures using MD simulations. A promising hit, shown in Figure 6 as compound 12, was discovered and validated on a UV radiation sensitivity cell-based assay [40]. The validated hit was termed NER inhibitor 01 (NERI01) has been shown to be effective in sensitizing colon cancer cells to UV radiation, which induces the same type of damage as cisplatin and its lesions are removed by ENR.

7.3. XPF-ERCC1 inhibitors

The final study focused on the more challenging problem of interfering with the ERCC1-XPF interaction. As shown in Figure 4, the two proteins have a very close interaction with each

http://dx.doi.org/10.5772/46014

other. A comparison of atomic fluctuations (as revealed by the corresponding B-factor values) between the unbound-XPF and the bound-XPF structures is shown in Figure 7. Almost all XPF residues are rigid in the bound case compared to the free structure. This indicates a massive interaction between ERCC1 and XPF in which almost every residue from XPF is either interacting or being affected by an interaction with ERCC1 residues. The most flexible regions in XPF include residues 828 to 835, 859 to 862, 878 to 882 and 892 to 905. These have almost no flexibility in the bound structure, demonstrating a contribution to binding with ERCC1.

The enthalpic contribution, as calculated by the MM-PBSA analysis, to the binding energy between the two proteins is exceptionally large (-123 kcal/mol). While the solvation energy contributed passively to the interaction (298 kcal/mol), compensation from the electrostatic and van der Waals interactions dominated the overall interaction (-238 kcal/mol and -184 kcal/mol, respectively). From these analyses we showed that ERCC1-residues shared ~50% of the total energy with PHE293 being the residue that contributes the most to the ERCC1-XPF interaction (-11 kcal/mol). On the XPF side, PHE894 has been found to contribute -7.7 kcal/mol to the binding energy. With the exception of ASP839 from XPF which disfavored the interaction by ~1 kcal/mol, the indicated residues favored the binding between ERCC1 and XPF. This allowed us to identify a binding site on the XPF surface that was used to identify putative inhibitors of this protein-protein interaction.

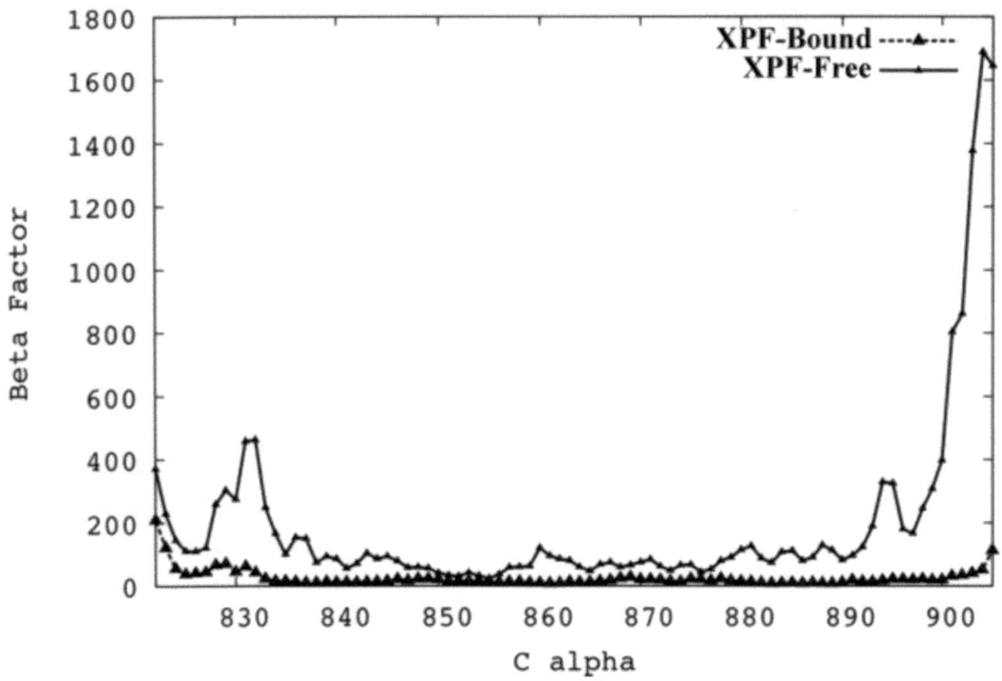

Figure 7. Flexibility of the XPF residues. Atomic fluctuations for the free and bound XPF proteins are shown here. Binding of ERCC1 to XPF considerably stabilized the protein, indicating a wide range of protein-protein interaction.

The screening methodology adopted the VS protocol shown in Figure 4 and used to screen the CN chemical library, NCI diversity set and DrugBank compounds for inhibitors of this interaction. A number of promising hits were experimentally validated and were very effective in disrupting the NER pathway and potentiating cisplatin efficacy. The most promising compounds with binding modes are shown in Figure 8.

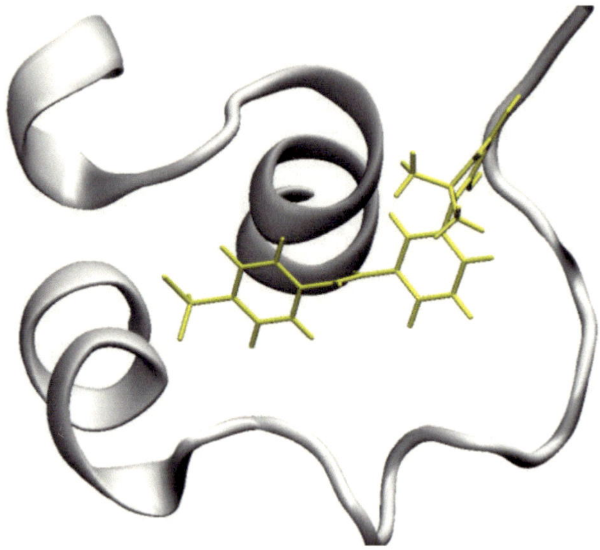

Figure 8. Binding mode of most promising XPF-ERCC1 inhibitor.

8. Conclusions

DNA damaging agents induce lesions into the genome aiming at preventing cancer cells from proliferating and invading the surrounding tissue. However, DNA repair pathways remove the induced damage and, hence, increase resistance to an otherwise efficacious treatment [1]. This approach has validated DNA repair enzymes as new molecular targets in the context of the battle against cancer. Nucleotide excision repair (NER) is a major DNA repair mechanism that removes mainly DNA lesions that distort the DNA helix or form bulky injuries to the genome. Among the most affected drugs with NER activity are platinum compounds such as cisplatin, the backbone for many treatments of solid tumors including testicular, bladder, ovarian, head and neck, cervical, lung and colorectal cancer. It has been demonstrated that NER is the major DNA repair mechanism that removes cisplatin-induced DNA damage, and that resistance to platinum-based therapy correlates with high expression of ERCC1, a major element of the NER machinery. Therefore, one way to improve such drugs and reduce their acquired resistance is by developing inhibitors that would regulate the NER machinery.

This chapter reviewed the state-of-the-art efforts that were made to identify inhibitors of the NER pathway. We discussed the various methods that were used toward this aim and illustrated the mode of action of the identified inhibitors. The earlier efforts were not focused on NER as a target. However, the first identified NER-inhibitors were discovered unintentionally. These efforts include the examples of finding the three drugs F11782 [33], UCN-01 (7-hydroxystaurosporine) [34] and Et743 as weak inhibitors of the NER activity. Recent studies exploited the fact that ERCC1 and its associated proteins XPA and XPF have a considerable correlation between resistance to cisplatin and their over-expression in cancer cells [19]. The latter studies were aimed at discovering specific inhibitors that target these interactions in the hope of disturbing their binding and hence reducing the NER activity. In this regard, we described the development of two different classes of NER inhibitors. The first class, represented by the lead compound NERI01 target the ERCC1-XPA interaction, while the second class represented by NERI02 targets the ERCC1-XPF interaction. Future directions of this research include the development of derivative structures for the identified hits and their optimization for improved drug-like properties and higher specificity to target their representative protein interactions. While great efforts have been done both *in silico* and *in vitro* to identify and validate novel inhibitors for the two mentioned NER targets, no *in vivo* studies have been performed on them yet. This is mainly due to the fact that the two proteins have been very recently recognized as druggable targets and no one in the past thought of regulating NER as a way to improve cancer therapy. However, we think that the studies presented here offer a proof-of-concept that inhibiting the interaction of ERCC1 with either XPA or XPF has a considerable impact on the NER mechanism and, therefore, enhances the efficacy of chemotherapeutic treatments that are associated with acquired resistance due to over expression of the NER elements. We hope that this chapter will be found of value to the researchers and clinicians interested in developing new drug candidates that can improve the efficacy of and reduce resistance against platinum treatments and other DNA damaging agents as a way to arrest tumor progression.

Acknowledgements

This research was supported by funding from NSERC, Alberta Cancer Foundation, Alberta Cancer Research Institute, Canadian Breast Cancer Foundation, Alberta Advanced Education and Technology and the Allard Foundation.

Author details

K. Barakat[1,2] and J. Tuszynski[3,4]

1 Department of Physics, University of Alberta, Canada

2 Department of Engineering Mathematics and Physics, Fayoum University, Fayoum, Egypt

3 Department of Physics, University of Alberta, Canada

4 Department of Oncology, University of Alberta, Canada

References

[1] Harper JW, Elledge SJ. The DNA damage response: ten years after. Mol Cell. 2007;28:739-45.

[2] Basu B, Yap TA, Molife LR, de Bono JS. Targeting the DNA damage response in oncology: past, present and future perspectives. Curr Opin Oncol. 2012;24:316-24.

[3] Barakat KH, Gajewski MM, Tuszynski JA. DNA polymerase beta (pol beta) inhibitors: A comprehensive overview. Drug Discov Today. 2012;17:913-20.

[4] Barakat KH, Torin Huzil J, Luchko T, Jordheim L, Dumontet C, Tuszynski J. Characterization of an inhibitory dynamic pharmacophore for the ERCC1-XPA interaction using a combined molecular dynamics and virtual screening approach. J Mol Graph Model. 2009;28:113-30.

[5] Rouillon C, White MF. The evolution and mechanisms of nucleotide excision repair proteins. Res Microbiol. 2011;162:19-26.

[6] Nouspikel T. DNA repair in mammalian cells : Nucleotide excision repair: variations on versatility. Cell Mol Life Sci. 2009;66:994-1009.

[7] Koberle B, Tomicic MT, Usanova S, Kaina B. Cisplatin resistance: preclinical findings and clinical implications. Biochim Biophys Acta. 2010;1806:172-82.

[8] Metzger R, Leichman CG, Danenberg KD, Danenberg PV, Lenz HJ, Hayashi K, et al. ERCC1 mRNA levels complement thymidylate synthase mRNA levels in predicting response and survival for gastric cancer patients receiving combination cisplatin and fluorouracil chemotherapy. J Clin Oncol. 1998;16:309-16.

[9] Handra-Luca A, Hernandez J, Mountzios G, Taranchon E, Lacau-St-Guily J, Soria JC, et al. Excision repair cross complementation group 1 immunohistochemical expression predicts objective response and cancer-specific survival in patients treated by Cisplatin-based induction chemotherapy for locally advanced head and neck squamous cell carcinoma. Clin Cancer Res. 2007;13:3855-9.

[10] Bellmunt J, Paz-Ares L, Cuello M, Cecere FL, Albiol S, Guillem V, et al. Gene expression of ERCC1 as a novel prognostic marker in advanced bladder cancer patients receiving cisplatin-based chemotherapy. Ann Oncol. 2007;18:522-8.

[11] Jun HJ, Ahn MJ, Kim HS, Yi SY, Han J, Lee SK, et al. ERCC1 expression as a predictive marker of squamous cell carcinoma of the head and neck treated with cisplatin-based concurrent chemoradiation. Br J Cancer. 2008;99:167-72.

[12] Rosenberg E, Taher MM, Kuemmerle NB, Farnsworth J, Valerie K. A truncated human xeroderma pigmentosum complementation group A protein expressed from an adenovirus sensitizes human tumor cells to ultraviolet light and cisplatin. Cancer Res. 2001;61:764-70.

[13] Tsodikov OV, Ivanov D, Orelli B, Staresincic L, Shoshani I, Oberman R, et al. Structural basis for the recruitment of ERCC1-XPF to nucleotide excision repair complexes by XPA. EMBO J. 2007;26:4768-76.

[14] Wood RD. DNA damage recognition during nucleotide excision repair in mammalian cells. Biochimie. 1999;81:39-44.

[15] de Laat WL, Jaspers NG, Hoeijmakers JH. Molecular mechanism of nucleotide excision repair. Genes Dev. 1999;13:768-85.

[16] Sung P, Bailly V, Weber C, Thompson LH, Prakash L, Prakash S. Human xeroderma pigmentosum group D gene encodes a DNA helicase. Nature. 1993;365:852-5.

[17] Sijbers AM, de Laat WL, Ariza RR, Biggerstaff M, Wei YF, Moggs JG, et al. Xeroderma pigmentosum group F caused by a defect in a structure-specific DNA repair endonuclease. Cell. 1996;86:811-22.

[18] Yano JK, Wester MR, Schoch GA, Griffin KJ, Stout CD, Johnson EF. The structure of human microsomal cytochrome P450 3A4 determined by X-ray crystallography to 2.05-A resolution. J Biol Chem. 2004;279:38091-4.

[19] Martin LP, Hamilton TC, Schilder RJ. Platinum resistance: the role of DNA repair pathways. Clin Cancer Res. 2008;14:1291-5.

[20] Kang S, Ju W, Kim JW, Park NH, Song YS, Kim SC, et al. Association between excision repair cross-complementation group 1 polymorphism and clinical outcome of platinum-based chemotherapy in patients with epithelial ovarian cancer. Exp Mol Med. 2006;38:320-4.

[21] Shirota Y, Stoehlmacher J, Brabender J, Xiong YP, Uetake H, Danenberg KD, et al. ERCC1 and thymidylate synthase mRNA levels predict survival for colorectal cancer patients receiving combination oxaliplatin and fluorouracil chemotherapy. J Clin Oncol. 2001;19:4298-304.

[22] Lord RV, Brabender J, Gandara D, Alberola V, Camps C, Domine M, et al. Low ERCC1 expression correlates with prolonged survival after cisplatin plus gemcitabine chemotherapy in non-small cell lung cancer. Clin Cancer Res. 2002;8:2286-91.

[23] Olaussen KA, Dunant A, Fouret P, Brambilla E, Andre F, Haddad V, et al. DNA repair by ERCC1 in non-small-cell lung cancer and cisplatin-based adjuvant chemotherapy. N Engl J Med. 2006;355:983-91.

[24] Cobo M, Isla D, Massuti B, Montes A, Sanchez JM, Provencio M, et al. Customizing cisplatin based on quantitative excision repair cross-complementing 1 mRNA expression: a phase III trial in non-small-cell lung cancer. J Clin Oncol. 2007;25:2747-54.

[25] Scheil-Bertram S, Tylus-Schaaf P, du Bois A, Harter P, Oppitz M, Ewald-Riegler N, et al. Excision repair cross-complementation group 1 protein overexpression as a predictor of poor survival for high-grade serous ovarian adenocarcinoma. Gynecol Oncol. 2010;119:325-31.

[26] Altaha R, Liang X, Yu JJ, Reed E. Excision repair cross complementing-group 1: gene expression and platinum resistance. Int J Mol Med. 2004;14:959-70.

[27] Ozkan M, Akbudak IH, Deniz K, Dikilitas M, Dogu GG, Berk V, et al. Prognostic value of excision repair cross-complementing gene 1 expression for cisplatin-based chemotherapy in advanced gastric cancer. Asian Pac J Cancer Prev. 2010;11:181-5.

[28] Sugasawa K, Ng JM, Masutani C, Iwai S, van der Spek PJ, Eker AP, et al. Xeroderma pigmentosum group C protein complex is the initiator of global genome nucleotide excision repair. Mol Cell. 1998;2:223-32.

[29] Li L, Elledge SJ, Peterson CA, Bales ES, Legerski RJ. Specific association between the human DNA repair proteins XPA and ERCC1. Proc Natl Acad Sci U S A. 1994;91:5012-6.

[30] Buchko GW, Isern NG, Spicer LD, Kennedy MA. Human nucleotide excision repair protein XPA: NMR spectroscopic studies of an XPA fragment containing the ERCC1-binding region and the minimal DNA-binding domain (M59-F219). Mutat Res. 2001;486:1-10.

[31] Saijo M, Kuraoka I, Masutani C, Hanaoka F, Tanaka K. Sequential binding of DNA repair proteins RPA and ERCC1 to XPA in vitro. Nucleic Acids Res. 1996;24:4719-24.

[32] Orelli B, McClendon TB, Tsodikov OV, Ellenberger T, Niedernhofer LJ, Scharer OD. The XPA-binding domain of ERCC1 is required for nucleotide excision repair but not other DNA repair pathways. J Biol Chem. 2010;285:3705-12.

[33] Barret JM, Cadou M, Hill BT. Inhibition of nucleotide excision repair and sensitisation of cells to DNA cross-linking anticancer drugs by F 11782, a novel fluorinated epipodophylloid. Biochem Pharmacol. 2002;63:251-8.

[34] Jiang H, Yang LY. Cell cycle checkpoint abrogator UCN-01 inhibits DNA repair: association with attenuation of the interaction of XPA and ERCC1 nucleotide excision repair proteins. Cancer Res. 1999;59:4529-34.

[35] Aune GJ, Furuta T, Pommier Y. Ecteinascidin 743: a novel anticancer drug with a unique mechanism of action. Anticancer Drugs. 2002;13:545-55.

[36] Wood RD, Robins P, Lindahl T. Complementation of the xeroderma pigmentosum DNA repair defect in cell-free extracts. Cell. 1988;53:97-106.

[37] Salles B, Rodrigo G, Li RY, Calsou P. DNA damage excision repair in microplate wells with chemiluminescence detection: development and perspectives. Biochimie. 1999;81:53-8.

[38] Perrin D, van Hille B, Barret JM, Kruczynski A, Etievant C, Imbert T, et al. F 11782, a novel epipodophylloid non-intercalating dual catalytic inhibitor of topoisomerases I and II with an original mechanism of action. Biochem Pharmacol. 2000;59:807-19.

[39] Wang Q, Fan S, Eastman A, Worland PJ, Sausville EA, O'Connor PM. UCN-01: a potent abrogator of G2 checkpoint function in cancer cells with disrupted p53. J Natl Cancer Inst. 1996;88:956-65.

[40] Barakat KH, Jordheim LP, Dumonte C, Tuszynski J. Virtual screening and biological evaluation of inhibitors targeting the XPA-ERCC1 interaction. Accepted in PLoS ONE. 2012.

[41] Jordheim LP, Barakat KH, Heinrich-Balard L, Matera E-L, Cros-Perrial E, Bouledrak K, et al. Small molecule inhibitors of ERCC1-XPF protein-protein interaction synergize alkylating agents in cancer cells. Submitted to Molecular Pharmacology. 2012.

[42] Lin JH, Perryman AL, Schames JR, McCammon JA. The relaxed complex method: Accommodating receptor flexibility for drug design with an improved scoring scheme. Biopolymers. 2003;68:47-62.

[43] Schames JR, Henchman RH, Siegel JS, Sotriffer CA, Ni H, McCammon JA. Discovery of a novel binding trench in HIV integrase. J Med Chem. 2004;47:1879-81.

[44] Markowitz MN, B.Y. Gotuzzo, F.; Mendo, F.; Ratanasuwan, W.; Kovacs, C.; Zhao, J.; Gilde, L.; Isaacs, R.; Teppler, H. Potent antiviral effect of MK-0518, novel HIV-1 integrase inhibitor, as part of combination ART in treatment-naive HIV-1 infected patients. 16th International AIDS Conference, Toronto, Canada. 2006.

[45] Babakhani A, Talley TT, Taylor P, McCammon JA. A virtual screening study of the acetylcholine binding protein using a relaxed-complex approach. Comput Biol Chem. 2009;33:160-70.

[46] Amaro RE, Schnaufer A, Interthal H, Hol W, Stuart KD, McCammon JA. Discovery of drug-like inhibitors of an essential RNA-editing ligase in Trypanosoma brucei. Proc Natl Acad Sci U S A. 2008;105:17278-83.

[47] Durrant JD, McCammon JA. Potential drug-like inhibitors of Group 1 influenza neuraminidase identified through computer-aided drug design. Comput Biol Chem. 2010;34:97-105.

[48] Durrant JD, Urbaniak MD, Ferguson MA, McCammon JA. Computer-aided identification of Trypanosoma brucei uridine diphosphate galactose 4'-epimerase inhibitors: toward the development of novel therapies for African sleeping sickness. J Med Chem. 2010;53:5025-32.

[49] K. Barakat, L. Jordheim, C. Dumontet, Tuszynski. J. Virtual screening and biological evaluation of inhibitors targeting the XPA-ERCC1 interaction. Molecular Cancer Therapeutics. Submitted Jan 2012

Chapter 21

The Molecular Epidemiology of DNA Repair Polymorphisms in Carcinogenesis

Paul W. Brandt-Rauf, Yongliang Li,
Changmin Long and Regina Monaco

Additional information is available at the end of the chapter

http://dx.doi.org/10.5772/53936

1. Introduction

There are well-established examples of highly penetrant mutations in genes that are directly involved in carcinogenesis and result in a high risk of cancer in the individuals who carry these mutations. Some of the best examples include syndromes of defective DNA repair, such as xeroderma pigmentosum [1]. However, these examples tend to be very rare and thus contribute minimally to the overall burden of cancer risk. Nevertheless, it has long been suspected that less penetrant susceptibility may be produced by much more common variants in the same cancer-related genes, for example, in the form of single nucleotide polymorphisms (SNPs), that presumably would be less disruptive and therefore produce more subtle effects on the function of the encoded proteins but which could contribute greatly to overall cancer attributable risk in populations due to their widespread occurrence [1]. Because several of these common polymorphisms occur in DNA repair proteins, many epidemiologic studies have examined their relationship to cancer risk [2-4].

These studies have looked at all different types of cancer, many different at-risk populations, several different DNA repair pathways, and a variety of polymorphisms at different sites [5-18]. The results to date at best have been inconsistent, conflicting and confusing with many examples of positive, negative or null associations between particular polymorphisms and particular cancers, even in multiple large meta-analyses of the data. For example, a very recent large, rigorous and systematic review of the literature on the involvement of DNA repair polymorphisms in human cancer reached the conclusion that because of the inconsistencies in the literature "none of the cancer genome-wide association studies (GWAs) published so far showed highly statistically significant associations for any of the common DNA repair gene variants" and "clarification of the discrepancies in the literature is needed." [4] It was suggested that one way to proceed would be that "gene/environment and gene/lifestyle interactions for carcinogenic mechanisms involving DNA repair should be investigated more systematically and with less classification error." [4] However, even in studies of populations with exposures to known environmental carcinogens and the cancers most closely associated with those exposures, the results of DNA repair polymorphism studies have not always been clear-cut; these inconsistencies may also be the result of poor exposure classification, multiple confounders and/or poor understanding of the exact mechanisms of DNA damage and/or repair [19-23]. In other words, what is needed is to study model systems where there are clear linkages between the exposure to the carcinogenic risk factor and the specific DNA damage that it produces with the DNA repair mechanisms that would correct those particular defects.

In environmental carcinogenesis studies of DNA repair polymorphisms, the majority of the work has focused on base excision repair (BER) or nucleotide excision repair (NER) pathways, since these are thought to play dominant roles in the repair of damage from exogenous carcinogens, including chemical carcinogens. In both of these pathways, numerous polymorphisms in numerous proteins that make up the DNA repair machinery have been examined. However, much of the focus has been on the particular proteins in the respective pathways that contain the most common polymorphic variants, in particular the x-ray cross complementing-1 (XRCC1) protein in BER and the xeroderma pigmentosum-D (XPD) protein in NER [24-38].

This is also understandable because of the critical roles that each of these proteins play in their respective pathways. For example, in BER the particular type of damage produced by exposure to a chemical carcinogen is usually recognized and removed by a specific DNA glycoslase. The BER apparatus includes numerous other proteins that complete the repair at the resultant abasic site once the damage is removed: apurinic/apyrimidinic endonuclease (APE1), poly(ADP-ribose) polymerase-1 (PARP-1), poly(ADP-ribose) polymerase-2 (PARP-2), DNA polymerase β (Pol β) and DNA ligase IIIα (Lig III). AP endonuclease is responsible for cleaving the phosphodiester bond at the abasic site created by the glycosylase. PARP-1 and to a lesser extent PARP-2 participate in the repair process by catalyzing ribosylation of a number of DNA-bound proteins, thereby decreasing the affinity of these proteins for DNA, and allowing the repair machinery to access the damaged site. Pol β, the polymerase involved in short patch repair, provides two essential activities, deoxyribophosphodiesterase activity which releases the 5' sugar phosphate group, and gap filling synthesis, where one nucleotide is added to the 3' OH. Finally, Lig III seals the nick in an ATP-dependent manner [39, 40]. The XRCC1 protein is critical to this process since it acts as a scaffold protein in this pathway and appears to enhance the activity of the other BER proteins. Although XRCC1 has not been demonstrated to contain enzymatic activity of its own, it is thus necessary for coordinating and regulating the early and late stages of BER through its protein interaction modules [41, 42].

XRCC1 is known to contain three common polymorphic sites that might be expected to have an effect on XRCC1 structure and function because they occur in or near important protein domains [11]. For example, the polymorphism at amino acid residue 194, which results in the substitution of a tryptophan for the normal arginine, occurs in the XRCC1 N-terminal domain from amino acid residues 1-195 that has been observed to mediate its interaction with the palm-thumb domain of Pol β [43]. A second polymorphism at amino acid residue 280, which results in the substitution of a histidine for the normal arginine, occurs in the region between the N-terminal domain and the BRCA1 carboxy terminal (BRCT1) domain of the protein and close to the nuclear localization signal site and thus could affect the relationship between these two critical domains and/or the protein's localization ability [44]. The third and most common polymorphism in XRCC1 occurs at amino acid residue 399, resulting in the substitution of a glutamine for the normal arginine, within the highly conserved BRCT1 domain from amino acid residues 315-403, which has been associated with the functioning of PARP1, PARP2 and APE1 [45].

Like BER, NER occurs in a series of steps: damage recognition, unwinding and demarcation of the DNA, excision of the single-stranded fragment containing the damaged site, and DNA re-synthesis. NER is accomplished primarily through the action of proteins of the xeroderma pigmentosum family of genes which are categorized into 7 different groups (A-G). XPC and XPE proteins are involved in recognition of different types of DNA damage. XPB and XPD are DNA helicases that function as subunits of the transcription factor IIH complex (TFIIH) to promote DNA bubble formation at the damaged site by unwinding the DNA as XPA complexes with replication protein A (RPA) for demarcation. XPF and XPG are structure-specific endonucleases for excision of the damaged site. Finally, replicative DNA polymerase and DNA ligase I complete the repair [46, 47]. XPD is one of the major players in NER and is essential for life [48, 49].

XPD is also known to contain at least two common polymorphic sites, namely at amino acid residues 312 (aspartic acid->asparagine) and 751 (lysine->glutamine) [50]. The 751 site is assumed to be particularly important for XPD function since it occurs in the C-terminal domain of the protein which has been suggested to interact with the p44 helicase activator protein of the TFIIH complex [51]; also, it is been shown that an XPD mutation that results in the loss of the final 17 C-terminal amino acids, including residue 751, results in the clinical disease phenotype of trichothiodystrophy [52].

In summary, an ideal system for investigating the role of DNA repair polymorphisms in carcinogenesis might be an exposure to a known chemical carcinogen that produces specific types of DNA damage that are repaired by the BER and/or NER pathways where the effects of common polymorphisms in XRCC1 and XPD on the damage and repair could be studied.

2. A model for the study of the epidemiology of dna repair polymorphisms in carcinogenesis

Such a potential model system for the study of the role of DNA repair polymorphisms in chemical carcinogenesis is provided by the known carcinogen vinyl chloride (VC) because considerable detail is available concerning the molecular biology of its pathogenic pathway which allows for careful study of the role of DNA damage and repair in the carcinogenic process in exposed human populations through the application of molecular epidemiologic approaches (Figure 1).

As noted, VC is a well-established animal and human carcinogen. It is most strongly associated with liver cancer, in particular the rare, sentinel neoplasm of angiosarcoma of the liver (ASL), a malignant tumor of the endothelial cells of the liver [53]. However, VC has also been identified as a cause of hepatocellular carcinoma (HCC), the corresponding malignant tumor of the parenchymal cells of the liver [54]. In addition, it has been associated with other malignancies, e.g., lung and brain, although these associations remain much more controversial. The most significant exposures to VC occur in the petrochemical and plastics industries because VC is used in the manufacture of polyvinyl chloride, one of most high-volume plastics in the world. For example, it is estimated that worldwide more than 2,200,000 workers are probably occupationally exposed to VC. General population exposures also occur primarily through the air and water. For example, elevated levels of VC have been found not only in the air near VC manufacturing and processing facilities but also in the vicinity of many hazardous waste sites and municipal landfills, either due to the direct disposal of VC or from the microbial degradation of other chlorinated solvents to form VC. In some cases, dangerously high levels have been detected in the air at some of these landfills [53]. General population exposures may also occur from tobacco smoke, drinking water from PVC pipe, and consumption of food and beverages from PVC packaging and bottles, although probably at much lower levels.

VC is a gas so the most significant exposures are respiratory. Following inhalation, absorption is rapid in humans and most subsequent metabolism occurs in the liver [53]. Phase I metabolism is primarily via the cytochrome P-450 isoenzyme 2E1 (CYP2E1) to generate the reactive intermediates chloroethylene oxide (CEO) and chloracetaldehyde (CAA) which are further metabolized in phase II reactions by glutathione-S-transferases (GSTs) and aldehyde dehydrogenase 2 (ALDH2) to end products for ultimate excretion. However, CEO and CAA can readily interact with cellular macromolecules, including DNA, to produce promutagenic effects. VC biotransformation to CEO probably occurs principally in hepatocytes, but the epoxide can also reach and react with adjacent sinusoidal lining cells, so that mutagenic effects can occur in parenchymal liver cells and non-parenchymal endothelial cells, providing a logical rationale for the association between VC exposure and ASL as well as HCC [55]. The major VC-associated liver DNA adduct is 7-(2-oxoethyl)guanine, comprising up to 98% of all adducts formed. However, this adduct is eliminated from the DNA with a very short half-life, principally by chemical depurination, and is not considered to be promutagenic. On the other hand, three etheno DNA adducts are also formed in much less abundance, but they are known to be promutagenic. These are: N^2,3-ethenoguanine (εG) ; 1,N^6-ethenoadenine (εA) ; and 3,N^4-ethenocytosine (εC) [56].

The promutagenic properties of etheno-DNA adducts that are not fully repaired by one or another of the DNA repair pathways have been well documented in experimental systems *in vitro*, as well as *in vivo* in bacterial and mammalian cells. The εA adduct generates A->T, A->G and A->C base changes; the εG adduct generates G->A base changes; and the εC adduct generates C->A and C->T base changes [55]. These experimental results are consistent with the tumor mutational spectra identified in exposed animals and humans in oncogenes and tumor suppressor genes. Of particular interest have been the A->T transversions at codons 179, 249 and 255 of the *TP53* tumor suppressor gene generated by εA adducts and the G->A transitions at codon 13 of the K-*ras* oncogene generated by εG adducts, because of their frequent occurrence in human ASLs from VC-exposed individuals but not in sporadic ASLs in individuals without VC exposure. In addition, other results suggest that these VC-associated mutations, particularly the codon 13 K-*ras* mutation, may be a relatively early event in VC carcinogenesis, and thus the occurrence of these mutations may be useful biomarkers of cancer risk in exposed individuals, as discussed below.

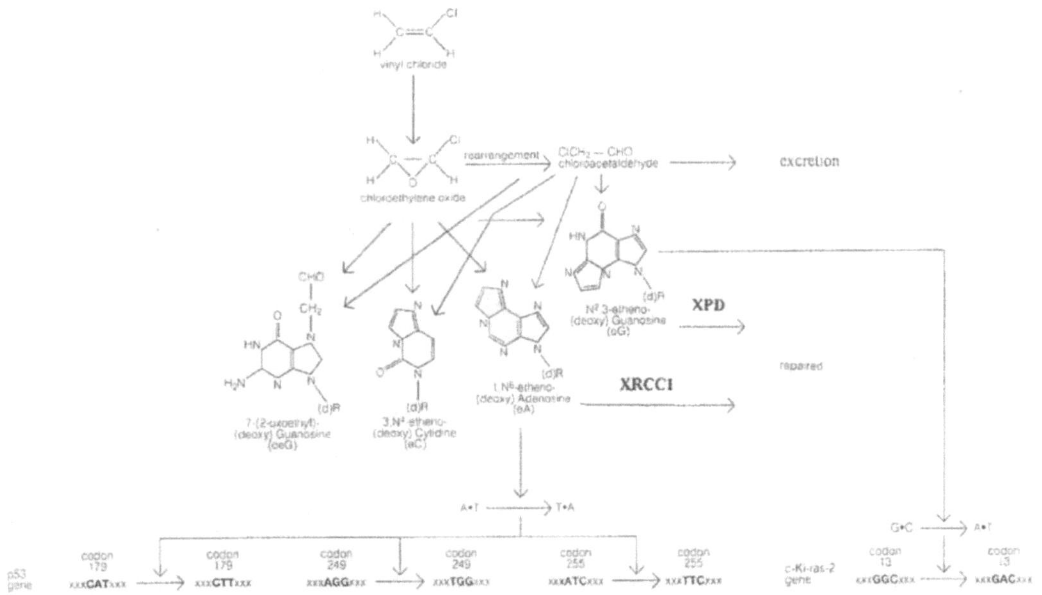

Figure 1. Proposed mechanism of VC-induced DNA damage and repair as a model system for the study of the effects of polymorphisms in BER and NER pathways.

The G->A transition at codon 13 of K-*ras* results in the substitution of an aspartic acid for the normal glycine at amino acid residue 13 in the encoded p21 protein product. This substitution is believed to be oncogenic, having been identified in other human tumors as well. The oncogenic mechanism of action of this substitution is thought to be through the production of a conformational change in p21 which may be responsible for altering its intrinsic GTPase activity, thus affecting signal transduction within the cell leading to uncontrolled growth and division [57]. Similarly, the A->T transversions at various codons of *p53* produce their corresponding amino acid substitutions in the encoded p53 protein product, all changes that have been shown to cause the protein to adopt its so-called "malignant" conformation with a concomitant loss of its normal tumor suppressor activity [57]. These protein changes provide a useful indicator of the pathogenic consequences of the occurrence of the corresponding mutations, as well as convenient intermediate biomarkers of VC effect to study the molecular epidemiology of VC carcinogenesis in exposed human populations, including the effects of polymorphisms in the relevant DNA repair pathways.

It has been shown that the mutant *ras*-p21 protein containing aspartic acid for glycine at amino acid residue 13 can be distinguished from the wild-type protein and other mutant *ras*-p21 proteins immunologically with a mouse monoclonal antibody specific for this protein. For cells in culture that contain the mutant *ras* gene, it is possible to use this monoclonal antibody to detect mutant *ras*-p21 expression in the cells by immunocytochemistry and in the extracellular supernatant by immunoblotting. In analogous situations *in vivo,* mutant Asp 13 *ras*-p21 can be detected in tumor tissue by immunohistochemistry and in the serum by immunoblotting of VC-exposed workers with ASLs known to contain the mutant *ras* gene but not in the serum of VC-exposed workers with ASLs that do not contain the mutation or in unexposed controls [57-59].

An analogous, although slightly more complicated situation occurs with p53. As noted, all of the VC-induced mutations in the *p53* gene have been shown to cause a similar conformational change in the encoded p53 protein that results in the exposure of a common epitope, which is normally not immunologically detectable in the wild-type protein. Thus, these mutant p53 proteins can be distinguished from wild-type p53 immunologically with a mouse monoclonal antibody that binds to this mutant-specific epitope. For cells in culture that contain the mutant *p53* genes, it is possible to use this monoclonal antibody to detect mutant p53 protein expression in the cells by immunocytochemistry and in the extracellular supernatant by immunoblotting or by enzyme-linked immunosorbent assay (ELISA). In the analogous situation *in vivo,* mutant p53 can be detected in the tumor tissue by immunohistochemistry and in the serum by immunoblotting or ELISA of VC-exposed workers with ASLs known to contain the mutant p53 genes but not of VC-exposed workers with ASLs that do not contain the mutations or in unexposed controls. In some cases of mutant p53-positive tumors, it is known that individuals can also develop an antibody response to the mutant p53 which can obscure the detection of the mutant p53 protein itself. However, it is also possible to detect these autoantibodies to mutant p53 using an ELISA. Thus, the detection in serum of mutant p53 protein and/or an antibody response to mutant p53 protein can be used together to best identify individuals who have a *p53* mutation in their tumors [57, 60, 61].

Based on the above evidence, it seems that these serum biomarkers for mutant *ras*-p21 and mutant p53 accurately reflect the occurrence of the corresponding DNA damage in the target tissue of VC-exposed workers. In addition, these biomarkers have been identified not only in VC-exposed workers with ASLs but also in VC-exposed workers with non-malignant (but potentially pre-malignant) angiomatous lesions and in VC-exposed workers without any apparent neoplastic disease [57, 62-64]. In a large cohort of French VC workers, the presence of these biomarkers was found to occur with a highly statistically significant dose-response relationship with regard to estimated, cumulative VC exposure, supporting the claim that the generation of the biomarkers was indeed the result of the exposure [65]. Similar results with these biomarkers have been noted in several other VC workers cohorts around the world [66-71]. To date in these various studies, at least five VC-exposed biomarker-positive workers without ASL have developed subsequent liver lesions presumed to be ASLs, also suggesting that these biomarkers may have predictive value for the subsequent occurrence of cancer.

However, at any given level of VC exposure, some workers will have none, one or both mutant biomarkers. One possible explanation for this inter-individual variability is genetic differences in the proteins that metabolize VC or repair the DNA damage it produces. Although polymorphisms in the proteins involved in metabolizing VC have been shown to have an effect, polymorphisms in DNA repair proteins have been found to be even more significant.

There are several potential mechanisms by which VC-induced adducts could be repaired before they have a chance to cause mutations. As noted above, the oxoethyl adduct is removed rapidly by chemical depurination. The potential repair of the etheno adducts, however, is more complicated and involves the BER and NER pathways.

For example, the 1,N^6-εA adducts are recognized and removed by 3-methyl adenine DNA glycosylase which is part of the BER pathway [55]. Likewise, the 3,N^4-ethenocytosine adducts are also repaired with high efficiency by BER via the thymine DNA glycosylase. Therefore, polymorphisms in the BER pathway that could decrease DNA repair efficiency, particularly the polymorphisms in XRCC1, might be expected to result in an increase in εA and εC adduct levels at any given level of exposure in VC-exposed individuals with a resultant increase in the VC-associated mutant biomarkers, particularly the mutant p53 biomarker. In contrast, the N^2,3-ethenoguanine adducts have been shown to be not very efficiently repaired by BER [56, 72]. Thus, if they are repaired, it is likely to be by a different DNA repair pathway such as NER. Therefore, polymorphisms in the NER pathway that could decrease DNA repair efficiency, particularly the polymorphisms in XPD, might be expected to result in an increase in εG adduct levels at any given level of exposure in VC-exposed individuals with a resultant increase in the VC-associated mutant biomarkers, particularly the mutant *ras*-p21 biomarker.

In fact in the aforementioned French VC worker cohort, we have been able to identify the effect of the XRCC1 polymorphisms on the occurrence of the mutant p53 biomarker, but not the mutant *ras*-p21 biomarker [73-75]. The difference in effect on the two biomarkers is expected, since, as noted the εA adducts that result in the mutant p53 biomarker are repaired efficiently by BER but the εG adducts that result in the mutant *ras*–p21 biomarker are not, so changes in XRCC1 might affect the former but should not affect the latter. Among the three XRCC1 polymorphisms, the most significant effect on the mutant p53 biomarker was attributable to the residue 399 polymorphism. In this case, individuals who were homozygous variant Gln-Gln at 399 had a statistically significant 1.9-fold risk of occurrence of the mutant p53 biomarker compared to homozygous Arg-Arg wild-type individuals, even after controlling for potential confounders including cumulative VC exposure, and the gene-environment interaction between the polymorphism and VC exposure appeared to be potentially supra-multiplicative [75]. Studies in other VC worker populations have found similar effects of the XRCC1 polymorphisms, particularly the 399 polymorphism, on the mutant p53 biomarker, as well as other biomarkers of DNA damage [76-79].

This is also consistent with various experimental results examining this model system. For example, molecular modeling of the BRCT1 domains of the normal and polymorphic forms of XRCC1 demonstrates that the 399 substitution produces significant conformational changes in this domain, including the loss of secondary structural features such as α-helices that can be critical for mediating protein-protein interactions that would allow XRCC1 to coordinate

BER [80]. Also, studies of lymphoblasts from individuals of different genotypes exposed *in vitro* to the reactive metabolites of VC showed that cells with the XRCC1 399 homozygous variant Gln-Gln genotype had an approximate 4-fold decrease in efficiency of repair of εA DNA adducts compared to cells with the homozygous wild-type Arg-Arg genotype [74, 81], resulting in an approximate 1.8-fold increase in mutation frequency in the polymorphic cells compared to the wild-type cells as determined by the hypoxanthine-guanine phosphoribosyltransferase (HPRT) assay [82]. Based on mutational spectrum studies in CAA-exposed human cell lines [83], the resultant increase in ▪ A DNA adducts would especially result in an increase in A->T transversions consistent with those found in the tumors of VC-exposed workers, as noted above.

Furthermore, in the French VC worker cohort, we have been able to identify the effect of the XPD polymorphisms on the occurrence of both mutant biomarkers, although the most marked and statistically significant effect was on the mutant *ras*-p21 biomarker, as expected [75]. In this case, individuals who were homozygous variant at either residue 312 or 751 had a statistically significant 2.6-3.0-fold increased risk of occurrence of the mutant *ras*–p21 biomarker compared to homozygous wild-type individuals, even after controlling for potential confounders including cumulative VC exposure. Furthermore, in the case of the residue 751 polymorphism, the gene-environment interaction between the polymorphism and VC exposure, as well as the gene-gene interaction between the XPD and CYP2E1 polymorphisms (which could increase VC metabolism to its promutagenic reactive metabolites and thus also increase etheno-DNA adducts at any given level of VC exposure with a resultant increase in the mutant biomarkers) appeared to be potentially multiplicative [75]. Once again, studies in other VC worker populations have found similar effects of the XPD polymorphisms on other biomarkers of DNA damage [77].

This is also consistent with various experimental results in this model system. For example, molecular modeling of the normal and polymorphic forms of XPD demonstrates that these substitutions produce discrete local conformational changes in the protein which affect its overall structure and could affect its function [82, 84], and, in particular, are projected to interfere with its protein-protein interactions and binding to other components of the TFIIH complex (Figure 2; adapted from Gibbons et al. [85]). Also, studies of lymphoblasts from individuals of different genotypes exposed *in vitro* to the reactive metabolites of VC showed that cells with the XPD 751 homozygous variant Gln-Gln genotype had an approximate 5-fold decrease in efficiency of repair of εG DNA adducts compared to cells with the homozygous wild-type Lys-Lys genotype [82], resulting in an approximate 4.8-fold increase in mutation frequency in the polymorphic cells compared to the wild-type cells as determined by the HPRT assay, even though there is no difference in the level of expression of the XPD protein among cells that are homozygous wild-type, heterozygous or homozygous polymorphic at this codon (Figure 3). Once again, based on mutational spectrum studies in CAA-exposed human cell lines [83], the resultant increase in ▪ G DNA adducts would especially result in an increase in G->A transitions consistent with those found in the tumors of VC-exposed workers.

A thorough understanding of the molecular biology and molecular epidemiology of VC carcinogenesis can provide the basis for new molecular approaches to the prevention of VC-induced cancers and potentially other cancers related to DNA-damaging agents. For example, one approach to secondary prevention could be based on "personalized prevention" derived from knowledge of the status of individual's DNA repair capability. Although little is currently known about methods for altering DNA repair activity, there is some evidence to suggest augmenting DNA repair may be possible. Several *in vitro* studies have shown that DNA repair processes can be increased by selenium-based compounds in response to radiation or chemically induced DNA damage [86]. More recently, a study in mice has suggested that selenocystine administration, although it did not protect against immediate DNA damage following ionizing radiation exposure, was nevertheless protective because it enhanced the rate of repair of the induced DNA damage [87]. In cohorts exposed to DNA damaging agents, determination of the dose of selenium compounds to provide an optimum effect on DNA repair could be based on the genetic status of the exposed individuals in terms of the presence of polymorphisms in key components of the repair apparatus, and the success of such interventions could be effectively monitored by following mutant biomarkers of DNA damage.

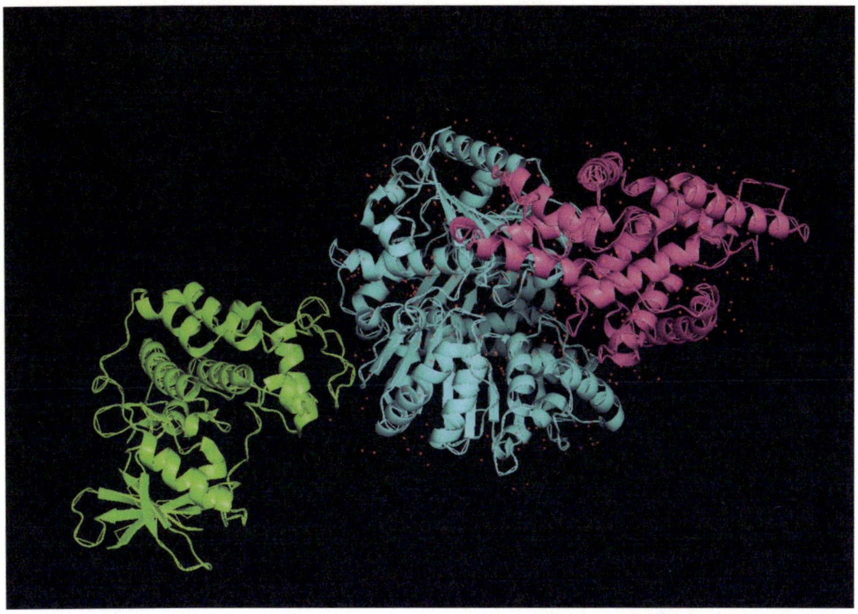

Figure 2. Protein backbone structures showing the proposed interaction effect of XPD (blue), cyclin H (pink) and cdk7 (green) in the TFIIH complex.

3. Conclusion

VC provides an instructive model for the study of the role of DNA repair polymorphisms in chemical carcinogenesis. A detailed understanding of the molecular biology of VC carcinogenesis has provided new ways of studying the molecular epidemiology of

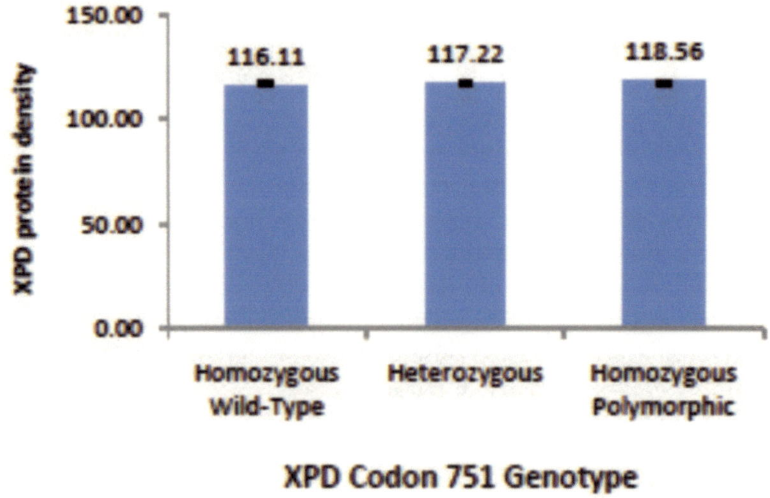

Figure 3. Levels of expression of the XPD protein in lymphocyte cell lines that are homozygous wild-type, heterozygous or homozygous polymorphic at codon 751.

VC carcinogenesis in exposed humans, which in turn may provide the basis for new approaches to the prevention and treatment of VC-related cancer. This model could also have much broader implications, since other potential carcinogenic exposures share some of the same molecular biologic pathways of damage and repair as VC similar molecular epidemiologic biomarkers could be useful for monitoring their carcinogenic process and the effect of altered susceptibility due to changes in DNA repair capability. Such studies in additional model systems would further help to define the exact significance of DNA repair polymorphisms in the development of human cancers.

Acknowledgements

This work was supported in part by grants to PWB-R from NIOSH, R01-OH04192 and R01-OH07590.

Author details

Paul W. Brandt-Rauf*, Yongliang Li, Changmin Long and Regina Monaco

*Address all correspondence to: pwb1@uic.edu

Division of Environmental and Occupational Health Sciences, School of Public Health, University of Illinois at Chicago, Chicago, USA

References

[1] Au WW (2006) Heritable Susceptibility Factors for the Development of Cancer. J. radiat. res. 47:B13-B17.

[2] Berwick M, Vineis P (2000) Markers of DNA Repair and Susceptibility to Cancer in Humans: An Epidemiologic Review. J. natl. cancer inst. 92:874-897.

[3] Goode EL, Ulrich CM, Potter JD (2002) Polymorphisms in DNA Repair Genes and Associations with Cancer Risk. Cancer epidemiol biomarkers prev. 11:1513-1530.

[4] Ricceri F, Matullo G, Vineis P (2012) Is There Evidence of Involvement of DNA Repair Polymorphisms in Human Cancer? Mutat. res. 736:117-121.

[5] Jiricny J, Nystrom-Lahti M (2000) Mismatch Repair Defects in Cancer. Curr. opin. genet. dev. 10:157-161.

[6] Hung RJ, Hall J, Brennan P, Boffetta P (2005) Genetic Polymorphisms in the Base Excision Repair Pathway and Cancer Risk: A HuGE Review. Am. j. epidemiol. 162:925-942.

[7] Weiss JM, Goode EL, Ladiges WC, Ulrich CM (2005) Polymorphic Variation in hOGG1 and Risk of Cancer: A review of the Functional and Epidemiologic Literature. Mol. carcinog. 42:127-141.

[8] Clarkson SG, Wood RD (2005) Polymorphisms in the Human XPD (ERCC2) Gene, DNA Repair Capacity and Cancer Susceptibility: An Appraisal. DNA repair 4:1068-1074.

[9] Hu Z, Ma H, Chen F, Wei Q, Shen H (2005) XRCC1 Polymorphisms and Cancer Risk: A Meta-Analysis of 38 Case-Control Studies. Cancer epidemiol. biomarkers prev. 14:1810-1818.

[10] Manuguerra M, Saletta F, Karagas MR, Berwick M, Vegila F, Vineis P, Matullo G (2006) XRCC3 and XPD/ERCC2 Single Nucleotide Polymorphisms and the Risk of Cancer: A HuGE Review. Am. j. epidemiol. 164:297-302.

[11] Tudek B (2007) Base Excision Repair Modulation as a Risk Factor for Human Cancers. Mol. aspects med. 28:258-275.

[12] Bugni JM, Han J, Tsai M, Hunter DJ, Samson LD (2007) Genetic Association and Functional Studies of Major Polymorphic Variants of MGMT. DNA repair 6:1116-1126.

[13] Qiu L, Wang Z, Shi X, Wang Z (2008) Associations between XPC Polymorphisms and Risk of Cancers: A Meta-Analysis. Eur. j. cancer 44:2241-2253.

[14] Wang F, Chang D, Hu F, Sui H, Han B, Li D, Zhao Y (2008) DNA Repair Gene XPD Polymorphisms and Cancer Risk: A Meta-Analysis Based on 56 Case-Control Studies. Cancer epidemiol. biomarkers prev. 17:507-517.

[15] Jiang J, Zhang X, Yang H, Wang W (2009) Polymorphisms of DNA Repair Genes: ADPRT, XRCC1, and XPD and Cancer Risk in Genetic Epidemiology. In: Verma M,

editor. Methods in Molecular Biology, Cancer Epidemiology, vol. 471. Totowa: Humana Press. pp. 305-333.

[16] Wilson DM, Kim D, Berquist BR, Sigurdson AJ (2011) Variation in Base Excision Repair Capacity. Mutat. res. 711:100-112.

[17] Ding D, Zhang Y, Yu H, Guo Y, Jiang L, He X, Ma W, Zheng W (2012) Genetic Variation of XPA Gene and Risk of Cancer: A Systematic Review and Pooled Analysis. Int. j. cancer 131:488-496.

[18] Gossage L, Perry C, Abbotts R, Madhusudan S (2012) Base Excision Repair Factors are Promising Prognostic and Predictive Markers in Cancer. Curr. mol. pharmacol. 5:115-124.

[19] Hulla JE, Miller MS, Taylor JA, Hein DW, Furlong CE, Omiecinski CJ, Kunkel TA (1999) Symposium Overview: The Role of Genetic Polymorphism and Repair Deficiencies in Environmental Disease. Toxicol. sci. 47:135-143.

[20] de Boer JG (2002) Polymorphisms in DNA Repair and Environmental Interactions. Mutat. res. 509:201-210.

[21] Belitsky GA, Yakubovskaya MG (2008) Genetic Polymorphism and Variability of Chemical Carcinogenesis. Biochemistry 73:543-554.

[22] Klaunig JE, Wang Z, Pu X, Zhou S (2011) Oxidative Stress and Oxidative Damage in Chemical Carcinogenesis. Toxicol. appl. pharmacol. 254:86-99.

[23] Simonelli V, Mazzei F, D'Errico M, Dogliotti E (2012) Gene Susceptibility to Oxidative Damage: From Single Nucleotide Polymorphisms to Function. Mutat. res. 736:104-116.

[24] Stern MC, Johnson LR, Bell DA, Taylor JA (2002) XPD Codon 751 Polymorphism, Metabolism Genes, Smoking, and Bladder Cancer Risk. Cancer epidemiol. biomarkers prev. 11:1004-1011.

[25] Shen M, Hung RJ, Brennan P, Malaveille C, Donato F, Placidi D, Carta A, Hautefeuille A, Boffetta P, Porru S (2003) Polymorphisms of the DNA Repair Genes XRCC1, XRCC3, XPD, Interaction with Environmental Exposures, and Bladder Cancer Risk in a Case-Control Study in Northern Italy. Cancer epidemiol. biomarkers prev. 12:1234-1240.

[26] Gao WM, Romkes M, Day RD, Siegfried JM, Luketich JD, Mady HH, Melhem MF, Keohavong P (2003) Association of the DNA Repair Gene XPD Asp312Asn Polymorphism with p53 Gene Mutations in Tobacco-Related Non-Small Cell Lung Cancer. Carcinogenesis 24:1671-1676.

[27] Terry MB, Gammon MD, Zhang FF, Eng SM, Sagiv SK, Paykin AB, Wang Q, Hayes S, Teitelbaum SL, Neugut AI, Santella RM (2004) Polymorphism in the DNA Repair Gene XPD, Polycyclic Aromatic Hydrocarbon-DNA Adducts, Cigarette Smoking, and Breast Cancer Risk. Cancer epidemiol. biomarkers prev. 13:2053-2058.

[28] Han J, Hankinson SE, Colditz GA, Hunter DJ (2004) Genetic Variation in XRCC1, Sun Exposure, and Risk of Skin Cancer. Br. j. cancer 91:1604-1609.

[29] Neumann AS, Sturgis EM, Wei Q (2005) Nucleotide Excision Repair as a Marker for Susceptibility to Tobacco-Related Cancers: A Review of Molecular Epidemiological Studies. Mol. carcinog. 42:65-92.

[30] Han J, Colditz GA, Liu JS, Hunter DJ (2005) Genetic Variation in XPD, Sun Exposure, and Risk of Skin Cancer. Cancer epidemiol. biomarkers prev. 14:1539-1544.

[31] Leng S, Cheng J, Zhang L, Niu Y, Dai Y, Pan Z, Li B, He F, Zheng Y (2005) The Association of XRCC1 Haplotypes and Chromosomal Damage Levels in Peripheral Blood Lymphocytes Among Coke-Oven Workers. Cancer epidemiol. biomarkers prev. 14: 1295-1301.

[32] Zhao XH, Jia G, Liu YQ, Liu SW, Yan L, Jin Y, Liu N (2006) Association Between Polymorphisms of DNA Repair Gene XRCC1 and DNA Damage in Asbestos-Exposed Workers. Biomed. environ. sci. 19:232-238.

[33] Long XD, Ma Y, Wei YP, Deng ZL (2006) The Polymorphisms of GSTM1, GSTT1, HYL1*2, and XRCC1, and Aflatoxin B1-Related Hepatocellular Carcinoma in Guangxi Population, China. Hepatol. res. 36:48-55.

[34] Neri M, Ugolini D, Dianzani I, Gemignani F, Landi S, Cesario A, Magnani C, Mutti L, Puntoni R, Bonassi S (2008) Genetic Susceptibility to Malignant Pleural Mesothelioma and Other Asbestos-Associated Diseases. Mutat. res. 659:126-136.

[35] Long XD, Ma Y, Zhou YF, Yao JG, Ban FZ, Huang YZ, Huang BC (2009) XPD Codon 312 and 751 Polymorphisms, and AFB1 Exposure, and Hepatocellular Carcinoma Risk. BMC cancer 9:400.

[36] Sterpone S, Cozzi R (2010) Influence of XRCC1 Genetic Polymorphisms on Ionizing Radiation-Induced DNA Damage and Repair. J. nucleic acids

[37] Toumpanakis D, Theocharis SE (2011) DNA Repair Systems in Malignant Mesothelioma. Cancer lett. 312:143-149.

[38] Zhang XH, Zhang X, Zhang L, Chen Q, Yang Z, Yu J, Fu H, Zhu YM (2012) XRCC1 Arg399Gln Was Associated with Repair Capacity for DNA Damage Induced by Occupational Chromium Exposure. BMC res. notes 5:263.

[39] Fortini P, Pascucci B, Parlanti E, D'Errico M, Simonelli V, Dogliotti E (2003) The Base Excision Repair: Mechanisms and Its Relevance for Cancer Susceptibility. Biochemie 85:1053-1071.

[40] Baute J, Depicker A (2008) Base Excision Repair and Its Role in Maintaining Genome Stability. Crit. rev. biochem mol. biol. 43:239-276.

[41] Thompson LH, West MG (2000) XRCC1 Keeps DNA from Getting Stranded. Mutat. res. 459:1-18.

[42] Caldecott KW (2003) XRCC1 and DNA Strand Break Repair. DNA repair 2:955-969.

[43] Marintchev A, Mullen MA, Maciejewski MW, Pan B, Gryk MR, Mullen GP (1999) Solution Structure of the Single-Strand Break Repair Protein XRCC1 N-Terminal Domain. Nat. struct. biol. 6: 884-893.

[44] Marintchev A, Robertson A, Dimitriadis EK, Prasad R, Wilson SH, Mullen GP (2000) Domain Specific Interaction in the XRCC1 Polymerase Beta Complex. Nucleic acids res. 28:2049-2059.

[45] Vidal AE, Boiteux S, Hickson ID, Radicella JP (2001) XRCC1 Coordinates the Initial and Late Stages of DNA Abasic Site Repair through Protein-Protein Interactions. EMBO j. 20:6530-6539.

[46] Nouspikel T (2009) DNA Repair in Mammalian Cells: Nucleotide Excision Repair: Variations in Versatility. Cell. mol. life sci. 66:994-1009.

[47] Bergoglio V, Magnaldo T (2006) Nucleotide Excision Repair and Related Human Diseases. Genome dyn. 1:35-52.

[48] Oksenych V, Coin F (2010) The Long Unwinding Road: XPB and XPD Helicases in Damaged DNA Opening. Cell cycle 9:90-96.

[49] Lehmann AR (2008) XPD Structure Reveals Its Secrets. DNA repair 7:1912-1915.

[50] Benhamou S, Sarasin A (2002) ERCC2/XPD Gene Polymorphisms and Cancer Risk. Mutagenesis 17:463-469.

[51] Bienstock RJ, Skovaga M. Mandavilli BS, Van Houten B (2003) Structural and Functional Characterization of the Human DNA Repair Helicase XPD by Comparative Molecular Modeling and Site-Directed Mutagenesis of the Bacterial Repair Protein UvrB. J. biol. chem.. 278:5309-5316.

[52] Botta E, Nardo T, Broughton BC, Marinoni S, Lehmann AR, Stefanini M (1998) Analysis of Mutations in the XPD Gene in Italian Patients with Trichothiodystrophy: Site of Mutation Correlates with Repair Deficiency, but Gene Dosage Appears to Determine Clinical Severity. J. hum. genet. 63:1036-1048.

[53] Agency for Toxic Substances and Disease Registry (2006) Toxicological Profile for Vinyl Chloride. Atlanta: US Department of Health and Human Services.

[54] Grosse Y, Baan R, Straif K, Secretan B, El Ghissassi F, Bouvard V, Altieri A, Cogliano V (2007) Carcinogenicity of 1,3-Butadiene, Ethylene Oxide, Vinyl Chloride, Vinyl Fluoride, and Vinyl Bromide. Lancet oncol. 8:679-680.

[55] Dogliotti E (2006) Molecular Mechanisms of Carcinogenesis by Vinyl Chloride. Ann. 1st super sanita 42:163-169.

[56] Cohen SM, Storer RD, Criswell KA, Doerrer NG, Dellarco VL, Pegg DG, Wojcinski ZW, Malarkey DE, Jacobs AC, Klaunig JE, Swenberg JA, Cook JC (2009) Hemangiosarcoma in Rodents: Mode-of-Action Evaluation and Human Relevance. Toxicol. sci. 111:4-18.

[57] Li Y, Asherova M, Marion MJ, Brandt-Rauf PW (1998) Mutant Oncoprotein Biomarkers in Chemical Carcinogenesis. In: Mendelsohn ML, Mohr LC, Peeters JP, editors.

Biomarkers – Medical and Workplace Applications. Washington: Joseph Henry Press. pp. 345-353.

[58] DeVivo I, Marion MJ, Smith SJ, Carney WP, Brandt-Rauf PW (1994) Mutant c-Ki-ras p21 Protein in Chemical Carcinogenesis in Humans Exposed to Vinyl Chloride. Cancer causes control 5:273-278.

[59] Li Y, Marion MJ, Asherova M, Coulibaly D, Smith SJ, Do T, Carney WP, Brandt-Rauf PW (1998) Mutant p21ras in Vinyl Chloride Exposed Workers. Biomarkers 3:433-439.

[60] Brandt-Rauf PW, Chen JM, Marion MJ, Smith SJ, Luo JC, Carney W, Pincus MR (1996) Conformational Effects in the p53 Protein of Mutations Induced during Chemical Carcinogenesis: Molecular Dynamic and Immunologic Analyses. J. protein chem. 15:367-375.

[61] Smith SJ, Li Y, Whitney R, Marion MJ, Partilo S, Carney WP, Brandt-Rauf PW (1998) Molecular Epidemiology of p53 Protein Mutations in Workers Exposed to Vinyl Chloride. Am. j. epidemiol. 147:302-308.

[62] Brandt-Rauf PW, Luo JC, Cheng TJ, Du CL, Wang JD, Marion MJ (2000) Mutant Oncoprotein Biomarkers of Vinyl Chloride Exposure: Application to Risk Assessment. In: Anderson D, Karakaya AE, Sram RJ, editors. Human Monitoring after Environmental and Occupational Exposure to Chemical and Physical Agents. Amsterdam: IOS Press. pp. 243-248.

[63] Brandt-Rauf PW, Luo JC, Cheng TJ, Du CL, Wang JD, Rosal R, Do T, Marion MJ (2002) Molecular Biomarkers and Epidemiologic Risk Assessment. Hum. ecol. risk assess. 8:1295-1301.

[64] Marion MJ, DeVivo I, Smith S, Luo JC, Brandt-Rauf PW (1996) The Molecular Epidemiology of Occupational Carcinogenesis in Vinyl Chloride Exposed Workers. Int. arch. occup. environ. health 68:394-398.

[65] Schindler J, Li Y, Marion MJ, Paroly A, Brandt-Rauf PW (2007) The Effect of Genetic Polymorphisms in the Vinyl Chloride Metabolic Pathway on Mutagenic Risk. J. hum. genet. 52:448-455.

[66] Trivers GE, Cawley HL, DeBenedetti VM, Hollstein M, Marion MJ, Bennett ML, Hoover ML, Prives CC, Tamburro CC, Harris CC (1995) Anti-p53 Antibodies in Sera of Workers Occupationally Exposed to Vinyl Chloride. J. natl. cancer inst. 87:1400-1407.

[67] Luo JC, Liu HT, Cheng TJ, Du CL, Wang JD (1998) Plasma Asp13-Ki-ras Oncoprotein Expression in Vinyl Chloride Monomer Workers in Taiwan. J. occup. environ. med. 40:1053-1058.

[68] Luo JC, Liu HT, Cheng TJ, Du CL, Wang JD (1999) Plasma p53 Protein and Anti-p53 Antibody Expression in Vinyl Chloride Monomer Workers in Taiwan. J. occup. environ. med. 41:521-526.

[69] Luo JC, Cheng TJ, Du CL, Wang JD (2003) Molecular Epidemiology of Plasma Oncoproteins in Vinyl Chloride Monomer Workers in Taiwan. Cancer detect. prev. 27:94-101.

[70] Mocci F, De Biasio AL, Nettuno M (2003) Anti-p53 Antibodies as Markers of Carcinogenesis in Exposures to Vinyl Chloride. G. ital. med. lav. ergon. 25:S21-S23.

[71] Mocci F, Nettuno M (2006) Plasma Mutant-p53 Protein and Anti-p53 Antibody as a Marker: An Experience in Vinyl Chloride Workers in Italy. J. occup. environ. med. 48:158-164.

[72] Dosanjh MK, Chenna A, Kim E, Fraenkel-Conrat H, Samson L, Singer B (1994) All Four Known Cyclic Adducts Formed in DNA by the Vinyl Chloride Metabolite Chloroacetaldehyde are Released by a Human DNA Glycosylase. Proc. natl. acad. sci. usa 91:1024-1028.

[73] Li Y, Marion MJ, Rundle A, Brandt-Rauf PW (2003) A common Polymorphism in XRCC1 as a Biomarker of Susceptibility for Chemically Induced Genetic Damage. Biomarkers 8:408-414.

[74] Li Y, Marion MJ, Zipprich J, Freyer G, Santella RM, Kanki C, Brandt-Rauf PW (2006) The Role of XRCC1 Polymorphisms in Base Excision Repair of Etheno-DNA Adducts in French Vinyl Chloride Workers. Int. j. occup. med. environ. health 19:45-52.

[75] Li Y, Marion MJ, Zipprich J, Santella RM, Freyer G, Brandt-Rauf PW (2009) Gene-Environment Interactions between DNA Repair Polymorphisms and Exposure to the Carcinogen Vinyl Chloride. Biomarkers 14:148-155.

[76] Wong RH, Du CL, Wang JD, Chan CC, Luo JC, Cheng TJ (2002) XRCC1 and CYP2E1 Polymorphisms as Susceptibility Factors of Plasma Mutant p53 Protein and Anti-p53 Antibody Expression in Vinyl Chloride Monomer-Exposed Polyvinyl Chloride Workers. Cancer epidemiol. biomarkers prev. 11:475-482.

[77] Zhu SM, Xia ZL, Wang AH, Ren XF, Jiao J, Zhao NQ, Qian J, Jin L, Christiani DC (2008) Polymorphisms and Haplotypes of DNA Repair and Xenobiotic Metabolism Genes and Risk of DNA Damage in Chinese Vinyl Chloride Monomer (VCM)-Exposed Workers. Toxicol. let. 178:88-94.

[78] Ji F, Wang W, Xia ZL, Zheng YJ, Qiu YL, Wu F, Miao WB, Jin RF, Qian J, Jin L, Zhu YL, Christiani DC (2010) Prevalence and Persistence of Chromosomal Damage and Susceptible Genotypes of Metabolic and DNA Repair Genes in Chinese Vinyl Chloride-Exposed Workers. Carcinogenesis 31:648-653.

[79] Wang Q, Ji F, Sun Y, Qiu YL, Wang W, Wu F, Miao WB, Li Y, Brandt-Rauf PW, Xia ZL (2010) Genetic Polymorphisms of XRCC1, HOGG1 and MGMT and Micronucleus Occurrence in Chinese Vinyl Chloride-Exposed Workers. Carcinogenesis 31:1068-1073.

[80] Monaco R, Rosal R, Dolan MA, Pincus MR, Brandt-Rauf PW (2007) Conformational Effects of a Common Codon 399 Polymorphism on the BRCT1 Domain of the X-Ray Cross-Complementing-1 Protein. Protein j. 26:541-546.

[81] Li Y, Long C, Lin G, Marion MJ, Freyer G. Santella RM, Brandt-Rauf PW (2009) Effects of the XRCC1 Codon 399 Polymorphism on the Repair of Vinyl Chloride Metabolite-Induced DNA Damage. J. carcinogen. 8:108-112.

[82] Brandt-Rauf PW, Li Y, Monaco R, Kovvali G, Marion MJ (2012) Plastics and Carcinogenesis: The Example of Vinyl Chloride. J. carcinogen. 11:50-60.

[83] Matsuda T, Yagi T, Kawanishi M, Matsui S, Takebe H (1995) Molecular Analysis of Mutations Induced by 2-Chloroacetaldehyde, the Ultimate Carcinogenic Form of Vinyl Chloride, in Human Cells Using Shuttle Vectors. Carcinogenesis 16:2389-2394.

[84] Monaco R, Rosal R, Dolan MA, Pincus MR, Freyer G, Brandt-Rauf PW (2009) Conformational Effects of a Common Codon 751 Polymorphism on the C-Terminal Domain of the Xeroderma Pigmentosum D Protein. J carcinogen. 8:93-97.

[85] Gibbons BJ, Brignole EJ, Azubel M, Murakami K, Voss NR, Bushnell DA, Asturias FJ, Kornberg RD (2012) Subunit Architecture of General Transcription Factor TFIIH. Proc. natl. acad. sci. usa 109:1949-1954.

[86] Valdiglesias V, Pasaro E, Mendez J, Laffon B (2010) In Vitro Evaluation of Selenium Genotoxic, Cytotoxic, and Protective Effects: A Review. Arch. toxicol. 84:337-351.

[87] Kunwar A, Jayakumar S, Bhilwade HN, Bag PP, Bhatt H, Chaubey RC, Priyadarsini KI (2011) Protective Effects of Selenocystine Against γ-Radiation-Induced Genotoxicity in Swiss Albino Mice. Radiat. environ. biophys. 50:271-280.

Chapter 22

Aspects of DNA Damage from Internal Radionuclides

Christopher Busby

Additional information is available at the end of the chapter

http://dx.doi.org/10.5772/53942

1. Introduction

In this chapter, there is insufficient space to exhaustively review the research which has been carried out on internal radionuclide effects. I hope only to highlight evidence which shows that internal radionuclides cannot be assessed by the current radiation risk model, and to suggest some research directions that may enable a new model to be developed, one which more accurately quantifies the real effects of such exposures. The biological effects of exposure to ionizing radiation have been studied extensively in the last 70 years and yet very little effort has gone into examining the health effects of exposure to internal incorporated radionuclides. This is curious, since the biosphere has been increasingly contaminated with novel man-made radioactive versions of naturally occurring elements which living creatures have adapted to over evolutionary timescales, and intuition might suggest that these substances could represent a significant hazard to health, one not easily or accurately modelled by analogy with external photon radiation (X-rays and gamma rays).

The question of the health effects of internal radionuclide exposures began to be asked in the early 1950s when there was widespread fallout contamination of food and milk from atmospheric nuclear tests. It quickly became the subject of disagreements between two committees of the newly formed International Commission on Radiological Protection (ICRP)[1]. The questions of the equivalence of internal and external radiation exposure, which were the basis of these disagreements, have still not been resolved. In the West, up to very recently, the whole spectrum of health effects from internal incorporated radionuclides has focused on animal studies of Radium, Plutonium and Strontium-90 and human retrospective studies of those individuals exposed to Radium-226 and Thorium-232 in the contrast medium "Thorotrast". These studies suffer from a number of problems which will be discussed.

Soviet scientists were more interested in internal radiation effects from fission-product radionuclides, but unfortunately their valuable studies have been difficult to access since they are published in Russian. In 1977 Gracheva and Korolev published a book summarising work in this area which was translated in India in 1980 as *Genetic Effects of the Decay of Radionuclides in* Cells [2]. This presented a wealth of interesting data relating to beta emitter genetic effects in various systems and drew attention to the distinction that must be made between external and internal radiation. This is important since the whole assessment of radiation in terms of health has been through the quantity "absorbed dose" and what can be called the bag-of-water model.

In this bag of water model, illustrated in Fig 1, the total energy transferred by the radiation to living tissue is diluted into a large mass, greater than a kilogram, as if the effects were uniform throughout the tissue being considered. In Fig 1 the tissue mass A represents an external irradiation by X-rays or gamma rays and here the effects are uniform across the tissue. But in the case B, for internal irradiation, it is clear that it is possible, for certain kinds of exposure, for tissue local to the source to receive very large amounts of radiation energy at the same overall energy transfer to the tissue mass.

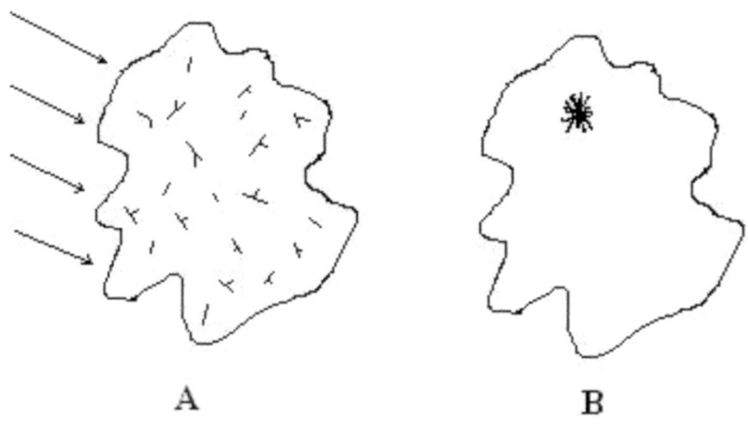

Figure 1. Comparing external and internal irradiation: the ICRP/ ICRU bag of water model. In case A, external radiation (X-rays or gamma rays) there are 20 events uniformly spaced throughout the tissue and the "absorbed dose" (see text) at any microscopic point is evenly distributed. In case B, for internal irradiation (here from a radioactive particle) there is a very large transfer of energy to a small tissue volume and the concept of "absorbed dose" does not apply.

Thus, in the historic and also the current system of radiation protection, those experts who assess radiation risk, who are termed *Health Physicists,* calculate the cumulative absorbed dose in Grays, i.e. in terms of the total energy in Joules imparted by the beta electron or alpha particle decays of the internal radionuclide contamination to one kilogram of tissue. For this calculation, the tissue is modelled as water. For example, those whose body contains 100 Bq of Strontium-90 are assessed, for the purposes of radiation protection, as having received a cumulative absorbed dose of 100 x w where w is the "cumulative (absorbed) dose coefficient", obtained from measurements of the biological half life of the Strontium in the body and the decay energy of each decay in Joules. This number **w** is to be found in a Table published by the ICRP. In the case of the Strontium-90 contaminated individual, if the person weighed 50 kg, then the mean activity concentration would be 2 Bq/kg. The resulting absorbed dose would then be $2 \times 2.8 \times 10^{-8}$ (this is the ICRP 72 dose coefficient [3]). In other words, the committed dose is 5.6×10^{-8} Sv (0.056 μSv). But can this be safely compared with a dose from a chest X-ray (40 μSv) or from natural background radiation (2500 μSv) or from a high dose acute exposure to gamma rays from an atomic bomb linearly scaled to zero dose (the current way of modelling radiation effects)? This chapter explores this question. It is one which has become increasingly necessary as serious health effects, including cancer and leukemia, have been reported in those exposed to internal radioactivity in areas contaminated by radionuclides released from nuclear sites, weapons testing fallout and accidents like Chernobyl and Fukushima, at very low conventionally calculated "absorbed doses".

The matter has been discussed in some detail since 1998 by the independent European Committee on Radiation Risk (ECRR) whose reports [4, 5] provide a methodology for assessing health effects through a system of weighting factors based on available data. As more and more evidence emerged after 1995 that something was very wrong with the ICRP absorbed dose approach to internal radiation, the UK government set up a Committee Examining Radiation Risk from Internal Emitters (CERRIE). Since there were (and are) political dimensions to the issue, the committee was composed of scientists and experts from the nuclear industry and the official radiation protection organisations in the UK. Unfortunately the 4-years process ended in acrimony, legal threats to member of the committee, and failure to agree a final report. Two reports were issued [6, 7]. However, there was agreement that there were reasonable concerns about the safety of employing "absorbed dose" for certain internal radionuclide situations, and similar concerns about the safety of the ICRP model were made in 2005 by the French IRSN [8]. The error factor that these discussions led to was believed by different ends of the CERRIE process to be between 10-fold and 1000-fold. More recently, the value put on this error factor by the retired Scientific Secretary of the ICRP at a meeting in Stockholm in 2009 was "two orders of magnitude". What this means, in our Strontium-90 case above, is that the dose from 100Bq contamination to the whole body is no longer 0.056μSv but may now be between 0.56μSv and 56μSv and the risk of fatal cancer is proportionately increased. To put this in perspective, the mean Sr-90 dose over the period 1959-1963 to individuals in the northern hemisphere was given as about 1 mSv [9]. The ICRP risk model gives a 0.45% per Sievert excess lifetime cancer risk. Epidemiological studies suggest that the cancer "epidemic" which began in the 1980s in areas of high rainfall and fallout is a consequence of the earlier fallout exposures [10]. The weighting of dose necessary to explain this is greater than 300 if calculated from the ICRP absolute risk factor of 0.05/Sv [5, 11]. Many other instances of anomalous health effects from exposure to internal radionuclides require hazard weighting factors of between 100-fold and more than 1000-fold, and these are consequences of mechanisms which will be presented.

2. Fundamental principles

Ionising radiation, however it is delivered, creates harmful effects by causing mutations in genetic material both at the somatic level (cellular DNA) and germ cell level (heritable mutations). The mutations are caused by alterations in the cellular DNA in the nucleus and in mitochondria. These are brought about by three mechanisms:

a. Direct ionisation of the DNA and subsequent chemical alteration of the bases to molecules which are not recognised as a coding signal.

b. Indirect ionisation of the DNA by reactive species produced by ionisation of water (called Reactive Oxygen Species ROS).

c. A mechanism termed "Genomic Instability" which is an inducible cell-cell signal consequence of the production of ROS in the cytoplasm (non-DNA region) of an irradiated cell. This process is communicable between cells in some way and even between individuals and has been termed the "bystander effect".

These mechanisms are well described in the literature and in textbooks, and the processes described here can be found in the reports of radiation protection agencies e.g. [12].

Ionising radiation always transfers its energy to matter in the form of structured tracks of charged particles. Photon radiation (gamma and X-radiation) is absorbed by matter mainly through Compton Effect, Photoelectron, and Pair-production. All these cause the creation of tracks of energetic electrons which carry the energy of the original photon and collide with molecules in the absorbing medium causing ionisation. The ionised fragments (in the case of living tissue mainly of water) then recombine or react with local molecular entities causing chemical changes in the molecular structure. Various chemical reactions take place e.g.

$H_2O\ (\text{radiation}) \rightarrow H_2O^{+} + e^{-}$

$H_2O^{+} + H_2O \rightarrow OH^{*} + H_3O^{+}$

The free radical OH* has an unpaired electron and is highly reactive; it will combine with local species including DNA if that is close to the track. If it reacts again with water species the result is a range of highly reactive fragments which are collectively described as Reactive Oxygen Species. The process can be written:

$H_2O\ (\text{radiation}) \rightarrow e_{aq}, H^{*}, H_2O_2, H_2, OH^{*}.$

The relative concentrations of the main ROS are [12]:

e_{aq} (hydrated electron) 45%

OH* (hydroxyl radical) 45%

H* (hydrogen radical) 10%

These reactive species attack molecules in the cell and cause damage; because it is an oxidising agent the OH* radical is likely to be the most effective DNA damaging agent, abstracting a hydrogen atom from the deoxyribose moiety of DNA yielding a highly reactive DNA radical. This will then rearrange or react with local molecules to produce a new molecule in the DNA coding sequence, the gene, a molecule which is unrecognizable to the coding transfer process and alters the message of the gene.

It seems that evolution has recognised the dangers of high levels of cellular ROS and has developed a process to deal with the threat to the species or to the organism. At the organism level the process involves firstly the existence of double strands of DNA which permit repair of ionisation damage to a base located on one strand by copying from the opposite strand. This type of lesion, termed a "point mutation" is a more likely result for chemical mutagenesis or random attack by ROS species present in the cell at some background concentration (as a by product of other chemical processes in the cell). In some cells, the result of DNA damage is programmed cell suicide, termed apoptosis. But at the organism level, one response is the induction of genomic instability, whereby a signal is switched on in the DNA resulting in increased levels of random mutagenesis built into cell replication of the damaged cell and also bystander cells. The exact purpose of this process, which is well documented, is uncertain [13]. If the damage is more extensive, involving locally multiply damaged sites (LMDS) or both strands, it becomes more difficult to accurately repair the material and either a fixed mutation or cell death results.

Internal exposure results from the radioactive decay of radionuclides incorporated into tissue through inhalation or ingestion. There are three principle types of decay which represent the majority of all internal exposures. Gamma decay, which produces fast electron tracks, β decay which also produces fast electron tracks, and alpha decay. In addition there are also short range electron tracks from Auger decays. The main internal nuclides of environmental and radiobiological importance are listed in Table 1.

Apart from effects at the nuclide (recoil, transmutation) β decay is indistinguishable from the fast (photoelectron) electron tracks produced from gamma and X-ray interactions. With β-decay, unstable elements change into elements with one greater atomic number Z and emit an electron in the process; they may also emit a gamma ray. Sometimes the daughter nuclide is also unstable and may further decay. An example is Strontium-90 which emits a β-particle of endpoint energy 546 keV (kiloelectron volts) and transmutes into Yttrium-90 which further emits a β–particle of endpoint energy 2280 keV and transmutes into stable Zirconium-90. There are several series decay sequences in which ten or more unstable nuclides are formed, one from another. An example is the natural α-emitter Uranium-238 which decays through twelve sequential unstable radionuclides until the sequence stops at stable Lead-206. Transmutation involving α-decay involves the change of the chemical element to one with Atomic Number Z four places lower on the Periodic Table. Thus U-238 emits an α-particle and decays to Thorium-234.

There is strong evidence that damage to DNA is the cause of the effects of ionising radiation. For example, experiments have been carried out with nuclides which have short range electron emissions (Auger emissions) or Tritium chemically incorporated into DNA precursors so that these elements become covalently bonded to the DNA. The measured harmful effects are up to 100-times greater than would be predicted from the "absorbed dose" showing that it is the ionisation in the DNA that is key to the destruction of the cell [14, 15]. Another argument is based on the effects of the weak β-emitter Tritium, as tritiated water HTO. The measured effects of Tritium exposure are not too different from that expected on the basis of the absorbed dose (although it may be higher, see below). But clearly the Tritium will be evenly distributed throughout the cell. Since the beta energy of Tritium is only 6 keV the electron track range will be less than 0.5 μ and the ionisations will occur in clusters, uniformly distributed in the cell but with no overlap. It is clear that only those clusters which are close to the DNA will have an effect on the DNA, and the great majority of the energy will be "wasted" in the cytoplasm. Thus for a Tritium dose modelled by ICRP as 1 mSv, only a very small fraction of the Tritium decays will contribute to the effect.

The main target DNA, in the cell nucleus, represents a very small fraction of the total material in the cell. In a 10 μ diameter cell (mass 520 pg) there is 6 pg of DNA made up of 2.4 pg bases, 2.3 pg deoxyribose, 1.2 pg phosphate. In addition, associated with this macromolecule are 3.1 pg of bound water and 4.2 pg of inner hydration water [16]. Since absorbed dose is given as Joules per kilogram, if it were possible to accurately target the DNA complex alone, a dose to the cell (mass 520 pg) of 1 milliJoule per kilogram (one milliGray, one milliSievert) would, if absorbed only by the DNA complex (6 pg), represent a dose of 520/6 = 87 mSv to the DNA. It is possible to imagine the DNA as an organ of the body, like the thyroid gland or the breast. If this is done, then there should be a weighting factor for its radiobiological sensitivity of 87 which would be based on spatial distribution of dose alone. Of course, for external photon irradiation, to a first approximation, tracks are generated at random in tissue. Therefore only a small proportion of these tracks will intercept the DNA but the interception will be mainly uniform, and the health effects from such external exposure may be assumed to be described by the averaging approach of "absorbed dose". This is not the case for internal exposures from radionuclide decays in a number of quite specific circumstances which will be described below (see [5]).

The calculations of "absorbed dose" also assume that the medium irradiated has uniform isotropic qualities with an absorption coefficient roughly equivalent to that of water. However the absorption of gamma radiation is proportional to the 4th power of the atomic number Z. It follows that the probability of absorption of gamma radiation will be location specific, and this is highly relevant to a number of high Z elements, either biologically necessary (Iodine, Z=53) or as contaminants (Uranium Z=92) [17].

Radionuclides are primarily chemical elements with the affinities and reactivities of the non-radioactive forms of these elements. They will therefore have quite specific biochemical pathways in the body and may accumulate at positions in cells as a result of their chemical group, valency, ionic volumes, charge etc. This will result in high local doses at sites where they accumulate. In addition, the decay of a nuclide attached to some cell structure or macromolecule will result in the alteration of the radionuclide into a different element with a different charge, with resultant recoil energy. This will always break the chemical bond and result in ionisation. Thus there will be local ionisation and this may be on some critical macromolecule like DNA. These localisation and transmutation effects were studied in the 1960s but no attempt has been made to incorporate them for radiation protection purposes.

http://dx.doi.org/10.5772/53942

The decay of a radionuclide attached chemically to the DNA is illustrated schematically in Fig 2.

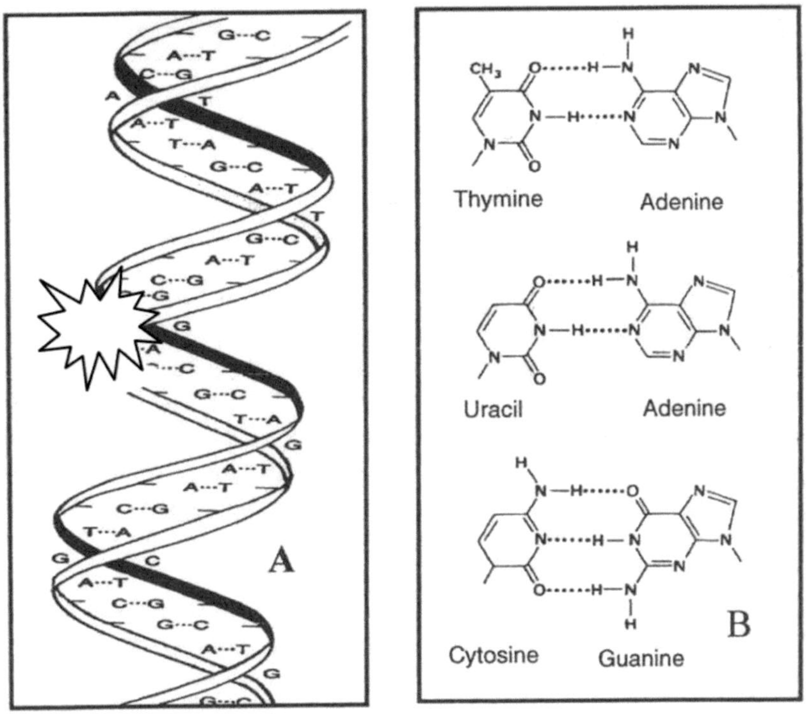

Figure 2. Certain radionuclides (Sr-90, Uranium) bind to DNA and when they decay cause (a) transmutation ionisation and (b) local electron emission ionisation (Auger, β particle) on or close to the critical target for radiation effects.

Cells have two phases of activity during their lifespan. They are mostly in a quiescent phase where DNA is not localised spatially. For a short period at the end of their lifespan, when they replicate, they are in a cell cycle phase. In this phase they are much more sensitive to irradiation. Therefore this repair replication phase represents a critical window for mutagenesis if it can be engineered. The radiation sensitivity of the repair replication phase has been studied extensively and it was suggested [18, 19] that two irradiation events separated by about 10-12 hours could represent an enhanced hazard since the first pushed quiescent cells into repair replication and the second damaged them during the sensitive 12 hour period. The idea is termed the Second Event theory. There is some evidence for it from work with split doses of X-rays. It will be discussed below.

3. Concerns about internal radionuclides

To summarise, the position is that the current assessment of harm from radiation exposure is based on a quantity which does not assume any structure in the tissue being irradiated. It does not distinguish between different radionuclides on the basis of their chemical properties except at the organ level (Iodine/ thyroid) and it does not include any weighting for chemical affinities for DNA, nor for transmutation effects. It does not consider the fractionation of doses within cell cycle repair times. Risk factors are based almost entirely on acute external gamma ray exposures. The main concerns are for radionuclides which are significant environmental contaminants and which are listed in Table 3.

3.1. Proximity effects on local doses

Since the genotoxic effects of radiation are mediated by ionisation and the local concentration of reactive oxygen species, it is firstly this local ionization density that is the proper measure of the effectiveness of a radiation exposure. The current risk model acknowledges this by weighting the highly ionizing α particle tracks by an arbitrary factor of 20. But of concern is the overlap of such tracks, and of electron tracks from β–decays or Auger electron showers with active DNA in the nucleus, and especially at the time when this is in some critical state, as in cell repair/division. For externally delivered photon radiation, it can be assumed (in the absence of high-Z photoelectron effects) that ionization is uniform across tissue. Under these circumstances it is only a matter of probability whether a cell is intercepted by a track or not. It has been calculated [20] that, at normal Natural Background levels, each cell in the body will, on the basis of probability, receive one hit per year (a hit being the traversal of the cell by an electron track). Of these hits, some small proportion will involve a track that intercepts the DNA and may cause damage. This damage, if it results in a point mutation, will be repaired before cell division. The ionisation density in a photoelectron track is assumed to be low. Therefore, for external exposure, a dose of 1 mSv to the whole body can be assumed to provide a dose of 1 mSv to the cell on average. At the cell level, this is not the case. A cell can be intercepted by a track or not. If not, then the cell dose is zero and there is no ionisation. If so, then the cell dose can be greater than 1 mSv. The dose to the DNA from such processes will again be either zero or some dose greater than 1 mSv.

For internal exposures, the probability of interception of the track is clearly a function of the distance of the nuclide from the DNA. In addition, internal exposures may be to α tracks which carry significantly more ionisation density. The range of most α tracks (which carry about of 5 MeV energy) is about 4 cell diameters and so, theoretically, the track dose to the cell from one decay is in the region of 500 mSv. The matter becomes serious when the nuclide is an alpha emitter but also has a high chemical affinity for DNA. This is the case for Uranium. Anomalous effects from internal nuclides have been known for a long time. Early studies of cell doses from Tritium were carried out by Apelgot [21] and Robertson and Hughes [22] and reviews of Tritium and of S-35 and P-32 studies are found in ref [2]. In order to emphasise the profound effects which can be identified in internal exposures, the case of Carbon-14 will be examined in greater detail below.

The cell dose from any decay is fairly simple to approximate on the basis of a continuous slowing down approximation and the assumption that the energy delivered along a track is a constant function of the track length. Electron track lengths in tissue for a range of energies are given in Table 1. These apply also to photoelectrons which have energies almost equal to the gamma photons that produced them. Assuming a cell diameter of 10 μ, the energy deposited in the cell is merely the decay energy divided by the track length in the cell. This is then converted into Joules (1 keV = 1.6 x 10^{-19} J) and divided by the mass of the cell in kg. For a 10 μ diameter cell this is 5.2 x 10^{-13} kg. For the Strontium-90 example, a single decay track will deposit approximately 1 mSv in each cell traversed by the track.

Energy (keV)	Range (cms)	*Linear energy transfer keV/μ	Examples (maximum β–energy, keV)
5	1.2 E-4	4	Tritium (5.7)
15	5.2 E-4	2.9	
20	8.6 E-4	2.3	
150	2.8 E-2	0.53	Sulfur-35 (167);Carbon-14 (155)
500	1.78 E-1	0.28	Strontium-90 (546) Caesium-137 (514) Iodine-131 (607) Caesium-134 (658) Barium-140 (168)
1000	4.42 E-1	0.22	Iodine-132 (1610,1210,1040) Barium-140 (1020,1010)
2000	9.92 E-1	0.201	Yttrium-90 (2280) Iodine-132 (2160)

* this is simply the loss of energy of the particle over unit distance

Table 1. Continuous slowing down range in muscle tissue for electrons in g cm^{-2} (values very similar to range in water) (from ICRU Report 35 Table 2.5 [23])

3.2. Calculating the spatial effect enhancement

The spatial effect enhancement is the probability of an ionisation track from an internal nuclide intercepting the DNA at some given level of ionisation density, compared with the probability of this happening from external radiation.

Thus we take the mutagenic event of interest to be associated with absorbed dose (energy per unit mass) in a volume element of a track which is coincident with active DNA in space and time. For nuclides with chemical affinity for DNA this ratio is clearly very large. In the limiting case of covalent binding it can be assumed that approximately half of the decays of the bound nuclide traverse the DNA, and in addition the *transmutation* of the nuclide causes a point ionisation at its position. In the limit this probability will be 1; for example, C-14 which is incorporated into one of the DNA bases will decay and change into Nitrogen. This will immediately destroy the purine or pyrimidine base which it is part of and will introduce a mutation which may or may not be repaired.

The probability of the interception of a charged particle track intercepting the DNA depends on the distance of the point source and the dimensions of the DNA target employed. The cross sectional diameter of one strand is about 0.3 nm but, in mitosis, various much larger condensed targets exist. The principle is the same, however: the probability of intercepting the target falls off rapidly with distance. The result for a condensed DNA target of cross section 0.1 x 1 μ is given in Fig 3. The calculation is given in Appendix A. The result confirms what is intuitively obvious: the effect of radionuclide decay in the cytoplasm is much less harmful than for nuclides bound to DNA. This is particularly significant for the α-emitters which have chemical affinity for DNA, Uranium (as UO_2^{++}) and, possibly, Plutonium.

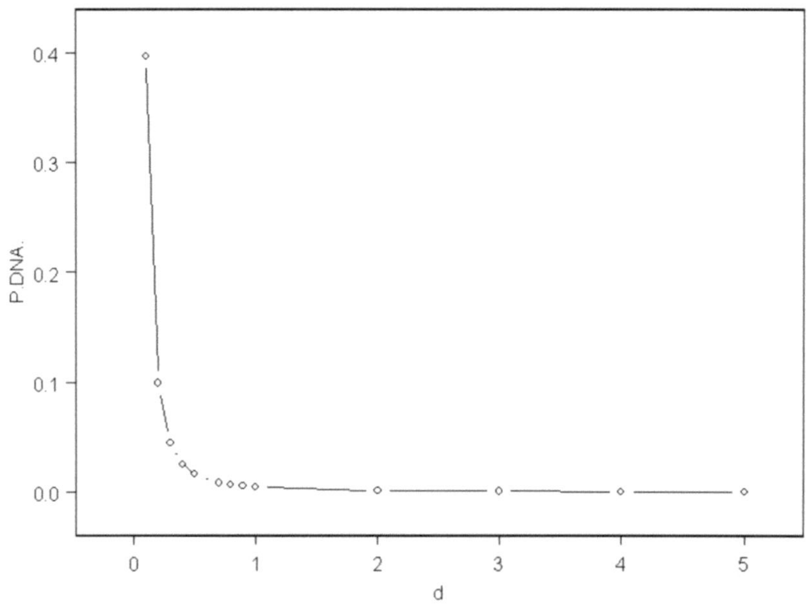

Figure 3. Approximate probability of a track interception of a DNA target modelled as a strip of 0.1 x 1 μ by distance in μ from target. In this model, the maximum probability is 0.5 for a nuclide located on the surface of a flat strip.

One other simple way to illustrate this spatial effect is merely to consider the tissue as two compartments, an organ A which may be called "DNA" and one B which may be called "everything else". The current ICRP risk model calculates the absorbed dose of any internal exposure by dividing the total decay energy by the mass. This would not distinguish between compartments A and B; both would receive the same dose. But as far as cancer is concerned (or other consequences of genetic damage) all the ionisation in compartment B is wasted. It has no effect. Therefore it is the dose to compartment A that is the cause of the effect. This would suggest that the spatial enhancement is at minimum the ratio MassB/MassA or about 90-fold. This assumes that *all* the DNA in the cell is a critical target which is unlikely to be the case. If the critical DNA represented even 1/10th of the total cellular DNA, the spatial enhancement from track interception alone would be 900-fold.

3.3. Double strand breaks

At natural background radiation levels, where there is one "hit" per cell per year, the Poisson probability of multiple tracks across the DNA strand is low. Most of the "hits" are repairable and the biological response is proportional to the dose. But it is believed on the basis of good evidence that genetic mutations result from multiply damaged sites [12]. If two adjacent DNA strands are broken, then repair is not possible since there is no template from which to copy the correct sequence. Ward et al. (1988) [16] compare DNA damage necessary to inactivate exposed cells between radiation and chemical mutagens. Table 2 lists some of the results:

Agent	DNA lesion	No of lesions per cell
Ionizing radiation	SSB	1000
	DSB	40
	Total LMDS	440
Benzo[a]pyrene 4,5 oxide	Carcinogenic adduct	100,000
methylnitrosourea	7-methylguanine	800,000
Aflatoxin	Carcinogenic adduct	10,000

Table 2. Yields of DNA damage necessary to kill 63% of exposed cells [16]

From Table 2 it is clear that ionizing radiation is more effective than the most powerful chemical carcinogens in causing genetic lesions to the DNA, but it is the double strand breaks (DSBs) and LMDS which are the most efficient processes. From simple kinetic theory it is clear that the probability of inducing double strand breaks or LMDS will increase as the number of tracks per unit time increases. At low background external doses this is very unlikely. But as the dose rate increases, so the likelihood of multiple tracks increases (for a discussion see [18]). This is not true for a number of internal exposure situations where multiple tracks can occur at very low doses, conventionally assessed. The first is exposure to particulates.

Radioactivity from releases from nuclear explosions, e.g. accidents like Chernobyl, or from weapons tests or Uranium weapons is partly in the form of sub-micron particulates which are respirable and can be translocated from the lung. Tissue near such particles will receive multiple tracks even though the dose, as assessed as energy per unit mass may be very low. Similar multiple track effects can occur close to high Z element particles whether they are intrinsically radioactive or not, e.g. platinum (catalysers), bismuth, gold (prostheses), due to secondary photoelectron conversion from natural background gamma radiation [7, 17]. The second is where a relatively immobilised nuclide has a sequential decay pathway and so there is more than one decay from approximately the same position. This situation is more genotoxic when the decays occur within the repair replication cycle; the Second Event [7] and this situation will be discussed separately.

Radionuclide	Half life (Decay product)	Decay	Reasons for concern	Other remarks
Tritium H3	12.32 y Helium-3	Low energy β	Ubiquitous; Discharged in large amounts by all nuclear sites and weapons tests; present as tritiated water and easily incorporated into body. Can be present as organically bound tritium which may accumulate in the body.	Evidence of serious genetic effects in invertebrate development at very low doses; short range of β decay causes high ionisation density.
Carbon-14	5730 y Nitrogen	β emitter	Discharged by nuclear sites, particularly reprocessing sites (Sellafield) and weapons tests. Incorporated into the carbon of the body	Doses by ingestion mainly of vegetables, milk, fish. Both Carbon and hydrogen (Tritium) make up the structure of living systems. Transmutes to a gas, nitrogen.
Sulphur-35	87 days Chlorine	β emitter	Discharged from nuclear sites. Concentrates in foods.	Sulphur also a part of internal macromolecules in living systems. Transmutes to a reactive gas, Chlorine
Strontium-90	28.9 y Yttrium-90	β emitter	Globally Widespread. Atmospheric test fallout, nuclear sites, accidents (Chernobyl, Fukushima); Group 2 affinity for DNA	Second event nuclide with daughter Y-90 of concern since it binds to DNA
Krypton-85	10.7 y Rubidium-85	β emitter	Very large amount routinely released from nuclear sites is building up in atmosphere.	Very soluble in fats and therefore can build up in body fat (beast tissue, lymphatic tissue) following inhalation
Barium-140	12 d Lanthanum -140	β emitter	Large quantities from nuclear weapons tests; Group 2 affinity for DNA	Second event emitter binds to DNA. Of concern in assessing effects of nuclear atmospheric tests and accidents
Iodine-131	8 days Xenon-131m	βγ emitter	Large amounts from accidents, licensed releases. Affinity for Thyroid and Thyroxine in circulating blood	Second event emitter with daughter Xe-131m short half life. Transmutes to a gas.
Tellurium-132	3.25 d Iodine-132	βγ emitter	Released in large amounts from accidents; daughter is Iodine 132	Second event series
Caesium-134	2 y Barium-134	βγ emitter	Released from nuclear explosions, accidents	Binds to muscle
Caesium-137	30 y Barium-137m	βγ emitter	Released from nuclear explosions, accidents, nuclear sites under licence	Binds to muscle; concerns over effects on heart in Chernobyl contaminated areas.

Radionuclide	Half life (Decay product)	Decay	Reasons for concern	Other remarks
Radium-226	1599 y Radon-222	α emitter	NORM Contamination near oil and gas processing sites; widely studied but problems with the studies (see text). Decays to Radon gas.	Group 2 Calcium seeker. Binds to DNA. Evidence of non-cancer reduction in lifespan in human studies.
Polonium-210	139d Lead-204	α emitter	Releases from nuclear sites; daughter of Lead 201 which can build up in environment as a result of contamination from NORM	
Uranium-238	4.5×10^9y Series	α emitter	Releases from nuclear sites; contamination from mining and processing; from weapons fallout and accidents; from battlefield weapons usage and testing. Widespread in the environment but generally not measured near nuclear sites	High Z photoelectron effects; binds to DNA; considerable evidence for its anomalous genotoxicity
Plutonium-239	2.4×10^4 y Uranium-23 5	α emitter	Releases from nuclear sites, weapons test fallout, widespread environmental contaminant	Binds to DNA (?) evidence for anomalous genotoxicity

Table 3. Internal radionuclides of concern

Third, if an alpha emitting nuclide is either randomly positioned near or chemically attracted to the DNA, there is a significant probability that the highly ionising track will traverse the two strands of the DNA and damage multiple sites. This is the origin of the high efficiency of alpha emitters which resulted in their being weighted by ICRP. Fourth, there are situations where dose is delivered by very low energy beta emitters; the best example is Tritium. Because dose is assessed as energy per unit mass, the very low decay energy of Tritium means that there is a large number of decays from different atoms of Tritium (90 tracks) to deliver the same dose as one 500 keV β decay from Caesium-137 or from the traversal of a cell by a 500 keV photoelectron track. This would suggest a mechanism backing the evidence (see below) that Tritium represents a greater mutagenic hazard than is calculated on the basis of its absorbed dose.

3.4. Summary of enhancement mechanisms; caveats over high dose studies

The target for radiation effects is the DNA, the nuclear DNA and the sensitivity to radiation varies depending on whether the cell is in quiescent phase or in repair replication. Within the 12 hour repair replication period there are other sensitive windows. The end point for radiation damage to the DNA can be genetic mutation leading to heritable damage (in germ cells) or cancer, but if the ionisation density is too great, or the sequential hits to close together then the cell will die. The interesting thing then is that this will *decrease the fixed mutation rate* and therefore *will decrease the cancer rate*. Thus we would not expect studies of high dose and high dose rate to elicit information which informs on low dose and low dose rate.

The dose/ dose rate response in cancer studies will inevitably have a complex character for this reason. This is clear from the results of retrospective studies of Radium and Thorotrast contamination, studies which have been influential in supporting the current radiation risk model, an issue with will be discussed further below. The key point is that, for certain internal exposure regimes, the ionisation density at the DNA and the damage to the DNA can be extremely high even though the absorbed dose, as calculated by the current methodology, may be extremely low.

The regions of internal and external dose, are illustrated in Fig 4.

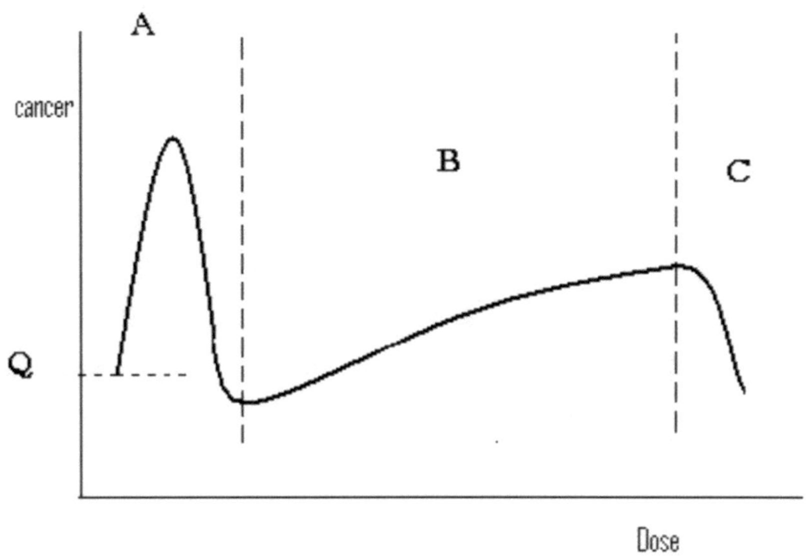

Figure 4. Regions of interest in a theoretically predicted dose response relation (see text and ECRR2010). Exactly this dose response is seen in infant leukemia rates after Chernobyl in Greece, Germany (3 dose regions) Wales, Scotland and Belarus (see [25]).

The analysis from ECRR 2010 [5] is described in Fig 4, the end point is assumed to be cancer rate. Q is the background rate. There are three regions. In the first region A, sensitive cells in repair replication are first mutated (positive slope) and then overwhelmed (negative slope). Next, in region B the cells in quiescent phase are mutated and eventually overwhelmed in C. This is also the organism response since at high doses C the organism suffers from non cancer causes of death which affect the cancer rates, reducing them as the dose increases. These responses are seen in many epidemiological and animal studies but are generally misinterpreted. Burlakova has made a special study of dose response relationships and has shown the type AB response for a wide range of objective markers of DNA damage and also whole organism end-points [24].The dose response is seen in, and most easily explained in, infant leukemia after internal radiation exposures. As the exposure increases, foetal death ensues at some point, and the leukemia rate in the infant falls [25]. If the dose response is assumed to be linear, and the low dose data points assumed to be data scatter, a line drawn between the background cancer rate Q and the peak in region B cuts the response line in such a way as to suggest that radiation is actually reducing cancer rate, the so-called hormesis theory. The analysis in ECRR2010 points out that this is a misinterpretation of the data.

From what has been discussed, it is possible to summarise the mechanisms that may lead to increased risk of damage to DNA, and indeed to decreased risk in the case of high local doses which will kill rather than fix mutations. The mechanisms are listed in Table 4 where enhancements from alpha emitters with affinity for DNA may deliver such high local doses as to inactivate the cell.

Mechanism	Range	Examples
Spatial location		
DNA affinity	0.1-100	Uranium, Strontium, Barium, Radium Plutonium?
Membrane affinity	?	Caesium, Potassium, Rubidium, Chlorine, Sodium
DNA incorporation	Very high	Tritium, Carbon-14
Particulates	10-1000	Uranium. Plutonium
Protein incorporation	?	Sulphur-35, Tritium, Carbon-14
Transmutation	5-100	All covalently bound internal nuclides e.g. Sulphur-35, Tritium, Carbon-14
Temporal location		
Critical cell lifespan phase interception by immobilised source	0.01-100	Strontium-90 , Tellurium-132, Tritium, Radium-226, particulates
Critical repair replication window interception	0.01-1000	Strontium-90 , Tellurium-132, Tritium, Radium-226, particulates
Fat soluble noble gases	?	e.g. Kr-85
High Atomic Number photoelectron amplification	U-238 100-1000	Uranium, Platinum, Gold, Bismuth, potentially all elements with Z"/>53

Table 4. Main mechanisms of enhancement of genetic hazard from internal irradiation (see ECRR2010).

4. Specific concerns and new research directions

4.1. Location enhancement and chemical affinity

Concern has been shown since the 1950s that radionuclides of Group 2 in the Periodic Table, notably Strontium-90 and Barium-140, may have high affinity for DNA. These elements exist in solution as dipositive ions which are known to concentrate in organs (bones, teeth) which have high phosphate concentrations. Calcium and Magnesium are also known to bind electrostatically to the DNA Phosphate backbone and to stabilise its conformation. It is therefore likely that Strontium, Barium and Radium also have such affinity. The concentration of the radiation risk establishment on Radium epidemiology has been based on an end-point of bone cancer because the nuclide concentrates in bone. The affinity for DNA has been overlooked.

In the 1960s, for the reason that it was believed that Strontium would bind to DNA, and because some experiments showed that this was the case, there was significant concern about Strontium-90 contamination of milk. Mouse experiments demonstrated effects on intrauterine foetal death [26], and studies on rats showed development effects from Sr-90 [27]. There were effects at very low doses from Sr-90 [28], and by 1970 the director of the UK Medical Research Council suggested that further interest be taken in research on Sr-90 [29]. However nothing was done. In 2004, the CERRIE committee unanimously called for there to be further research into the effects of exposure to Sr-90 [6]. Also classified with these Group 2 is Uranium which exists in solution as the dipositive ion UO_2^{++} the Uranyl ion. This has very high affinity for DNAP [30] which led to its introduction as a chromosome stain for electron microscopy as early as 1960 [31].

The most necessary research is to measure the affinity of Strontium, Radium and Uranyl ion for chromosomes *in vivo*. Owing to the high opacity of Uranium there are certainly potential electron microscope methods for examining its location in cells *in vivo*. It might be possible to employ autoradiography to measure the affinity constants in vivo for Ra-226, Sr-90 and Ba-140. Affinity constants for DNAP can be easily measured *in vitro* for Strontium, Barium and Radium but this does not appear to have been done.

Animal studies of Radium and Uranium have assumed that the end point must be bone cancer or leukemia, and that only high doses will cause cancer. Effects at low doses have been assumed to be random scatter. It is suggested that low dose animal studies be undertaken with lifespan observation of all possible conditions to resolve this issue.

1. *There is the question of membrane affinity. If certain ions congregate at certain* membranes, the local ionisation density from radioactive decay will be higher than if these were uniformly distributed in cytoplasm. Experiments with the nuclide Sodium-22 by Petkau showed a supralinear dose response and effects at very low doses as calculated by using the total solution volume as a denominator [32]. If such effects occur *in vivo* there are a number of critical membranes which might be destroyed from internal radionuclide ions. Experiments *in vitro* might involve K-40, and Cs-137.

2. *DNA is made from Carbon, Oxygen, Hydrogen and Nitrogen. Carbon-14 and* Tritium can both therefore become covalently bonded into the molecule, and Tritium can easily exchange with labile hydrogen atoms on -SH, -OH and –NH moieties. The resultant decay will result in the total internal rearrangement or local reaction resulting in permanent alteration of the molecule. This will produce a point mutation with 100% efficiency. The electrons from the decay or reactive species created during the trans-

mutations through abstraction of protons from water may damage other local DNA leading to LMDS or DSBs. In the case of C-14, the transmutation to N-14 will totally destroy the molecule since the two elements have different valency, outer electron structure, and reactivity. Owing to the long half-life of C-14, experiments on its genetic effects have been difficult to carry out. Nevertheless, some studies have been published which show that these transmutation effects dominate the hazards of C-14 and Tritium incorporation (see below).

4.2. Particulates

The problem of the anisotropy of dose from internal "hot particles" was raised by Tamplin in the 1980s [33]. It was discussed by CERRIE and was the subject of a review by Charles et al in 2003 [34]. Since the 1950s, there has been a new class of internal radionuclide exposure which has not existed throughout evolution. This is the sub-micron or nanometre diameter radioactive particle. Particles below 1μ diameter can be inhaled and translocated from the lung to the lymphatic system. They are created in nuclear explosions, from power station accidents, from nuclear site releases and from Uranium weapons on battlefields. Depending on their nuclide composition they can produce very high local doses to tissue in which they become immobilised, but may also, depending on their diameter and composition, produce lower doses. Two concerns are Uranium and Plutonium oxide particles. Both contaminated large areas of land in Europe after Chernobyl. Both are resuspended from coastal sediments where contamination exists e.g. the Baltic Sea and the Irish Sea and plutonium from this latter source has been measured in coastal autopsy specimens [35], sheep faeces, and childrens teeth [36]. The well known Seascale child leukemia cluster [37] was discussed by the authorities [40] who dismissed the idea that the leukemia was caused by inhalation of plutonium and uranium on the basis that the doses to the lymphatic system were below natural background [38, 39]. However, the methodology employed diluted the particulate energy into a lymphatic system modelled as several kilograms of tissue [38] rather than the tracheobronchial lymph nodes which weigh about then grams and which are known to be the origin of leukemia in some animals.

The problem with the hot particle issue is that there will be a range of local energies (local dose) which will have either little effect (A), a genetic effect (B) or a killing effect (C). This was pointed out in 1986 following Chernobyl [41] and the idea is illustrated in Fig 5. Regions A to C will have dimensions resulting (a) from the activity and composition of the particle and (b) from its diameter. A particularly interesting case is that of a weakly radioactive particle like U-238 produced from battlefield use of Uranium weapons, so called depleted Uranium. Such a particle may be more carcinogenic than the much more radioactive plutonium particles found in the Irish Sea and epidemiology seems to bear this out. Of interest also is the photoelectron amplification of natural background radiation by internal high atomic number particles like Uranium-238, but also other elements (see below). It is not sufficient to dispute the hazards from particulates by pointing out that they will have such high activities that cells will be killed rather than mutated e.g. [34, 6].

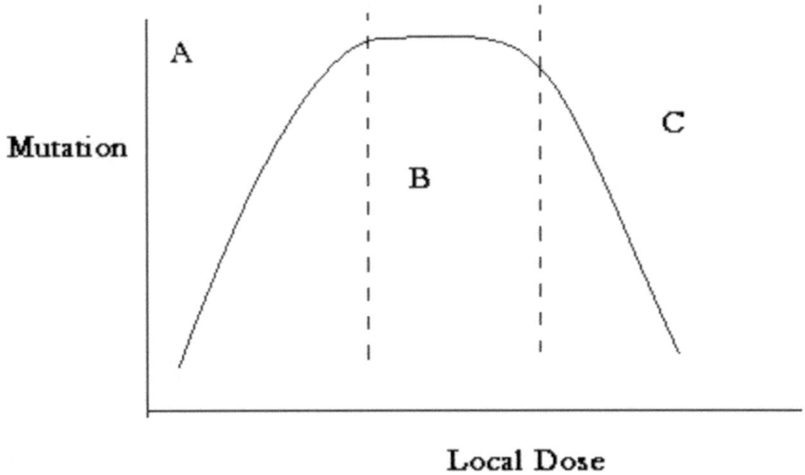

Figure 5. Effects in cells local to "hot particles" (see text).

4.3. Protein and DNA incorporation and transmutation

The inactivation of key enzymes or DNA by incorporation through biosynthesis of radionuclide substituted precursors is a matter that seems to have been entirely overlooked in radioprotection. The environmental contamination nuclides which will inactivate biological molecules are those from which they are constituted, namely Carbon (C-14), Hydrogen (Tritium), and Sulfur (S-35). Some results for C-14 and Tritium will be briefly presented. There is an important experiment which shows the contribution of transmutation to the lethal effects of C-14. Apelgot and Latarjet [42, 43] incorporated C-14 into the cells of the bacteria *e.coli* by culturing in a medium containing 2-14C-thymidine. The samples were stored at -196 C, The specific activity of the 2-^{14}C thymidine was 166 MBq/milliMol. The experiments continued for a year. To evaluate the role of the β-radiation, a control non-radioactive bacteria sample was stored in the presence of 2-^{14}C thymidine in such a way that the radioactivity per cm^3 of this suspension was the same as the study sample. From a comparison of the results, the authors concluded that the predominant lethal effect was from transmutation with an efficiency of 160-times that which would be obtained from the β-radiation. Similar results have been obtained from studies of C-14 by Anderson and Person [44, 45] who put the hazard coefficient relative to β–radiation at 10-fold. These authors studied the mutagenic effect of C-14 and compared transmutation with external X-ray doses. Pluchennik [46, 47] studied the mutagenic effect of C-14 decay in *Chlorella* grown in a medium containing a single carbon source with different fractions of C-14. The number of mutants from the C-14 rose rapidly at low fractions and quickly saturated due to killing effects; the data showed that the mutagenic effect considerably exceeded that due to external radiation. Other research carried out in the 1960s has largely confirmed this generalisation [2].

The genetic effects of incorporation of C-14 are of concern since the atmospheric nuclear tests in the 1950s and 1960s greatly increased the C-14 in the atmosphere. The genetic hazard to man was first pointed out by Totter et al [48] in 1958 and also by Pauling [49]. A number of studies were carried out on different systems. These include onion bulbs [50, 51] grown in an atmosphere of $^{14}CO_2$ resulting in chromosome aberrations, micronuclei and elongated cells. Onion bulbs were also studied by Friedkin and Atchison [52] who compared chromosome aberration in the roots between labelled thymidine (incorporated in DNA) and thymine (not incorporated). The frequency of aberrations was 3.95% for the thymidine but only 0.43% for the thymine, showing that the effect of transmutation was 9-times that of the β –radiation. A study of the effect of the C-14 position in the thymidine [53] showed quite clearly that it was transmutation that was the cause of the effects.

Kuzin et al [54, 55] compared the transmutational component of C-14 incorporation with external γ radiation in the broad bean. The amount of chromosomal aberration in 2 days was found to be 25-times per rad for the transmutational component. Other studies on drosophila [56, 57] give results which suggest that the mutagenic efficiency of C-14 is about three times that of chronic external γ radiation. Valuable reviews of effects from Tritium and Sulphur-35 are presented in [2].

Tritium has been increasing in the biosphere since the nuclear atmospheric testing. The main form in which it exists is tritiated water (HTO) but the nuclide also is incorporated into carbon compounds e.g. CH_3T and this is termed organically bound Tritium. Tritium is also employed for radioactively labelling compounds in chemical, medical and biochemical research. Tritium has a half-life of 12.6 years and radiates low energy β-particles (0-18 keV) and when incorporated in a molecule it transmutes to Helium with molecular restructuring and ionisation and realises a recoil energy of 0-3 keV. These events convey a high probability of destruction or inactivation of the parent molecule. If this is a macromolecule, local restructuring may alter the tertiary folding structure and inactivate the entire molecule. Thus the effects of Tritium are amplified in the ratio of the molecular mass to the Tritium mass, which may be by orders of magnitude. The question of whether these results show enhancement of effect relative to externally calculated absorbed dose does not seem to have been addressed either for lethality or mutation. Experiments with very low dose exposures of Tritium to invertebrates have identified significant developmental effects [58]. Tritium is also of interest as a pseudo-second event nuclide (see below) owing to the fact that the number of events associated with unit dose is far greater than the mean event number associated with background gamma radiation.

4.4. Temporal location: The second event theory

It is well known that dividing cells are more sensitive to radiation than quiescent cells. Once cells are committed to division, they enter the active part of the cell cycle, during which DNA repair takes place followed by cell division. It is therefore clear that any damage or signal which moves cells from quiescence into the repair replication sequence puts the cells into a condition where a second damaging event will carry an enhanced risk of mutation or lethality. This is the basis of the Second Event Theory [18, 19]. This postulates that split doses to the cell DNA, separated by 10-12 hours, will represent an enhancement of hazard. The sequence is vanishingly unlikely for external natural background irradiation but exceedingly likely for a number of specific internal sequential emitters. These include exposure regimes involving Sr-90/Y-90, Te-132/I-132 and various others. They include hot particles (since there are continuous releases of tracks from these) and also Tritium which, due to its very low decay energy, produces many more tracks per unit dose than natural background radiation.

The probabilities of second event processes occurring can be calculated but depend on basic assumptions. A paper by Cox and Edwards of the UK National Radiological Protection Board [59] concluded that the cell dose enhancements were finite but low. However it was pointed out that there were major faults in the cell dimensions employed in this study [60]. Clearly, the enhancement is a function of the location of the Second Event nuclide, the factor increasing sharply as the critical volume is reduced. For location on the DNA the potential enhancement becomes enormous. Table 5 shows results for Sr90/Y90. A number of studies have indeed shown anomalous genetic hazard from Sr-90/Y-90 [7, 18]. However, since Strontium also binds to DNA it carries enhancement from other mechanisms. An interesting experiment which suggests that there are 2nd event effects from Sr-90/Y90 was a comparison of the genetic damage effectiveness of Sr-90 and the singly decaying Sr-89 on yeast suspensions at the same doses. The results showed that the Sr90 was four-times as genetically damaging as the Sr89 for the same dose [61]. Further support comes from cell culture experiments with split doses of X-rays which show an enhancement of effect for split dose regimes during the repair replication period [18, 62, 63]. In view of the important implications this has for medical X-ray and radiology the question should be examined by further research. Such research might include (a) split dose research on living animals, e.g drosophila, zebra fish, (b) comparison of sequential decay effects from indentical elements with different decay sequences e.g. Sr-90/Y-90 vs. Sr-89.

External dose comparison	2nd Event enhancement probability [19]	Cox and Edwards (2000)[59] Cox Edwards and Simmonds (2004) [6]
1 mGy	30	1.3
0.1 mGy	200	*8.6*
0.01 mGy	1900	*82*
0.001 mGy	9400	*407*
1 atom per g of tissue	5×10^9	

Table 5. Second Event Enhancements for Sr-90/Y-90 (From Busby 1998 [19])

http://dx.doi.org/10.5772/53942

4.5. Secondary photoelectron effects

The quantity employed in radiation protection, *absorbed dose*, is defined as D = ΔE /ΔM. Hitherto, the mass into which the energy has been diluted is that of living tissue; ICRU provide tables of absorption coefficients for different living tissue, adipose, bone, muscle etc. which can be employed for calculations involving doses, but generally all these denominator quantities have the absorption characteristics of water (H_2O) (ICRU35 1984). The absorption of electromagnetic (photon) radiation is due to a number of processes, the main three being pair-production, Compton scattering and photoelectron production. For elements of atomic number greater than about 30, and for photon energies of less than about 500 keV, the photoelectric effect predominates. Even for the low atomic number elements that make up living systems, there is fairly quantitative conversion of incident photon radiation below 200 keV (and induced photon radiation from second order and third order processes) into photoelectrons. These are fast electrons which are indistinguishable from beta radiation and have the energy of the incident photon minus their binding energy (which is generally far less than the incident photon energy and can be ignored). The absorption of photon radiation by elements is proportional to the fourth or fifth power of the atomic number Z. Thus the predominant absorber in water is the Oxygen atom Z=8 and it is reasonable to give the effective atomic number of water as 7.5. Of course, there are elements in tissue with higher atomic numbers, but interestingly, apart from Iodine (Z=53) few elements with Z>26 (Iron, Fe).The incorporation of high Z elements into living systems would generally be harmful since it would increase the radiation dose, and therefore such developments have been lost though evolutionary selection. Iodine is an exception, but it should be noted that the main sites for radiation damage in terms of sensitivity are the main sites for Iodine concentration, the thyroid gland and the blood. It has been suggested that the metabolic and cell repair status controls exercised by the thyroid gland are the reason why Iodine has been incorporated into living systems and is employed as a kind of radiation-repair control mechanism [17].

A problem in radiation protection arises when high Z elements are incorporated into living tissue, since the enormously greater absorption of photon radiation by such material will result in enhanced doses to tissues adjacent to the high Z material. The problem was first addressed in 1947 in relation to X-rays of bone [64] and has been studied in the past in relation to prostheses. More recently, interest has shifted to the use of high Z material to enhance photon radiotherapies for tumour destruction where it has been shown to be effective. Gold nanoparticles have been successfully employed (and patented) for radiotherapy enhancement [65].

Despite this knowledge, the enhancement of photon radiation by high Z contaminants has not been addressed in radiation protection. The situation may have arisen out of the fact that prosthetic materials are not intrinsically radioactive and contamination from high Z elements like Lead (Z=82) are considered under the heading of chemical toxicity. The issue was raised in 2005 [66, 67]. It was pointed out that there are two circumstances where the Secondary Photoelectron Effect (SPE) would have significant radiological implications. These are (a) for high Z elements that bind to DNA and (b) for internal high Z particulates. In the latter case, the effect will increase as the particle size is reduced, since for massive high Z contamination e.g. prostheses, most of the photoelectrons are wasted inside the bulk material. The emergence of the photoelectrons into tissue is a function of the mean electron path in the material, and the absorbed dose in local tissue is a function of the electron range and thus its energy.

The radiological implications of the idea emerged in considering the anomalous health effects of Depleted Uranium weapons and were presented to the CERRIE Committee in 2003 and the UK Ministry of Defence in 2004 although nothing was done. More recently there have been attempts to quantify the effects for particles through Monte Carlo modelling [68, 69], but these have not generally been very credible treatments or able to cope with the small volumes of complex media involved, and the results have been far removed from the few experimental data published [70, 65].

The particular concern is for the element Uranium, since this has been employed since 1991 as a weapon; the Depleted Uranium (DU) penetrators, used from the 1991 Persian Gulf War onward, produce a fallout comprising sub-micron Uranium Oxide particles which are environmentally mobile and respirable. Uranium has another quality which makes it of interest in SPE; as the uranyl ion UO_2^{++} it has a very high affinity for DNA phosphate: some 10^{10} M^{-1} [30]. This affinity has been known since the 1960s when it was first employed as an electron microscope stain for imaging chromosomes [31].

The SPE is therefore likely here to cause enhanced photoelectron ionization at the DNA due to enhanced absorption of natural background radiation (or medical X-rays). A similar process occurs with the Platinum chemotherapeutic agent cisplatin which binds to the DNA and acts as an antenna for background radiation and radiotherapy beams.

For SPE phantom radioactivity in other elements of high atomic number, the tissue doses are enhancements of the incident photon dose at the point of the atom or particle being considered. Due to the complex interactions these local doses must be determined by experiment. However, these experiments are straightforward and involve X-irradiation of high Z element contaminated tissue at different doses. In principle, this development suggests that the internalization of any high Z particle which is biologically long-lived will cause continuous irradiation of local tissue cell populations, which would represent a carcinogenic hazard. This has implications for those employing prosthetic materials and also for the dispersion of high Z particles (Tungsten, Platinum, Bismuth, Lead) in the environment. It also suggests that it may be of interest to examine tumours for the presence of high Z particles at their centre. Table 6 lists a number of potentially hazardous SPE elements.

Finally it should be pointed out that physical modelling through Monte Carlo codes is unlikely to establish useful data and certainly should not be employed as an attempt to dismiss the importance of the proposed mechanism.

Nevertheless, a FLUKA Monte Carlo model of the absorption by nanoparticles of Gold and Uranium carried out by [71] Elsaesser *et al* 2007 graphically confirmed the effect. The results for photoelectron track production following absorption of 100 keV photons is shown in Fig 6 below. Enhancement factor in this calculation for the 10nm Uranium particle relative to water was approximately 8000.

http://dx.doi.org/10.5772/53942

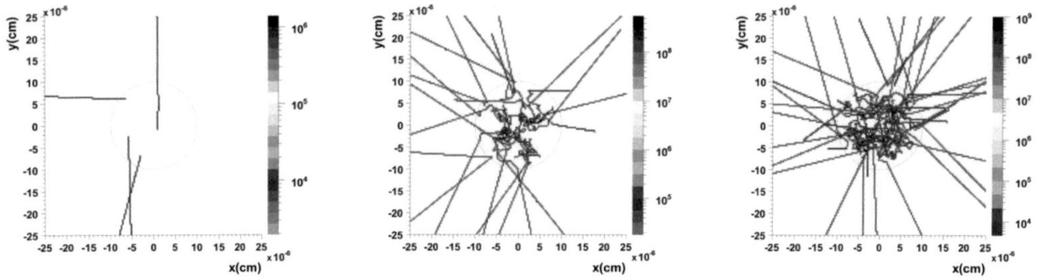

Figure 6. Photoelectron tracks emerging from (left to right) 10 nm particles of water (Z=7.5), Gold (Au; Z =79) and Uranium (U;Z=92) after irradiation with 100keV photons. Monte Carlo (FLUKA code) analysis. Track numbers are in proportion to the 4th power Z law (tracks are shown as projections on a flat plane). Note that the model uses 1000 incident photons for Au and U but 10,000 for water [71]

Material	Z	Z^4/tissue	Source	Note
U	92	22642	Weapons particles, nuclear fuel cycle, atomic and thermonuclear bomb tests	Binds to DNA; known to cause cancer in animals and genomic damage at very low concentrations
Th	90	20736	Incandescent mantles Contrast media	Highly insoluble
Bi	83	14999	General contaminant	Insoluble
Pb	82	14289	General contaminant	Toxic; SH binding
Hg	80	12945	General contaminant	Toxic; enzyme binding
Au	79	12310	Prostheses; colloid used for rheumatism	Friction particles may travel in body; inert and insoluble
Pt	78	11698	Vehicle catalysers, general contaminant	Inert and insoluble
W	74	9477	Weapons; general particle contaminant	Associated with child leukemia cluster Fallon Nevada; known to cause genomic damage and cancer in animals.
Ta	73	8975	Capacitors	
I	53	2493	Thyroid, blood plasma	Radiation sensitivity

Table 6. Biologically significant environmental contaminants and materials exhibiting phantom radioactivity through the Secondary Photoelectron Enhancement (SPE) of natural background and medical X-rays

4.6. Fat soluble radioactive noble gases

The nuclide Krypton-85 has been released to the biosphere continuously since 1945 and increasingly from nuclear energy processes. With a half-life of 10.7 y and a β decay of 672 keV the concentration in the atmosphere has been building up to the extent that liquid air is now significantly radioactive. The assessment of harm from Kr-85 has generally been associated with skin doses from β decays in air. However Krypton (and Radon) are far more soluble in fats than in water and this water/oil partition driven equilibrium might cause build up of these nuclides in lymphatic tissue as a result of equilibria in the lung.

5. Conclusions and recommendations.

5.1. Epidemiology: Uranium effects

The current radiation risk position, that of the ICRP and its associated organisations, has been adequately reviewed by Harrison and Day [72]. With regard to the questions raised in the present overview, the only useful discussion in this paper, as in the CERRIE majority report [6], is the belief that the application of external risk models to internal exposures is supported by epidemiological studies of Thorotrast and Radium. It is therefore worth briefly looking more closely at these.

5.2. Radium and thorotrast studies: Re-examining the data

The increasing pressure brought to bear on the ICRP risk model focuses intensely on the arguments about internal and external radiation exposure rehearsed in the previous section. The ICRP and the radiation protection agencies have to concede much of the science, but fall back on the epidemiology. The problem is, very little human epidemiologic research has been done on internal radionuclide exposures. There are, however, two sets of studies which are said to broadly support the arguments that the current risk model is correct. These are the studies of individuals medically treated with Radium and Thorotrast. The studies originally were carried out because of doubt over the use of the external based risk model to deal with internal radionuclide exposures at a time when internal exposures from alpha emitters like plutonium were increasing in proportion to the development of the A-Bombs and H-Bombs. All of these studies were of roughly the same type. A group of individuals was formalised and then records were traced, or the individuals themselves were traced to see what the number of cancers were. The end point was always cancer, since the project was to see if the ICRP cancer risk model was accurate for these internal exposures. The medical and other (e.g. laboratory) exposures to Radium had been largely before 1960; e.g radium clock dial painters, and there were many of these who had survived from the period when they were employed. In addition there were individuals who had been exposed to Ra-224 as a treatment for various illnesses. There had been a fashion to treat syphilis, hypertension, gout, infectious polyarthritis, "muscular rheumatism", anaemia, epilepsy and multiple sclerosis [29] with radium. Then there were many individuals who had been injected with the substance Thorotrast, an X-ray contrast medium based on the nuclide Th-232, the daughter of which is Ra-228. So these are all internal radium exposures. What was reported in studies was that the cancer yields, mainly of liver cancer, bone cancer, and leukaemia could be roughly related to the exposures and that the yield was not too far away from the yield predicted by the

http://dx.doi.org/10.5772/53942

ICRP external type of risk model, i.e. the A-Bomb survivors. These studies are the last remaining defence that the current risk agencies can mobilise. There are a number of fatal problems with all the radium studies:

- The study groups were assembled long after the exposures and so not all those who had been exposed were in the study group: only the survivors. Many were dead. This biased the samples.
- A number of published studies give sufficient data to show that there was a high rate of death in the early period before the groups were assembled.
- The doses were not isotropic; for Thorotrast, the material was stored in depots in parts of the body where cells were quite resistant to radiation.

In addition, the doses were very large, so these studies were not of low dose chronic exposure but were in fact high dose internal chronic exposure.

Some of these problems were raised in 1970 in relation to the pioneering work by Robley Evans. Evans was a physicist and was concerned with the question of physical dosimetry of small quantities of internal emitters. Writing in the *British Journal of Cancer* in 1970, JF Loutit [29] took issue with the methodology of the Radium studies and pointed out that the massive bone marrow damage resulting from Radium exposure (which had been reported by many authors before Evans) would result in a very large excess death rate from a range of diseases. Loutit wrote that the limiting hazard from internally retained radium acquired occupationally being bone cancer needed to be reconsidered. He pointed out that evidence already existed in the 1930s from the work of Martland that those with substantial body burdens of radium had considerable life shortening and that the associated pathology had not been clarified. Loutit re-examined the radium dial case reports and found that internal radium had a profound effect on the bone marrow, best described as leukopenic anemia. This identifies one source of increased risk from non cancer illness and death which would have removed individuals from Radium and Thorotrast study groups. Indeed, the problem with all these studies is that they exclude about half of the exposed population who may have been lost to the researchers but are very likely to have died of cancer or a range of non cancer illnesses. In the better reported studies, where more data is made available, it is possible to see that this is indeed the case. An example is Wick et al. (1983) who examined cancer in Ra-224 patients. I have reduced the data from a diagram in this paper to produce the graph in Fig 7 which shows the percentage dead in the age group at exposure by the period between exposure and death. It is clear from the trend that for all the groups, the most deaths will have occurred in the first five years in individuals that were not in the study group.

This Ra-224 study by Wick et al. [73] is of the exposure group of German patients who were treated between 1948 and 1975 with Ra-224 for ankylosing spondylitis. There were 1501 total patients, among them 69 were missing and 433 were dead. What did they die of? We don't hear. But 3 of them developed bone cancer, 5 developed leukemia, and 6 bone marrow failure (cf Loutit above). This tiny cancer yield may approximate to the range predicted by the ICRP model (assuming that the dose could be accurately described) but what about the missing people? What about the 433 who died? If they died of conditions caused by the stress on their immune system (bone marrow failures and silent bone marrow problems) then the cancer yield is not a proper representation of the effects of the radium exposures on this group. And the cancer yield to produce an approximation to the ICRP risk predictions for leukemia is lower than in the control group. Addition of a handful of cases from the missing individuals or a handful of pre-leukemic immune-compromised individuals from the 633 dead would have a profound effect on the outcome of the study.

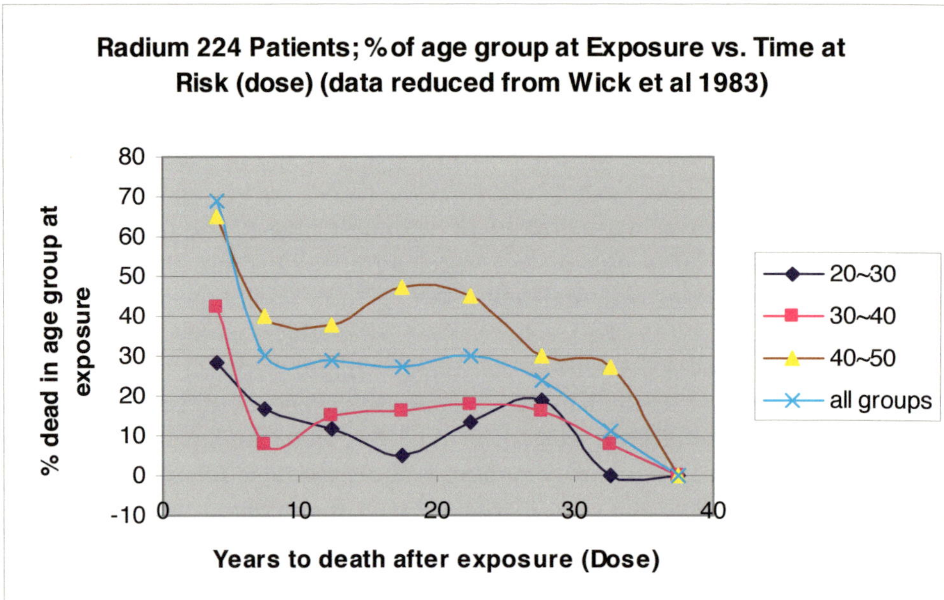

Figure 7. Percentage of each age group at exposure plotted against years to death from exposures in the Ra-224 study of Wick et al 1983. [73]

A similar picture is found in the thorotrast studies, where it is possible to see enough data. For example, in the paper by Mori et al 1983, 282 Japanese war wounded ex-servicemen thorotrast cases are followed up [74]. There were deaths from liver cancer, cirrhosis of the liver and also blood diseases. But in 170 deaths in the group, 42% were from cancer and 37% from other causes. There was no dose response for the cancers and the cancer yield was about 20-times greater than expected from ICRP. But the most interesting aspect is that from analysis of this group, the death rate was very high and the age at death very low compared with all Japanese populations. This is missed in the report since the method employed was to choose sick pathology controls from a hospital pathology records sample. I have compared their age specific death rates with all-Japan. Plots of the survival curves in the females in this group show that 100% were dead by age 75 compared with 65% for the equivalent all-Japan population. Results are given in Fig 8.

http://dx.doi.org/10.5772/53942

Of course, about 40% of these study group women died of cancer: the effects of the thorotrast. But note that the others died from something else; they didn't live to a ripe old age nor did they live as long as the all Japan population. This is clear from the survival curves in Figure 8 which show almost a 20 years age effect in the women. For men, the shift was about 9 years (my unpublished results, not shown).

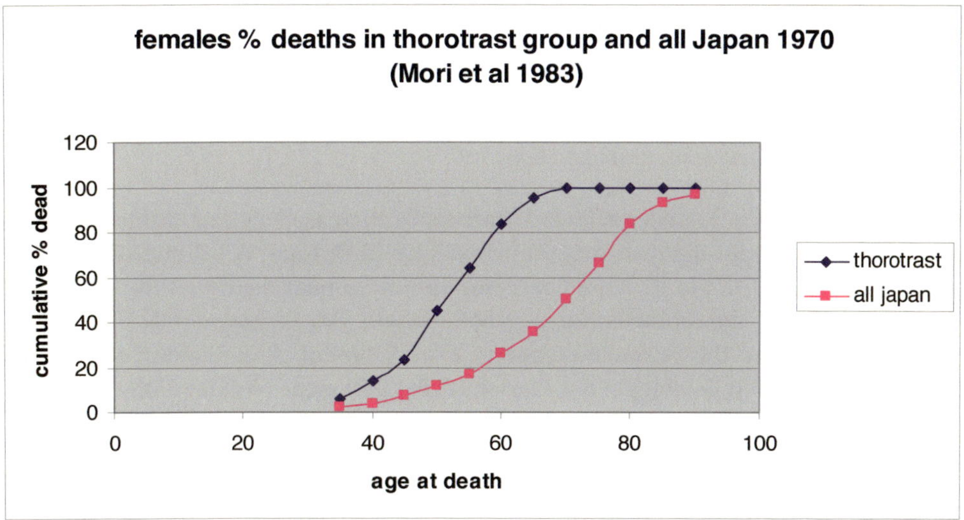

Figure 8. Survival curves for female thorotrast patients studied by Mori et al 1983 compared with all Japan. Data reduced from tables in Mori et al 1983 [74] and Japanese government publications.

The conclusions of this brief account of the re-examinations of the radium and thorotrast studies show that they cannot be used as indicators for low dose chronic risk to internal radionuclides. Apart from the fact that the doses were (like the A-Bomb doses) very large, the main fatal flaw was and is that confounding causes of death make the cancer yield conclusions unsafe. Loutit 1970 makes the point that the damage to the bone marrow would be likely to occur in the case of the weapons-fallout component Strotium-90, and he urged the research community to concentrate on examining risk from that nuclide, an exhortation which the research community entirely failed to take notice of. Loutit was a Medical Research Council MRC (Harwell) director.

5.3. Uranium

The anomalous health effects of exposure to Uranium, especially in the form of particulates, have been increasingly clear in the last 10 years. The radiobiological evidence is reviewed in ECRR2009 [75] and there is insufficient space here to do more than note that the current risk external radiation based model cannot begin to explain or predict what is found empirically. Despite the massive evidence including studies by nuclear industry and military scientists, the agencies ICRP, UNSCEAR, BEIR et al persist in their assertions that the observed effects cannot be due to Uranium. Most recently there have been studies of French Uranium workers showing leukemia and lymphoma excess, lung cancer excess and heart disease at doses which are too low by some 2000-times to explain them on the basis of current risk models [76, 77, 78]. There is an urgent need to carry out research into this issue. The effects of photoelectron amplification can easily be examined by studies involving varying external X-ray doses at different concentrations of Uranium particulates and molecular Uranyl ion in cell culture and animal studies. There is no routine measurement of Uranium in the vicinity of nuclear sites. This should also be remedied.

5.4. other epidemiological evidence

5.4.1. Childhood cancer near nuclear installations

There have been reports in peer reviewed journals of increased risk of childhood leukemia and non Hodgkin lymphoma near many nuclear sites in Europe. A list and discussion may be found in ECRR2010. Child leukemia excesses are found near nearly all the sites that have been examined [5]. e.g the reprocessing sites at Sellafield [37] Dounreay UK [79] and La Hague (France) [80] near the Atomic Weapons Establishment Aldermaston (UK) [81], the Atomic Energy Research Establishment Harwell (UK) [82], near Hinkley Point nuclear power station (UK) [83] and recently near all the combined nuclear sites in Germany (KiKK study) [84] and near all the combined nuclear sites in France [85], GB, and Switzerland.

The radiation risk community [86, 87] basing calculations on the ICRP risk model have worked out the dose ranges and say they cannot be more than a few microSieverts, well below Natural Background. The ICRP risk model predicts an excess risk of 0.05 cancers per Sievert. 100 microSieverts is 1/10,000 th (10^{-4} of a Sievert). An Excess Absolute Risk of 0.05/Sv is Excess Relative Risk (ERR) of 5E-8 per μSv. This, divided by the spontaneous risk of 3E-4 for 0-4 y old children, is 1E-3 per 6 microSv. But there are twice as many child leukemias as are expected: a doubling of risk: the ERR observed in the KiKK study was ~ERR=1. So ICRP predicts a 1000-fold lower risk than found in the KiKK study.)

The ICRP does not give a risk factor for childhood leukaemia but to define a difference between external and internal exposure we can employ the Excess Relative Risk based on the obstetric X-ray studies analysed by Wakeford and Little [88]. This gives an Excess Relative Risk of 50/Sv and based on the 40/Sv Obstetric X-rays results of Alice Stewart.

Stewart found a 40% excess risk after an X-ray dose of 10 mSv [88]. That would suggest a 4% increase after 1 mSv, 0.4% after 100 μSv. But we are seeing a 100% increase at this level. The error is now 100/0.4 = 250-fold.

5.4.2. Infant leukemia after Chernobyl

Five different groups [89-93] reported a statistically significant increase in infant leukemia in 5 different countries of Europe in those children who were in the womb at the time of the Chernobyl Caesium-137 fallout as measured by whole body monitoring. The effect was also reported from the USA [94]. Thus the Chernobyl exposure is the only explanation for the in-

http://dx.doi.org/10.5772/53942

crease. This occurred and was reported from Greece, Germany, Scotland, Wales, Belarus, USA and the error this shows in the ICRP model was the subject of two peer reviewed papers in 2000 [92] and 2009 [25]. Using the Alice Stewart relation between dose and leukemia above, the error is about 400-fold (depending on the country) [25]. Using the ICRP model it is upwards of 1000-fold. This analysis is most relevant since it unequivocally supports the causal relation revealed by the nuclear site child leukemias yet in this case fission product internal radiation can be the only cause.

5.4.3. *Cancer following Chernobyl in Northern Sweden*

The study by Martin Tondel found a 11% increase in cancer for every 100 kBq/sq metre of Cs-137 from Chernobyl [95]. It is possible to calculate that 100 kBq/m^2 Cs-137 including a further 100kBq/ m^2 of Cs-134 if reduced exponentially due to rain washout to rivers and lakes with half life of 6 months would give a committed effective dose of about 1 mSv. The ICRP model [96] predicts an Excess Relative Risk of 0.45 per Sv, so the ICRP expected excess relative risk, including a Dose Rate Reduction Factor of 2 (as used by ICRP) is 0.0225%. The error in ICRP model defined by Tondel's result is thus 490-fold.

5.4.4. *Human sex ratio at birth perturbed by low doses of internal fission-product ionising radiation*

Studies by Hagen Scherb and Kristina Voigt [97] show clear and highly statistically significant alterations in the human sex ratio at birth (the number of boys born to girls) after (a) atmospheric bomb testing, (b) Chernobyl and (c) near nuclear facilities. Effects are shown to be local, European (several countries were studied) and global, supporting earlier evidence of increases in infant mortality during the period of atmospheric weapons testing [98, 99]. Sex ratio has been accepted as a measure of genetic damage with the preferential killing of one or other sex depending on the type of exposure (mothers or fathers). According to Scherb and Voigt, millions of babies were killed *in utero* by these effects [100]. A recent reanalysis of the sex ratio effect in Hiroshima reveals the effect in those populations also [101], evidence which was overlooked by the USA researchers through poor epidemiology and questionable decisions. This evidence objectively confirms the serious genotoxic effect of internal ionising radiation on germ cells and the exquisite sensitivity of humans and other living creatures to releases from Uranium fission. The ICRP does not consider such effects nor are they included in any assessment of harm.

5.4.5. *Cancer and genotoxic effects in Iraq following DU exposure*

A series of studies of the population of Fallujah Iraq shown [102- 104] to have been exposed to Uranium following the 2003-2004 battles have revealed extremely high rates of congenital malformations at birth and cancer and leukemia/lymphoma in adults. The studies also draw attention to significant sex ratio effects at birth beginning after 2004. These results, and the increases in genotoxic effects in the offspring of Gulf veterans support and are supported by the other sets of observations reviewed above which show that inhaled Uranium nanoparticles represent a very serious hazard which is entirely overlooked by ICRP.

5.4.6. Chernobyl effects as reported in the Russian peer-reviewed literature

The effects of the Chernobyl accident exposures have been reported in the Russian language peer review literature since 1996. These results have been reviewed by Busby and Yablokov 2006 [105] Yablokov et al 2010 [106] and Busby et al 2011 [107] but have been largely ignored by ICRP. They constitute a very large body of peer reviewed work which show that the effects of the Chernobyl accident exposures are massive and extremely serious [108]. They range from cancer and leukemia to heart disease especially in children together with a range of illnesses which can be best described by the term premature ageing [108]. They include congenital transgenerational diseases and are reported in animals and plants which cannot be affected by the kind of psychological processes (radiophobia) which have been employed by the radiation risk establishment to account for the early reports coming out of the affected territories. In addition, there are objective measurements of serious biological harm to humans and other living creatures affected by the exposures. The germline mutations found by minisatellite tests [109] in humans were also associated with real morphological effects and fitness loss in birds [110] and were shown to have caused significant sex ratio changes in the birds and also population loss [111] which is in agreement with the findings of Scherb and Voigt and the infant mortality findings [98, 99]. The implications for the understanding of the historic effects of the nuclear project on human health are alarming.

5.5. Summary and conclusions

The current radiation risk model is insecure for internal radionuclide effects. Massive evidence exists from epidemiology and also published studies of the effects of internal radionuclide exposures that the effects of location, chemical binding or affinity, temporal decay patterns and transmutation of internal radionuclides can have much greater genetic or lethal effects on cells than are predicted by the absorbed dose model. These data have been published since the 1950s but ignored for the purpose of radioprotection. Many critical research issues should have been pursued but have not been. It is recommended that those issues and research studies highlighted in this contribution are seen as a priority.

Appendix

Calculating the probability of a track interception with DNA as a function of distance of the point source

The model is given in Fig 9 and Fig 10. It locates the source at the centre of a sphere S radius r distance d from the DNA which is modelled as a cylinder of length 2R. We put $r<D$. Any decay which intercepts an infinitesimal strip of area A on the DNA cross section can be mapped onto a small area B on the surface of the sphere S. The required probability assumes that the decay can be in any direction. It is thus equal to the area B / total area of the sphere.

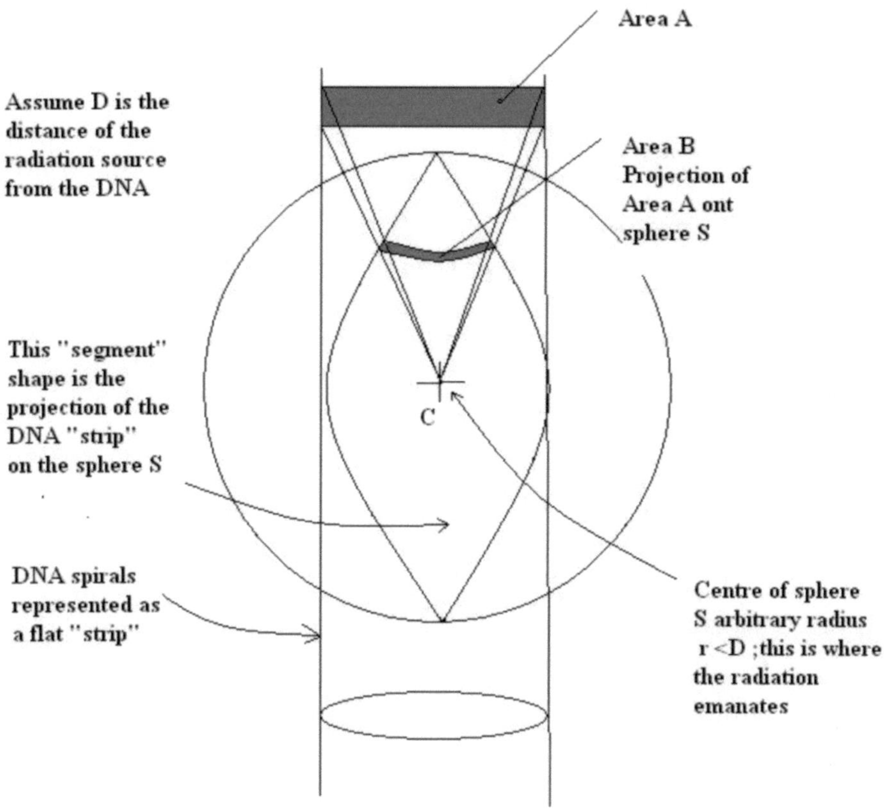

Figure 9. Model

From Fig 2, tan θ = R/d; θ = arctan (R/d)

Length of arc A = 2rθ = 2arctan (R/d)

d′ = d/cos θ; θ = arctan (R/d′) = arctan ((Rcos α)/d)

Area B (Fig 1) = 2rθ. rdα = 2r^2 arctan((Rcos α)/d)

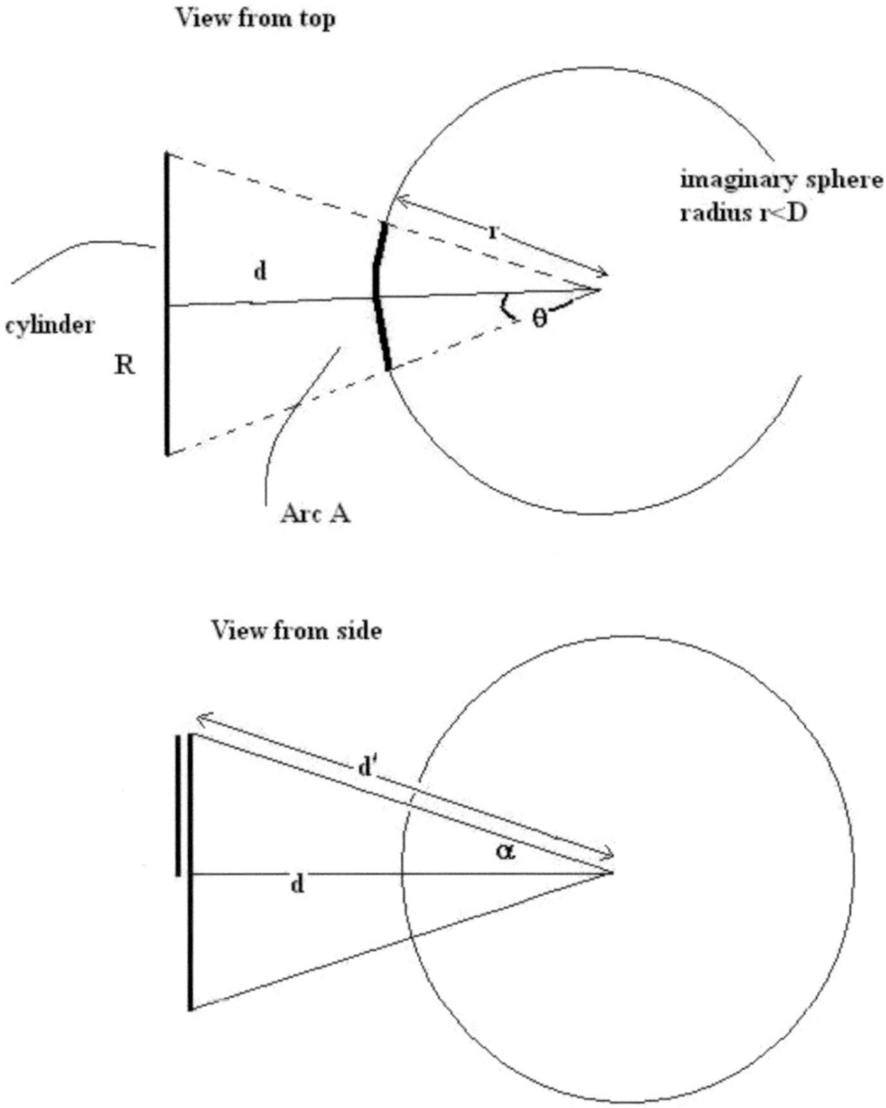

Figure 10. Model from top and side

Area B (Fig 1) = $2r\theta.\ rd\alpha = 2r^2 \arctan((R\cos\alpha)d)$

Whole area of segment =

$$4r^2\int_0^{\pi/2} \arctan((R\cos\alpha)/d)d\alpha$$

And the required probability is this divided by the surface area of the sphere $4\pi r^2$

$$P\ (DNA) = \frac{1}{\pi}\int_0^{\pi/2} \arctan((R\cos\alpha)/d)d\alpha$$

http://dx.doi.org/10.5772/53942

Author details

Christopher Busby

Jacobs University, Bremen, Germany

References

[1] Caufield, K. (1989), *Multiple Exposure: Chronicles of the Radiation Age* (London: Secker and Warburg).

[2] Gracheva LM and Korolev VG (1980) *Genetic effects of the decay of radionuclides in cells.* Edited by I.A.Zacharov. Calcutta: Oxonian Press PVT

[3] ICRP Publication 72 (1996) Age-dependent Doses to the Members of the Public from Intake of Radionuclides Part 5, Compilation of Ingestion and Inhalation Coefficients. Amsterdam: Elsevier

[4] ECRR2003 (2003) *2003 recommendations of the European Committee on Radiation Risk-The health effects of ionizing radiation at low dose--Regulator's edition.* Busby C.C editor with Bertell R, Yablokov A, Schmitz Feuerhake I and Scott Cato M (Brussels: ECRR-2003) Translations of the above into French Japanese Russian and Spanish (see www.euradcom.org for details)

[5] ECRR2010 (2010) *The 2010 Recommendations of the European Committee on Radiation Risk. The Health Effects of Ionizing Radiation at Low Doses and Low Dose Rates.* Eds. Busby C, Yablolov AV, Schmitz Feuerhake I, Bertell R and Scott Cato M Brussels: ECRR; Aberystwyth Green Audit

[6] CERRIE (2004) Report of the Committee Examining Radiation Risk from Internal Emitters (CERRIE) *Chilton, UK: National Radiological Protection Board*

[7] Busby CC, Bramhall R and Dorfman P (2004) *CERRIE Minority Report 2004: Minority Report of the UK Department of Health/ Department of Environment (DEFRA) Committee Examining Radiation Risk from Internal Emitters (CERRIE)* Aberystwyth: Sosiumi Press

[8] IRSN (2005) Les consequences sanitaire des contaminations internes chroniques par les radionucleides. Ed:-F.Paquet Rapport DRPH/2005-20 Fontenay aux Roses: Institut de Radioprotection et de Surete Nucliare

[9] UNSCEAR, (1977) *Sources and Effects of Ionising Radiation,* Report to the General Assembly, with annexes, (New York, United Nations).

[10] Busby, C. (1994), Increase in Cancer in Wales Unexplained, BMJ, 308: 268.

[11] Busby C.C (2002). 'High Risks at low doses.' Proceedings of 4th International Conference on the Health Effects of Low-level Radiation: Keble College Oxford, Sept 24 2002. (London: British Nuclear Energy Society).

[12] BEIR V (1990) BEIR (Committee on Biological Effects of Ionising Radiation), (1990) The Health Effects of Exposure to Low Levels of Ionising Radiation, BEIR V, (Washington: National Academy Press).

[13] Mothershill C and Seymour C (2012) Human and environmental health effects of low doses of radiation. In *Fukushima—What to expect. Proceedings of the 3rd International Conference of the European Committee on Radiation Risk, Lesvos, Greece May 5/6 2009* Eds Busby C, Busby J, Rietuma D and de Messieres M. Brussels, Belgium: ECRR

[14] Baverstock, K.F. & Charlton, D.E. 1988. *DNA Damage by Auger Emitters*. Taylor and Francis, London

[15] Hofer KG (1998) Biophysical aspects of Auger Processes- a review. *Acta Oncol.*35 798-96

[16] Ward, J.F., Limoli, P., Calabro-Jones, P. & Evans, W.F. 1988. Radiation vs.chemical damage to DNA. In: Nygard, O.F., Simic, M. & Cerutti, P. (eds.), Anticarcinogenesis and Radiation Protection. Plenum, New York.

[17] Busby Chris and Schnug Ewald (2008) Advanced biochemical and biophysical aspects of uranium contamination. In: (Eds) De Kok, L.J. and Schnug, E. *Loads and Fate of Fertilizer Derived Uranium.* Backhuys Publishers, Leiden, The Netherlands, ISBN/EAN 978-90-5782-193-6.

[18] Busby, C.C. (1995), *Wings of Death: Nuclear Pollution and Human Health* (Aberystwyth: Green Audit)

[19] Busby, C.C.(1998), 'Enhanced mutagenicity from internal sequentially decaying beta emitters from second event effects.' In 'Die Wirkung niedriger Strahlendosen- im kindes-und Jugendalter, in der Medizin, Umwelt ind technik, am Arbeitsplatz'. Proceedings of International Congress of the German Society for Radiation Protection. Eds: Koehnlein W and Nussbaum R. Muenster, 28 March 1998 (Bremen: Gesellschaft fur Strahlenschutz)

[20] Goodhead DT (1991) Biophysical features of radiation at low dose and low dose rate. In CB Seymour and C Mothershill (Eds) New Developments in fundamental and applied radiobiology London: Taylor and Francis.

[21] Apelgot S and DBuguesne M (1963) Energie dissipee par le Tritium dans les microorganisms. *Int.J.Radiation Biol.* 7 (1) 65-74

[22] Robertson JS and Hughes WL (1959) Intranuclear irradiation with Tritium labeled thymidine. In: Proc 1st National Biophysical Conference Columbus Ohio 278-283

[23] ICRU 35 (1984) Radiation Dosimetry: Electron Beams with energies between 1 and 50MEv. Bethesda MD USA: ICRU

[24] Burlakova E B; Goloshchapov A N, Zhizhina G P, Konradov A A, (2000) New aspects of regularities in the action of low doses of low level irradiation. In Low Doses of Ra-

diation—Are They Dangerous? Burlakova E B, Ed.; Nova Science Publishers: New York, NY, USA,

[25] Busby C.C. (2009) Very Low Dose Fetal Exposure to Chernobyl Contamination Resulted in Increases in Infant Leukemia in Europe and Raises Questions about Current Radiation Risk Models. International Journal of Environmental Research and Public Health.; 6(12):3105-3114. http://www.mdpi.com/1660-4601/6/12/3105

[26] Luning, K. G., Frolen, H., Nelson, A., and Ronnbaeck, C. (1963), `Genetic Effects of Strontium-90 Injected into Male Mice', Nature, No 4864 197: 304-5.

[27] Smirnova, E. I. and Lyaginska, A. M. (1969), `Heart Development of Sr-90 Injured Rats', in Y. I. Moskalev and Y. I. Izd (eds.), Radioaktiv Izotopy Organizs (Moscow: Medizina), 348

[28] Stokke, T., Oftedal, P. and Pappas, A. (1968), `Effects of Small Doses of Radioactive Strontium on the Rate Bone Marrow', Acta Radiologica, 7: 321-9.

[29] Loutit J F (1970), Malignancy from Radium. Brit.J.Cancer 24(2) 17-207

[30] Nielsen, P.E, Hiort, C., Soennischsen, S.O., Buchardt, O., Dahl, O. & Norden, B. 1992. DNA binding and photocleavage by Uranyl VI salts. J. Am. Chem. Soc. 114: 4967-4975.

[31] Huxley, H.E. & Zubay, G. 1961. Preferential staining of nucleic acid containing structures for electron microscopy. Biophys. Biochem. Cytol. 11: 273.

[32] Petkau A (1980) Radiation carcinogenesis from a membrane perspective *Acta Physiologica Scandinavica* suppl. 492. 81-90

[33] Tamplin AR and Cochran TB (1974) Radiation standards for hot particles. A report on the inadequacy of existing radiation standards related to exposures of man to insoluble particles of plutonium and other alpha emitting hot particles. Washington, USA: Natural Resources Defence Council

[34] Charles MW, Mill AJ and Darley P (2003) Carcinogenic risk from hot particles. J.Radiol.Prot. 23 5-28

[35] Popplewell, DS, Ham GJ, Dodd NJ, Shuttler SD (1988) 'Plutonium and Cs-137 in autopsy tissues in Great Britain' Sci. Tot. Environment 70 321-34

[36] Priest, N. D., O'Donnell, R.G., Mitchell, P. I., Strange, L., Fox, A., Henshaw, D. L., and Long, S. C. (1997), 'Variations in the concentration of plutonium, strontium-90 and total alpha emitters in human teeth collected within the British Isles', Science of the Total Environment, 201, 235-243.

[37] Beral V E. Roman, and M. Bobrow (eds.) (1993), Childhood Cancer and Nuclear Installations (London: British Medical Journal).

[38] Independent Advisory Group (1984), Investigation of the Possible Increased Incidence of Cancer in West Cumbria, The Black Report, (London: HMSO).

[39] Royal Society (2001) The Health Effect of Depleted Uranium Weapons Vol 1 London: Royal Society

[40] COMARE, (1996) The Incidence of Cancer and Leukaemia in Young People in the Vicinity of the Sellafield Site in West Cumbria: Further Studies and Update since the Report of the Black Advisory Group in 1984, COMARE 4th Report (Wetherby: Department of Health).

[41] Hohenemser C, Deicher M, Hofsass H, Lindner G, Recknagel E and Budnick J (1986) Agricultural impact of Chernobyl: a warning. *Nature* 321 817

[42] Apelgot S (1968) Effect letal de la disintegration des atomes radioactifs (3H, 14C, 32P) incorpres dans bacteria. In: Biological Effects of Transmutation and decay of incorporated Radioisotopes. Vienna: IAEA 147-163

[43] Apelgot S and Latarjet R (1962) Marquage d'un acide deoxyribonucleique bacterien par le radiophosphore, le radiocarbone at le tritium: comparison des effets letaux. Biochim et Biophys Acta 55(1) 40-55

[44] Andersen FA and Person S (1971) Incorporation of 14C labeled precursors into *e.coli* The lethal and mutagenic effects. *Radiation Res.* Abstr. 47 (1) p261

[45] Andersen FA and Person S (1973) Incorporation of 14C labeled precursors into *e.coli* The lethal and mutagenic effects. *Radiation Res.* Abstr. 21 (1) p4

[46] Pluchnnik G (1965) Mutagenyii protsess u khorelly pri assimilatsii radioaktivnoi uglekiskoty (mutagenic process in Chlorella during assimilation of radioactive carbon dioxide) *Genetika* 1(5) 19-25)

[47] Pluchennik G (1966) Comparative study of mutagenic effects of incorporated isotopes of the most important organogenic elements. Report 1. Mutagenic effects of incorporated 14C from the example of reversion to autotrophy of diploid yeasts that are homozygous in relation to mutations for adenine requirement. (Russian) *Genetika* 2(5) 117-124

[48] Totter IR, Zerle MR and Hollister H (1958) Hazards to man of Carbon-14. *Science* 128 1490-1495

[49] Pauling L (1958)Genetic and somatic effects of Carbon-14 *Science* 128 1183-1186

[50] Beal JM (1950) Chromosome aberrations in onion roots from plants grown in an atmosphere containing 14-CO_2. *Amer.J.Botany* 37 660-661

[51] Beal M and Scully NJ (1950) Chromosome aberrations in onion roots from plants grown in an atmosphere containing 14-CO_2. *Botan.Gas*112 232-235

[52] McQuade HA, Friedkin M and Atchison AA (1956) Radiation effects of thymidine 2-^{14}C. 1. Uptake of thymidine 2-^{14}C and thymine 2-^{14}C in the onion root tip. 2. Chromosomal aberrations caused by thymidine 2-^{14}C. and thymine 2-^{14}C in the onion root tip. *Expt.Cell.Res.* 11 (2) 249-264

[53] McQuade HA and Friedkin M (1960) Radiation effects of thymidine ^{3}H and thymidine ^{14}C. *Expt.Cell.Res.* 21(1) 118-125

[54] Kuzin AM (1962) Biological effects of increased concentrations of ^{14}C in the atmosphere (Russian) in *Radiation Genetics* Izd-vo AN SSSR Moscow 274-278

[55] Kuzin AM (1962) Effectiveness of biological action of ^{14}C when incorporated in live cells. In *Radionatsionnaya Genetika* Izd-vo AN SSSR Moscow 267-273

[56] Purdom CE (1965) Genetic effect of incorporated ^{14}C in *D.MelanogasterMutation Res.* 2(2) 156-167

[57] Kuzin AM, Glembotskii Ya M, Lapkin Yu A (1964) Mutagenic efficiency of incorporated Carbon 14. (Russian) *Radiobiologiya* 4(6) 804-809

[58] Jha AM, Dogra Y, Turner A and Millward GE (2005) Impact of low doses of tritium on the marine mussel *myrtilis edulis*. Genotoxic effects and tissue specific bioconcentrations. *Mutat.Res* 56(1) 47-57

[59] Cox R and Edwards A (2000) Commentary on the Second Event Theory of Busby *Int.J.Radiat.Biol* 76(1) 119-125

[60] Busby C.,(2000), 'Response to Commentary on the Second Event Theory by Busby' *International Journal of Radiation Biology* 76 (1) 123-125

[61] Gracheva LM and Shanshiashvili TA (1983) Genetic effects of decay of radionuclide products of fission of nuclear fuel II.Lethal and mutagenic effects on the mutation of cells of the yeast *saccharomyces cerevisiae* induced by Sr-90 and Sr-89. *Genetika* (Moscow) 9/4 532-5

[62] Miller RC and Hall EJ (1978) X-ray dose fractionation and oncogenic transformations in culture mouse embryo cells. *Nature* 272 58-60

[63] Borek C and Hall EJ (1974Rffects of split doses of X-rays on Neoplastic transformation of single cells *Nature* 252 499-501

[64] Speirs, F.W. 1949. The influence of energy absorption and electron range on dosage in irradiated bone. *Brit. J. Radiol.* 22: 521-533.

[65] Hainfeld, J.F., Slatkin, D.N. & Smilowitz, H.M. 2004. The use of gold nanoparticles to enhance radiotherapy in mice. *Phys. Med. Biol.* 49: N309-N315.

[66] Busby CC (2005) Does uranium contamination amplify natural background radiation dose to the DNA? *European J. Biology and Bioelectromagnetics*. 1 (2) 120-131

[67] Busby CC (2005) Depleted Uranium Weapons, metal particles and radiation dose. *European J. Biology and Bioelectromagnetics*. 1(1) 82-93

[68] Pattison J E, Hugtenburg R P, Green S, (2009) Enhancement of natural background gamma-radiation dose around uranium micro-particles in the human body. J.Royal http://rsif.royalsocietypublishing.org/content/early/2009/09/23/rsif.2009.0300.abstract

[69] Eakins, JS, Jansen J. Th. M. and Tanner R. J. (2011) A Monte Carlo analysis of possible cell dose enhancements effects by Uranium microparticles in photon fields Radiation Protection Dosimetry (2011), Vol. 143, No. 2–4, pp. 177–180 doi:10.1093/rpd/ncq398

[70] Regulla, D.F., Hieber, L.B. & Seidenbusch, M. 1998. Physical and biological interface dose effects in tissue due to X-ray induced release of secondary radiation from metallic gold surfaces. *Radiat. Res.* 150: 92-100

[71] Elsaesser A, Busby C, McKerr G and Howard CV (2007) Nanoparticles and radiation. EMBO Conference: Nanoparticles. October 2007 Madrid

[72] Harrison J and Day P (2008) Radiation doses and risks from internal emitters. *J Radiol.Prot.* 28 137-159

[73] Wick RR, Chmelevsky,D and Goessner W (1984) Risk to bone and haematopoetic tissue in ankylosing spondilitis patients. In W.Goessner, GB Gerber , U Hagen and A Luz. Eds *The radiobiology of radium and thorotrast.* Munich Germany: Urban and Schwartzenberg

[74] Mori T, Kumatori T, Kato Y, Hatakeyama S, Kamiyama R, Mori W, Irie H, Maruyama T and Iwata S (1983) Present status of medical study of thorotrast patients in Japan. Pp123-135 . In W.Goessner, GB Gerber , U Hagen and A Luz. Eds *The radiobiology of radium and thorotrast.* Munich Germany: Urban and Schwartzenberg

[75] ECRR2009 (2009) The health effects of exposure to Uranium. Brussels: ECRR (www.euradcom.org)

[76] Guseva Canu I, Laurier D, Caër-Lorho S, Samson E, Timarche M, Auriol B, Bérard P, Collomb P, Quesned B, Blanchardone E (2010) Characterisation of protracted low-level exposure to uranium in the workplace: A comparison of two approaches. *International Journal of Hygiene and Environmental Health* 213 (2010) 270–277

[77] Guseva Canu, Irina, Garsi, Jerome-Philippe, Cae°r-Lorho Sylvaine, Jacob SophieCollomb, Philippe, Acker Alain, Laurier Dominique (2012) Does uranium induce circulatory ? First results from a French cohort of uranium workers *Occup. Envir. Med.* OEM Online First, published on March 3, 2012 as 10.1136/oemed-2011-100495

[78] Guseva Canu I, Jacob S Cardis E, Wild P Cae°r –Lorho S, Auriol B, Garsi JP, Tirmarche M, Laurier D (2010) Uranium carcinogenicity in humans might depend on the physical and chemical nature of uranium and its isotopic composition: results from pilot epidemiological study of French nuclear workers. Cancer Causes Control DOI 10.1007/s10552-011-9833-5

[79] Urquhart T D, Black R T, Muirhead M T, et al., (1991) Case-control study of leukaemia and non-Hodgkins lymphoma in children in Caithness near the Dounreay nuclear installation. British Medical Journal; 302:687-692.

[80] Viel J-F, Poubel D, Carre A, (1995) Incidence of leukaemia in young people and the La Hague nuclear waste reprocessing plant: a sensitivity analysis. Statistics in Medicine, 14, 2459-2472.

[81] Busby C, and M. Scott Cato, (1997)`Death Rates from Leukemia are Higher than Expected in Areas around Nuclear Sites in Berkshire and Oxfordshire', *British Medical Journal*, 315 (1997): 309

[82] Busby C, and M. Scott Cato, (1997)`Death Rates from Leukemia are Higher than Expected in Areas around Nuclear Sites in Berkshire and Oxfordshire', British Medical Journal, 315 (1997): 309

[83] Bowie C, Ewings P D, (1988) Leukaemia incidence in Somerset with particular reference to Hinkley Point, Taunton: Somerset Health Authority.

[84] Kaatsch P, Spix C, Schulze-Rath R, Schmiedel S, Blettner M, (2008) Leukaemias in young children living in the vicinity of German nuclear power plants. Int J Cancer 122 , pp. 721-726.

[85] Sermage-Faure Claire, Laurier Dominique, Goujon-Bellec Stéphanie, Chartier Michel, Guyot-Goubin, Aurélie, Rudant Jérémie, Hémon Denis, Clavel Jacqueline (2012) Childhood leukemia around French nuclear power plants—The geocap study, 2002–2007 International Journal of Cancer Volume 131 (5) E769–E780 DOI: 10.1002/ijc.27425

[86] COMARE (Committee on Medical Aspects of Radiation in the Environment), (1986) The Implications of the New Data on the Releases from Sellafield in the 1950s for the Conclusions of the Report on the Investigation of a Possible Increased Incidence of Cancer in West Cumbria, COMARE 1st Report (London: HMSO).

[87] NRPB, (1995) Risks of leukaemia and other cancers in Seascale from all sources of ionising radiation NRPB R-276 (Chilton: NRPB).

[88] Wakeford R and Little MP (20030) Risk coefficients for childhood cancer after intrauterine irradiation. A review. Int.J.Rad.Biol. 79 293-309

[89] Michaelis J, Kaletsch U, Burkart W and Grosche B, (1997) Infant leukaemia after the Chernobyl Accident Nature 387, 246.

[90] Petridou E, Trichopoulos D, Dessypris N, Flytzani V, Haidas S, Kalmanti M, Koliouskas D, Kosmidis H, Piperolou F, Tzortzatou F, (1996) Infant Leukaemia after in utero exposure to radiation from Chernobyl, Nature, 382:25, 352.

[91] Gibson B E S, Eden O B, Barrett A, et al., (1988) Leukaemia in young children in Scotland, The Lancet, 630

[92] Busby, C. C. and Cato, M. S. (2000), 'Increases in leukemia in infants in Wales and Scotland following Chernobyl: evidence for errors in risk estimates' Energy and Environment 11(2) 127-139 92 Busby C.C. and Cato M.S. (2001) 'Increases in leukemia in infants in Wales and Scotland following Chernobyl: Evidence for errors in statutory risk estimates and dose response assumptions'. International Journal of Radiation Medicine 3 (1) 23

[93] Busby C.C. (2009) Very Low Dose Fetal Exposure to Chernobyl Contamination Resulted in Increases in Infant Leukemia in Europe and Raises Questions about Current

Radiation Risk Models. International Journal of Environmental Research and Public Health.; 6(12):3105-3114. http://www.mdpi.com/1660-4601/6/12/3105

[94] Mangano J, (1997) Childhood leukaemia in the US may have risen due to fallout from Chernobyl, British Medical Journal, 314: 1200.

[95] Tondel M, Hjalmarsson P, Hardell L, Carisson G, Axelson A, (2004) Increase in regional total cancer incidence in Northern Sweden. *J Epidem. Community Health.* 58 1011-1016.

[96] ICRP, (2007) *The 2007 recommendations of the International Commission on Radiological Protection*. ICRP 103 Orlando USA: Elsevier

[97] Scherb H and Voigt K (2010) The human sex odds ratio at birth after the atmospheric bomb tests, Chernobyl, and in the vicinity of nuclear facilities. Env.Sci.Pollut.Res. Int 18 (5) 697-707

[98] Sternglass E J, (1971) Environmental Radiation and Human Health, in Proceedings of the Sixth Berkeley Symposium on Mathematical Statistics and Probability, ed. J. Neyman (Berkeley, Calif.: University of California Press).

[99] Whyte R K, (1992) First Day Neonatal Mortality since 1935: A Re-examination of the Cross Hypothesis, *British Medical Journal*, 304: 343-6.

[100] Scherb H and Voigt K (2011) in Busby C, Busby J, Rietuma D and de Messieres M Eds. (2011) Fukushima: What to Expect. Proceedings of the 3rd International Conference of the European Committee on Radiation Risk May 5/6th Lesvos Greece. Brussels: ECRR; Aberystywth UK: GreenAudit

[101] Padmanabhan VT (2011) in Busby C, Busby J, Rietuma D and de Messieres M Eds. (2011) Fukushima: What to Expect. Proceedings of the 3rd International Conference of the European Committee on Radiation Risk May 5/6th Lesvos Greece. Brussels: ECRR; Aberystywth UK: GreenAudit

[102] Alaani Samira, Tafash Muhammed, Busby Christopher, Hamdan Malak and Blaurock-Busch Eleonore (2011) Uranium and other contaminants in hair from the parents of children with congenital anomalies in Fallujah, Iraq Conflict and Health 2011, 5:15 doi:10.1186/1752-1505-5-15

[103] Busby, Chris; Hamdan, Malak; Ariabi, Entesar. (2010) Cancer, Infant Mortality and Birth Sex-Ratio in Fallujah, Iraq 2005–2009. Int. J. Environ. Res. Public Health 7, no. 7: 2828-2837. doi:10.3390/ijerph7072828

[104] Alaani S, Al Fallouji M, Busby C and Hamdan M (2012) Pilot study of congenital rates at birth in Fallujah, Iraq, 2010 *J. Islam. Med. Assoc. N. Amer*. Sept 1st 2012

[105] Busby C, Yablokov A V (2006, 2009) *ECRR 2006. Chernobyl 20 years On. The health Effects of the Chernoby lAccident* Aberystwyth: Green Audit

[106] Yablokov A V, Nesterenko V B, Nesterenko A V, (2009) Chernobyl: Consequences of the Catastrophe for people and the environment. Annals of the New York Academy of Sciences. Vol 1181 Massachusetts USA: Blackwell

[107] Busby C, Busby J, Rietuma D and de Messieres M Eds. (2011) Fukushima: What to Expect. Proceedings of the 3rd International Conference of the European Committee on Radiation Risk May 5/6th Lesvos Greece. Brussels: ECRR; Aberystwyth UK: Green-Audit

[108] Malko M V, (1998) Chernobyl accident: the crisis of the international radiation community in Imanaka T: Research activities about the radiological consequences of the Chernobyl NPS accident and social activities to assist the sufferers of the accident. (Kyoto University: Research Reactor Institute).

[109] Dubrova Y E, Nesterov V N, Jeffreys A J et al., (1997) Further evidence for elevated human minisatellite mutation rate in Belarus eight years after the Chernobyl accident. Mutation Research 381 267-278.

[110] Ellegren H, Lindgren G, Primmer C R, Moeller A P, (1997), Fitness loss and Germline mutations in Barn Swallows breeding in Chernobyl, *Nature* 389/9, 583-4.

[111] Møller AP, Bonisoli-Alquati A, Rudolfsen G, Mousseau TA (2012) Elevated Mortality among Birds in Chernobyl as Judged from Skewed Age and Sex Ratios. PLoS ONE 7(4): e35223. doi:10.1371/journal.pone.0035223

Chapter 23

Radiosensitization Strategies Through Modification of DNA Double-Strand Break Repair

Yoshihisa Matsumoto, Shoji Imamichi,
Mikoto Fukuchi, Sicheng Liu, Wanotayan Rujira,
Shingo Kuniyoshi, Kazuki Yoshida,
Yasuhiro Mae and Mukesh Kumar Sharma

Additional information is available at the end of the chapter

http://dx.doi.org/10.5772/54684

1. Introduction

DNA double-strand break (DSB) is considered most critical type of DNA damage. In eukaryote, DSB is repaired mainly through non-homologous end-joining (NHEJ) and homologous recombination (HR). Our understanding on the molecular mechanisms of these DNA repair mechanisms has been greatly deepened in the last two decades.

In NHEJ, DSB is first recognized by Ku protein (Fig.1 (1)), heterodimer consisting of Ku70 and Ku86 (also known as Ku80), which in turn recruits DNA-PK catalytic subunit (DNA-PKcs) (Fig.1 (2)). The comprex consisting of Ku70, Ku86 and DNA-PKcs is termed DNA-dependent protein kinase (DNA-PK). When the DSB are not readily ligatable, processing takes place prior to ligation (Fig.1 (3)). Processing might involve a number of enzymes depending on the shape of each DNA end and compatibility of two ends to be ligated: Artemis nuclease, DNA polymerase μ/λ, polynucleotide kinase/phosphatase (PNKP), Aprataxin (APTX) and Aprataxin and PNKP-like factor (APLF, also known as PALF, C2orf13 or Xip1). DSBs are finally joined by DNA ligase IV, which is in tight association with XRCC4 (Fig.1 (4)). XRCC4-like factor (XLF, also known as Cernunnos), is essential at this step, especially when two ends are not compatible.

In HR, a complex consisting of Mre11, Rad50 and Nbs1, termed MRN complex, is thought to play two important roles in the initial stage (Fig.1 (1')): recruitment of ATM (Fig.1 (2'')) and resection of one of the strands (Fig.1 (2')). ATM is a protein kinase structurally similar to DNA-PKcs. Although ATM is thought to phosphorylate a great number of proteins as revealed by phosphoproteomic analyses, the phosphorylation of histone H2AX at Ser139 is thought one of the most important events, triggering signal transduction cascade involving mediator protein like MDC1 and ubiquitin ligases like RNF8 and RNF168. As Mre11 bears 5′-3′ exonuclease activity, MRN resects one of the DNA strands to generate single-stranded DNA (ssDNA), which serves as a probe for the search for homology. Replication protein A (RPA) binds to ssDNA (Fig.1 (2′)) and facilitate the formation of Rad51 filament in cooperation with BRCA2, PALB2, Rad52 and Rad51 paralogues (Fig.1 (3′)). RPA also recruites ATRIP, which in turn recruits ATR, another protein kinase structurally related to DNA-PK and ATM (Fig.1 (3″)). ATR phosphorylate checkpoint kinase Chk1 to initiate signal transduction pathway leading to cell cycle checkpoints. Rad51 promotes strand exchange between homologous sequences (Fig.1 (4′)). Template-dependent strand synthesis is proceeded by replication machinery including PCNA and DNA polymerase δ and ε (Fig.1 (5′)). Finally, the junction of two DNA molecules (Holliday's junction) are resolved by nucleases Mus81-Eme1, ERCC1-XPF or SLX1-SLX4 (Fig.1 (6′)). Alternatively, synthesized strand aneals with opposite end of DSB, detaches from the temprate strand, followed by synthesis and ligation of complementary strand (synthesis-dependent strand anealing; SDSA, not shown here).

Here, we will overview approaches to radiosensitization through the modification of DSB repair enzymes.

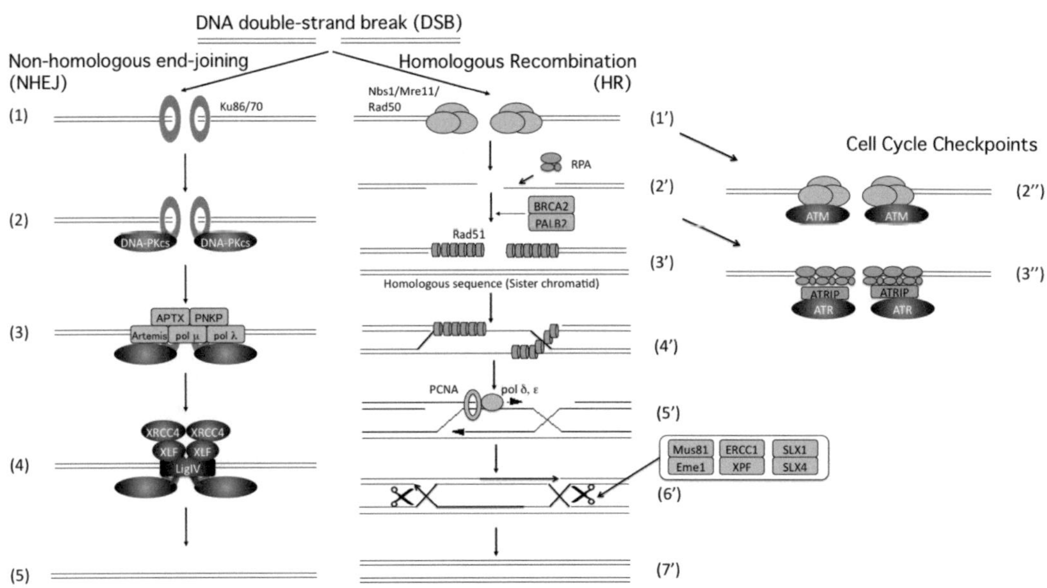

Figure 1. DNA double-strand break repair mechanisms.

2. DNA-PK, ATM and ATR kinases as targets for radiosensitizer

2.1. DNA-PK

DNA-PK was initially found in the extracts of HeLa cell, rabbit reticulocyte, Xenopus egg and sea urchin egg (Walker et al., 1985) and was purified from Hela cell nuclei as a 300-350 kDa protein, which is now called DNA-PKcs (Carter et al., 1990; Lees-Miller et al., 1990). Later it was found that Ku is an essential component of DNA-PK (Dvir et al., 1992, 1993; Gottlieb and Jackson, 1993). Furthermore, it was also shown that DNA-PK requires binding of DNA-PKcs to DNA ends via Ku to be activated, suggesting its possible role in sensoring DSBs (Gottlieb and Jackson, 1993). Ku86 was shown to be equivalent to XRCC5 (X-ray repair cross complementing) gene product, which is missing in X-ray sensitive rodent cell lines including *xrs*-5, -6, XR-V9B and XR-V15B (Taccioli et al., 1994; Smider et al., 1994). Subsequently, DNA-PKcs was found to correspond to XRCC7, which is deficient in *scid* mouse as well as several radiosensitive cultured human and rodent cell lines (Kirchgessner et al., 1995; Blunt et al., 1995; Peterson et al., 1995; Lees-Miller et al., 1995). DNA-PK is abundant in human cells and its activity can be measured using synthetic peptides derived from p53 (Lees-Miller et al., 1992), enabling extensive studies on its biochemical properties even before molecular cloning of DNA-PKcs.

First reported selective inhibitor of DNA-PK is OK-1035, 3-cyano-5-(4-pyridyl)-6-hydrazonomethyl- 2-pyridone (Fig.2 A), which was found by screening of more than 10,000 microbial extracts and synthetic compounds (Take et al., 1995). IC_{50} (50% inhibitory concentration) on DNA-PK was 8 μM, which was more than 50-fold lower than that on other seven kinases examined, although it was reported to be much higher, *i.e.*, 100 μM, in others' study (Stockley et al., 2001). OK-1035 was shown to suppress adriamycin-induced p21 expression in cultured human carcinoma cell at concentrations 500 - 2000 μM (Take et al., 1996) and also to retard the repair of DSB measured by neutral single cell gel electrophoresis (comet) assay (Kruszewski et al., 1998).

Sequence of DNA-PKcs revealed its similarity to phosphatidylinositol 3-kinase (PI3K) (Hartley et al., 1995). This study also that fungal metabolite wortmannin (Fig.2 B), which had been known as an inhibitor of PI3K, could inhibit DNA-PK (Hartley et al., 1995). IC_{50} of wortmannin is reported to be 0.016 μM and 0.12 μM (Sarkaria et al., 1998; Izzard et al., 1999). It was also shown that wortmannin binds covalently to DNA-PKcs and functions as non-competitive, irreversible inhibitor of DNA-PK (Sarkaria et al., 1998; Izzard et al., 1999). Expectedly, a number of studies have demonstrated radiosensitizing effects of wortmannin but there is a concern whether the observed radiosensitization was really due to inhibition of DNA-PK. In this regard, some studies showed that radiosensitization by these compounds could be observed even in DNA-PKcs-deficient cells (Rosenzweig, et al., 1997; Hosoi et al., 1998), indicating that radiosensitization by these compounds was not solely due to inhibition of DNA-PK. In addition to ATM discussed next, PI3K-Akt pathway, which might be even more sensitive to wortmannin, might be important to sustain cell survival after irradiation. On the other hand, there are also studies showing that radiosensitization was not observed in DNA-PKcs deficient cells (Chernikova, et al., 1999; Hashimoto, et al., 2003). These studies argue that, even if wortmannin affect PI3K or other kinase more potently than DNA-PK, the radiosensitizing effect might be mainly due to inhibition of DNA-PK.

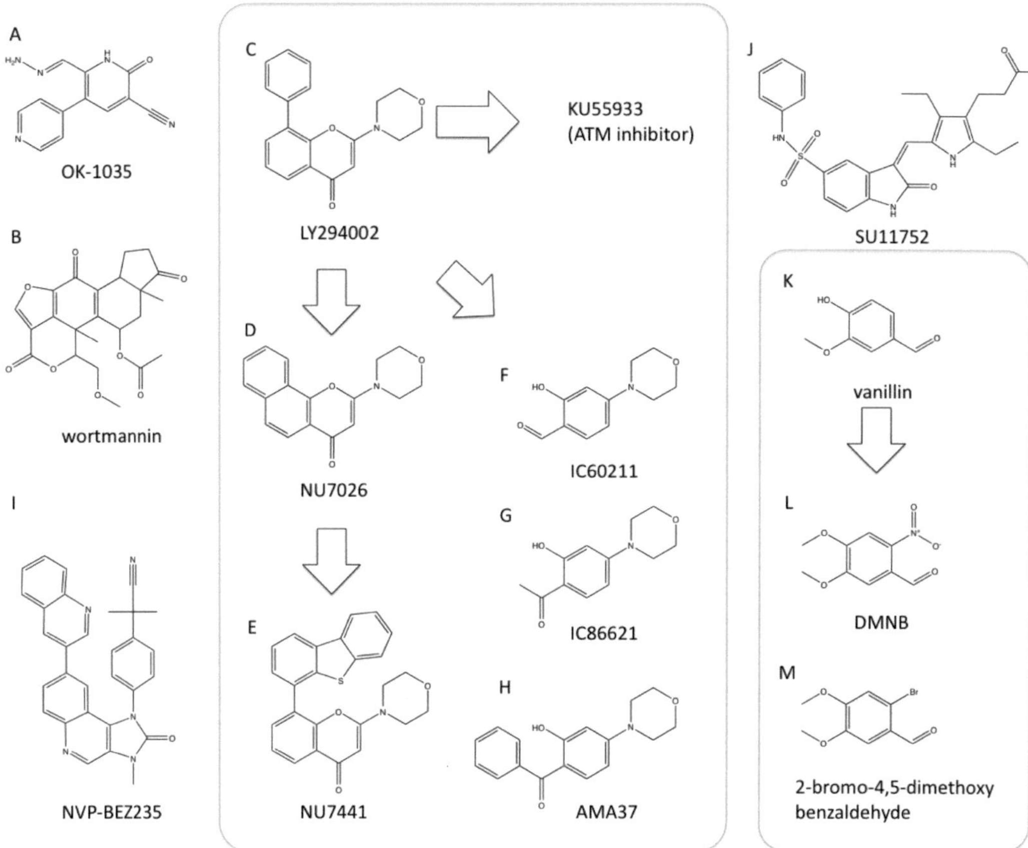

Figure 2. Strucuture of DNA-PK inhibitors.

Another PI3K inhibitor LY294002, 2-(4-morpholinyl)-8-phenyl-4H-1-benzopyran-4-one (Fig.2 C) was also shown to inhibit DNA-PK. In contrast to wortmannin, LY294002 competes with ATP (Izzard et al., 1999). IC_{50} of LY294002 is reported to be 6 μM (Izzard et al., 1999). LY294002 was used as a leading compound to explore more potent and selective inhibitors of DNA-PK. NU7026, 2-(morpholin-4-yl)-benzo[h]chromen4-one (Fig.2 D), was found as selective inhibitor of DNA-PK (Veuger et al., 2003). IC_{50} of NU7026 was 0.23 μM for DNA-PK, 13 μM for PI3K and >100 μM for ATM and ATR (Veuger et al., 2003). NU7026 sensitized cultured cells toward radiation in a manner dependent on DNA-PK (Veuger et al., 2003). Synthesis and screening of chromen-4-one library resulted in identification of NU7441 (Fig.2 E), 8-dibenzothiophen-4-yl-2-morpholin-4-yl-chromen-4-one (Leahy et al., 2004; Hardcastle et al., 2005). IC_{50} of NU7441 was 0.014 μM for DNA-PK, 5.0 μM for PI3K and >100 μM for ATM and ATR (Leahy et al., 2004). NU7441 sensitized cultured cells toward radiation and etoposide in a manner dependent on DNA-PK at 0.5 μM (Zhao et al., 2006). Screening of the derivatives of LY294002 also lead to the identification of other selective inhibitors of DNA-PK; IC60211 (Fig.2 F, 2-Hydroxy-4-morpholin-4-yl-benzaldehyde, IC_{50}: 0.43 μM), IC86621 (Fig.2 G, 1-(2-Hydroxy-4-morpholin-4-yl-phenyl) -ethanone, IC_{50}: 0.12 - 0.17 μM), AMA37 (Fig.2 H, 1-(2-Hydroxy- 4-morpholin-4-yl-phenyl)-phenyl-methanone, IC_{50}: 0.27 μM) (Kashishian et al., 2003; Knight et al., 2004).

It was recently reported that NVP-BEZ235 (Fig.2 I, 2-methyl-2-(4-(3-methyl-2-oxo-8-(quinolin-3-yl)-2,3-dihydro-1H -imidazo[4,5-c]quinolin-1-yl)phenyl)propanenitrile), which had been initially identified as a dual inhibitor for PI3K and mammalian target of rapamycin (mTOR) (Maira et al., 2008), inhibited DNA-PK, ATM and ATR and sensitizes cells to ionizing radiation (Toledo et al., 2011; Mukherjee et al., 2012). NVP-BEZ235 sensitized the cultured cells to radiation and inhibited DSB repair, as shown by persistence of 53BP1 foci, to a greater extent than NU7026 and KU55933 (Mukherjee et al., 2012). NVP-BEZ235 sensitized ATM-deficient cells, i.e., fibroblast from ataxia telangiectasia patient, and also DNA-PKcs-deficient human glioma cell M059J (Mukherjee et al., 2012), which could be due to dual inhibition of DNA-PK and ATM. Moreover, inhibition of *in cellulo* phosphorylation mediated by DNA-PK and ATM was achieved at low concentration, *i.e.*, 0.1 - 0.5 μM, while the similar extent of inhibition was achieved at 10 μM (Mukherjee et al., 2012).

Screening of a three-substituted indoline-2-one library lead to identification of SU11752 (Fig. 2 J) as selective DNA-PK inhibitor (IC_{50}: 0.13 μM) (Ismail, et al., 2004). Vanillin, 4-hydroxy-3-methoxybenzoaldehyde (Fig.2 K), was found to inhibit DNA-PK albeit at a relatively high concentration, i.e., IC_{50} 1500 μM (Durant and Karran, 2003). Screening of library of vanillin derivatives lead to finding of more potent inhibitors, 4,5-dimethoxy-2-nitrobenzaldehyde (DMNB, Fig.2 L) and 2-bromo-4,5- dimethoxybenzaldehyde (Fig.2 M), whose IC_{50} were 15 μM and 30 μM, respectively (Durant and Karran, 2003).

DNA-PK can be inhibited by homopolymeric phosphorythioate oligonucleotides, suramin and heparin (Hosoi et al., 2002). Inhibitory activities of homopolymeric phosphorothioate oligonucleotides on DNA-PK were independent of base composition but were dependent on length. IC_{50} decreased as length increased: 0.975 μM for 12 mer and 0.013 μM for 36 mer (Hosoi et al., 2002). IC_{50} of suramin and heparin were 1.7 μM and 0.27 μg ml^{-1}, respectively (Hosoi et al., 2002). Suramin sensitized cultured human cancer cell toward ionizing radiation but not to ultraviolet radiation (Hosoi et al., 2004). Furthermore, suramin did not affect the radiation sensitivity of *scid* cells, which are deficient in DNA-PK, indicating that radiosensitizating effects of suramin were mediated through inhibition of DNA-PK (Hosoi et al., 2004).

Single chain antibody variable fragment (scFv) is another approach to achieve specific inhibition of DNA-PK. ScFv was initially generated from existing murine monoclonal antibody 18-2, expressed in *E. coli* and introduced into the cell by microinjection (Li et al., 2003). The epitope of scFv 18-2 was mapped within 2001-2025 region, which is outside of kinase domain and thus ScFv 18-2 inhibited DNA-PK activity only modestly (Li et al., 2003). Nevertheless, microinjection of scFv 18-2 resulted in the inhibition of NHEJ, indicated by persistence of γ-H2AX foci and sensitized cells toward ionizing radiation (Li et al., 2003). However, the use of scFv as clinical radiosensitization might be difficult without a method to deliver it efficiently into the cell nucleus. ScFv 18-2 conjugated with nuclear localization signal was developed

(Xiong et al., 2009). In more recent study, scFv was conjugated with folate and introduced into the cell nucleus via folate receptor-mediated endocytosis and exhibited radiosensitization in terms of clonogenic survival (Xiong et al., 2012). Another study screened a phage-displayed library of humanized scFv and identified a new antibody against DNA-PKcs, anti-DPK3-scFv (Du et al., 2010). Transfection of cDNA of anti-DPK3-scFv into human cancer cells resulted in increased radiosensitivity with decreased repair capability (Du et al., 2010). It also sensitized transplanted tumor on mice toward radiation (Du et al., 2010).

2.2. ATM

ATM, ataxia-telangiectasia mutated, was identified as the gene responsible for the genetic disorder ataxia telangiectasia, showing similarity to PI3K (Savitsky et al., 1995). Subsequently similarity between ATM and DNA-PKcs, suggesting ATM might also be a protein kinase rather than a lipid kinase (Hartley et al., 1995). ATM was shown to be a protein kinase, which is activated by DNA damage and phosphorylates p53 at Ser15 (Banin et al., 1998; Canman et al., 1998).

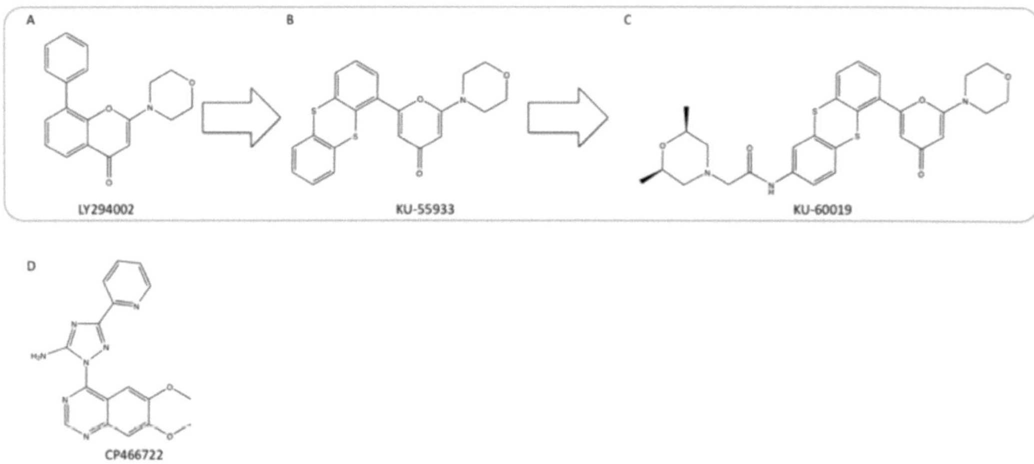

Figure 3. Structure of ATM inhibitors.

Like DNA-PK, ATM was also shown to be inhibited by wortmannin with IC_{50} of 0.15 μM (Sarkaria et al., 1998). It was also shown that administration of wortmannin to cultured cell phenocopies the defect of ataxia telangiectasia cell, *e.g.*, defective accumulation of p53 (Price and Youmell, 1996) and radioresistant DNA synthesis, which is thought to reflect defective G1/S- or S-phase checkpoint (Hosoi et al., 1998; Sarkaria et al., 1998). Caffeine, which was known to abrogate cell cycle checkpoint, was shown to inhibit ATM and ATR (Sarkaria et al., 1999; Hall-Jakson et al., 1999). IC_{50} for ATM and ATR was 200 μM and 1,100 μM, respectively (Sarkaria et al., 1999).

Selective inhibitors were found from the small molecule library of LY294002 derivatives (Hickson, et al., 2004; Hollick et al., 2007). Among them KU-55933, 2-morpholin-4-yl-6-

thialanthren-1-yl-pyran-4-one (Fig.3 B) showed inhibition of ATM with IC_{50} of 0.013 μM (Hickson, et al., 2004). IC_{50} values for other PI3K-related kinases were greater than 1.8 μM, which is approximately 200-fold higher than that for ATM (Hickson, et al., 2004). As in the case of DNA-PK inhibitors, morpholine group is important for inhibitory activity, as KU-58050, in which morpholine group was replaced by piperidine group was much less effective: IC_{50} was 300 μM (Hickson, et al., 2004). KU-55933 inhibited *in cellulo* phosphorylation of ATM substrates, *e.g.*, p53 at Ser15 and histone H2AX at Ser139, 10 μM induced by ionizing radiation, but not that induced by ultraviolet irradiation (Hickson, et al., 2004). Even at lower concentration, *i.e.*, 0.3 μM, the inhibition of p53 phosphorylation was significant, although there was trace amount of residual phosphorylation (Hickson, et al., 2004). It was also shown that KU-55933 sensitized cultured cell to ionizing radiation and to radiomimetic compounds, *e.g.*, etoposide and doxorubicin but did not alter the sensitivity of fibroblast from ataxia telangiectasia patients to ionizing radiation (Hickson, et al., 2004). Futhermore, KU-55933 was found to suppress HIV infection (Lau et al., 2005).

Modification of KU-55933 lead to identification of KU-60019 (Fig.3 C), 2-((2R, 6S)-2, 6-Dimethyl-morpholin-4-yl)-N-[5-(6-morpholin-4- yl-4-oxo-4H-pyran-2-yl)-9H-thioxanthen-2-yl]-acetamideas a more potent inhibitor of ATM (Golding et al., 2009). IC_{50} of KU-60019 for ATM was 0.0063 μM, whereas IC_{50} values for DNA-PKcs and ATR were 1.7 μM and >10 μM, respectively (Golding et al., 2009). KU-60019 mostly abolished ionizing radiation-induced phosphorylation of p53 at Ser15 and Chk2 at Thr68 at 1 to 3 μM, whereas > 10 μM concentration of KU-55933 was required to obtain similar extent of inhibition (Golding et al., 2009). KU-60019 at 1 μM showed similar extent of radiosensitization to KU-55933 at 10 μM (Golding et al., 2009).

Independent screening of chemical library lead to identification of CP466722, 2-(6,7-dimethoxyquinazolin-4-yl)-5- (pyridin-2-yl)-2H-1,2,4-triazole-3-amine, as a novel inhibitor of ATM (Rainey, et al., 2008). CPP466722 inhibited in cellolo phoshorylation of ATM at Ser1981, SMC1 at Ser957 and Chk2 at Thr68 but not affected the phosphorylation events, which are thought to be mediated through other PI3K-related kinases (Rainey, et al., 2008). CPP466722 sensitized cultured cells to radiation to a similar extent to KU-55933 (Rainey, et al., 2008).

CGK733 was reported to be a dual inhibitor of ATM and ATR, but the report was retracted thereafter because of fabrication. Even after the retraction, CGK733 was marketed as an inhibitor of ATM and ATR and several studies used CGK733 to show the involvement of ATM and/or ATR in response to DNA damage caused by a variety of agents. On the other hand, however, there is a report that this compound did not affect ATM and ATR kinase as shown, respectively, by ionizing radiation-induced phosphorylation of ATM at Ser1981 and Chk2 at Thr 68 and by ultraviolet radiation-induced phosphorylation of Chk1 at Ser317 (Choi et al., 2011, and references therein).

2.3. ATR

ATR was initially identified as a molecule structurally related to human ATM and yeast Rad3 (Cimprich et al, 1996; Keegan et al., 1996). ATR was then shown to be a protein kinase, which is capable of phosphorylating itself and p53 at Ser15 (Canman et al., 1998). ATR is thought to be a sensor of single-stranded DNA (ssDNA), binding to RPA (Replication Protein A) via ATRIP (ATR-interacting protein) (Zou and Elledge, 2003).

Despite of its structural similarity to DNA-PKcs, ATM and PI3K, ATR appeared refractory to wortmannin inhibition: IC_{50} of wortmannin for ATR was 1.8 μM, which was 10- to 100-fold higher than that for DNA-PKcs and ATM (Sarkaria et al., 1998). Selective inhibitors of ATR emerged recently.

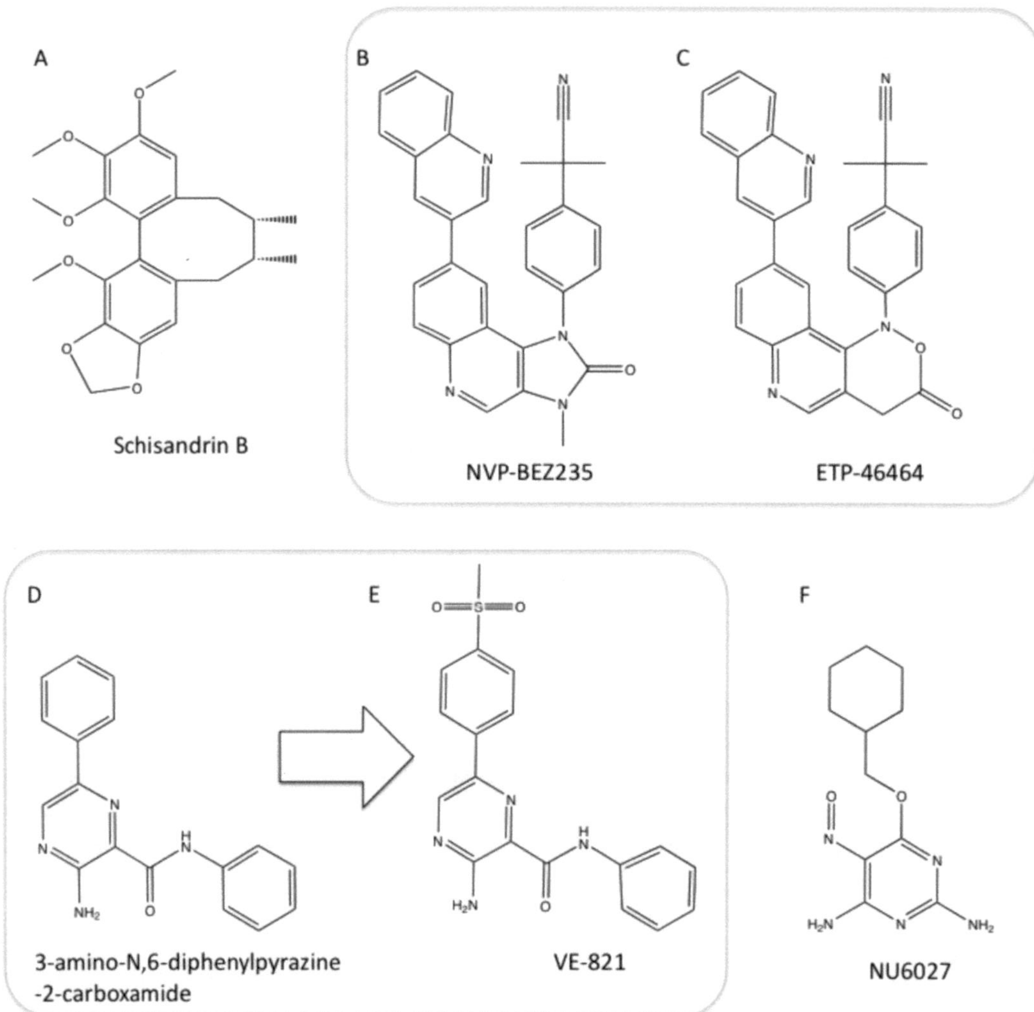

Figure 4. Structure of ATR inhibitors

Schisandrin B is an active ingredient of *Fructus schisandrae*, which has been used in traditional Chinese medicine to treat hepatitis and myocardial disorders (Fig.4 A). Schisandrin B was found to inhibit ATR (Nishida et al., 2009). IC_{50} of Schisandrin for ATR and ATM were, respectively, 7.25 μM and 1,700 μM and DNA-PK, PI3K and mTOR were not inhibited up to ~100 μM (Nishida et al., 2009). Schisandrin B sensitized cultured human cells to ultraviolet radiation and ionizing radiation at concentrations 1 - 30 μM (Nishida et al., 2009). Sensitization was not observed in cells from Seckel patient, who harbor mutation in ATR gene (Nishida et al., 2009), showing that the sensitizing effect is mediated through ATR.

Library of 623 compounds, which had exhibited some inhibitory effects on PI3K, was screened for their effects on *in cellulo* phosphorylaiton of H2AX stimulated by ATR-activating domain of TopBP1 (Toledo et al., 2011). This screening identified NVP-BEZ235 (Fig.4 B) and ETP-46464 (Fig.4 C) (Toledo et al., 2011). Whereas NVP-BEZ235 also inhibited DNA-PK and ATM (see above), ETP-464 did not affect DNA-PK and ATM (Toledo et al., 2011). These compounds mostly inhibited the phosphorylation *in cellulo* of H2AX and other ATR substrates, *e.g.*, Chk1, even at 0.1 - 0.5 μM (Toledo et al., 2011).

High throughput screening of ATR by *in vitro* kinase assay identified 3-amino-N,6-diphenylpyrazine-2-carboxamide (Charrier et al., 2011). IC_{50} of this compounds for ATR was 0.62 μM, whereas that for ATM and DNA-PK was > 8 μM (Charrier et al., 2011). Then the derivatives of this compound were synthesized and subjected to test for ATR inhibition. VE-821, 3-amino-6-(4-(methylsulfonyl)phenyl)-N-phenylpyrazine-2-carboxamide, was found as most potent and selective inhibitor of ATR (Charrier et al., 2011). IC_{50} of VE-821 for ATR was 0.026 μM, whereas that for ATM and DNA-PK was > 8 μM and 4.4 μM, respectively (Charrier et al., 2011).

NU6027, 2,6-diamino-4-cyclohexyl-methyloxy-5-nitroso-pyrimidine, was initially developed as an inhibitor of cyclin- dependent kinases (CDKs) (Arris et al, 2000). NU6027 was recently found, however, to inhibit ATR more potently than CDK2 (Peasland et al., 2011). NU6027 inhibited *in cellulo* phosphorylation of Chk1 at Ser345 with IC_{50} of 6.7 μM, whereas autophosphorylation of DNA-PKcs at Ser2056 and ATM at Ser1981 were not affected at 10 μM (Peasland et al., 2011). NU6027 sensitized cultured cells to hydroxyurea and cisplatin, but this effect was not observed in ATR-knocked down cells, showing that sensitization was mediated through ATR (Peasland et al., 2011).

It might be added that p53-deficient cells, than p53-proficient cells, exhibited greater extent of sensitization toward ionizing radiation and other DNA damaging agents by ATR inhibitors NVP-BEZ235, ETP-46464 (Toledo et al., 2011), VE-821 (Reaper et al., 2011) and NU6027 (Peasland et al., 2011). This could be due to simultaneous inactivation of two checkpoint pathways mediated through ATM and ATR, respectively, the former of which involves p53. As most of cancer cells lose p53 function, inhibition of ATR might be a promising approach to achieve selective killing of cancer cells, minimizing the effects to surrounding normal cells.

3. Other DSB repair enzymes as targets for radiosensitizer

3.1. MRN complex

Mirin, Z-5-(4-hydroxybenzylidene)-2-imino-1,3-thiazolidin-4-one (Fig.5), was identified in a screen for smalll molecules inhibiting MRN-ATM pathway (Dupre et al., 2009). Restriction enzyme-digested plasmid was added to cell-free extract prepared from *Xenopus laevis* egg in 96-well format and the phosphorylation of H2AX-mimicking peptide was quantified. Approximately 10,000 compounds, which had exhibited inhibition of p53 activity or inteference with mitosis and spindle dynamics, were subjected to screen. Mirin inhibited H2AX phosphorylation in *Xenopus laevis* egg cell free extract with an IC_{50} of 66 μM and also autophosphorylation of ATM at Ser1981 in human cells within 25 - 100 μM range (Dupre et al., 2009). Mirin inhibited nuclease activity of Mre11, but did not affect DNA binding or DNA tethering activity of MRN complex (Dupre et al., 2009). Mirin also abrogated G2/M checkpoint, reduced homologous recombination and showed radiosensitizing effects in cultured human cells within 25 - 100 μM range (Dupre et al., 2009).

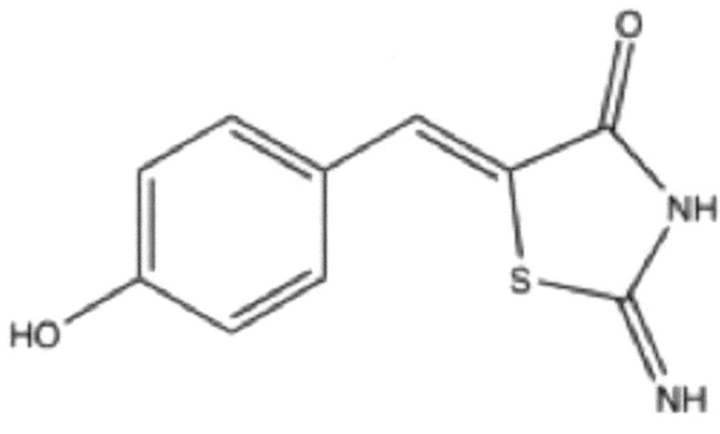

Figure 5. Structure of Mirin.

3.2. DNA ligase IV

Inhibitors of DNA ligases were searched in a database of 1.5 million commercially available low molecular weight chemicals by computer-aided drug design approach based on crystal structure of DNA ligase I (Chen et al., 2008). In this approach, L82 ((E)-2-((2-(2-((3,5-dibromo-4-methylphenyl)amino)ethyl)hydrazono)methyl)-4-nitrophenol, Fig.6 A), inhibiting DNA ligase I, L67 ((E)-4-chloro-5-(2-(4-hydroxy-3-nitrobenzylidene)hydrazinyl)pyridazin-3(2H)-one, Fig.6 B), inhibiting DNA ligases I and III, and L189 ((E)-6-amino-5-(benzylideneamino)-2-mercaptopyrimidin-4-ol, Fig.6 C), inhibiting DNA ligases I, III and IV, were identified. None of them inhibited the activity of T4 ligase (Chen et al., 2008). Kinetic alalysis indicated that, whereas L82 is non-competitive inhibitor, L67 and L189 competes with DNA substrate (Chen et al., 2008). L67 sensitized cultured human cancer cells to methylmethansulfonate at 3 μM (Chen et al., 2008). Similarly, L189 sensitized cultured human cancer cells to ionizing radiation at 20 μM (Chen et al., 2008). It might be noted that the sensitizing effects of L67 and L189 were not observed in non-cancer cells, suggesting is selective effects on cancer cells (Chen et al., 2008). These compounds can be a leading compounds for the development of more potent and/ or more selective inhibitors of DNA ligases.

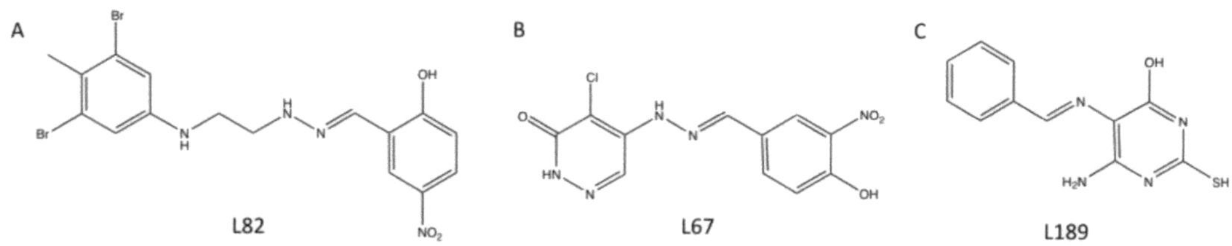

Figure 6. Strucutre of DNA ligase inhibitors.

3.3. DPYD as a new target

Gimeracil, 5-chloro-2,4-dihydroxypyridine (Fig.7), is an inhibitor of dihydropyrimidine dehydrogenease (DPYD) and used as a component of oral anti-cancer medicine S-1, in order to suppress degradation of 5-fluorouracil. The results of clinical trial of concurrent chemoradiotherapy using S-1 suggested possible radiosensitizing effect of S-1. Gimeracil increased radiosensitivity of cultured human cancer cells of various origin within 200 – 5,000 μM, being maximal within 1,000 – 5,000 μM range (Takagi et al., 2010). Cell lines deficient for DNA-PKcs or Ku86 were sensitized by gimeracil to radiation even to a greater extent than respective control cells (Takagi et al., 2010). On the other hand, radiosensitiztion was not observed in cell lines deficient for XRCC3, NBS1 or FANCD2 (Takagi et al., 2010). These observations collectively suggested that gimeracil exert radiosensitizing effects through inhibition of HR-mediated DSB repair. Gimeracil reduced the frequency of homologous recombination of chromosomal substrate including the restriction site of I-SceI by approximately 15% (Takagi et al., 2010). Gimeracil reduced the formation of ionizing radiation-induced foci of Rad51 and RPA but increased that of Nbs1, Mre11, Rad50 and FancD2 (Sakata et al., 2011). This observation suggested that gimeracil might have inhibited the step after strand resection by Mre11-Rad50-Nbs1 complex but before the loading of RPA and Rad51 onto single-stranded DNA. Although the role of DPYD in HR has not been described, treatment with siRNA for DPYD sensitized cells to ionizing radiation to a similar extent to gimeracil and also diminished the radiosensitization by gimeracil (Sakata et al., 2011). These results collectively indicate that gimeracil exerts radiosensitizing effects through inhibition of DPYD, which might have a novel role in HR.

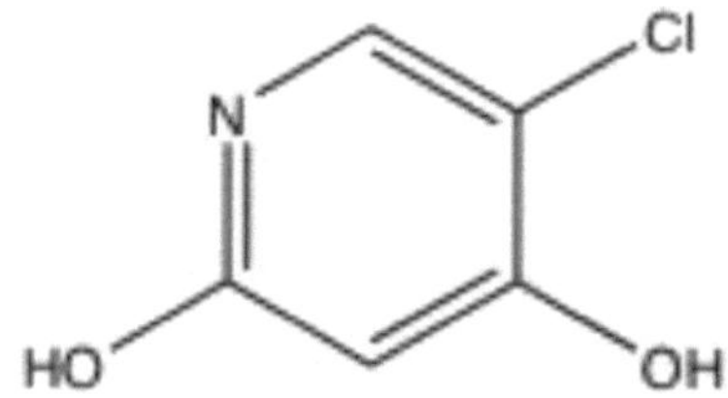

Figure 7. Structure of gimeracil.

4. Radiosensitization by hyperthermia

Hyperthermia, heating parts of body at 40 - 45 °C, has been used to treat cancer mostly combined with ionizing radiation. Hyperthemia is known to sensitize cells to ionizing radiation, inhibiting the repair of DNA damages including DSBs, but the molecular mechanism of radiosensitization by hyperthermia has remaind to be clarified.

Effects of hyperthermia on DNA polymerases α and β have been studied for a long time. These studies suggested that DNA polymerase β was sensitive to hyperthermia and its inactivation was correlated to radiosensitization as well as to cell killing (Spiro et al., 1982). Later it was reported that DNA polymerase β knocked out cells or overexpressed cells exhibited radiosensitization by hyperthermia indifferent from control cells (Raaphorst et al., 2004). Elucidation of DSB repair mechanisms through NHEJ and HR provided clues to the mechanisms of radiosensitization by hyperthermia.

Among essential factors in NHEJ, Ku is shown to be affected by hypethermia. Purified DNA-PK lost its activity upon incubation at 44°C for 5 - 30 min (Matsumoto et al., 1997). When DNA-PKcs and Ku were heated separately, heating of Ku, but not DNA-PKcs, lead to decrease in DNA-PK activity, suggesting that Ku, rather than DNA-PKcs, is heat sensitive component (Matsumoto et al., 1997). Inactivation of DNA-PK activity by hyperthermia was observed also *in cellulo, i.e.,* when culture cells were heated at 44 – 47°C (Burgman et al., 1997; Ihara et al., 1999; Umeda et al., 2003). It might be noted, however, that the extent of the loss of DNA-PK was greatly different between mouse, hamster and human cell, being greatest in mouse and least in human (Umeda et al. 2003). In murin cells, significant loss of DNA-PK activity was observed at lower tempertures, *i.e.,* 41°C or 42°C (our unpublished observations). DNA-PK activity could be restored by mixing the lysate of heated cells with the lysate of DNA-PKcs-deficient cells, but not with Ku86-deficient cells, indicating that *in cellulo* inactivation of DNA-PK by hyperthermia might be also due to the property of Ku rather than DNA-PKcs (Ihara et al., 1999). Moreover, Ku was identified as constitutive heat shock element-binding factor, CHBF, whose activity was lost by hyperthermia, allowing the binding of HSF1 (Kim et al., 1995). DNA binding activity of Ku correlated with extent of radiosensitization by hyperthermia (Burgman et al., 1997). Reduced solubility of Ku in aquaous buffer after hyperthermia was also reported, which might reflect aggregation (Beck and Dynlacht, 2001). However, the hypothesis that radiosensitization by hyperthermia is due to inactivation of Ku or DNA-PK has been challenged by genetic studies, showing that cells deficient for Ku or DNA-PKcs could be radiosensitized by hyperthermia to a similar extent or even to a greater extent than control cells (Kampinga et al., 1993; Raaphorst et al., 1993; Woudstra, et al, 1999, Raaphorst et al., 2004), although there are studies, in contrast, showing no or reduced radiosensitization in Ku- or DNA-PKcs-deficient cells (Iliakis and Seaner, 1990; O'Hara et al., 1995). Moreover, chicken lymphocyte DT40 derivative lacking Ku70 and Rad54, therefore, deficient in both of NHEJ and HR, still showed radiosensitization by hyperthermia (Raaphorst et al., 2004; Yin et al., 2004).

There is also accumulating studies on the effects of hyperthermia on MRN complex. It was initially found that Mre11, Rad50 and Nbs1 exported from nucleus to cytoplasm upon hyperthemia at 42.5°C or 45.5°C (Zhu et al., 2001; Seno and Dynlacht, 2004). This nuclear export of MRN complex increased when cells were irradiated prior to hyperthermia (Zhu et al., 2001; Seno and Dynlacht, 2004). Similar phonomenon was observed in mild hyperthermia at 41.1°C (Xu et al., 2002). However, in a recent study, inhibition of nuclear export of MRN complex by leptomycin B did not diminish radiosensitization by hyperthermia at 45.5°C for 10 min (Dynlacht et al., 2011). It was also shown, nevertheless, that ATLD cells, which have mutated in Mre11, did not show radiosensitization by hyperthermia at 41.5°C for 2 hrs or at 45.5°C for 10 min (Dynlacht et al., 2011). On the other hand, radiosensitization by hyperthermia was observed in NBS cells and Rad50-knocked down cells (Dynlacht et al., 2011). Exonuclease activity of Mre11 was decreased to ~10% by 42.5°C treatment for 15 min (Dynlacht et al., 2011). These results collectively indicate Mre11 as target for radiosensitization by hyperthermia.

Hyperthermia is shown to affect BRCA1 and BRCA2. Heating cultured human cancer cells at 42°C for 1 - 2 hrs or more decreased the amount of BRCA1 (Ma et al., 2003). It might be caused by protein degradation, but various inhibitors of proteases, so far as tested, failed to suppress the decrease of BRCA1 (Ma et al., 2003). Alternatively, it might be caused by protein aggregation and reduced solubility in aqueous buffers. It was also shown that BRCA1 deficient cells were sensitive to hyperthermia (Ma et al., 2003). Recent study reported the degradation of BRCA2 induced by mild hyperthermia at 41°C to 42.5°C (Krawczyk et al., 2011). Rad54-deficient ES cells and cells treated with XRCC3 siRNA were not radiosensitized by mild hyperthermia (Krawczyk et al., 2011). Furthermore, mild hyperthermia showed synthetic lethality with PARP-1 inhibitor oraparib, like BRCA2 deficient cancer cells (Krawczyk et al., 2011). These data collectively indicated BRCA2 as a major target of mild hyperthermia.

Obviously, hyperthermia inactivates many enzymes and induces aggregation of many proteins. In this regard, hyperthermia is not specific on certain enzyme, unlike inhibitors described above. However, susceptiblity to inactivation by hyperthermia might be greatly different among proteins. The extent of radiosensitization by hyperthermia can be greatly infuluenced by many factors, *e.g.*, cell type, genetic background, physiological conditions, heating temperature, duration of heating, sequence of heating and radiation and the interval between them. Further studies would be required to examine the effects of hyperthermia on various repair enzymes and and its relationship to radiosentizing effects under various conditions.

5. Concluding remarks and future perspectives

Because of great advances in our understanding of the moleuclar mechanisms of DSB repair in past two decades, extensive studies have been done to achieve radiosensitization by modification of DSB repair molecules. Especially, a number of inhibitors have been developed for DNA-PK, ATM and ATR protein kinases. We saw here that preceeding studies on DNA-PK and on PI3K greatly facilitated the studies on ATM and ATR. It might be underscored that LY294002, preexisting inhibitor of PI3K, served as a leading compound and enabled the finding of potent and specific inhibitors like NU7441 and KU-55933.

Studies toward the clinical application of these compounds are underway. Preclinical studies of pharmacokinetics and metabolism in mice were conducted for NU7026 and NU7441. In the case of NU7026, the radiosensitizing effect on cultured cancer cell was marginal upon the treatment at 10 μM for 2 hrs and could be increased by extending the treatment time up to 24 hrs (Nutley et al., 2005). On the other hand, however, NU7026 underwent rapid plasma clearance in mice, presumably because of oxidation and ring opening of morpholino group (Nutley et al., 2005). It was estimated that NU7026 should be administered four times per day at 100 mg/kg intraperitoneally in order to obtain radiosensitization (Nutley et al., 2005). In the case of NU7441, the radiosensitizating effect on cultured cancer cell could be obtained by treatment at 1 μM for 1 hr (Zhao et al., 2006). The concentration of NU7441 required for radiosensitization could be maintained within tumor tissues for more than 4 hrs at nontoxic dose (Zhao et al., 2006). The administration of etoposide and NU7441 to mice bearing human tumor xenografts synergistically delayed tumor growth, indicating the chemosensitizing effect of NU7441 *in vivo* (Zhao et al., 2006). Studies are still going on to obtain compounds with better characteristics, *e.g.*, higher aquaous solubility (Cano et al., 2010).

Search for inhibitors of enzymes other than protein kinases has been difficult due to the absence of assay system suitable for highthroughput screening. However, inhibitors of other enzymes, *i.e.*, Mre11 nuclease and DNA ligase IV have been developed, although few at present. Now these compuonds are obtained, more potent and specific inhibitors can be obtained by molecular evolution as in the case of DNA-PK, ATM and ATR protein kinases. Additionally, search for other inhibitors will be greatly facilitated by an aid of computer-based structural prediction and drug designing.

In addition to use of each chemicals alone, use of two or more chemicals together to inhibit two pathways of DSB repair or one of them with other repair mechanisms, which is called synthetic lethality approach, will be promising. Successful example is shown in the treatment of cancers arisen in the carriers of BRCA2 mutation with PARP-1 inhibitors. When PARP-1, which is essential for single-strand break (SSB) repair, is inactivated, SSB is converted to DSB, which requires BRCA2 to be repaired. As BRCA2 mutation is heterozygotic, normal cells retain BRCA2 function. On the other hand cancer cells have lost BRCA2 function and, therefore, shows extreme sensitivity to increased sensitivity to converted DSBs. This is instructive also to find a means to discriminate cancer cells and normal cells. As described in the previous section, although hyperthemia is not an approach to target a certain molecule specifically, it did show synthetic lethal effects with PARP-1 inhibitor. These examples underscores the importance of the choice of agents based on the thorough consideration of biological characteristics and genetic background of each cancer and patient. In addition to continuing persuit for the new radiosensitizing agents, extensive studies would be necessary regarding combinatorial approach and personalized medicine.

Note

We apologize for not citing many important literatures because of space limitation.

Acknowledgements

Our study was supported in part by Grant-in-Aid for Scientific Research from the Ministry of Education, Culture, Sport, Science and Technology of Japan to YM. MKS is supported by Takeda Science Foundation, Japan Society for Promotion of Sciences and Tokyo Biochemistry Research Foundation.

Author details

Yoshihisa Matsumoto, Shoji Imamichi, Mikoto Fukuchi, Sicheng Liu, Wanotayan Rujira, Shingo Kuniyoshi, Kazuki Yoshida, Yasuhiro Mae and Mukesh Kumar Sharma

Research Laboratory for Nuclear Reactors, Tokyo Institute of Technology, Tokyo, Japan

References

[1] Arris, C.E., Boyle, F.T., Calvert, A.H., Curtin, N.J., Endicott, J.A., Garman, E.F.,Gibson, A.E., Golding, B.T., Grant, S., Griffin, R.J., Jewsbury, P., Johnson, L.N., Lawrie, A.M., Newell, D.R., Noble, M.E., Sausville, E.A., Schultz, R. & Yu, W. (2000) Identification of novel purine and pyrimidine cyclin-dependent kinase inhibitors with distinct molecular interactions and tumor cell growth inhibition profiles. *J. Med. Chem.*, 43: 2797-2804.

[2] Banin, S., Moyal, L., Shieh, S.-Y. Taya, Y., Anderson, C. W., Chessa, L., Smorodinsky, N. I., Prives, C., Reiss, Y., Shiloh, Y., & Ziv, Y. (1998) Enhanced phosphorylation of p53 by ATM in response to DNA damage. *Science*, 281:1674-1677.

[3] Beck, B.D. & Dynlacht, J.R. (2001) Heat-induced aggregation of XRCC5 (Ku80) in nontolerant and thermotolerant cells. *Radiat. Res.*, 156: 767-774.

[4] Blunt, T.; Finnie,N.; Taccioli, G.; Smith, G.; Demengeot, J.; Gottlieb, T.; Mizuta, R.; Varghese, A.; Alt, F.; Jeggo, P. & Jackson, S.P. (1995) Defective DNA-dependent protein

kinase activity is linked to V(D)J recombination and DNA repair defects associated with the murine scid mutation. *Cell,* 80: 813-823.

[5] Burgman, P., Ouyang, H., Peterson, S., Chen, D.J. & Li, G.C. (1997) Heat inactivation of Ku autoantigen: possible role in hyperthermic radiosensitization. *Cancer Res.,* 57: 2847-2850.

[6] Canman, C. E., Lim, D.-S., Cimprich, K. A., Taya, Y., Tamai, K., Sakaguchi, K., Appella, E., Kastan, M. & Siliciano, J. D. (1998) Activation of the ATM kinase by ionizing radiation and phosphorylation of p53. *Science,* 281: 1677-1679.

[7] Cano, C., Barbeau, O.R., Bailey, C., Cockcroft, X.-L., Curtin, N.J., Guggan, H., Frigerio, M., Golding, B.T., Hardcastle, I.R., Hummersone, M.G., Knights, C., Menear, K.A., Newell, D.R., Richardson, C.J., Smith, G.C.M., Spittle, B. & Griffin, R.J. (2010) DNA-dependent protein kinase (DNA-PK) inhibitors. Synthesis and biological activity of quinolin-4-one and pyridopyrimidin-4-one surrogates for the chromen-4-one chemotype. *J. Med. Chem.,* 53: 8498-8507.

[8] Carter, T., Vancurova, I., Sun, I., Lou, W. & DeLeon, S. (1990) A DNA-activated protein kinase from HeLa cell nuclei. *Mol. Cell. Biol.,* 10: 6460-6471.

[9] Charrier, J.D., Durrant, S.J., Golec, J.M.C., Kay, D.P., Knegtel, R.M.A., MacCormick, S., Mortimore, M., O'Donnell, M.E., Pinder, J.L., Reaper, P.M., Rutherford, A.P., Wang, P.S.H., Young, S.C. & Pollard, J.R. (2011) Discovery of potent and selective inhibitors of ataxia telangiectasia mutated and Rad3 related (ATR) protein kinase as potential anticancer agents. *J. Med. Chem.,* 54: 2320-2330.

[10] Chen, X., Zhong, S., Zhu, X., Dziegielewska, B., Ellenberger, T., Wilson, G.M., MacKerell, A.D. & Tomkinson, A.E. (2008) Rational design of human DNA ligase inhibitors that target cellular DNA replication and repair. *Cancer Res.,* 68: 3169-3177.

[11] Chernikova, S.B., Wells, R.L. & Elkind, M.M. (1999) Wortmannin sensitizes mammalian cells to radiation by inhibiting the DNA-dependent protein kinase-mediated rejoining of double-strand breaks. *Radiat. Res.,* 151: 159-166.

[12] Choi, S., Toledo, L.I., Fernandez-Capetillo, O. & Bakkenist, C.J. (2011) CGK733 does not inhibit ATM or ATR kinase activity in H460 human lung cancer cells. *DNA Repair,* 10: 1000-1001.

[13] Cimprich, K.A., Shin, T.B., Keith, C.T. & Shreiber, S.L. (1996) cDNA cloning and gene mapping of a candidate human cell cycle checkpoint protein. *Proc. Natl. Acad. Sci. USA,* 93: 2850-2855.

[14] Dvir, A., Peterson, S.R., Knuth, M.W., Lu, H. & Dynan, W.S. (1992) Ku autoantigen is the regulatory component of a template-associated protein kinase that phosphorylates RNA polymerase II. *Proc. Natl. Acad. Sci. USA,* 89: 11920 -11924

[15] Dvir, A., Stein, L.Y., Calore, B.L. & Dynan,W.S. (1993) Purification and characterization of a template-associated protein kinase that phosphorylates RNA polymerase II. *J. Biol. Chem.,* 268: 10440-10447.

[16] Du, L., Zhou, L.-J., Pan, X.-J., Wang, Y.-X., Xu, Q.-Z., Yang, Z.-H., Wang, Y., Liu, X.-D., Zhu, M.-X. & Zhou, P.-K. (2010) Radiosensitization and growth inhibition of cancer cells mediated by an scFv antibody gene against DNA-Pkcs in vitro and in vivo. *Radiat. Oncol.*, 5: 70.

[17] Dupre, A., Boyer-Chatenet, Sattler, R.M., Modi, A.P., Lee, J.-H., Nicolette, M.L., Kopelovih, L., Jasin, M., Baer, R., Paull, T.T. & Gautier, J. (2009) A forward chemical genetic screen reveals an inhibitor of the Mre11-Rad50-Nbs1 complex. *Nat. Chem. Biol.*, 4: 119-125. (Corringendum Vol. 5, pp.1)

[18] Durant, S. & Karran, P. (2003) Vanillins – a novel family of DNA-PK inhibitors. *Nucleic Acids Res.*, 31: 5501-5512.

[19] Dynlacht, J.R., Batuello, C.N., Lopez, J.T., Kim, K.K. & Turchi, J.J. (2011) Identification of Mre11 as a target for heat radiosensitization. *Radiat. Res.*, 176: 323-332.

[20] Golding, S.E., Rosenberg, E., Valerie, N., Hussaini, I., Frigerio, M., Cockcroft, X.F., Chong, W.Y., Hummersone, M., Rigoreau, L., Menear, K.A., O'Connor, M., Povirk, L., van Meter, T. & Valerie, K. (2009) Improved ATM kinase inhibitor KU-60019 radiosensitizes glioma cells, compromises insulin, AKT and ERK prosurvival signaling, and inhibits migration and invasion. *Mol. Cancer Ther.*, 8: 2894-2902.

[21] Gottlieb, T.M. & Jackson,S.P. (1993) The DNA-dependent protein kinase: requirement for DNA ends and association with Ku antigen. *Cell*, 72:.131-142.

[22] Griffin, R.J., Fontana, G., Golding, B.T., Guiard, S., Hardcastle, I.R., Leahy, J.J.J., Martin, N., Richardson, C., Rigoreau, L., Stockley, M. & Smith, G.C.M. (2005) Selective benzopyranone and pyramido[2,1-a]isoquinolin-4-one inhibitors of DNA-dependent protein kinase: synthesis, structure-activity studies, and radiosensitization of a human tumor cell line in vitro. *J. Med. Chem.*, 48: 569-585.

[23] Hall-Jackson, C.A., Cross, D.A.E., Morrice, N. & Smythe, C. (1999) ATR is a caffeine-sensitive, DNA-activated protein kinase with a substrate specificity distinct from DNA-PK. *Oncogene*, 18: 6707-6713.

[24] Hartley, K.; Gell, D.; Smith, C.; Zhang, H.; Divecha, N.; Connelly, M.; Admon, A.; Lees-Miller, S.; Anderson, C. & Jackson, S. (1995) DNA-dependent protein kinase catalytic subunit: a relative of phosphatidylinositol 3-kinase and the ataxia telangiectasia gene product. *Cell*, 82: 849-856.

[25] Hardcastle, I.R., Cockcroft, X., Curtin, N.J., El-Murr, M. D., Leahy, J.J.J., Stockley, M., Golding, B.T., Rigoreau, L., Richardson, C., Smith, G.C.M. & Griffin, R.J. (2005) Discovery of potent chromen-4-one inhibitors of the DNA-dependent protein kinase (DNA-PK) using a small-molecule library approach. *J. Med. Chem.*, 48: 7829-7846.

[26] Hashimoto, M., Rao, S., Tokuno, O., Yamamoto, K., Takata, M., Takeda, S. & Utsumi, H. (2003) DNA-PK: the major target for wortmannin-mediated radiosensitization by the inhibition of DSB repair via NHEJ pathway. *J. Radiat. Res.*, 44: 151-159.

[27] Hickson, I., Zhao, Y., Richardoson, C.J., Green, S.J., Martin, N.M.B., Orr, A.I., Reaper, P.M., Jackson, S.P., Curtin, N.J. & Smith, G.C.M. (2004) Identification and characterization of a novel and specific inhibitor of the ataxia-telangiectasia mutated kinase ATM. *Cancer Res.*, 64: 9152-9159.

[28] Hollick, J.J., Rigoreau, L.J.M., Cano-Soumillac, C., Cockcroft, X., Curtin, N.J., Frigerio, M., Golding, B.T., Guiard, S., Hardcastle, I.R., Hickson, I., Hummersone, M.G., Menear, K.A., Martin, N.M.B., Matthews, I., Newell, D.R., Ord, R., Richardson, C.J., Smith, G.C.M. & Griffin, R.J. (2007) Pyranone, thiopyranone, and pyridone inhibitors of phosphatidylinositol 3-kinase related kinases. Structure-activity relationships for DNA-dependent protein kinase inhibition, and identification of the first potent and selective inhibitor of the ataxia telangiectasia mutated kinase. *J. Med. Chem.*, 50: 1958-1972.

[29] Hosoi, Y., Matsumoto, Y., Enomoto, A., Morita, A., Green, J., Nakagawa, K., Naruse, K. & Suzuki, N. Suramin sensitizes cells to ionizing radiation by inactivating DNA-dependent protein kinase. *Radiat. Res.* 162: 308-314 (2004).

[30] Hosoi, Y., Matsumoto, Y., Tomita, M., Enomoto, A., Morita, A., Sakai, K. Umeda, N., Zhao, H.-J., Nakagawa, K., Ono, T. & Suzuki, N. (2002) Phosphorothioate oligonucleotides, suramin and heparin inhibit DNA-dependent protein kinase activity. *Brit. J. Cancer*, 86: 1143-1149.

[31] Hosoi, Y., Miyachi, H., Matsumoto, Y., Ikehata, H., Komura, J., Ishii, K., Zhao, H.J., Yoshida, M., Takai, Y., Yamada, S., Suzuki, N. & Ono, T. (1998) A phosphatidylinositol 3-kinase inhibitor wortmannin induces radioresistant DNA synthesis and sensitizes cells to bleomycin and ionizing radiation. *Int. J. Cancer*, 78: 642-647.

[32] Ihara, M., Suwa, A., Komatsu, K., Shimasaki, T., Okaichi, K., Hendrickson, E.A. & Okumura, Y. (1999) Heat sensitivity of double-stranded DNA-dependent protein kinase (DNA-PK) activity. *Int. J. Radiat. Biol.*, 75: 253-258.

[33] Iliakis, G. & Seaner, R. (1990) A DNA double-strand break repair-deficient mutant of CHO cells shows reduced radiosensitization after exposure to hyperthermic temperatures in the plateau phase of growth. *Int. J. Hyperthermia*, 6: 801-812.

[34] Ismail, I.H., Marternsson, S., Moshinsky, D., Rice, A., Tang, C., Howlett, A., McMahon, G. & Hammarste, O. (2004) SU11752 inhibits the DNA-dependent protein kinase and DNA double-strand break repair resulting in ionizing radiation sensitization. *Oncogene*, 23: 873-882.

[35] Izzard, R.A., Jackson, S.P. & Smith, G.C.M. (1999) Competitive and noncompetitive inhibition of the DNA-dependent protein kinase. *Cancer Res.*, 59: 2581-2586.

[36] Kamping, H.H., Kanon, B., Konings, A.W.T., Stackhouse, M.A. & Bedford, J.S. (1993) Thermal radiosensitization in heat- and radiation-sensitive mutants of CHO cells. *Int. J. Radiat. Biol.*, 64: 225-230.

[37] Kashishian, A., Douangpanya, H., Clark, D., Schlachter, S.T., Eary, C.T., Schiro, J.G., Huang, H., Burgess, L.E., Kesicki, E.A. & Halbrook, J. (2003) DNA-dependent protein kinase inhibitors as drug candidates for the treatment of cancer. *Mol.Cancer Ther.*, 2: 1257-1264.

[38] Keegan, K.S., Holzman, D.A., Plug, A.W., Christenson, E.R., Brainerd, E.E., Flaggs, G., Bentley, N.J., Taylor, E.M., Meyn, M.S., Moss, S.B., Carr, A.M., Ashley, T. & Hoekstra, M.F. (1996) The Atr and Atm protein kinases associate with different sites along meiotically paring chromosomes. *Genes Dev.*, 10: 2423-2437.

[39] Kim, D., Ouyang, H., Yang, S.H., Nussenzweig, A., Burgman, P. & Li, G.C. (1995) A constitutive heat shock element-binding factor is immunologically identical to the Ku autoantigen. *J. Biol. Chem.*, 270: 15277-15284.

[40] Kirchgessner, C.; Patil, C.; Evans, J.; Cuomo, C.; Fried, L.; Carter, T.; Oettinger, M. & Brown, M. (1995) DNA-dependent kinase (p350) as a candidate gene for the murine SCID defect. *Science,* 267: 1178-1183.

[41] Knight, Z,A., Chiang, G.G., Alaimo, P.J., Kenski, D.M., Ho, C.B., Coan, K., Abraham, R.T. & Shokat, K.M. (2004) Isoform-specific phosphoinositide 3-kinase inhibitors from an arylmorpholine scaffold. *Bioorg. Med. Chem.*, 12: 4749-4759.

[42] Krawczyk, P.M., Eppink, B., Essers, J., Stap, J., Rodermond, H., Odijk, H., Zelensky, A., van Bree, C., Stalpers, L.J., Buist, M.R., Soullie, T., Rens, J., Verhagen, H.J., O'Connor, M.J., Franken N.A., ten Hagen, T.L., Kanaar, R. & Aten, J.A. (2011) Mild hyperthermia inhibits homologous recombination, induces BRCA2 degradation, and sensitizes cancer cells to poly (ADP-ribose) polymerase-1 inhibition. *Proc. Natl. Acad. Sci. USA,* 108: 9851-9856.

[43] Kruszweski, M., Wojewódzka, M., Iwaneńko, T, Szumiel, I. & Okuyama, A. (1998) Differential inhibitory effect of OK-1035 on DNA repair in L5178Y murine lymphoma sublines with functional or defective repair of double strand breaks. *Mutat. Res.*, 409: 31-36.

[44] Lau, A., SwinBank, K.M., Ahmed, P.S., Taylor, D.L., Jackson, S.P., Smith, G.C.M. & O'Connor, M.J. (2005) Suppression of HIV-1 infection by a small molecule inhibitor of the ATM kinase. *Nat. Cell Biol.,* 7: 493-500.

[45] Leahy, J.J.J., Golding, B.T., Griffin, R.J., Hardcastle, I.R., Richardson, C., Rigoreau, L. & Smith, G.C.M. (2004) Identification of a highly potent and selective DNA-dependent protein kinase (DNA-PK) inhibitor (NU7441) by screening of chromenone libraries. *Bioorg. Med. Chem. Lett.*, 14: 6083-6087.

[46] Lees-Miller, S.P., Chen,Y.-R. & Anderson,C.W. (1990) Human cells contain a DNA-activated protein kinase that phosphorylates simian virus 40 T antigen, mouse p53, and the human Ku autoantigen. *Mol. Cell. Biol.*, 10: 6472-6481.

[47] Lees-Miller, S., Godbout, R., Chan, D., Weinfeld, M., Day III, R., Barron, G. & Allalunis-Turner, J. (1995). Absence of p350 subunit of DNA-activated protein kinase from a radiosensitive human cell line. *Science,* 267: 1183-1185.

[48] Lees-Miller, S., Sakaguchi, K., Ullrich, S., Appella, E. & Anderson, C. (1992) Human DNA-activated protein kinase phosphorylates serines 15 and 37 in the amino-terminal transactivation domain of human p53. *Mol. Cell. Biol.,* 12: 5041-5049.

[49] Li, S., Takeda, Y., Wragg, S., Barrett, J., Phillips, A. & Dynan, W.S. (2003) Modification of the ionizing radiation response in living cells by an scFv against the DNA-dependent protein kinase. *Nucleic Acids Res.,* 31: 5848-5857.

[50] Ma, Y.X., Fan, S., Yuan, R., Meng, Q., Gao, M., Goldberg, I.D., Fuqua, S.A., Pestell, R.G. & Rosen, E.M. (2003) Role of BRCA1 in heat shock response. *Oncogene,* 22: 10-27.

[51] Maira, S.M., Stauffer, F., Brueggen, J., Furet, P., Schnell, C., Fritsch, C., Brachmann, S., Chene, P., De Pover, A., Schoemaker, K., Fabbro, D., Gabriel, D., Simonen, M., Murphy, L., Finan, P., Sellers, W. & Garcia-Echeverria, C. (2008) Identification and characterization of NVP-BEZ235, a new orally available dual phosphatidylinositol 3-kinase/ mammalian target of rapamycin inhibitor with potent in vivo antitumor activity. *Mol. Cancer Ther.,* 7: 1851-1863.

[52] Matsumoto, Y., Suzuki, N., Sakai, K., Morimatsu, A., Hirano, K. & Murofushi, H. (1997) A possible mechanism for hyperthermic radiosensitization mediated through hyperthermic lability of Ku subunits in DNA-dependent protein kinase. *Biochem. Biophys. Res. Commun.,* 234: 568-572.

[53] Mukherjee, B., Tomimatsu, N., Amancherla, K., Camacho, C.V., Pichamoorthy, N. & Burma, S. (2012) The dual PI3K/mTOR inhibitor NVP-BEZ235 is a potent inhibitor of ATM- and DNAPKcs-mediated DNA damage responses. *Neoplasia,* 14: 34-43.

[54] Nishida, H., Tatewaki, N., Nakajima, Y., Magara, T., Ko, K.M., Hamamori, Y. & Konishi, T. (2009) Inhibition of ATR protein kinase activity by schisandrin B in DNA damage response. *Nucleic Acids Res.,* 37: 5678-5689.

[55] Nutley, B.P., Smith, N.F., Hayes, A., Kelland, L.R., Brunton, L., Golding, B.T., Smith, G.C.M., Martin, N.M.B., Workman, P., & Raynaud, F.I. (2005) Preclinical pharmacokinetics and metabolism of a novel prototype DNA-PK inhibitor NU7026. *Brit. J. Cancer,* 93: 1011-1018.

[56] O'Hara, M.D., Pollard, M.D., Wheatley, G., Regine, W.F., Mohiuddin, M. & Leeper, D. B. (1995) Thermal response and hyperthermic radiosensitization of scid mouse bone marrow CFU-C. *Int. J. Radiat. Oncol. Biol. Phys.,* 31: 905-910.

[57] Peasland, A., Wang, L.-Z., Rowling, E., Kyle, S., Chen, T., Hopkins, A., Cliby, W.A., Sarkaria, J., Beale, G., Edmondson, R.J. & Curtin, N.J. (2011) Identification and evaluation of a potent novel ATR inhibitor NU6027, in breast and ovarian cancer cell lines. *Brit. J. Cancer,* 105: 372-381.

[58] Peterson, S., Kurimasa, A., Oshimura, M., Dynan, W., Bradbury, E. & Chen, D. (1995) Loss of the catalytic subunit of the DNA-dependent protein kinase in DNA double-strand-break-repair mutant mammalian cells. *Proc. Natl. Acad. Sci. USA*, 92: 3171-3174.

[59] Price, B.D. & Youmell, M.B. (1996) The phosphatidylinositol 3-kinase inhibitor wortmannin sensitizes murine fibroblast and human tumor cells to radiation and blocks induction of *p53* following DNA damage. *Cancer Res.*, 56: 246-250.

[60] Raaphorst, G.P., Maude-Leblanc, J. & Li, L. (2004) Evaluation of recombination repair pathways in thermal radiosensitization. *Radiat. Res.*, 161: 215-218.

[61] Raaphorst, G.P., Thakar, M. & Ng, C.E. (1993) Thermal radiosensitization in two pairs of CHO wild-type and radiation-sensitive mutant cell lines. *Int. J. Hyperthrmia*, 9: 383-391.

[62] Raaphorst, G.P., Yang, D.P. & Niedbala, G. (2004) Is DNA polymerase beta important in thermal radiosensitization? *Int. J. Hyperthermia*, 20: 140-143.

[63] Rainey, M.D., Charlton, M.E., Stanton, R.V. & Kastan, M.B. (2008) Transient inhibition of ATM kinase is sufficient to enhance cellular sensitivity to ionizing radiation. *Cancer Res.*, 68: 7466-7474.

[64] Reaper, P.M., Griffiths, M.R., Long, J.M., Charrier, J.-D., MacCormick, S., Charlton, P.A., Golec, J.M.C. & Pollard, J.R. (2011) Selective killing of ATM- or p53-deficient cancer cells through inhibition of ATR. *Nat. Chem. Biol.*, 7: 428-430.

[65] Rosenzweig, K.E., Youmell, M.B., Palayoor, S.T. & Price, B.D. (1997). Radiosensitization of human tumor cells by the phosphatidylinositol3-kinase inhibitors wortmannin and LY294002 correlates with inhibition of DNA-dependent protein kinase and prolonged G2-M delay. *Clin. Cancer Res.*, 3: 1149-1156.

[66] Sakata, K., Someya, M., Matsumoto, Y., Tauchi, H., Kai, M., Toyota, M., Takagi, M., Hareyama, M. & Fukushima, M. (2011) Gimeracil, an inhibitor of dihydropyrimidine dehydrogenase, inhibits the early step in homologous recombination. *Cancer Sci.*, 102: 1712-1716.

[67] Sarkaria, J.N., Busby, E.C., Tibbetts, R.S., Roos, P., Taya, Y., Karnitz, L.M. & Abraham, R.T. (1999) Inhibition of ATM and ATR kinase activities by the radiosnsitizing agent, caffeine. *Cancer Res.*, 59: 4375-4382.

[68] Sarkaria, J.N., Tibbetts, R.S., Busby, E.C., Kennedy, A.P., Hill, D.E. & Abraham, R.T. (1998) Inhibition of phosphoinositide 3-kinase related kinases by the radiosensitizing agent wortmannin. *Cancer Res.*, 58: 4375-4382.

[69] Savitsky, K.; Bar-Shira, A.; Gilad, S.; Rotman, G.; Ziv, Y.; Vanagaite, L.; Tagle, D.A.; Smith, S.; Uziel, T.; Sfez, S.; Ashkenazi, M.; Pecker, I.; Frydman, M.; Harnik, R.; Patanjali, S.R.; Simmons, A.; Clines, G.A.; Sartiel, A.; Jaspers, N.G.J.; Taylor, A.M.R.; Arlett, C.F.; Miki, T.; Weissmn, S.M.; Lovett, M.; Collins, F.S. & Shiloh,Y. (1995) A single ataxia telangiectasia gene with a product similar to PI-3 kinase. *Science*, 268: 1749-1753.

[70] Seno, J.D. & Dynlacht, J.R. (2004) Intracellular redistribution and modification of proteins of Mre11/Rad50/Nbs1 DNA repair complex following irradiation and heat-shock. *J. Cell. Physiol.*, 199: 157-170.

[71] Smider, V., Rathmell, W.K., Lieber,M.R. & Chu,G. (1994) Restoration of X-ray resistance and V(D)J recombination in mutant cells by Ku cDNA. *Science*, 266: 288-291.

[72] Spiro, I.J., Denman, D.L. & Dewey, W.C. (1982) Effect of hyperthermia on CHO DNA plymerase alpha and beta. *Radiat. Res.*, 89: 134-149.

[73] Stockley, M., Clegg, W., Fontana G., Golding, B.T., Martin, N., Rigoreau, L.J., Smith, G.C., & Griffin, R.J. (2001) Synthesis, crystal structure determination, and biological properties of the DNA-dependent protein kinase (DNA-PK) inhibitor 3-cyano-6-hydrazonomethyl-5-(4-pyridyl)prid-[1H]-2-one (OK-1035). *Bioorg. Med. Chem. Lett.*, 11: 2837 -2841.

[74] Taccioli, G.E., Gottlieb, T.M., Blunt, T., Priestley, A., Demengeot, J., Mizuta, R., Lehmann, A.R., Alt, F.W., Jackson, S.P. & Jeggo, P.A. (1994) Ku80: product of the *XRCC5* gene and its role in DNA repair and V(D)J recombination. *Science*, 265: 1442-1445.

[75] Takagi, M., Sakata, K., Someya, M., Tauchi, H., Iijima, K., Matsumoto, Y., Torigoe, T., Takahashi, A., Hareyama, M. & Fukushima, M. (2010) Gimeracil sensitizes cells to radiation via inhibition of homologous recombination. *Radiother. Oncol.*, 96: 259-266.

[76] Take, Y., Kumano, M., Hamano, Y., Fukatsu, H., Teraoka, H., Nishimura, S. & Okumura, A. (1995) OK-1035, a selective inhibitor of DNA-dependent protein kinase. *Biochem. Biophys. Res. Commun.*, 215: 41-47.

[77] Take, Y.; Kumano, M.; Teraoka, H.; Nishimura, S. & Okuyama, A. (1996) DNA-dependent protein kinase inhibitor (OK-1035) suppresses p21 expression in HCT116 cells containing wild-type p53 induced by adriamycin. *Biochem. Biophys. Res. Commun.*, 221: 207-212.

[78] Toledo, L.I., Murga, M., Zur, R., Soria, R., Rodriguez, A., Martinez, S., Oyarzabal, J., Pastor, J., Bischoff, J.R. & Fernandez- Capetillo., O. (2011) A cell-based screen identifies ATR inhibitors with synthetic lethal properties for cancer-associated mutations. *Nat. Struct. Mol. Biol.*, 18: 721-727.

[79] Veuger, S.J., Curtin, N.J., Richardson, C.J., Smith, G.C.M. & Durkacz, B.W. (2003) Radiosensitization and DNA Repair Inhibition by the Combined Use of Novel Inhibitors of DNA-dependent Protein Kinase and Poly(ADP-Ribose) Polymerase-1. *Cancer Res.*, 63: 6008-6015.

[80] Walker, A.I., Hunt, T., Jackson, R.J. & Anderson, C.W. (1985) Double-stranded DNA induces the phosphorylation of several proteins including the 90 000 mol. wt. heat-shock protein in animal cell extracts. *EMBO J.*, 4: 139-145.

[81] Woudstra, E.C., Konings, A.W.T., Jeggo, P.A. & Kampinga, H.H. (1999) Role of DNA-PK subunits in radiosensitization by hyperthermia. *Radiat. Res.*, 152: 214-218.

[82] Xiong, H., Lee, R.J., Haura, E.B., Edwards, J.G., Dynan, W.S. & Li, S. (2012) Intranuclear delivery of a novel antibody-derived radiosensitizer targeting the DNA-dependent protein kinase catalytic subunit. *Int. J. Radiat. Oncol. Biol. Phys.*, 83: 1023-1030.

[83] Xiong, H., Li, S., Yang, Z., Burgess, R.B., & Dynan, W.S. (2009) E. coli expression of a soluble, active single-chain antibody variable fragment containing a nuclear localization signal. *Protein Expr. Purif.*, 66: 172-180.

[84] Xu, M., Myerson, R.J., Straube, W.L., Moros, E.G., Lagroye, I., Wang, L.L., Lee, J.T. & Roti Roti, J.L. (2002) Radiosensitization of heat resistant human tumour cells by 1 hour at 41.1°C and its effect on DNA repair. *Int. J. Hyperthermia*, 18: 385-403.

[85] Yin, H.-L., Suzuki, Y., Matsumoto, Y, Tomita, M, Furusawa, Y, Enomoto, A, Morita, A, Aoki, M, Yatagai, F, Suzuki, T, Hosoi, Y, Ohtomo, K & Suzuki N. (2004) Radiosensitization by hyperthermia in chicken B lymphocyte cell line DT40 and its derivatives lacking non-homologous end-joining and/or homologous recombination pathways of DNA double-strand break repair. Radiat Res 162: 433-441.

[86] Zhao, Y., Thomas, H.D., Matey, M.A., Cowell, I.G., Rihardson, C.J., Griffin, R.J., Calvert, A.H., Newell, D.R., Smith, G.C.M. & Curtin, N.J. (2006) Preclinical evaluation of a potent novel DNA-dependent protein kinase inhibitor NU7441. *Cancer Res.*, 66: 5354-5362.

[87] Zhu, W.-G., Seno, J.D., Beck, B.D. & Dynlacht, J.R. (2001) Translocation of MRE11 from the nucleus to the cytoplasm as a mechanism of radiosensitization by heat. *Radiat. Res.*, 156: 95-102.

[88] Zou, L & Ellege, S.J. (2003) Sensing DNA damage through ATRIP recognition of RPA-ssDNA complex. *Science*, 300: 1542-1548.